A Lange Medical Book

PEDIATRICS ON CALL

Edited by

Charles A. Pohl, MD
Clinical Associate Professor of Pediatrics
Associate Dean for Student Affairs and Career Counseling
Jefferson Medical College of Thomas Jefferson University
Philadelphia, Pennsylvania

Series Editor
Leonard G. Gomella, MD
The Bernard W. Godwin, Jr., Professor of Prostate Cancer
Chairman, Department of Urology
Jefferson Medical College of Thomas Jefferson University
Philadelphia, Pennsylvania

Lange Medical Books/McGraw-Hill
Medical Publishing Division

New York   Chicago   San Francisco   Lisbon   London   Madrid
Mexico City   Milan   New Delhi   San Juan
Seoul   Singapore   Sydney   Toronto

Pediatrics On Call

3 4 5 6 7 8 9 0   IBT/IBT   0 9 8

ISBN: 0-07-143655-3
ISSN: 1556-6927

Notice

This book was set in Helvetica by International Typesetting and Composition.
The editors were Janet Foltin, James F. Shanahan, Robert Pancotti, and Patrick Carr.
The production supervisor was Sherri Souffrance.
The index was prepared by Michael Ferreira.
The art manager was Charissa Baker.
IBT Global was printer and binder.

This book is printed on acid-free paper.

INTERNATIONAL EDITION ISBN 0-07-110501-8
Copyright © 2006. Exclusive rights by The McGraw-Hill Companies, Inc., for manufacture and export. This book cannot be reexported from the country to which it is consigned by McGraw-Hill. The International Edition is not available in North America.

To the girls in my life . . . especially Emma and Annie . . .
and
To Donald R. Pohl, MD, my pediatrician and dad.
Thanks for all of your love and support!

Contents

Associate Editors

Clara A. Callahan, MD
Clinical Associate Professor of Pediatrics
Vice Dean for Academic Affairs
Jefferson Medical College of Thomas Jefferson University
Philadelphia, Pennsylvania

J. Carlton Gartner, Jr., MD
Professor of Pediatrics
Jefferson Medical College of Thomas Jefferson University
Pediatrician-in-Chief
Alfred I. duPont Hospital for Children
Wilmington, Delaware

Kathleen Kilroy Bradford, MD
Assistant Professor of Pediatrics
University of North Carolina School of Medicine
Chapel Hill, North Carolina

Contributors

Sheeja K. Abraham, MD
Assistant Professor of Pediatrics
Division of Pediatric Gastroenterology
Jefferson Medical College of Thomas Jefferson University
Philadelphia, Pennsylvania

Ellen Arch, MD
Staff Physician/Clinical Geneticist
Alfred I. duPont Hospital for Children
Wilmington, Delaware

Magdy William Attia, MD
Associate Professor of Pediatrics
Jefferson Medical College of Thomas Jefferson University
Philadelphia, Pennsylvania

Jeanne Marie Baffa, MD
Clinical Associate Professor of Pediatrics
Jefferson Medical College of Thomas Jefferson University
Pediatric Cardiologist
The Nemours Cardiac Center
Alfred I. duPont Hospital for Children
Wilmington, Delaware

Mara L. Becker, MD
Pediatric Rheumatology Fellow
Alfred I. duPont Hospital for Children
Wilmington, Delaware

Caroline D. Boyd, MD
Pediatric Critical Care Fellow
Alfred I. duPont Hospital for Children
Wilmington, Delaware

Kathleen Kilroy Bradford, MD
Assistant Professor of Pediatrics
University of North Carolina School of Medicine
Chapel Hill, North Carolina

B. Randall Brenn, MD
Assistant Professor of Anesthesiology and Pediatrics
Jefferson Medical College of Thomas Jefferson University
Senior Staff Anesthesiologist
Alfred I. duPont Hospital for Children
Wilmington, Delaware

AnneMarie C. Brescia, MD
Attending Physician
Division of Rheumatology
Alfred I. duPont Hospital for Children
Wilmington, Delaware

Robert P. Brislin, DO
Staff Attending Anesthesiologist
Department of Anesthesiology and Critical Care Medicine
Children's Hospital of Philadelphia
Philadelphia, Pennsylvania

Michael P. Carboni, MD
Clinical Assistant Professor
Division of Pediatric Cardiology
Duke University Medical Center
Durham, North Carolina

Aaron S. Chidekel, MD
Assistant Professor of Pediatrics
Jefferson Medical College of Thomas Jefferson University
Philadelphia, Pennsylvania

Maria Childers, MD
Assistant Professor of Pediatrics
Jefferson Medical College of Thomas Jefferson University
Philadelphia, Pennsylvania

Esther K. Chung, MD, MPH
Assistant Professor of Pediatrics
Jefferson Medical College of Thomas Jefferson University
Pediatrician
Alfred I. duPont Hospital for Children
Philadelphia, Pennsylvania

Sandra Como-Fluehr, MSN, RN, APRN, BC
Pain Management Nurse Specialist
Department of Anesthesiology and Critical Care Medicine
Alfred I. duPont Hospital for Children
Wilmington, Delaware

Deborah M. Consolini, MD
Assistant Professor of Pediatrics
Jefferson Medical College of Thomas Jefferson University
Pediatrician
Alfred I. duPont Hospital for Children
Wilmington, Delaware

Steven P. Cook, MD, FACS, FAAP, FRSM
Clinical Assistant Professor
Department of Otolaryngology/Head and Neck Surgery
Jefferson Medical College of Thomas Jefferson University
Chief, Division of Pediatric Otolaryngology
Alfred I. duPont Hospital for Children
Wilmington, Delaware

Andrew T. Costarino, Jr., MD
Professor of Anesthesiology and Chairman of Pediatrics
Jefferson Medical College of Thomas Jefferson University
Philadelphia, Pennsylvania

Kate Cronan, MD
Associate Professor
Department of Pediatrics
Jefferson Medical College of Thomas Jefferson University
Philadelphia, Pennsylvania

Shermine Dabbagh, MD
Chief, Division of Pediatric Nephrology
Alfred I. duPont Hospital for Children
Wilmington, Delaware

Parul P. Dand, MD
Pediatrician
Shah Associates
Lexington Park, Maryland

Allan R. De Jong, MD
Director, Children at Risk Evaluation (CARE) Program
Alfred I. duPont Hospital for Children
Wilmington, Delaware

Ellen S. Deutsch, MD, FACS, FAAP
Associate Professor of Otolaryngology and Pediatrics
Alfred I. duPont Hospital for Children
Wilmington, Delaware

Joan S. Dipalma, MD
Attending Physician
Division of Pediatric Gastroenterology
Alfred I. duPont Hospital for Children
Wilmington, Delaware

Maureen F. Edelson, MD
Medical Director of Blood Bank
Department of Laboratory Medicine
Alfred I. duPont Hospital for Children
Wilmington, Delaware

Gary A. Emmett, MD, FAAP
Clinical Associate Professor of Pediatrics
Director of General Pediatrics
Jefferson Medical College of Thomas Jefferson University
Philadelphia, Pennsylvania

T. Ernesto Figueroa, MD, FAAP, FACS
Chief, Division of Pediatric Urology
Alfred I. duPont Hospital for Children
Wilmington, Delaware

Christopher N. Frantz, MD
Chief, Division of Hematology/Oncology
Alfred I. duPont Hospital for Children
Wilmington, Delaware

J. Carlton Gartner, Jr., MD
Professor of Pediatrics
Jefferson Medical College of Thomas Jefferson University
Pediatrician-in-Chief
Alfred I. duPont Hospital for Children
Wilmington, Delaware

Michael H. Goodman, MD
Chief, Division of Neurology
Alfred I. duPont Hospital for Children
Wilmington, Delaware

Gregory C. Griffin, MD
Attending Physician
Division of Pediatric Hematology/Oncology
Alfred I. duPont Hospital for Children
Wilmington, Delaware

Louis H. Guernsey, Jr., MD
Pediatric Pulmonologist
Alfred I. duPont Hospital for Children
Wilmington, Delaware

Hazel Guinto-Ocampo, MD, FAAP
Attending Physician
Division of Emergency Medicine
Alfred I. duPont Hospital for Children
Wilmington, Delaware

Jason B. Hann-Deschaine, MD
Appoquinimink Pediatrics
Townsend, Delaware

James H. Hertzog, MD
Pediatric Intensivist
Department of Anesthesiology and Critical Care Medicine
Alfred I. duPont Hospital for Children
Wilmington, Delaware

Laszlo Hopp, MD
Associate Professor
Division of Nephrology
Alfred I. duPont Hospital for Children
Wilmington, Delaware

Laura S. Inselman, MD
Pediatric Pulmonologist
Medical Director of Pulmonary Function Laboratory
Alfred I. duPont Hospital for Children
Wilmington, Delaware

Elizabeth P. Ives, MD
Urology Resident
Thomas Jefferson University Hospital
Philadelphia, Pennsylvania

Bruce Kaiser, MD
Pediatric Nephrologist
Alfred I. duPont Hospital for Children
Wilmington, Delaware

Susanne Kost, MD
Associate Professor
Division of Emergency Medicine
Alfred I. duPont Hospital for Children
Wilmington, Delaware

Kelly R. Leite, DO
Assistant Professor of Pediatrics
Assistant Director, Pediatric Residency Program
Penn State College of Medicine
Hershey, Pennsylvania

James Jeffrey Malatack, MD
Director of Diagnostic Referral Service
Pediatric Medical Liver Transplantation Program
Alfred I. duPont Hospital for Children
Wilmington, Delaware

Keith J. Mann, MD
Associate Director, Pediatric Residency Program
Alfred I. duPont Hospital for Children
Wilmington, Delaware

Stephen J. McGeady, MD
Associate Professor of Pediatrics
Division of Allergy, Asthma, and Immunology
Jefferson Medical College of Thomas Jefferson University
Chief, Division of Pediatric Allergy, Asthma, and Immunology
Alfred I. duPont Hospital for Children
Wilmington, Delaware

Charles P. McKay, MD
Director, Bone and Mineral Program
Division of Pediatric Nephrology
Alfred I. duPont Hospital for Children
Wilmington, Delaware

Robin E. Miller, MD
Attending Physician
Division of Pediatric Hematology/Oncology
Alfred I. duPont Hospital for Children
Wilmington, Delaware

Linda Muir, MD
Pediatric Gastroenterologist
Sacred Heart Medical Center
Providence Physician Services
Spokane, Washington

Ursula Nawab, MD
Neonatology Fellow
Thomas Jefferson University Hospital
Philadelphia, Pennsylvania

Robert C. O'Reilly, MD, FACS
Pediatric Otolaryngologist
Alfred I. duPont Hospital for Children
Wilmington, Delaware

Raj Padman, MD
Chief, Division of Pulmonology
Director, Cystic Fibrosis Program
Alfred I. duPont Hospital for Children
Wilmington, Delaware

Scott Penfil, MD
Director, Pediatric Critical Care Training Program
Alfred I. duPont Hospital for Children
Wilmington, Delaware

Melanie Pitone, MD, FAAP
Attending Physician
Division of Pediatric Emergency Medicine
Alfred I. duPont Hospital for Children
Wilmington, Delaware

Charles A. Pohl, MD
Clinical Associate Professor of Pediatrics
Associate Dean for Student Affairs and Career Counseling
Jefferson Medical College of Thomas Jefferson University
Philadelphia, Pennsylvania

Amanda Pratt, MD
Assistant Professor
Division of Pediatric Emergency Medicine
University of Medicine and Dentistry of New Jersey—Robert
Wood Johnson Medical School
New Brunswick, New Jersey

Erin Preston, MD
Instructor of Pediatrics
Jefferson Medical College of Thomas Jefferson University
Philadelphia, Pennsylvania

James S. Reilly, MD, MS, FACS
Professor of Otolaryngology and Pediatrics
Jefferson Medical College of Thomas Jefferson University
Philadelphia, Pennsylvania

Steven B. Ritz, MD
Attending Cardiologist
The Nemours Cardiac Center
Alfred I. duPont Hospital for Children
Wilmington, Delaware

Marianne Ruby, MD, FACOG
Clinical Instructor
Division of Reproductive Endocrinology
Jefferson Medical College of Thomas Jefferson University
Philadelphia, Pennsylvania

Jean M. Russell, RN, BSN, CRNI
IV Therapy Coordinator
Department of Nursing
Alfred I. duPont Hospital for Children
Wilmington, Delaware

Richard J. Scarfone, MD, FAAP
Associate Professor of Pediatrics
University of Pennsylvania School of Medicine
Philadelphia, Pennsylvania

Steven M. Selbst, MD
Professor of Pediatrics and Vice Chair for Education
Jefferson Medical College of Thomas Jefferson University
Pediatric Residency Program Director
Alfred I. duPont Hospital for Children
Wilmington, Delaware

Glenn Stryjewski, MD, MPH
Department of Anesthesia and Critical Care
St. Christopher's Hospital for Children
Philadelphia, Pennsylvania

Shamim Tejani, PharmD
Clinical Pharmacy Coordinator
Alfred I. duPont Hospital for Children
Wilmington, Delaware

Andrew W. Walter, MS, MD
Associate Professor of Pediatrics
Division of Pediatric Hematology/Oncology
Jefferson Medical College of Thomas Jefferson University
Philadelphia, Pennsylvania

Rhonda S. Walter, MD
Acting Chief, Division of Developmental Medicine
Alfred I. duPont Hospital for Children
Wilmington, Delaware

Philip Wolfson, MD
Professor of Surgery
Jefferson Medical College of Thomas Jefferson University
Philadelphia, Pennsylvania

Ejaz Yousef, MD
Clinical Assistant Professor
Division of Allergy and Immunology
Jefferson Medical College of Thomas Jefferson University
Philadelphia, Pennsylvania

Preface

I am grateful to be able to bring you the first edition of *Pediatrics On Call.* The "on-call" series of which this book is a part is based on a concept applied by Tricia Gomella, MD, in her book, *Neonatology: Basic Management, On Call Problems, Diseases, and Drugs.* The books in this series reflect how clinicians typically approach and manage patients; that is, patients usually present with a specific complaint or problem, which necessitates an evaluation and action rather than a specific diagnosis. *Pediatrics On Call* is designed to aid the practitioner and serve as a learning resource to housestaff and students, enabling them to better understand medical conditions in children and provide the necessary tools to initiate the evaluation and care of these young patients.

It would be remiss not to acknowledge those who have made this book possible. The staff at McGraw-Hill, especially Janet Foltin and Donna Frassetto, have been supportive and patient. All three associate editors, Drs. Callahan, Gartner, and Bradford, have devoted significant effort as well as endless attention to detail to ensure academic integrity. The contributors have provided medical expertise and insight while giving up valuable personal time. And finally I must acknowledge and thank our pediatric patients, who have been our teachers through the years.

Charles A. Pohl, MD
Philadelphia, Pennsylvania
December 2005

Common Abbreviations and Acronyms

The following are common abbreviations used in medical records and in this edition.

/: per
< : less than, younger than
> : more than, older than
≥ : more than or equal to
≤ : less than or equal to
↓ : decrease(d)
↑ : increase(d)
→ : leads to
ABCs: airway, breathing, and circulation
ABG: arterial blood gas
ABPA: allergic bronchopulmonary aspergillosis
ACE: angiotensin-converting enzyme
ACLS: advanced cardiac life support
ACTH: adrenocorticotropic hormone
ADH: antidiuretic hormone
ADP: adenosine diphosphate
AG: anion gap
AIDS: acquired immunodeficiency syndrome
ALT: alanine aminotransferase
ALTE: apparent life-threatening event
AM: morning
AME: apparent mineralocorticoid excess
ANA: antinuclear antibody
ANC: absolute neutrophil count
AP: anteroposterior

APIGN: acute postinfectious glomerulonephritis
APRV: airway pressure release ventilation
APTT: activated partial thromboplastin time
ARDS: acute respiratory distress syndrome
ARF: acute rheumatic fever; acute renal failure
AST: aspartate aminotransferase
ATN: acute tubular necrosis
ATP: adenosine triphosphate
AV: atrioventricular
β-HCG: beta human chorionic gonadotropin
BiPAP: bilevel positive airway pressure
BM: bowel movement
BP: blood pressure
BUN: blood urea nitrogen
Ca: calcium
CaO_2: arterial oxygen content
cap: capsule
CBC: complete blood count
CF: cystic fibrosis
CHF: congestive heart failure
Cl: chloride
CMV: cytomegalovirus
CNS: central nervous system
COX-2: cyclooxegenase-2
CPAP: continuous positive airway pressure

CPK: creatine phosphokinase
CPP: central perfusion pressure
CPR: cardiopulmonary resuscitation
CPS: child protective services
CRP: C-reactive protein
CSF: cerebrospinal fluid
CT: computed tomography
CVA: costovertebral angle
CVP: central venous pressure
D_5W: 5% dextrose in water
DAT: direct antiglobulin test
DC: direct current
DDAVP: desmopressin acetate
DDH: developmental dysplasia of the hip
DHEAS: dehydroepiandrosterone sulfate
DIC: disseminated intravascular coagulation
DiSIDA: 2,6-diisopropylacetanilido-iminodiacetic acid
DKA: diabetic ketoacidosis
dL: deciliter
DM: diabetes mellitus
DMSA: dimercaptosuccinic acid
Do_2: oxygen delivery
E coli: Escherichia coli
EBV: Epstein-Barr virus
ECFV: extracellular fluid volume
ECG: electrocardiogram
EDTA: ethylenediamine tetra-acetic acid
EEG: electroencephalogram
EENT: eyes, ears, nose, throat
ELISA: enzyme-linked immunosorbent assay
EMLA: eutectic mixture of local anesthetics
EMS: emergency medical services
ENT: ear, nose, throat
EPAP: expiratory positive airway pressure
EPI: epinephrine
ERCP: endoscopic retrograde cholangiopancreatography
ESR: erythrocyte sedimentation rate

ET: endotracheal
$ETco_2$: end-tidal carbon dioxide
ETT: endotracheal tube
FAO: fatty acid oxidation
FE_{Mg}: fractional excretion of magnesium
FHH: familial hypocalciuric hypercalcemia
Fio_2: fraction of inspired oxygen
FSGS: focal segmental glomerulosclerosis
FTT: failure to thrive
FUO: fever of unknown origin
FWLS: fever without localizing signs
g: gram
GABHS: group A β-hemolytic streptococcus
GCS: Glasgow Coma Scale
G-CSF: granulocyte colony-stimulating factor
GERD: gastroesophageal reflux disease
GFR: glomerular filtration rate
GGTP: gamma-glutamyl transpeptidase
GI: gastrointestinal
GM-CSF: granulocyte-macrophage colony-stimulating factor
G6PD: glucose-6-phosphate dehydrogenase
GRA: glucocorticoid remediable aldosteronism
GU: genitourinary
h: hour
H: hydrogen
HCG: human chorionic gonadotropin
HCl: hydrochloric acid
HCO_3: bicarbonate
Hct: hematocrit
HEENT: head, eyes, ears, nose, and throat
HFOV: high-frequency oscillatory ventilation
Hgb: hemoglobin
HIDA: hepato-iminodiacetic acid

HIPAA: Health Insurance Portability and Accountability Act
HIV: human immunodeficiency virus
HLA: human leukocyte antigen
HMWK: high-molecular-weight kininogen
HPF: high-power field
HR: heart rate
HSP: Henoch-Schönlein purpura
HUS: hemolytic uremic syndrome
IBD: inflammatory bowel disease
ICP: intracranial pressure
ICU: intensive care unit
I:E ratio: inspiratory-to-expiratory ratio
Ig: immunoglobulin
IM: intramuscular
IN: intranasal
INR: international normalized ratio
I&O: intake and output
IO: intraosseous
IPAP: inspiratory positive airway pressure
IPH: idiopathic pulmonary hemorrhage
ISI: international sensitivity index
ITP: idiopathic thrombocytopenic purpura
IU: International Unit
IUGR: intrauterine growth retarded
IV: intravenous
JNA: juvenile nasopharyngeal angiofibroma
JRA: juvenile rheumatoid arthritis
K: potassium
Kcal: kilocalorie
KCl: potassium chloride
kg: kilogram
KUB: [X-ray examination of] kidneys, ureters, and bladder
L: liter
LCPD: Legg-Calvé-Perthes disease
LDH: lactate dehydrogenase
LGA: large for gestational age

LP: lumbar puncture
LR: lactated Ringer solution
m: meter
MAOI: monoamine oxidase inhibitor
MAP: mean arterial pressure
max: maximum
MBS: modified barium swallow
MCD: minimal change disease
mcg: microgram
mcL: microliter
MCL: midclavicular line
MCV: mean corpuscular volume
MDI: metered dose inhaler
Mg: magnesium
mg: milligram
min: minute
mL: milliliter
mm: millimeter
mm Hg: millimeters of mercury
mmol: millimole
mo: month
mOsm: milliosmole
MRA: magnetic resonance angiography
MRCP: magnetic resonance cholangiopancreatography
MRI: magnetic resonance imaging
MSUD: maple syrup urine disease
Na: sodium
NC: nasopharyngeal carcinoma
NG: nasogastric
NGU: nongonoccocal urethritis
NH_4Cl: ammonium chloride
NICU: neonatal intensive care unit
NIF: negative inspiratory force
NP: nasopharyngeal
NPO: nothing by mouth (*nulla per os*)
NS: normal saline
NSAIDs: nonsteroidal anti-inflammatory drugs
OI: oxygenation index
O&P: ova and parasites
OS: intraosseous

OSAS: obstructive sleep apnea syndrome

OTC: over-the-counter

PA: posteroanterior

PA_{CO_2}: peripheral alveolar carbon dioxide content

Pa_{CO_2}: peripheral arterial carbon dioxide content

Pa_{O_2}: peripheral arterial oxygen content

PALS: pediatric advanced life support

P_B: barometric pressure

PCP: phenylcyclohexyl piperidine

PDA: patent ductus arteriosus

PEEP: positive end-expiratory pressure

P/F ratio: Pa_{O_2}-to-Fi_{O_2} ratio

PFIC: progressive familial intrahepatic cholestasis

pg: picogram

PICU: pediatric intensive care unit

PID: pelvic inflammatory disease

PIP: positive inspiratory pressure

PMN: polymorphonuclear neutrophil

PO: by mouth (*per os*)

PPD: purified protein derivative

PPI: protein pump inhibitor

ppm: parts per million

PR: by rectum (*per rectum*)

prn: as often as needed (*pro re nata*)

PRVC: pressure-regulated volume control

PSV: pressure support ventilation

PT: prothrombin time

PTH: parathyroid hormone

PTT: partial thromboplastin time

PVNS: pigmented villonodular synovitis

q: every

q6h: every 6 hours

q8h: every 8 hours

q15min: every 15 minutes

RAP: recurrent abdominal pain

RBC: red blood cell

RDW: red blood cell distribution width index

RE: retinol equivalent

RMSF: Rocky Mountain spotted fever

RPR: rapid plasmin reagin (test)

RR: respiration rate

RSV: respiratory syncytial virus

RTA: renal tubular acidosis

s: second

SCFE: slipped capital femoral epiphyses

SCIWORA: spinal cord injury without radiographic abnormality

SGA: small for gestational age

SIADH: syndrome of inappropriate secretion of antidiuretic hormone

SIDS: sudden infant death syndrome

SIMV: synchronized intermittent mandatory ventilation

SLE: systemic lupus erythematosus

sp gr: specific gravity

SPECT: single-photon emission computed tomography

Sp_{O_2}: functional oxygen saturation; pulse oximetry

SQ: subcutaneous

SSRIs: selective serotonin reuptake inhibitors

STD: sexually transmitted disease

SVT: supraventricular tachycardia

$T_{1/2}$: half-life

T_3: triiodothyronine

T_4: thyroxine

tab: tablet

TAR: thrombocytopenia—absent radius

tbsp: tablespoon

TIBC: total iron-binding capacity

TMP-SMX: trimethoprim-sulfamethoxazole

TORCH: toxoplasmosis, other (congenital syphilis and viruses), rubella, cytomegalovirus, and herpes simplex virus

TPN: total parenteral nutrition

TRALI: transfusion-related acute living injury

tsp: teaspoon

UDP: uridine diphosphate

UTI: urinary tract infection

UV: ultraviolet

VC: vital capacity

VCUG: voiding cystourethrogram

V/Q: ventilation-perfusion

VSD: ventricular septal defect

VT: ventricular tachycardia

V_T: tidal volume

VUR: vesicoureteral reflux

vWD: von Willebrand disease

vWF: von Willebrand factor

WBC: white blood cell

wk: week

wt: weight

w/w: weight; percent weight

XLH: X-linked hypophosphatemic (rickets)

y: year

I. On Call Problems

1. ABDOMINAL DISTENTION

I. Problem. An 8-month-old boy is brought to the pediatrician because of abdominal distention.

II. Immediate Questions

A. What are the vital signs? Because infants are diaphragmatic breathers, distention may impair respiratory function and cause tachypnea. Massive distention can compromise cardiac output, resulting in hypotension and tachycardia. Fever suggests infection, such as peritonitis or pneumonia, which can cause distention from adynamic ileus.

B. Is abdomen usually distended? Abdominal distention resulting from obesity and fecal retention occurs gradually, whereas that from intestinal obstruction is more rapid.

C. Is there associated pain or discomfort? Acute intestinal obstruction and inflammatory conditions are accompanied by pain. Distention that develops more slowly may be painless.

D. Has there been any vomiting? Vomiting, particularly bilious or feculent, is a frequent sign of intestinal obstruction.

E. When was the most recent bowel movement? What is patient's usual bowel pattern? Complete obstruction and adynamic ileus are usually associated with lack of bowel movements. Constipation is associated with infrequent or difficult passage of stool.

F. Has patient previously been well? Organomegaly, tumors, and ascites often occur in chronically ill children who have diminished activity, failure to thrive, and fever.

G. Does patient void normally? Is there any diminution in urine output? Distention may occur from hydronephrosis, obstructed bladder, polycystic kidney, or urinary ascites. Intestinal obstruction and ascites frequently produce hypovolemia.

H. If an adolescent girl, has patient had regular periods? Giant ovarian cysts and pregnancy may cause abdominal distention.

III. Differential Diagnosis. Distention may be caused by obesity, gas within or outside the GI tract, ascites, feces, a large mass, and, in adolescent females, pregnancy. As a mnemonic remember the **6 F's:** **F**at, **F**latus, **F**luid, **F**eces, **F**earsome-sized masses, and **F**etus.

A. Obesity. Strikingly increased incidence in United States; however, the abdomen in infants and children may be normally protuberant until puberty.

B. Gas

1. **Intestinal obstruction.** The more distal the obstruction, the greater is the distention.
   a. **Causes in neonates.** Intestinal atresia, meconium ileus, meconium plug.
   b. **Causes in older children.** Incarcerated hernias, intussusception, midgut volvulus, Meckel diverticulum, adhesions from previous surgery.
2. **Adynamic (paralytic) ileus.** Intestine dilates from accumulated gas and fluid when there is diminished peristaltic activity. Seen with infectious or inflammatory conditions of the abdomen (eg, necrotizing enterocolitis), systemic infections (eg, UTIs, pneumonia), hypokalemia, and following surgical manipulation of intra-abdominal organs.
3. **Pneumoperitoneum.** Abdomen can distend from free air or sequestered fluid accompanying peritonitis.
   a. **Causes in neonates.** Necrotizing enterocolitis, spontaneous gastric perforation.
   b. **Causes in older children.** Perforated peptic ulcer, Meckel diverticulum.
4. **Excessive air in GI tract.** Infants and children may swallow large quantities of air with feeding or crying.

C. **Ascites.** Nonpurulent fluid in peritoneal cavity. May be serous, chylous, urinary, biliary, or bloody.
1. **Serous.** From increased splanchnic capillary hydrostatic pressure, and decreased plasma oncotic pressure. **Causes:** Hepatobiliary (cirrhosis, biliary atresia, other causes of portal hypertension), cardiac (congestive heart failure, constrictive pericarditis), or peritoneal (infectious, from tuberculosis or bacteria producing peritonitis; intra-abdominal tumors).
2. **Chylous.** From congenital malformation of lymphatic channels, lymphatic obstruction due to abdominal or mediastinal masses, or traumatic disruption.
3. **Urinary.** From fluid retention in renal failure, decreased plasma protein with nephrotic syndrome, and direct extravasation of urine with obstructive uropathy.
4. **Biliary.** From perforated gallbladder or common bile duct.
5. **Bloody.** From trauma.

D. **Constipation.** Most often functional; may also be mechanical (from an anteriorly displaced anus), neurologic (with defects of the spinal cord), metabolic (associated with hypokalemia and hypothyroidism), or a result of Hirschsprung disease.

E. **Masses.** May represent enlarged organ (liver, spleen, kidney, bladder), tumor (neuroblastoma, Wilms tumor, hepatoblastoma, ovarian tumors), or cyst (ovarian, omphalomesenteric, mesenteric).

F. **Pregnancy.** In adolescent girls.

IV. Database

A. Physical Exam Key Points

1. **Vital signs.** Tachypnea suggests respiratory compromise, whereas hypotension and tachycardia are associated with poor venous return or hypovolemia. Fever may occur with infectious processes.

2. **Lungs.** Shallow breathing occurs with compression of diaphragm. Auscultate for pneumonia.

3. **Abdomen**

   a. **Inspection.** A protuberant abdomen from obesity is uniformly rounded, with the umbilicus buried. An everted umbilicus indicates increased intra-abdominal pressure. Distention from ascites is most marked in the hypogastric area when upright; flanks bulge when supine. When ascites is severe, skin is shiny, with prominent veins. Distention caused by abdominal masses may be asymmetric. Diastasis rectus (midline protrusion from xiphoid to umbilicus) is a normal variant.

   b. **Auscultation.** Bowel sounds are high pitched in early obstruction, diminished with adynamic ileus and peritonitis.

   c. **Percussion.** Differentiate air (tympany) from fluid and solid structures (dull). Free intra-abdominal air causes loss of normal dullness on percussion of the liver. Free fluid produces shifting dullness, percussible in the flanks when patient is supine and moving to dependent side when in lateral decubitus position.

   d. **Palpation.** Abdomen may be rigid from peritonitis or tense from ascites. Note location, size, consistency, and movability of masses (retroperitoneal masses do not move with respiration). Stool can often be identified by its deformability. A fluid wave from ascites is demonstrated by tapping the flank with the right hand and receiving an impulse with the left hand on the opposite flank while an assistant presses downward along the midline.

4. **Rectal exam.** Check for imperforate anus and fecal impaction. Tenderness may imply peritonitis. Functional obstruction from Hirschsprung disease may be explosively decompressed.

5. **Hernias.** Assess groin and umbilicus.

6. **Intake and output.** Check for fluid retention or dehydration.

B. Laboratory Data

1. **CBC.** Leukocytosis or left shift suggests infection; anemia may be associated with intra-abdominal bleeding.

2. **Serum electrolytes, BUN, creatinine, liver function tests.** Hypokalemia can cause an ileus. Elevated bilirubin and transaminases can identify hepatic disease. Elevated BUN and creatinine indicate renal failure.

3. **ABGs.** Respiratory acidosis implies hypoventilation from distention. Metabolic acidosis accompanies intestinal ischemia (eg, with severe necrotizing enterocolitis).

TABLE I–1. IDENTIFICATION OF ASCITIC FLUID

Fluid	Color	Characteristics
Serous		
Transudate	Clear yellow	Sp gr < 1.020, protein < 2.5 g/dL, serum:ascites albumen > 1.1
Exudate	Turbid	Sp gr > 1.020, protein > 3 g/dL serum:ascites albumen < 1.1, elevated leukocyte count
Chyle	Milky white[a]	Triglycerides < 1000 mg/dL, leukocytes 1000–5000 cells/mm^3, 70–90% lymphocytes
Urine	Clear yellow	Creatinine 5–10 mg/dL
Bile	Green, golden yellow	Bilirubin 100–400 mg/mL
Pus	Purulent	Many leukocytes, bacteria on Gram stain and culture

[a] Clear yellow in neonates who have never been fed.

> 4. **Paracentesis.** If ascites is present, insert butterfly needle in left lower quadrant and aspirate. Fluid is readily identified as serous, chyle, urine, bile, or pus (Table I–1). Serous fluid may be transudate (from increased hydrostatic pressure) or exudate (from inflammatory process).
> 5. **β-HCG.** Measure in any patient who may be pregnant.
> C. **Radiographic and Other Studies**
> 1. **Chest and abdominal x-rays.** Chest x-ray may show limited lung volumes from increased intra-abdominal pressure or pneumonia as a cause of ileus. Upright chest x-ray is the best view for detecting pneumoperitoneum. Abdominal x-rays will demonstrate intestinal obstruction, fecal retention, and adynamic ileus. A mass is suggested by a paucity of intestinal loops in a particular area; ascites is seen as generalized haziness.
> 2. **GI contrast x-rays.** May be indicated if there is evidence of obstruction.
> 3. **Ultrasonography.** Can characterize abdominal masses and is very sensitive in detecting fluid; can also differentiate free fluid, loculated fluid, and fluid in a cyst.
> 4. **CT scan.** Provides excellent anatomic detail of enlarged intra-abdominal organs and other masses.
> V. **Plan.** If respiration or perfusion is impaired, provide urgent resuscitation. Perform intubation with positive pressure ventilation and give IV fluid therapy if needed, even while diagnostic workup is carried out. Specific treatment depends on cause of distention.
> A. **Obstruction.** Insert NG tube to suction, usually followed by surgery. Exceptions include meconium ileus, meconium plug, and intussusception, which may be treated successfully with contrast enemas. Hirschsprung disease may be managed with decompressive enemas until surgery is performed.
> B. **Adynamic ileus.** Usually temporary; treat underlying cause.

    C. Pneumoperitoneum. A surgical emergency with peritonitis; administer IV fluids and antibiotics while preparing patient for surgery.

    D. Ascites. Aspirate only if there is respiratory compromise or pain, because this measure is only temporary (fluid will reaccumulate). If fluid is removed too rapidly, hypovolemia and hypotension may result.

       1. Serous. Salt and fluid restriction, diuretics, and rarely, if intractable, peritoneovenous shunting. Definitive management of transudative and exudative ascites requires treatment of underlying condition (cirrhosis, constrictive pericarditis, peritonitis).

       2. Biliary. Surgical drainage and alleviation of biliary obstruction.

       3. Urinary. Decompression and drainage of obstruction.

       4. Chylous. Reduce flow through obstructed or perforated lymphatic channels by withholding oral intake with TPN initially, then implement low-fat diet enhanced with medium-chain triglycerides. Surgery if no response.

    E. Constipation. Rectal irrigations followed by comprehensive bowel management program. If Hirschsprung disease is suspected, order barium enema and rectal biopsy to confirm.

    F. Masses. Enlarged intra-abdominal organs are treated by managing underlying condition. Urinary obstruction is decompressed. Abnormal masses are resected.

VI. Problem Case Diagnosis. The 8-month-old boy with abdominal distention had a history of delayed passage of meconium and infrequent bowel movements. He presented with respiratory distress and poor perfusion and had a massively distended, tympanitic abdomen. Rectal exam yielded an explosive output of stool and gas with decompression. Contrast enema and rectal biopsy confirmed Hirschsprung disease.

VII. Teaching Pearl: Question. Why do infants who are born with congenital obstruction of the intestine usually have no significant abdominal distention at the time of birth?

VIII. Teaching Pearl: Answer. Before birth, the GI tract does not contain air; thus, even with complete obstruction distention is rare. Over 24–48 hours, distention develops as air is swallowed, with the degree of distention being proportional to how far down in the intestine the obstruction is located. If an infant's abdomen is distended at birth, consider something other than simple mechanical obstruction (ie, meconium peritonitis or intra-abdominal fluid).

REFERENCES

Fischer AC. Ascites. In Mattei P, ed. *Surgical Directives: Pediatric Surgery.* Lippincott Williams & Wilkins, 2003:505–510.

Jordan MR, Ziai M. Abdominal masses. In Ziai M, ed. *Bedside Pediatrics.* Little Brown, 1983:407–410.

Riazi J, Dale JT, Ziai M. Ascites. In Ziai M, ed. *Bedside Pediatrics*. Little Brown, 1983:359–372.

2. ABDOMINAL PAIN

I. Problems
  A. A 14-month-old boy is brought to the emergency department with abdominal pain of 6 hours' duration.
  B. A 15-year-old girl is brought to the pediatrician because of lower abdominal pain that has lasted 2 days.

II. Immediate Questions
  A. How old is patient? Many conditions that cause abdominal pain are age specific. Necrotizing enterocolitis only occurs in early infancy, midgut volvulus is most common in the first year, intussusception is seen mostly in toddlers, appendicitis is rare in the newborn and increases in frequency through adolescence, and many gynecologic disorders are seen only in girls after puberty.
  B. Where is the pain located? Gastroenteritis and most types of functional abdominal pain are centrally located; pain of appendicitis begins centrally and then migrates to the right lower quadrant; gallbladder and hepatic pain occurs in the right upper quadrant and may radiate to the back or right shoulder; pain from the stomach, duodenum, and pancreas occurs in the epigastrium; pain from the small intestine is central; pain from the large intestine occurs in the hypogastrium; pain from the spleen is felt in the left upper quadrant and may radiate to the left shoulder; pain from the kidneys or ureters is often felt in the flank and may radiate to the groin; and pain from the ovaries or fallopian tubes occurs in the ipsilateral lower quadrant.
  C. What is the quality of the pain? Visceral pain, produced by distention of a hollow organ or stretching of the capsule of a solid organ, is colicky and dull (eg, intestinal obstruction, early appendicitis, ureteral calculus, hepatitis). Parietal pain involves inflammation of the peritoneum and is sharp, well localized, and exacerbated by movement (eg, appendicitis in its later stages, necrotic intestine, perforated viscus).
  D. Duration of pain? Gastroenteritis and mesenteric adenitis start gradually and plateau over hours. Appendicitis starts gradually and classically increases in severity until perforation occurs. Urinary calculi, ovarian torsion, and ruptured ovarian cyst are sudden in onset and severe from the outset. Pain of intussusception is intermittent over hours and sometimes days. Functional pain is most frequently chronic.
  E. Has patient had this pain before? Functional abdominal pain is most likely to be recurrent. However, volvulus and even appendicitis may be self-limited on several occasions and then recur with full-blown manifestations.

F. Are there associated GI symptoms? Individuals with significant intra-abdominal pathology are rarely hungry. Nausea, vomiting, and a change in bowel habits often accompany GI conditions such as gastroenteritis, appendicitis, and intestinal obstruction. Bilious vomiting is indicative of obstruction and possibly volvulus. Vomiting preceding pain is most characteristic of gastroenteritis. Copious diarrhea is typical with enteric infections, and severe constipation itself can be the cause of the pain.

G. Urinary symptoms? UTIs are associated with dysuria, frequency, and urgency; calculi may produce dysuria and hematuria.

H. Symptoms from other organ systems? Abdominal pain in children is frequently a manifestation of extra-abdominal disease (eg, pharyngitis, otitis, pneumonia). Intussusception frequently follows a viral illness.

I. Is there a history of trauma? Abdominal injuries may be a source of pain.

J. In postpubertal girls, when was the last period? Is there a history of sexual intercourse? Vaginal discharge? Consider pelvic inflammatory disease (PID), mittelschmerz, and ectopic pregnancy, depending on gynecologic history.

K. Fever? With appendicitis, there is typically afebrile or low-grade fever until perforation; with viral conditions and peritonitis, temperature may be highly elevated.

L. Chronic systemic illnesses? Children with sickle cell disease may have abdominal pain from a crisis; those with diabetes can have abdominal pain associated with ketoacidosis. Leukemia may produce typhlitis during periods of severe leukopenia. Inflammatory bowel disease can cause abdominal pain during periods of exacerbation.

III. Differential Diagnosis. Because both acute and chronic abdominal pain are extremely common in children, the challenge is to identify the relatively few patients with significant medical and surgical illnesses that require treatment. In a survey of children with acute abdominal pain in the emergency department, 86% had self-limited disease and only 1% required surgical intervention. Diagnostic probabilities are age dependent.

A. Patients Older Than 3 Years of Age

1. Appendicitis. The most common cause of abdominal pain that requires surgery in children older than age 2 years; prototype of the so-called acute abdomen. Early diagnosis is most important, because perforation may occur 36–48 hours after onset.

2. Mesenteric lymphadenitis. Usually a diagnosis of exclusion when no other cause is found or a normal appendix is seen during exploration for presumptive appendicitis. Considered to be viral in origin. Pain is more generalized, with fewer peritoneal signs than in appendicitis. Leukocyte count usually is normal.

3. **Gastroenteritis.** May be caused by a virus or *Salmonella, Shigella, Campylobacter,* or *Yersinia.* Vomiting and diarrhea precede pain. Tenesmus and blood in stool may be noted, but peritonitis is absent. Stool cultures are usually diagnostic.

4. **Meckel diverticulitis.** Presentation is similar to appendicitis but is much less common, and pain is not as localized to the right lower quadrant. Diagnosis is rarely made before surgery.

5. **Intestinal obstruction.** Causes in older children include Meckel diverticulum that twists or telescopes, and adhesions from previous surgery.

6. **Constipation.** Frequent cause of acute or recurrent pain in children. Usually functional but may be due to Hirschsprung disease, an anteriorly displaced anus, defects of the spinal cord, or metabolic abnormalities (ie, hypokalemia, hypothyroidism).

7. **Inflammatory bowel disease.** Ulcerative colitis or Crohn disease is frequently accompanied by pain; either condition may also give rise to toxic megacolon. Crohn disease may appear as acute ileitis (10% of cases) and have a presentation similar to appendicitis.

8. **Typhlitis.** Occurs in immunosuppressed patients (eg, leukemia) when leukocytes < 1000/mm^3. Involves terminal ileum and right colon and is probably infectious.

9. **Biliary colic, cholecystitis.** Gallstones are most common in adolescent girls; may also occur in children with hemolytic anemias and those who have received long-standing TPN.

10. **UTI.** Cystitis is usually associated with dysuria, frequency, and urgency; pyelonephritis with fever and flank tenderness.

11. **Urinary calculus.** May produce excruciating "writhing" pain in flank or abdomen as well as hematuria.

12. **Ovarian cyst.** Rare before puberty. May produce pain when it bleeds, ruptures, or twists. Torsion is a surgical emergency.

13. **PID.** Salpingitis or tuboovarian abscess is common among adolescent girls.

14. **Mittelschmerz.** Ovulatory bleeding can cause peritoneal irritation; occurs midway in cycle.

15. **Ectopic pregnancy.**

16. **Primary peritonitis.** May occur in normal children (especially girls 2–6 years of age) but is more common in patients with nephrotic syndrome or cirrhosis, or after splenectomy. Bacterial infection; probably hematogenous source.

17. **Other systemic illnesses.** Abdominal pain may accompany other acute and chronic conditions (eg, lower lobe pneumonia, hepatitis, Henoch-Schönlein purpura, hemolytic uremic syndrome, sickle cell disease, porphyria, diabetes).

18. **Recurrent abdominal pain (RAP).** Occurs in 10% of children. Most cases are functional (ie, no structural or biochemical

basis is found); 5–10% have one of the causes listed above. Emotional stress may contribute. Abdominal pain is more likely to be functional if it is intermittent, centrally located, not associated with meals, vomiting, a change in bowel habits, or jaundice; if it does not awaken patient from sleep; if patient is not ill; and if growth and development are normal.

    a. Possible mechanisms. Increased gastric acid, intestinal hyperactivity, spasm of abdominal wall muscles.

    b. Irritable bowel syndrome. This form of RAP occurs in older children and adolescents and is characterized by pain with diarrhea or constipation. Pain is often relieved by defecation.

B. Patients Younger Than 3 Years of Age

    1. Necrotizing enterocolitis. Inflammatory condition of the intestine. Occurs almost exclusively in premature infants and can progress to necrosis and perforation.

    2. Colic. Recurrent inconsolable crying during the first 3–4 months in infants who are otherwise healthy. Occurs mostly at night. Episodes are characterized by knees drawn up to the abdomen.

    3. Midgut volvulus. Associated with intestinal malrotation. May occur at any age but is most common during first year. Patient may present initially with bilious vomiting; early recognition is crucial to prevent intestinal necrosis.

    4. Intussusception. Telescoping of one portion of the intestine into another, usually ileocolic. Most common in children aged 6 months to 2 years. Usually idiopathic (ie, no pathologic lead point).

IV. Database

    A. Physical Exam Key Points. Most patients can be diagnosed clinically, without need for sophisticated tests. Critical question is: Does patient require urgent surgery or can more leisurely evaluation take place? It is controversial whether analgesics will mask the findings of abdominal disease. Many surgeons maintain they cannot adequately assess patients who have received narcotics, although recent studies suggest otherwise. A compromise may be to administer a single dose of analgesia if it is decided to observe patient and then reassess when medication wears off. If surgery is definitely planned, pain relief may be provided.

    1. General appearance. Note overall appearance, how patient moves about, and whether he or she "looks sick." Writhing with intermittent crying and drawing the knees up suggests colicky pain; lying still in fetal position is more indicative of peritonitis.

    2. Vital signs. Children with nonperforated appendicitis rarely have a high fever; significant fever suggests a viral syndrome or peritonitis.

3. **EENT, lungs.** Because abdominal pain, particularly in young children, may be caused by extra-abdominal conditions, check for conditions such as otitis, pharyngitis, and pneumonia.
4. **Abdomen**
   a. **Inspection.** Distention may be associated with intestinal obstruction or peritonitis. Note scars from previous surgery.
   b. **Auscultation.** Hyperactive bowel sounds accompany many nonsurgical causes of abdominal pain (eg, gastroenteritis). High-pitched sounds are associated with early obstruction. Diminished or absent sounds are indicative of peritonitis.
   c. **Percussion.** If abdomen is distended, tympany signifies gas; dullness occurs with fluid or solid organs. Loss of liver dullness may indicate pneumoperitoneum.
   d. **Palpation.** The most important part of the exam. As a rule, involuntary guarding signifies peritonitis and warrants surgical intervention. Beginning in the area most remote from the pain, palpate, first gently and then deeply. Watch for wincing (implies significant tenderness). Ask if patient feels pain in the area being palpated or somewhere else. Instead of testing for rebound, ask patient to puff out the abdomen and then suck it in; pain during this maneuver implies peritoneal irritation.
5. **Rectal exam.** Unnecessary to perform in all cases, because yield is low and exam is traumatic. Useful for feeling a mass, diagnosing fecal retention, and as an alternative to pelvic exam in young girls.
6. **Pelvic exam.** Often deferred, even in adolescent girls, because similar information may be obtained from rectal exam with patient supine or from ultrasound. Cervical motion tenderness and cervical cultures are positive in PID.
7. **Skin.** Jaundice is a manifestation of hepatobiliary disease. Some causes of abdominal pain are associated with characteristic rashes (eg, Henoch-Schönlein purpura).
B. **Laboratory Data**
   1. **CBC and differential.** Leukocytosis and left shift are usual findings with appendicitis. Children with chronic illnesses (eg, inflammatory bowel disease) are often anemic. If marked neutropenia (WBCs < 1000/mm^3), consider typhlitis.
   2. **Serum electrolytes, glucose, BUN, creatinine.** If significant vomiting, check electrolytes and hydration status. BUN and creatinine are elevated in hemolytic uremic syndrome. Glucose is elevated in diabetic patients whose abdominal pain is associated with ketoacidosis.
   3. **Bilirubin, AST, ALT, alkaline phosphatase.** Elevated in hepatobiliary disease.
   4. **Amylase, lipase.** Elevated in pancreatitis (lipase is more specific).

5. **Urinalysis and culture.** UTIs are associated with WBCs in urine and a positive culture; calculi produce hematuria. (Presence of a few WBCs or RBCs is also consistent with appendicitis adjacent to ureter or bladder.) Urine sediment is often abnormal in Henoch-Schönlein purpura.

6. **β-HCG.** Exclude ectopic pregnancy in postpubertal girls with lower abdominal pain.

7. **Cervical culture.** Obtain if PID is suspected.

8. **Stool culture.** If diarrhea is prolonged or associated with blood or elevated fecal leukocytes, check for *Campylobacter, Yersinia, Salmonella, Shigella,* and *Clostridium difficile.*

9. **ESR.** Nonspecific, but usually elevated in inflammatory bowel disease.

C. **Radiographic and Other Studies.** Imaging studies are unnecessary in most children with abdominal pain, because diagnosis can be established clinically.

1. **Chest and abdominal x-rays.** Chest x-ray may reveal lower lobe pneumonia; an upright chest film is the best view for detecting pneumoperitoneum. Abdominal x-rays are usually nonspecific but will show intestinal obstruction, stool with constipation, and occasionally a radiopaque urinary calculus or an appendiceal fecalith. Pneumatosis intestinalis (air in the wall of the intestine) is the hallmark of necrotizing enterocolitis. In patients with inflammatory bowel disease, a much dilated transverse colon suggests toxic megacolon.

2. **Ultrasonography.** Often useful if pain is localized. The best imaging study for gynecologic causes of abdominal pain (eg, ovarian torsion, ovarian cysts, PID with tuboovarian abscess). May identify inflamed appendix when diagnosis is unclear.

3. **CT scan.** Provides excellent anatomic detail of entire abdomen. Considered 95% accurate in diagnosing appendicitis. Typhlitis may be diagnosed and followed to identify necrosis and perforation. Because significant radiation exposure is involved, use only when necessary.

4. **GI contrast x-rays.** Immediately obtain an upper GI series for bilious vomiting if midgut volvulus is suspected. Upper and lower GI contrast studies are useful in patients with obstruction or inflammatory bowel disease.

5. **Upper and lower GI endoscopy.** Useful in patients with inflammatory bowel disease.

6. **Diagnostic laparoscopy.** If the cause of persistent abdominal pain cannot be identified by other means, intra-abdominal organs can be viewed directly with a laparoscope. If patient has right lower abdominal pain, the appendix should be removed even if it appears normal; in many cases the pain will resolve.

V. **Plan**

A. **Overall Plan.** The vast majority of children with abdominal pain have self-limited conditions that will resolve without medical treatment and thus require only reassurance. It is more important to ascertain whether surgery is required than to arrive at a precise preoperative diagnosis. If findings are equivocal, a period of observation or further imaging studies can be helpful.

B. **Surgical Intervention.** Children identified with acute surgical abdominal conditions should undergo surgery without delay.

1. **Preoperative measures.** These can be instituted while the operating room is being prepared and include IV hydration, broad-spectrum antibiotics, and, if there is obstruction or significant vomiting, NG suction.

2. **Volvulus and torsion.** Midgut volvulus and ovarian torsion require the most urgent surgery, because even a brief delay can result in necrosis.

3. **Appendicitis.** Almost all children with appendicitis should undergo surgery promptly. An exception is the relatively few in whom perforation occurred days ago and who present with a walled off, well-localized infection without peritonitis. In such cases, broad-spectrum antibiotics and possible percutaneous drainage (if there is an abscess), followed by an interval appendectomy 6–8 weeks later, may lower the complication rate.

4. **Intussusception.** In most children with intussusception, the intestine can be reduced with air or liquid contrast by an experienced radiologist; if unsuccessful, surgery is required.

VI. **Problem Case Diagnoses**

A. The 14-month-old boy with abdominal pain had ileocolic intussusception, seen on an air-contrast enema. It was successfully reduced and he was discharged the following day.

B. The 15-year-old girl with right lower quadrant abdominal pain underwent ultrasonography, which showed normal ovaries and an acutely inflamed appendix that was subsequently removed.

VII. **Teaching Pearl: Question.** Why does the pain in most children with appendicitis start out centrally and then "move" to the right lower abdomen?

VIII. **Teaching Pearl: Answer.** The initial pain in appendicitis is caused by distention. Stretch receptors in the wall of the appendix transmit through the same visceral nerves that supply the T10 dermatome, located around the umbilicus. As the inflammation progresses to involve the serosa, the parietal peritoneum transmits somatic pain, which is well localized to the site of the appendix, usually the right lower quadrant.

REFERENCES

Bagnell PC. Clinical evaluation of gastrointestinal symptoms in children. In Goldbloom RB, ed. *Pediatric Clinical Skills,* 2nd ed. Churchill Livingstone, 1997:219–238,

Berkowitz ID, Shapiro JR. Abdominal pain. In Ziai M, ed. *Bedside Pediatrics.* Little Brown, 1983:395–405.

Gillis DA. Surgical assessment of the child's abdomen. In Goldbloom RB, ed. *Pediatric Clinical Skills,* 2nd ed. Churchill Livingstone, 1997:239–257.

Mattei P. Abdominal pain. In Mattei P, ed. *Surgical Directives: Pediatric Surgery.* Lippincott Williams & Wilkins, 2003:781–786.

3. ACIDOSIS

I. **Problem.** An 8-year-old girl with a long-standing history of poorly controlled asthma presents with severe respiratory distress. An albuterol nebulizer and 100% oxygen are immediately administered. ABG levels show pH of 7.20, $Paco_2$ of 64, and Pao_2 of 284. Bicarbonate (HCO_3) level is 22 mEq/L.

II. **Immediate Questions**

A. **What is patient's mental status?** A patient who has impaired mental status may be "tiring out" from breathing yet still have inadequate ventilation. Consider endotracheal intubation if there is not an immediate response to therapy.

B. **What are patient's other vital signs? Is patient in shock? What is the volume status?** Typically, patients with respiratory acidosis are both tachycardic and tachypneic in an effort to "blow off" excessive CO_2. Bradycardia or bradypnea may represent a near-arrest situation requiring urgent intervention and possible endotracheal intubation. Shock exists when metabolic demands of the body are not being met; this leads to lactic acidosis (metabolic). Initial therapy should virtually always include fluid resuscitation to correct hypovolemia.

C. **What are patient's oxygen saturation and Pao_2 values?** Although elevated $Paco_2$ is indicative of respiratory failure, inadequate oxygenation can more rapidly lead to cardiac arrest and requires immediate attention.

D. **Are breath sounds inaudible, unequal, or absent?** Patients without audible breath sounds may be so "tight" that they are unable to move air. In this situation, aerosolized medications may be ineffective because of inadequate delivery to distal bronchioles. Consider other modalities to deliver medications (IV or SQ). Be prepared for patient to "crash" quickly. Consider the possibility of a spontaneous pneumothorax when breath sounds are unequal or unilaterally absent.

E. **What medications has patient received?** Narcotics are a common cause of respiratory depression.

F. **Does patient have a history or signs and symptoms consistent with sepsis or sepsis syndrome?** Inadequate tissue perfusion secondary to septic shock can cause metabolic acidosis.

G. **Is acidosis primarily respiratory, primarily metabolic, mixed, or compensated?**

1. **Respiratory acidosis**

a. **Defect.** Respiratory acidosis is caused by inadequate alveolar ventilation (eg, from medications that depress respiration, neuromuscular disorders, or increased CO_2 production), or by ineffective gas exchange (eg, from airway obstruction, bronchoconstriction, or alveolar disease).

b. **Laboratory manifestation.** Increased Pa_{CO_2}; decreased pH.

c. **Compensation.** Normal respiratory response to hypercapnia is to increase alveolar ventilation (through increased minute ventilation, respiratory rate, and depth of breaths). In addition to serum buffers (primarily proteins), renal compensatory mechanisms (increased HCO_3 reabsorption) may be present after 24–36 hours.

d. **Evaluate pH in conjunction with Pa_{CO_2}.** In general, pH will decrease by .008 for every 1 torr by which Pa_{CO_2} is > 40 (eg, Pa_{CO_2} of 60 is 20 torr > 40; pH would be expected to decrease by $20 \times .008 = .16$, as follows: serum pH = $7.40 - .16 = 7.24$). If pH is above the calculated number, then there is some degree of metabolic compensation; if below it, then there is a metabolic acidosis in addition to respiratory acidosis.

2. **Metabolic acidosis**

a. **Defect.** Increased acid accumulation or decreased extracellular HCO_3.

b. **Laboratory manifestation.** Decreased serum pH; decreased serum HCO_3.

c. **Compensation.** Increasing minute ventilation causes a decreased Pa_{CO_2}, which causes pH to increase; cells exchange extracellular H^+ for intracellular Na^+ and K^+. The kidneys compensate more slowly by excreting H^+ and generating HCO_3. The degree of **respiratory compensation** can be estimated by the following formula:

$$Pa_{CO_2} = 1.5 \, (HCO_3) + 8 + 2$$

d. **Classification. Anion-gap (AG) metabolic acidosis** occurs with increased endogenous production of acid, as in lactic acidosis or diabetic ketoacidosis. The AG can be estimated by the following formula:

$$AG = [Na^+] - ([Cl^-] + [HCO_3])$$

Normal AG is 11 ± 4, although there are several exceptions. AG acidosis can exist even with a normal AG in patients who are severely hypoalbuminemic or those who have pathologic paraproteinemias. For every 1 g/dL decrease in albumin, AG decreases by 2.5–3 mmol. Pathologic paraproteinemias lower AG because immunoglobulins are largely cationic. AG may not reflect an underlying acidosis in a patient with significant alkalemia (pH > 7.5). In these circumstances, albumin is more negatively charged, which increases unmeasured anions.

III. **Differential Diagnosis.** In acutely ill patients, metabolic and respiratory acidosis commonly coexist.

  A. **Respiratory Acidosis.** There are many possible causes of respiratory acidosis, including airway obstruction (foreign bodies, tongue displacement, laryngospasm, congenital malformations or airway malacia, severe bronchospasm), respiratory center depression (general anesthesia, sedatives, narcotics, CNS injury or ischemia, drugs or toxins, and electrolyte disorders), increased CO_2 production (sepsis, seizures, malignant hyperthermia, shivering, hypermetabolic states, overfeeding with TPN), neuromuscular diseases (spinal cord injuries, Guillain-Barré syndrome, myasthenia gravis, polymyositis, spinal muscular atrophy, muscular dystrophy, infantile botulism), intrinsic pulmonary disease (obstructive and restrictive conditions such as in chondrodystrophies, acute lung injury, acute respiratory distress syndrome [ARDS], pulmonary edema), extrinsic pulmonary disease (hemothorax, pneumothorax, flail chest, pleural effusions, obesity), and issues related to mechanical ventilation (obstructed endotracheal tube, inadequate ventilatory support, permissive hypercapnia).

  B. **Metabolic Acidosis.** May be associated with a normal or an increased AG. This division greatly facilitates diagnosis.

    1. **Elevated AG acidosis.** Causes include lactic acidosis (tissue hypoxia, shock, cardiac arrest, sepsis, hematologic emergencies), ketoacidosis (diabetes, alcohol induced, starvation), renal failure (uremic metabolic acidosis), and toxins (salicylates, methanol, ethylene glycol).

    2. **Normal AG metabolic acidosis.** Usually the result of HCO_3 loss from bowel or kidneys but can occur from treatment with exogenous acids (eg, HCl). Normal AG acidoses are subcategorized on the basis of K^+ level.

      a. **Hypokalemia.** Associated with diarrhea, ureteral diversion, proximal renal tubular acidosis (RTA), type I RTA and hyperalimentation.

      b. **Hyperkalemia.** Can be found in hyperaldosterone states, ammonium chloride (NH_4Cl) administration, and type IV distal RTA.

      c. Differential diagnosis includes:

        i. GI loss of HCO_3 (from diarrhea, ileostomy, proximal colostomy, ureteral conduit).

        ii. Renal loss of HCO_3 (proximal RTA, carbonic anhydrase inhibitor).

        iii. Renal tubular disease (acute tubular necrosis, chronic tubulointerstitial disease, distal RTA types I and IV, hypoaldosteronism, aldosterone inhibitors).

> > **iv.** Medications (NH_4Cl, HCl, hyperalimentation, dilutional acidosis).

IV. Database. Clinical manifestations of acute respiratory acidosis and acute ventilatory failure are the same. They depend on the absolute increase in $Paco_2$, rate of rise of $Paco_2$, and severity of associated hypoxemia.

A. Physical Exam Key Points

1. **General appearance.** Mottled, cool, or clammy skin may indicate sepsis, a common cause of metabolic acidosis in the ICU setting. Fever typically also is present

2. **Vital signs.** Is there tachycardia, bradycardia, hypertension, hypotension, or any cardiac dysrhythmia? Peripheral vasodilatation? If present, reevaluate current support and check mechanical ventilator settings if patient is intubated.

3. **CNS.** There may be somnolence or obtundation, anxiety or confusion, psychosis, tremors, headache, or papilledema. In the absence of direct CNS injury, presence of these findings indicates inadequate cerebral perfusion or oxygenation, or both.

4. **Lungs.** Listen for decreased breath sounds, stridor, rales, crackles, or wheezes. *If metabolic acidosis is present,* compensatory mechanisms include deep, rapid respirations (Kussmaul breathing).

5. **Cardiovascular findings.** Cardiogenic shock may cause acidosis. Acidosis by itself may cause arrhythmias, reduce myocardial contractility, and decrease responsiveness to catecholamines.

6. **HEENT.** Tracheal shift may indicate tension pneumothorax; jugular venous distention is seen with tension pneumothorax or cardiac tamponade. Fetor hepaticus (halitosis of fruity odor) may suggest hepatic failure or diabetic ketoacidosis.

7. **Abdomen.** Distention, tenseness, involuntary guarding, or other peritoneal signs may indicate acute abdomen as the initial cause of acidosis.

B. Laboratory Data

1. **ABGs.** Follow serial values to assess effects of treatment and identify need for intubation. Pulse oximetry is a valuable noninvasive tool to assess oxygenation. Measurement of end-tidal CO_2 can also be a reliable noninvasive tool to assess adequacy of ventilation.

2. **CBC.** Leukocytosis or leukopenia may indicate sepsis. High hemoglobin and hematocrit values may indicate dehydration; thrombocytopenia is usually associated with severe sepsis or DIC, or both.

3. **Electrolytes.** Calculate the AG. In non-AG metabolic acidosis, evaluate K^+ and Cl^-. Look for evidence of renal failure.

    4. Lactate. Increases in all forms of shock. Indicates anaerobic metabolism from inadequate tissue perfusion.

    5. Glucose and ketones. Increases may indicate diabetic ketoacidosis.

  C. Radiographic and Other Studies

    1. Chest x-ray. Look for pulmonary edema, infiltrates, pneumothorax, size of cardiac silhouette (increased with congestive heart failure or pericardial effusion), and endotracheal tube position.

    2. ECG. Evaluate for arrhythmias.

V. Plan. Appropriate treatment depends on identifying underlying cause of the acidosis.

  A. Respiratory Acidosis. If patient is oversedated with narcotics or benzodiazepines, consider administration of specific antidote. Electrolyte abnormalities (eg, hypokalemia, hypophosphatemia, hypocalcemia) may lead to muscular weakness and should be rapidly corrected. If patient has a neuromuscular disorder, noninvasive ventilation, such as continuous or bilevel positive airway pressure (CPAP or BiPAP), may be helpful. Extrinsic pulmonary disease (eg, pneumothorax, pleural effusion) should be treated specifically. Foreign bodies will require removal. Severe bronchoconstriction, as in asthma, should be aggressively treated with β-agonists, steroids, ipratropium, and possibly magnesium. Endotracheal intubation and mechanical ventilation should be considered if mental status is abnormal, if patient appears to be "tired" from the high work of breathing, if there is poor response to initial therapies, or if oxygenation is compromised.

  B. Metabolic Acidosis. Treat non-AG metabolic acidosis by replacing volume losses. Use isotonic fluid with low Cl^- content. Specific treatments exist for most causes of AG metabolic acidosis. These may include insulin for diabetic ketoacidosis; dialysis for renal failure; fluids, inotropes, pressors, and antibiotics for septic shock. Use of HCO_3 for lactic acidosis is controversial; if warranted, HCO_3 therapy can be guided by the following formula:

Body weight (kg) $\times$ 0.40 (volume of distribution of bicarbonate) $\times$ (24 $-$ HCO_3]) = Total mEq HCO_3

Give 50% of this amount in the first 12 hours by adding HCO_3 to a solution of D_5W.

VI. Problem Case Diagnosis. The 8-year-old patient had respiratory acidosis from inadequate ventilation secondary to reactive airway disease. She was given continuous aerosolized albuterol, intermittent aerosolized ipratropium bromide, and IV steroids. After minimal improvement, inhaled heliox (70%) was begun. Over the next several hours, she improved and heliox was discontinued. Ipratropium was stopped and albuterol was slowly weaned over the next 1–2 days.

Patient was discharged to home with instructions to continue albuterol and steroids.

VII. Teaching Pearl: Question. What is the significance of the absence of wheezing in the presence of respiratory distress or respiratory acidosis?

VIII. Teaching Pearl: Answer. Absence of wheezing may indicate that patient is extremely "tight" and unable to move enough air to cause a wheeze. *Beware of the "silent chest."*

REFERENCES

Rogers MC, Helfaer MA. *Handbook of Pediatric Intensive Care.* Williams & Wilkins, 1999.
Schrier RW. *Renal and Electrolyte Disorders,* 3rd ed. Little, Brown, 1986.

4. AIRWAY DEVICES

I. Problem. A 3-year-old boy who was recently admitted from the emergency department with respiratory distress has a room-air pulse-oximetry reading of 89%.

II. Immediate Questions

A. Is patient truly hypoxic or is the pulse-oximetry reading an artifact of measurement? Motion and improper oximeter probe placement may lead to falsely low readings. If pulse tracing is strong and corresponds to the heart rate, and the reading remains low, provide oxygen and examine patient.

B. What is patient's ventilation and hemoglobin saturation state? Pulse oximeters reflect only oxygenation and do not measure ventilation. Altered hemoglobin saturation states (eg, methemoglobin and carboxyhemoglobin) may lead to false oximeter readings.

C. How severe and prolonged has hypoxia been? This decision must be made early in the evaluation, always assessing and correcting airway, breathing, and circulation (ABCs) initially.

III. Differential Diagnosis

A. Airway Obstruction. In the lower airway, consider asthma; in the upper airway, choanal atresia.

B. Decreased Diffusion of Gas From Alveoli to Capillaries. Includes pneumonia and aspiration.

C. Abnormal Cardiopulmonary Blood Flow. Includes cyanotic congenital heart disease and pulmonary embolus.

D. Alteration in Neuromuscular Control of Respiration. Includes drugs and muscular dystrophy.

IV. Database

A. Physical Exam Key Points. Observation of general appearance (including level of alertness) is important. Evaluate for cyanosis, airway patency, respiratory rate and effort, and cardiac abnormalities. Listen for snoring, stridor, wheezing, rales, and adequacy of air movement.

B. Laboratory Data

    1. Pulse oximetry.

    2. ABGs. Consider ABGs with co-oximetry if an altered hemoglobin saturation state is suspected.

C. Radiographic and Other Studies. Obtain based on history and physical exam findings.

V. Plan

A. Oxygen Administration

    1. Administer oxygen to any seriously ill or injured patient with potential respiratory insufficiency, even if pulse-oximetry readings are normal, and to any mildly to moderately ill child whose readings are low (< 93%).

    2. Use caution in children whose respiratory drive is dependent on hypoxia, such as an infant with ductal-dependent congenital heart lesion (eg, hypoplastic left heart syndrome) or a child with chronic respiratory illness.

    3. Use best-tolerated method of oxygen delivery that effectively maintains adequate oxygenation. For example, consider risk of increased agitation and respiratory distress when attempting to attach a cannula or mask to child. Humidified oxygen is preferred, when possible, to avoid drying mucosa.

    4. Allow alert children to assume preferred position, as they will naturally optimize their air entry and minimize work of breathing.

B. Oxygen Delivery

    1. "Blow-by" oxygen

        a. Provides sidestream oxygenation through wide-bore tubing or a mask directed toward child's face and is generally best tolerated when held by parent.

        b. Amount of oxygen provided is highly variable but is usually accepted by child.

    2. Nasal cannula

        a. Consists of a small-diameter tube with two short curved prongs that enter nares; tubing may loop about ears or be taped to cheeks. It is relatively comfortable and allows child to eat and talk. Effective for infants who are obligate nasal breathers and for children who require only low levels of supplemental oxygen.

        b. Maximum flow rate is 3 L/min; flows above this rate do not deliver increased oxygen and only serve to irritate nasal mucosa.

        c. Percentage of supplemental oxygen delivered (generally < 30%) is highly dependent on minute ventilation and degree of nasal breathing and is obviously lessened in children who have nasal congestion or are crying.

   d. Remember when placing prongs into nares that curves should point back and not up, and that tubing poses a strangulation hazard if looped completely around child's neck.

3. Simple face mask

   a. Consists of a clear mask with two open side ports that allow for exhalation and air entry if oxygen flow is insufficient.

   b. Set inspiratory flow at 6–10 L/min; this will provide 35–60% Fio_2, depending on respiratory rate.

4. Partial rebreathing mask

   a. Consists of a simple face mask attached to a reservoir bag that contains oxygen and oxygen-rich expired gas.

   b. With each breath, patient pulls air from the bag rather than room air, allowing Fio_2 of 50–60% (assuming adequate flow to the bag). Bag should be inflated at all times, requiring flow rate of 10–12 L/min.

5. Nonrebreathing mask

   a. A simple face mask and reservoir bag with valves added. One valve covers one side port of the face mask with a simple flap that prevents inspiration of room air; the other valve covers the reservoir bag so that expired air cannot enter bag. One side port of the face mask is intentionally left open in case oxygen flow is accidentally discontinued, so that mask does not completely obstruct air entry.

   b. Patient pulls 100% oxygen from the reservoir bag, which must remain adequately inflated to function properly. With an adequate seal and adequate flow to the bag (10–15 L/min), this system is capable of delivering Fio_2 of up to 90%.

6. Oxygen hoods and tents

   a. Hoods. Consider for younger, less mobile, or sleeping patients. Made of clear hard or soft plastic, hoods cover patient's head and upper body but allow access to rest of body. They are well tolerated by young infants. With a flow of 10–15 L/min, Fio_2 of 80–90% may be achieved if hood is not disturbed.

   b. Tents. Made of clear soft plastic but have limited usefulness as they may impede access to and visualization of patient, especially when condensation forms on inner surface.

C. Relief of Airway Obstruction. Pediatric airway is proportioned such that a small degree of swelling or inflammation may significantly obstruct air entry, and proportions of tongue and lymphoid tissue may lead to obstruction even in the absence of disease. When physical exam suggests upper airway obstruction and basic life support measures (eg, head-tilt, jaw-thrust maneuvers) fail to relieve obstruction, consider airway adjuncts for use under certain circumstances.

D. Airway Adjuncts

 1. Nasopharyngeal (NP) airway

   a. A soft rubber or plastic tube with a proximal flange that serves as a conduit for air through an obstructed nasopharynx.

   b. Uses. Conscious or unconscious patients; may be particularly useful in neurologically impaired children with poor pharyngeal tone.

   c. Contraindications to use. Include epistaxis, nasal polyps, and suspected cribriform plate fracture.

   d. Steps to insertion

   i. Choose correct size, with diameter approximating that of nares, and length approximating distance from tragus of ear to tip of nose.

   ii. Apply topical vasoconstrictor to nares and lubricant to tube.

   iii. Insert tube straight back into nares such that angled side faces turbinates.

   iv. Assess fit and effect. With proper fit, nares should not blanch and tip should be just visible behind uvula. If tube is too long, the end may cause gagging or reflex laryngospasm or bradycardia through vagal stimulus.

   v. Reassess frequently. NP airways are narrow and likely to become obstructed with secretions, and require frequent reassessment. Long-term use may contribute to mucosal irritation and sinus obstruction.

 2. Oropharyngeal airway

   a. Consists of a hard, hollow, molded plastic device with a bite block and flange that serves to position tongue and open oropharynx for air entry.

   b. Cautions. Will induce gagging and vomiting and should not be used in conscious patients.

   c. Steps to insertion

   i. Choose correct size. With flange at the incisors, tip should reach angle of mandible. If too short, may push tongue back and worsen obstruction; if too long, may cause gagging or reflex laryngospasm or bradycardia through vagal stimulus.

   ii. Depress tongue with a tongue blade and insert airway, concave side against tongue, under direct visualization. Have suction ready in case of vomiting.

   iii. Assess response and patient tolerance. If improved, airway may be taped in place. If obstruction persists, consider a different size or attempt more definitive airway control.

 3. Suctioning. In many cases, upper airway obstruction is related directly to secretions and may be alleviated with suctioning.

a. **Types**
   i. **Flexible suction catheters.** Better for mucus and thin secretions than are tips. Used for NP and artificial airway suction.
   ii. **Rigid plastic (Yankauer) tips.** Better for particulate matter than are catheters. Attached via wide-bore tubing to portable or wall suction units. Wall suction is more powerful, up to −300 mm Hg.
b. **Regulation of suctioning.** Set at −80 to −120 mm Hg; may be adjusted at the source or by varying occlusion of side port of catheter tip.
c. **Intervals of suction.** Limit to 20–30 seconds to avoid irritation and potential vagal stimulus.

E. **Bag-Mask Ventilation.** Indicated when patient is unable to maintain adequate oxygenation or ventilation with spontaneous breathing.
   1. **Types**
      a. **Self-inflating bags.** May be used without an oxygen or airflow source, but some varieties contain a valve that prohibits free flow of oxygen unless positive pressure is delivered via the bag.
      b. **Flow-inflating bags (also known as anesthesia or Mapleson circuits).** Require an oxygen or air source to inflate the bag, and allow continuous administration of oxygen even when positive pressure is not applied. These systems also allow a better feel for lung compliance, although they can be technically more difficult to use.
   2. **Technique**
      a. Choose ventilation face mask based on patient's facial size. Mask opening should completely cover patient's nose and mouth, without pressing on eyes.
      b. Ensure that inflatable rim is inflated to allow airtight seal.
      c. Hold mask firmly against patient's face with thumb and index finger encircling base, allowing remaining fingers to support patient's mandible. Avoid pressing on soft tissue under the mandible, which could potentially occlude airway.
      d. Squeeze attached resuscitator bag with sufficient pressure to inflate patient's chest. In some cases (eg, with poor lung compliance or large body habitus), two-person technique may be necessary; one person to hold mask and maintain a good seal, and the other to squeeze resuscitator bag.
   3. **Potential complications.** Bag-mask ventilation may cause gastric distention and pneumothorax.

VI. **Problem Case Diagnosis.** During physical exam, the 3-year-old patient was found to have rales at the right base of the lung and was diagnosed with pneumonia. He tolerated oxygen via simple face mask, and oxygenation status improved.

VII. Teaching Pearl: Question. A patient with an upper airway obstruction requires an appropriately sized NP airway but one cannot be located. What can be substituted?

VIII. Teaching Pearl: Answer. A shortened endotracheal tube may be substituted for an NP airway. Remove the end 15-mm adapter piece, trim the tube to length from the proximal end (tragus to tip of nose), firmly reinsert the 15-mm adapter, and insert the tube into the nasopharynx. The endotracheal tube is slightly more rigid than the usual NP airways and may not become occluded as easily, although it is potentially more damaging to tissues.

REFERENCES

Hazinski MF, Zartsky AL, eds. Airway, ventilation, and management of respiratory distress and failure. In: *Pediatric Advanced Life Support Provider Manual.* American Heart Association, 2002:81–126.

Scarfone R. Airway adjuncts, oxygen delivery, and suctioning the upper airway. In: Henretig F, King C, eds. *Textbook of Pediatric Emergency Procedures.* Williams & Wilkins, 1997:101–118.

5. ALKALOSIS

I. **Problem.** A 3-week-old male infant has progressively worsening projectile emesis (nonbilious and nonbloody). On physical exam, the infant is tachycardic and lethargic, and has weight loss and slight abdominal distention with a palpable right upper quadrant mass.

II. **Immediate Questions**

A. **What do physical exam findings say about patient's hydration status?** Vital sign changes (tachycardia) coupled with mental status exam and weight loss indicate severe dehydration in this infant due to hypovolemia from repeated emesis. Immediate attention is required.

B. **What do electrolyte findings indicate?** Electrolyte findings for this infant include Na^+ of 131 mEq/L, K^+ of 2.1 mEq/L, Cl^- of 88 mEq/L, and bicarbonate (HCO_3) of 30 mEq/L. This patient has hypochloremic, hypokalemic metabolic alkalosis caused by loss of gastric fluid (primarily H^+ and Cl^- ions). Because of the gastric outlet obstruction, there is no contribution to the ongoing fluid losses by pancreatic, intestinal, or biliary fluid. To compensate for Cl^- losses, there is concomitant urinary Na^+ and HCO_3 loss. If this condition persists, extracellular volume deficits will continue and renal compensation will occur, with urinary excretion of K^+ and H^+ in efforts to preserve Na^+ and subsequently maintain extracellular volume.

C. **What are initial concerns in immediate management of this patient?** Although emesis may ultimately require surgical intervention, hydration and electrolyte status are the primary concerns in initial management. Replacing fluid losses through adequate hydration and correction of electrolyte alterations should be the first steps in resuscitation of this infant. If fluid status is not addressed, infant may progress to a state of hypovolemic shock or symptomatic hypokalemia.

III. **Differential Diagnosis.** Confirm alkalosis (defined as pH > 7.44) *and* determine whether primary etiology is respiratory (decrease in PCO_2) or metabolic (increase in HCO_3).

A. **Respiratory Alkalosis.** Caused by a primary decrease in PCO_2 and seen in patients with hyperventilation (anxiety, fever, high altitude, salicylates, mechanical ventilation, sepsis, pneumonic processes, CNS disorders, hyperthyroidism) and urea cycle disorders.

B. **Metabolic Alkalosis.** Caused by elevation in serum HCO_3, which can be caused by a net loss of H^+, gain of HCO_3, or loss of extracellular fluid volume. A useful classification is based on urine Cl^- levels.

1. **Saline responsive.** Involves urine Cl^- levels < 10 mEq/L, which indicates renal reabsorption of Cl^- has occurred and patient will respond to saline replacement. Examples include vomiting (eg, pyloric stenosis), nasogastric (NG) suctioning, cystic fibrosis, congenital Cl^--wasting diarrhea, posthypercapnia, and Cl^--deficient formula intake.

2. **Saline resistant.** Involves urine Cl^- levels > 20 mEq/L. Examples include diuretic therapy, Bartter syndrome, Gitelman syndrome, hypokalemia, milk-alkali syndrome, excess mineralocorticoid production or ingestion (Cushing syndrome, hyperaldosteronism, adrenogenital syndrome, steroids, licorice, chewing tobacco).

IV. **Database.** History of presenting symptoms and medications provides the most useful information. Remember that alkalosis is not a primary disorder; usually it is secondary to an underlying disease process that must be identified and treated to correct the acid-base disturbance.

A. **Physical Exam Key Points**

1. **General appearance**. Is patient intubated or is an NG tube in place? Is patient alert, lethargic, febrile, or cachectic? Is there associated atypical facies ("moon facies") or weight loss?

2. **Respirations.** Is patient tachypneic?

3. **Cardiovascular.** Is there tachycardia? Regular rhythm?

4. **GI.** Are abdominal masses ("olive") or peristaltic wave present?

B. **Laboratory Data**

1. **ABGs.** Confirm pH > 7.44 and determine if primary disturbance is respiratory or metabolic (PCO_2 or HCO_3).

2. **Electrolytes and calcium.** Evaluate K^+ and Cl^- status; pattern may be suggestive of diagnosis (ie, hypochloremic, hypokalemic alkalosis seen with pyloric stenosis; hypokalemic

alkalosis seen with Bartter syndrome). Low Ca^{2+} levels are noted in milk-alkali syndrome.

3. Spot urine electrolytes. Help to determine type of metabolic alkalosis and future management (ie, response to Cl^- and fluid replacement).

4. Ammonia. Respiratory alkalosis, caused by stimulation of the respiratory center by hyperammonemia, is a frequent yet subtle clue to a urea cycle disorder.

5. Sweat test. Without adequate nutritional supplementation of Na^+ and Cl^-, infants with cystic fibrosis can have extracellular fluid losses resulting in loss of more Cl^- than HCO_3.

6. Salicylate level. Overdose from salicylate ingestion can cause mixed respiratory alkalosis with metabolic acidosis (high pH, low P_{CO_2}, and low HCO_3).

C. Radiographic and Other Studies

1. Chest x-ray. Pneumonic processes (pneumonia) resulting in hyperventilation may contribute to respiratory alkalosis. Patients with *Pneumocystis carinii* pneumonia, in particular, classically present with hypoxemia and respiratory alkalosis.

2. Upper GI and ultrasound scans. In the setting of progressive nonbilious emesis in an infant, it is necessary to rule out hypertrophic pyloric stenosis diagnosed by the classic "string sign" on upper GI series and increased length and thickness of pylorus on ultrasound.

V. Plan. Treatment is dependent on type of alkalosis and underlying cause. Alkalosis is a sign of a disorder and not the disease itself.

A. Volume Expansion. Give isotonic crystalloid solution for replacement of fluid losses as well as for maintenance. If hypokalemia is present, replace K^+ with a chloride salt (KCl); there are safety limitations to KCl infusions.

B. Metabolic Alkalosis

1. If patient is receiving diuretic therapy, consider temporarily discontinuing diuretics.

2. Chloride-resistant alkalosis can be treated with a carbonic anhydrase inhibitor (acetazolamide), which blocks proximal tubule reabsorption of HCO_3.

3. Treatment with HCl or ammonium chloride can be considered if alkalosis is severe (pH > 7.55) despite volume replacement or in cases with cardiac arrhythmias. Calculate H^+ ion deficit as follows:

$$H^+ \text{ ion deficit} = 0.3 \times \text{Weight (kg)} \times (\text{Measured } HCO_3 - \text{Desired } HCO_3 \text{ [mEq/L]})$$

C. Respiratory Alkalosis

1. Rarely life threatening, but underlying cause must be treated.

2. If patient is mechanically ventilated, consider reducing minute ventilation by reducing ventilator rate, inspiratory volume, or pressure. Adequate sedation may be required if a patient-triggered ventilator mode of ventilation is used.

VI. Problem Case Diagnosis. The 3-week-old infant was diagnosed with hypertrophic pyloric stenosis. Laboratory tests showed hypochloremic, hypokalemic alkalosis; and a thickened pylorus was visualized on abdominal ultrasound.

VII. Teaching Pearl: Question. What disorder and test must be considered in an ill-appearing, lethargic neonate with respiratory alkalosis?

VIII. Teaching Pearl: Answer. Urea cycle disorder and ammonia level must be considered; obtain serum ammonia level.

REFERENCES

Andreoli TE, Carpenter CJ, Bennett JC, Plum F, eds. *Cecil's Essentials of Medicine,* 4th ed. Saunders, 1997:198–202, 810–811.

Brewer ED. Disorders of acid-base balance. *Pediatr Clin North Am* 1990;37:429–447.

Gennari FJ. *Maxwell and Kleeman's Clinical Disorders of Fluid and Electrolyte Metabolism.* McGraw-Hill, 1994:957–989.

Hay WW, Groothuis JR, Hayward AR, Levin MJ, eds. *Current Pediatric Diagnosis and Treatment,* 12th ed. Appleton & Lange, 1995:705, 934–935, 1180–1189.

Urea Cycle Disorder Conference Group. Consensus statement from a conference for the management of patients with urea cycle disorders. *J Pediatr* 2001;138:51–55.

6. ALTERED MENTAL STATUS

I. Problem. A 9-year-old boy is brought to the emergency department after being found unresponsive by his parents.

II. Immediate Questions

A. Is patient breathing spontaneously? What are the vital signs? Rapid evaluation and support of airway, breathing, and circulation (ABCs) are the initial management priorities. All patients should receive 100% oxygen via face mask. Comatose patients who are apneic or have lost their protective airway reflexes require assisted ventilation with a bag-valve-mask device or endotracheal intubation. If head injury is suspected, immediately immobilize the cervical spine using in-line manual stabilization or placement of a cervical spine collar. Spine immobilization must then be maintained during airway management and endotracheal intubation. Patients in shock require rapid IV access, IV fluids, and possibly inotropic support after airway and breathing are controlled.

B. What is patient's level of consciousness?

1. Altered states of consciousness include:

a. Confusion. Impaired cognition manifested by disorientation, memory deficits, or difficulty following commands.

b. Delirium. Disconnection of ideas with disorientation, fearfulness, agitation, and irritability. Hallucinations may be present.

      c. Lethargy. Minimally reduced wakefulness with attention deficit. Easily distracted but able to communicate verbally or by gesture.

      d. Obtundation. Decreased alertness and interest in environment. Patient spends more time sleeping, and drowsiness persists when awakened.

      e. Stupor. Responsive only to vigorous, repeated, or painful stimulation and return to unresponsiveness when left alone.

      f. Coma. Complete unresponsiveness.

    2. Glasgow Coma Scale (GCS). This tool provides a more reliable method for describing level of consciousness (see Appendix F, p. 765).

  C. What is patient's dextrose level? Hypoglycemia is a common cause of altered mental status and is readily detected by bedside determination. Timely glucose administration to hypoglycemic patients can be lifesaving.

  D. Is drug overdose suspected? Does patient have small pupils? Consider administering IV naloxone for opiate overdose.

  E. Pertinent Historical Information

    1. Is there a history of witnessed or suspected trauma?

    2. Does patient have fever?

    3. What is the probability of poisoning, ingestion, or overdose?

    4. What are the associated symptoms (eg, headache, seizures, diplopia, weakness, vomiting, bloody diarrhea, abdominal pain)?

    5. Is there a contributing past medical history (eg, seizure disorder, brain tumor, ventricular shunt, sickle cell disease, metabolic disorder, diabetes, liver disease, renal failure)?

III. Differential Diagnosis. Altered mental status may have structural, medical, or functional causes. Common etiologies according to age are presented in Table I–2.

  A. Structural Causes. Tend to result in asymmetric or focal neurologic findings, particularly affecting pupillary response, extraocular movements, and motor response to pain.

    1. Trauma. Typically involves a shearing mechanism (diffuse axonal injury) from rapid deceleration. Shearing forces can rupture blood vessels and result in epidural, subdural, or intraparenchymal hemorrhage. When suspected mechanism of injury does not fit extent of patient's injuries, always consider inflicted trauma or child abuse.

    2. Tumor. Symptoms such as headache, vomiting, or focal neurologic deficit are typically present for weeks to months. Altered mental status can result from seizures, intracranial hypertension, or cerebral edema.

    3. Cerebrovascular event. Hemorrhagic and ischemic strokes occur with the same frequency in children. A ruptured arteriovenous malformation is the most common cause of hemorrhagic

TABLE I–2. COMMON CAUSES OF ALTERED MENTAL STATUS BY AGE

Age	Cause
Infant	Abuse
	Inborn errors of metabolism
	Infection
	Metabolic alterations
	Seizure
Child	Abuse or trauma
	Infection
	Intussusception
	Seizure
	Toxin
Adolescent	Psychiatric
	Seizure
	Toxin
	Trauma

stroke in children. Ischemic and thrombotic strokes occur most commonly in children with sickle cell disease and congenital heart defects; less commonly in children with hypercoagulable states, metabolic disorders, vasculitis, and other vascular abnormalities. Patients with hemorrhagic strokes tend to present with altered mental status and headache whereas those with ischemic strokes present with focal neurologic deficits.

4. **Hydrocephalus.** Infants present with increased head circumference, thin scalp with distended veins, and bulging fontanel. Other nonspecific symptoms such as irritability, poor feeding, and vomiting may be present. Sunset sign (decreased upward gaze), which results from weakness of cranial nerve VI, may be present.

   a. **Communicating.** Occurs when CSF is not absorbed by arachnoid villi as a result of infection or hemorrhage.

   b. **Noncommunicating.** Occurs when congenital malformations or acquired tumors block normal CSF circulation.

5. **Infection.** Contiguous spread of middle ear or sinus infection can lead to an epidural abscess in older children and adolescents.

B. **Medical Causes.** Include any process that decreases delivery of substrate to the brain. Pupils are generally equal and reactive, and neurologic exam is nonfocal.

1. **Infection.** Fever, irritability, lethargy, and vomiting are common presenting symptoms.

   a. **Meningitis.** Infants and young children often have nonspecific symptoms. Headache and neck stiffness may not be present in children younger than 2 years of age.

b. **Encephalitis.**
c. **Subdural empyem a.** May occur secondary to meningitis or from direct extension of otitis media or sinusitis. Seizures occur in two thirds of patients.
d. **Sepsis.** Can cause shock from circulating inflammatory mediators.

2. **Poisoning or overdose.** Poisoning or overdose from many substances can cause altered mental status (Table I–3). Because many drugs and toxins are not detectable on serum and urine screening tests, a high index of suspicion must be maintained. Some ingested substances cause a specific constellation of signs (toxidrome), which aids in diagnosis and management. Table I–4 summarizes common toxidromes.

3. **Seizure.** Children can present in the postictal state without a witnessed seizure. Seizures may be followed by a transient period of paralysis (Todd paralysis) usually affecting one side of the body, which may lead to a false suspicion of a structural etiology.

4. **Metabolic alterations.** Hyperglycemia or hypoglycemia, electrolyte (Na^+ or Ca^{2+}) abnormalities, and inborn errors of metabolism can cause altered mental status.

5. **Intussusception.** Occasionally, patients with intussusception can present with profound lethargy (presumably due to release of cytokines from the entrapped bowel wall) with little or no history of abdominal complaints.

TABLE I–3. SUBSTANCES THAT CAN CAUSE POISONING OR OVERDOSE ASSOCIATED WITH COMA

Amphetamines
Anticholinergics
Barbiturates
Benzodiazepines
Carbamazepine
Carbon monoxide
Clonidine
Cocaine
Ethanol
Gamma hydroxybutyrate (GHB)
Haloperidol
Narcotics
Phencyclidine (PCP)
Phenothiazines
Phenytoin
Salicylates
Selective serotonin reuptake inhibitors (SSRIs)
Tricyclic antidepressants

TABLE I-4. TOXIDROMES

Toxidrome	Mental Status	Pulse	RR	BP	Pupil Size	Skin	Temp	Specific Management
Opioid	Depressed	Low	Low	Low	Pinpoint	Normal	↓	Naloxone
Sedative hypnotic	Depressed	Low	Low	Low	Normal	Normal	Normal	Flumazenil (controversial)
Sympathomimetic	Agitated	High	Normal	High	↑	Diaphoretic	↑	Benzodiazepines
Cholinergic	Agitated	High or low	Normal	High or low	↑	Diaphoretic	Normal	Atropine, pralidoxime
Anticholinergic	Agitated or delirium	High	High or low	High or low	↑	Dry	↑	Physostigmine, benzodiazepines

↑ = increased; ↓ = decreased; BP = blood pressure; RR = respiratory rate; temp = temperature.

      6. Hemolytic uremic syndrome (HUS). HUS secondary to infection with *E coli* O157:H7 can cause lethargy, seizures, or coma from uremia.

  C. Functional Cause. Consider functional cause, especially when all organic causes have been ruled out.

IV. Database

  A. Physical Exam Key Points

    1. Level of consciousness. Assess using GCS.

    2. Ocular and motor responses. Assess the following to help determine whether illness has a structural or medical cause. Asymmetry points to a structural lesion.

      a. Pupillary size. Normal or asymmetric?

      b. Pupillary reflex. Fixed or reactive?

      c. Extraocular movements. Normal, asymmetric, or absent?

      d. Motor response to pain. Decorticate, decerebrate, or flaccid?

    3. Respiratory pattern. Identification of abnormal patterns can help differentiate structural from medical causes of altered mental status.

      a. Cheyne-Stokes respiration. Implies dysfunction of structures deep in both cerebral hemispheres or diencephalon; usually seen in metabolic encephalopathy.

      b. Central neurogenic hyperventilation. May occur with lesions of midbrain and pons.

      c. Cluster breathing. May result from primary or secondary brainstem lesions.

      d. Ataxic breathing. May result from primary disruption of medullary respiratory centers.

    4. Toxidromes (see Table I–4).

    5. Neurologic findings. Perform a thorough neurologic exam.

    6. Smell of patient's breath. May reveal alcohol intoxication or diabetic ketoacidosis.

    7. Signs of trauma. Boggy scalp swelling, Battle sign, raccoon eyes, retinal hemorrhages, hemotympanum, bruises, hematomas.

    8. Abdomen. Tenderness and palpable sausage-shaped mass are consistent with intussusception.

  B. Laboratory Data

    1. Glucose. Rapid bedside serum glucose determination immediately identifies hypoglycemia or hyperglycemia.

    2. Serum electrolytes. Reveal whether seizures are induced by electrolyte abnormalities (eg, Na^+ and Ca^{2+}), as well as presence of acidosis (bicarbonate) or uremia (BUN and creatinine).

    3. Liver function tests. Reveal presence of hepatic failure.

    4. Serum ammonia. Elevated level is associated with common inborn errors of metabolism.

    5. Serum or urine drug screening. Although limited, can identify potential toxins.

      6. Anticonvulsant drug levels. Obtain in patients with known seizure disorder.

      7. CBC, differential, blood and urine cultures. Obtain in febrile patients or whenever sepsis or CNS infection is suspected. CBC is also helpful in evaluation of patients with sickle cell disease or suspected HUS.

      8. Cerebrospinal fluid evaluation (cell count, chemistry, and culture). Obtain whenever CNS infection or sepsis is suspected.

      9. Guaiac test for occult blood. Stool may reveal occult GI bleeding in patients with intussusception or HUS.

  C. Radiographic and Other Studies

    1. CT scan of head. Obtain emergently whenever increased intracranial pressure or presence of a structural lesion is suspected, especially before performing lumbar puncture to avoid risk of cerebral herniation. Obtain in all patients with altered mental status of unclear etiology.

    2. Abdominal obstruction series. Helpful in screening for intussusception; if highly suspected, air or barium enema reduction is necessary.

    3. Skeletal survey. Obtain in children younger than 3 years of age who may have suffered inflicted injuries or child abuse.

    4. ECG. May be helpful in management of certain ingested substances or toxins.

V. Plan. Figure I–1 depicts a systematic approach to a patient with altered mental status.

  A. Initial Management

    1. Support ABCs: secure airway, administer 100% oxygen, and obtain IV access.

    2. Immobilize cervical spine in patients with known or suspected history of head injury.

    3. Assess GCS; if < 8, perform endotracheal intubation.

    4. Assess for signs of herniation (dilated nonreactive pupil, papilledema, posturing) or increased intracranial pressure (Cushing triad of hypertension, bradycardia, irregular respirations). If present, prevent hypercarbia and fever, maintain euvolemia, consider administration of mannitol or normal saline, and obtain emergent CT scan of head and neurosurgical consultation.

    5. Perform rapid bedside glucose determination. If glucose is ≤ 40, administer IV dextrose.

  B. Specific Treatment

    1. Narcotic overdose. If suspected, administer naloxone.

    2. Head injury or focal neurologic finding. Obtain CT scan of head and neurosurgical consultation.

    3. Metabolic alterations. Correct metabolic and electrolyte abnormalities and acidosis.

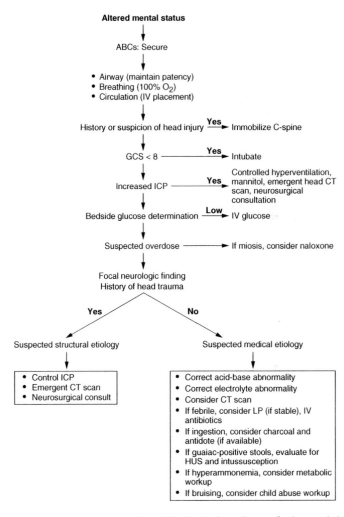

Figure I–1. Management algorithm for a child with altered mental status. (C-spine = cervical spine; GCS = Glasgow Coma Scale; HUS = hemolytic uremic syndrome; ICP = intracranial pressure; LP = lumbar puncture.)

   4. **Poisoning or overdose.** If suspected, administer charcoal (if
      indicated and ingestion occurred within 1 hour) and antidote if
      available.
   5. **Fever, CNS infection, or sepsis.** Perform a lumbar puncture if
      patient is stable and does not have signs of increased intracra-
      nial pressure. Administer antibiotics if considering bacterial
      CNS disease or sepsis.
   6. **Hyperammonemia.** Consider workup for metabolic disorder.
   7. **Guaiac-positive stools.** Evaluate for intussusception or HUS.

VI. Problem Case Diagnosis. The 9-year-old boy was breathing spon-
     taneously with a rate of 40 breaths/min and appeared dehydrated on
     admission to the emergency department. He was given 100% oxy-
     gen via face mask, and IV access was obtained. Rapid bedside
     blood glucose determination showed a critically high value, and sub-
     sequent venous blood gas and serum electrolyte determination
     showed diabetic ketoacidosis. Patient was rehydrated and started on
     an insulin infusion.

VII. Teaching Pearl: Question. What clues help differentiate a functional
      from an organic cause of altered mental status?

VIII. Teaching Pearl: Answer. Organic causes of altered mental status
       need to be excluded first. However, patients feigning unresponsive-
       ness will have increased heart rate with painful stimuli, may resist eye
       opening, and will avoid hitting the face when their hand is allowed to
       drop to it.

REFERENCES

Nelson DS. Coma and altered level of consciousness. In Fleisher GR, ed. *Textbook
   of Pediatric Emergency Medicine.* Lippincott Williams & Wilkins, 2000:165–176.
King D, Avner JR. Altered mental status. In Isaacman DJ, ed. Neurologic emergencies. *Clin Pediatr Emerg Med* 2003;4:171–178.

7. ANAPHYLACTIC REACTION

   I. Problem. Fifteen minutes after receiving an IV infusion of ampicillin,
      a 10-year-old boy with meningitis develops urticaria and wheezing,
      and the nurse reports that he "doesn't look good."

   II. Immediate Questions
       A. Is this anaphylaxis? If anaphylaxis is present, assess airway,
          breathing, and circulation (ABCs) while administering epineph-
          rine, 0.01 mL/kg of body weight. Consider other causes if ana-
          phylaxis is not present (Table I–5).
       B. What are the vital signs? Tachycardia is a common finding in
          children and is most often due to hypoxia, fear, or a compensatory

TABLE I–5. CONDITIONS TO CONSIDER IN DIFFERENTIAL DIAGNOSIS

Aspiration of foreign body
Asthma exacerbation
Flushing syndromes
Hereditary angioedema
Mastocytosis (high tryptase level when child is well)
Panic attack
Septic shock
Vasovagal syncope[a]

[a] Lack of pruritus in presence of slow pulse rate and low BP distinguishes vasovagal reaction from anaphylaxis.

response to evolving hypotension. Hypotension is an ominous sign, although normal BP does not rule out anaphylaxis.

C. Is patient well oriented and able to communicate? Mental confusion suggests poor cerebral perfusion. Inability to speak, dysphonia, hoarseness, or stridor could indicate upper airway obstruction from laryngospasm or laryngeal edema.

D. What medication(s) did patient receive?

1. Obtain the following information about suspected medication(s) immediately:
   a. Dose.
   b. Duration of use.
   c. Temporal relationship of symptoms with medication administration.
2. Common medications causing anaphylaxis are listed in Table I–6. Any medicine suspected of causing anaphylaxis must be stopped immediately.

E. Special Questions

1. Is there a previous history of anaphylaxis? If yes, reaction is more likely a repeat episode.
2. History of asthma? If yes, increases chances of mortality from anaphylaxis.
3. Are there any associated symptoms?
   a. **Dermatologic.** Pruritus and hives; *severe reaction can occur in the absence of skin manifestation.*
   b. **Respiratory.** Sneezing and nasal congestion, hoarseness, stridor, chest tightness, and wheezing.
   c. **GI.** Tingling sensation and feeling of fullness in mouth, nausea, vomiting, diarrhea, and abdominal pain.
   d. **Neurologic.** Dizziness, sense of impending death.

TABLE I–6. COMMON CAUSES OF ANAPHYLAXIS

- **Drugs**
  Allergen extracts
  Amphotericin B
  Antibiotics (penicillin and related antibiotics)
  Aspirin
  Blood products
  General anesthetics
  Neomycin
  Radiographic contrast medium
  Vaccines
  Vancomycin
- **Food**
  Fish and shellfish
  Peanuts
  Tree nuts
- **Others**
  Exercise
  Insect venom
  Latex

III. **Differential Diagnosis.** Anaphylaxis may involve one or several organ systems, including skin, upper and lower airways, and cardiovascular, GI, and neurologic systems. Because of this multisystem involvement, anaphylaxis must be distinguished from other disease processes occurring at these sites. Table I–5 lists conditions sharing some symptoms with anaphylaxis.

IV. **Database**
  A. **Physical Exam Key Points**
    1. **Vital signs.** Continue checking, with special attention to heart rate and BP.
    2. **Skin.** Look for flushing; pharyngeal, periorbital, or facial edema; profuse rhinorrhea; urticaria; angioedema; and generalized flushing.
    3. **Lungs.** Listen for wheezing, stridor, or dyspnea.
    4. **Neurologic and cardiovascular findings.** Monitor for impaired mental status and syncope.
  B. **Laboratory Data.** *Treatment of anaphylaxis should never be withheld while awaiting laboratory confirmation.*
    1. **Serum tryptase.** Elevated in anaphylaxis. Must be drawn between 1 and 6 hours of onset (2 mL of blood in red- or gold-top tube).
    2. **Urine *N*-methyl-histamine.** Elevated in anaphylaxis. Remains elevated for several hours after a reaction and can be measured by 24-hour urine sample.

        3. CBC. Check for hemoconcentration.
    C. Radiographic and Other Studies. Order as clinically indicated.

V. Plan
  A. Initial Management
    1. Continually assess and support ABCs as needed.
    2. Acute severe anaphylactic reaction requires immediate discontinuation of allergen. Apply tourniquet proximal to antigenic site if secondary to IM and SQ injection. Remember to remove tourniquet once patient is stable.
    3. Establish IV access.
    4. Close monitoring in an intensive care setting for 12–24 hours is required for anaphylactic shock. Relapse of anaphylaxis can occur hours after initial presentation.
    5. Further acute management is outlined in Figure I–2. Therapy should be guided by a board-certified allergist.
  B. Long-term Follow-up and Prevention
    1. Patients who have experienced anaphylaxis should be evaluated by an allergist.
    2. **Self-injected epinephrine.** Patients and their families should receive correct instruction on use of an autoinjectable epinephrine delivery device.
    3. Provide a list of drug(s) to avoid.
    4. Suggest that patient wear a medical alert bracelet.

VI. Problem Case Diagnosis. The 10-year-old patient had an anaphylactic reaction to ampicillin.

VII. Teaching Pearl: Question. Six hours after the initial reaction described in the opening problem statement, the 10-year-old patient develops an episode of tachycardia with shortness of breath. Is this a continuation of the same problem or more likely another "allergic reaction"?

VIII. Teaching Pearl: Answer. Several hours after the initial symptoms of anaphylaxis resolve, symptoms can recur without additional exposure to the inciting agent. This phenomenon, called a *biphasic reaction,* occurs in about 6% of patients with anaphylaxis.

REFERENCES

Sicherer SH. How to recognize and manage anaphylaxis. *J Res Dis Pediatr* 2003;5:191–198.

Uram R. What every pediatrician must know about anaphylaxis and anaphylactoid reactions. *Pediatr Ann* 2000;29:737–742.

Wyatt R. Anaphylaxis. How to recognize, treat and prevent potentially fatal attacks. *Postgrad Med* 1996;100:87–90, 96–99.

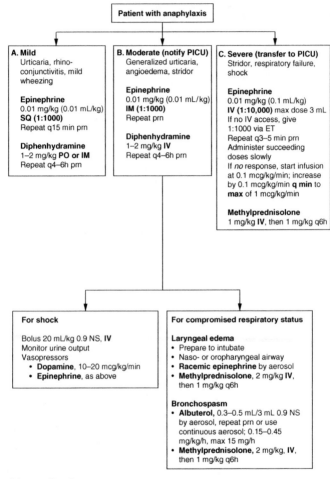

Figure I-2. General approach to management of anaphylaxis. (ACE = angiotensin-converting enzyme; ET = endotracheal; NS = normal saline; PICU = pediatric intensive care unit.)

8. ANEMIA

I. **Problem.** An 18-month-old boy is admitted for evaluation of pallor associated with a hemoglobin level of 6.5 g/dL.

II. **Immediate Questions**
- **A. What are the vital signs?** With no hypotension or severe tachycardia, transfusion therapy is not emergently indicated.
- **B. Is patient symptomatic?** In the absence of congestive heart failure, syncope, presyncope, or hemodynamic compromise, transfusion therapy is not emergently indicated.
- **C. Is there evidence of acute or recent blood loss (eg, hematemesis, melena, or hematochezia)?** GI blood loss can be divided into acute or chronic, upper GI and lower GI. Acute upper GI blood loss is more often life-threatening than lower GI blood loss.
- **D. History of hematuria?** Long-standing hematuria can cause iron deficiency anemia. Hemoglobinuria is found in hemolytic anemias with brisk intravascular hemolysis.
- **E. What medication(s) does patient take?** Aspirin and NSAIDs may lead to GI blood loss. Chemotherapy drugs, immunosuppressives, folate antagonists (trimethoprim-sulfamethoxazole), anticonvulsants (carbamazepine, valproate, dilantin), and anti-inflammatory drugs (phenylbutazone) may cause marrow suppression or aplasia. Penicillin, sulfonamides, or oxidants may cause hemolysis. Alcohol, isoniazid, and trimethoprim may cause maturation defects.
- **F. Is there significant organ dysfunction or active inflammatory disease?** Severe liver, kidney, adrenal, and thyroid dysfunction cause anemia. Rheumatoid arthritis, systemic lupus erythematosus, inflammatory bowel disease, vasculitides, and chronic osteomyelitis are associated with anemia of chronic disease.
- **G. How old is patient?** Nutritional iron deficiency is never responsible for anemia in term infants before 6 months of age or in premature infants before doubling birthweight. In the newborn period, anemia often results from recent blood loss, isoimmunization, congenital hemolytic anemia, or congenital TORCH infection. Anemia first detected at ages 3–6 months is likely congenital (initially not detected because of fetal hemoglobin).
- **H. Gender and ethnicity?** Consider glucose-6-phosphate dehydrogenase (G6PD) deficiency in male patients and those of Mediterranean and African origin; thalassemia syndromes in those of Mediterranean and Asian origin; hemoglobin S and C in those of African origin.
- **I. Neonatal history?** Jaundice in the newborn period suggests hemolytic anemia (hereditary spherocytosis or G6PD deficiency).
- **J. Dietary history and milk intake?** An excessive volume of cow's milk in a toddler (> 24 oz/day) commonly results in iron deficiency. Goat's milk is deficient in folate.
- **K. Other medical problems that may cause pseudoanemia?** Conditions associated with excess total body water (eg, congestive

heart failure) may cause pseudoanemia. In the setting of increased plasma volume, anemia may be made more apparent.

L. History or family history of anemia, splenomegaly, jaundice, thalassemia, sickle cell anemia, or G6PD deficiency? Patients with hereditary disorders of RBCs usually present nonacutely.

M. History of autoimmune disease or immunodeficiency? May be associated with direct Coombs-positive hemolytic anemias or anemia of chronic disease.

III. Differential Diagnosis. CBC with differential, visualization of peripheral smear, RBC indices, and reticulocyte count are essential and show where anemia results from decreased RBC production, blood loss, or increased RBC destruction.

A. Pancytopenia. All cell lines (hemoglobin, platelets, and WBCs) are decreased. Usually the result of marrow invasion, failure, or suppression caused by drugs, metastatic tumor, hematologic malignancies, and inflammatory diseases. Bone marrow failure (aplastic anemia) may be idiopathic.

B. Low Mean Corpuscular Volume (MCV) Anemias. Iron deficiency is the most common etiology, especially in menstruating girls and toddlers. Hypochromic, microcytic RBCs; target cells; basophilic stippling; marked anisocytosis; and poikilocytosis are seen with thalassemias. Lead poisoning, sideroblastic anemia, and anemia of chronic disease are also associated with low MCV. Red blood cell distribution width index (RDW) is normal in thalassemia trait but high in iron deficiency.

C. Normal MCV Anemias. Anemia of chronic disease is most common. Other etiologies include acute blood loss; chronic infections; collagen vascular diseases; malignancies; kidney, liver, thyroid, and adrenal dysfunction; and transient erythroblastopenia of childhood.

D. High MCV Anemias. Folate and vitamin B_{12} deficiencies are most common. Vitamin B_{12} deficiency may be secondary to pernicious anemia, bacterial overgrowth, ileal disease, and (rarely) dietary deficiency (eg, vegan diet). Folate deficiency is associated with dietary deficiency (eg, goat's milk diet), pregnancy, hyperthyroidism, and hemolytic anemias. Consider malabsorption if there is no obvious cause of folate deficiency. Peripheral smear demonstrates hypersegmented neutrophils and nucleated RBCs. Increased MCV may result from a markedly increased reticulocyte count.

E. Anemias With Increased Reticulocyte Count. Indicates bone marrow that is producing RBCs faster than normal, usually to compensate for loss of RBCs with a shortened life span or from acute blood loss. Reticulocytes appear 24–48 hours after significant acute blood loss. Causes include autoimmune hemolytic anemias and congenital hemolytic anemias (sickle cell anemia, thalassemias). Correction of a deficit (eg, iron deficiency) also leads to transient reticulocytosis.

IV. Database
  A. Physical Exam Key Points
  1. **Vital signs.** Check for hypotension. Patient may be *orthostatic* (decrease in systolic BP of 10 mm Hg or increase in heart rate of 20 beats/min 1 minute after sudden movement from supine to standing position), suggesting acute blood loss.
  2. **Skin.** Petechiae or purpura may be seen with thrombocytopenia in bone marrow failure or infiltration, hemolytic uremic syndrome, thrombotic thrombocytopenic purpura, or autoimmune hemolytic anemia. Telangiectasia, palmar erythema, and jaundice may indicate liver disease. Isolated jaundice suggests hemolysis. Lack of pink coloration of palmar creases indicates severe anemia.
  3. **Face.** Frontal bossing and prominence of maxillary and malar bones are seen with bone marrow hyperplasia in thalassemia major and severe congenital hemolytic anemias.
  4. **Eyes.** Retinal vessel tortuosity, microaneurysms, and hemorrhages can be present in patients with sickle S and C hemoglobinopathies.
  5. **Oropharynx.** Glossitis in vitamin B_{12} or iron deficiency; angular stomatitis with iron deficiency.
  6. **Heart.** Flow murmurs are common in anemia.
  7. **Abdomen.** Splenomegaly is associated with hemolysis, thalassemias, chronic leukemias, lymphomas, and acute leukemias. Ascites, hepatomegaly, and splenomegaly suggest liver disease (portal hypertension).
  B. Laboratory Data
  1. **Peripheral smear.** Note size and shape of RBCs and WBCs, and presence of platelets.
  2. **Reticulocyte count.** The most important laboratory test after peripheral smear.
     a. **Increased.** Indicates either an appropriate response to anemia or shortened RBC survival through blood loss or hemolysis.
     b. **Low.** With anemia, indicates that marrow is responding inappropriately to nutritional deficiency, marrow failure, or marrow replacement.
     c. **Very low (< 0.2%).** Seen with congenital pure red cell aplasia and transient erythroblastopenia of childhood.
  3. **Iron and total iron-binding capacity (TIBC) or transferrin.** Consider checking ferritin (reflects iron stores or an inflammatory process) in patients with microcytic anemia. Patients with iron deficiency anemia have low iron and normal or elevated TIBC or transferrin; ferritin is generally low but can be normal or high in response to inflammation. Very low MCV (< 70) and normal iron and TIBC suggest thalassemia. Increased hemoglobin A_2 on hemoglobin electrophoresis occurs with β-thalassemia trait.

Acute and chronic illnesses can dramatically affect iron and TIBC, making their utility in diagnosis of anemia low. If the question of iron deficiency requires definite diagnosis, a bone marrow exam with iron stains is indicated in children 4 years of age or older (by which time they have accumulated stainable iron in bone marrow). A trial of iron therapy can be both diagnostic and therapeutic in many patients.

4. **Guaiac test for occult blood.** Stool may reveal occult GI bleeding.
5. **Vitamin B$_{12}$ and folate.** Order these tests prior to transfusion if deficiency is suspected. In folate deficiency secondary to malnutrition, serum folate may be normal after one or two well-balanced meals; consider checking RBC folate level.
6. **Haptoglobin and urine hemosiderin.** Low haptoglobin indicates acute hemolysis. A positive urine hemosiderin, which tests for heme in shed renal tubular cells, indicates hemolysis; this may have occurred weeks earlier.
7. **Direct and indirect Coombs test.** Indicates that hemolysis is mediated by antibody. Direct Coombs test measures presence of antibody or complement, or both, on the RBC; indirect Coombs test detects antibody in plasma directed at the RBC. The direct Coombs test is more valuable in evaluating immuno-hemolytic disease; the indirect Coombs is of value as a blood-banking procedure. Detection of an antibody in plasma but not on the RBC suggests an alloantibody (usually IgG) rather than an autoantibody.
8. **Platelet count.** Elevated in early iron deficiency or transient erythroblastopenia of childhood. Decreased in folate and vitamin B$_{12}$ deficiency, severe iron deficiency, and with marrow replacement.

C. **Radiographic and Other Studies.** Order as clinically indicated.

V. **Plan**
   A. **Anemia With Hemodynamic Compromise or Complications**
      1. If patient is hemodynamically unstable, transfuse immediately.
      2. If evidence of acute bleeding, stop bleeding and obtain adequate IV access (anticipating need for transfusion).
   B. **Anemia Without Hemodynamic Compromise or Complications.** Proceed with workup in an orderly fashion. Laboratory testing is not always diagnostic, and bone marrow biopsy may be indicated.
   C. **Iron Deficiency Anemia.** Alter patient's diet as indicated to prevent recurrence or persistence. Sample stools for occult blood, especially in children older than 2–3 years of age; if positive, source of blood loss must be found. Heavy menstrual losses are most common cause of iron deficiency in young women. Iron stores are replenished with 6 mg/kg/day of elemental iron divided into 2 or 3 doses. Treatment is continued for at least 3 months after normalization of CBC to ensure adequate stores.

   D. **Folate Deficiency.** Usually due to dietary insufficiency.
      Supplement 1 mg folate PO daily. Folate, 1 mg daily, is also given
      for chronic hemolytic anemias to meet increased needs in replac-
      ing RBCs.
   E. **Vitamin B$_{12}$ Deficiency.** Inadequate dietary intake and true per-
      nicious anemia occur rarely in children. More likely causes of vita-
      min B$_{12}$ deficiency in children and adolescents include bacterial
      overgrowth, ileal disease, postsurgical gastrectomy, and ileal
      resection. Vitamin B$_{12}$ is replaced by administration of 100 mcg IM
      daily for 2 weeks, then 60–100 mcg IM every 4 weeks.
   F. **Hemolytic Anemia.** With elevated reticulocyte count and no obvi-
      ous source of blood loss, consider a destructive process. Brisk
      ongoing hemolysis results in elevation of total and indirect biliru-
      bin and increased LDH without concomitant increase in AST or
      ALT. Immune-mediated processes are diagnosed using Coombs
      test. Ill patients with a microangiopathic smear may have hemolytic
      anemia associated with hemolytic uremic syndrome or thrombotic
      thrombocytopenic purpura, or disseminated intravascular coagu-
      lation (DIC). Low platelets and fibrinogen, elevated PT and PTT,
      and fibrin degradation products indicate DIC. Inherited disorders
      (thalassemia, sickle cell anemia, or an enzymopathy) must be
      ruled out. The possibility of paroxysmal nocturnal hemoglobinuria
      and Wilson disease should be considered in cases with unclear
      etiology.
   G. **Anemia of Chronic Disease.** Usually a diagnosis of exclusion.
      There is no specific diagnostic test for this disorder; treatment is
      that of underlying disease.

VI. **Problem Case Diagnosis.** Review of systems and past medical,
    social, dietary, and family history for the 18-month-old boy were
    benign. Physical exam findings were normal except for pallor,
    decrease in visible scleral vessels, and lack of pink color in palmar
    creases. CBC showed normal WBC count and differential, elevated
    platelet count, normal MCV and RDW, and normal RBC morphology.
    Reticulocyte count was 0.1%. Results of bone marrow biopsy
    demonstrated absence of all erythroid precursors except the most
    primitive line. Patient was transfused expectantly when the hemoglo-
    bin level dropped to 5 g/dL and reticulocyte count remained at 0.1%.
    Seven weeks later, after a second transfusion, the reticulocyte count
    was 8%. The CBC normalized without recurrence of anemia. Patient
    was diagnosed with transient erythroblastopenia of childhood.

VII. **Teaching Pearl: Question.** What bedside trick can help in the diag-
     nosis of cold agglutinin hemolytic anemia?

VIII. **Teaching Pearl: Answer.** In a patient with pallor and dark urine,
      rotate a tube of the patient's anticoagulated blood at room tempera-
      ture and after chilling to look for large RBC aggregates termed
      bedside cold agglutinins. This form of hemolytic anemia is most

commonly associated with *Mycoplasma pneumoniae* or Epstein-Barr virus infection. If transfusion is indicated, keep all skin surfaces of patient very warm (and warm blood as it is transfused) to prevent pathologic IgM antibody from binding to the RBC surface, with resultant complement fixation and hemolysis.

REFERENCES

Hermiston ML, Mentzer WC. A practical approach to the evaluation of the anemic child. *Pediatr Clin North Am* 2002;49:877–891.
Nathan DG, Orkin SH, Ginsburg D, Loot AT. *Nathan and Oski's Hematology of Infancy and Childhood,* 6th ed, Vol 1. Saunders, 2003.
Segal GB, Hirsh MG, Feig SA. Managing anemia in a pediatric office practice: Part 2. *Pediatr Rev* 2002;23:111–122.

9. APNEA AND APPARENT LIFE-THREATENING EVENT

I. Problems

A. A 3-month-old male infant is brought to the emergency department after he reportedly stopped breathing at home. His mother states that he suddenly began gasping and choking and then became limp and lost color. When EMS personnel arrived, the infant was alert and in no apparent distress.

B. A 3-year-old boy with a history of snoring and chronic congestion is rushed to the emergency department in the middle of the night after he reportedly stopped breathing at home. He has a cold, but no fever, and was asleep at the time of the episode. Now he is awake, but sleepy. His color is good, but he is congested and mouth breathing.

II. Immediate Questions

A. Who is providing the history? Determine if the episode can be characterized as truly life threatening, frightening, or a variant of normal respiration. Obtaining an accurate history may be difficult because the person who observed the episode is usually untrained, often a frightened family member.

B. Was breathing movement present? How can event be categorized?

   1. Apparent life-threatening event (ALTE). An episode that is frightening to observer and is characterized by a combination of apnea, color change, marked change in muscle tone, choking, and gagging. In many cases, observer believes the episode was life threatening and in some instances believes infant or child has died. Because any relationship between ALTE and sudden infant death syndrome (SIDS) is unproven, the term "near-miss SIDS" or "aborted SIDS" should be avoided.

   2. Central apnea. Absence of airflow at nose or mouth *and* no respiratory efforts.

3. **Obstructive apnea.** Absence of airflow at nose or mouth despite continued respiratory efforts.
4. **Obstructive sleep apnea syndrome (OSAS).** A disorder of sleep consisting of prolonged partial upper airway obstruction, or episodic obstructive apnea, or both, that affects gas exchange during sleep as well as sleep architecture and quality. Adenotonsillar hypertrophy is the most common cause in children. Children who are obese and those with craniofacial syndromes (eg, midfacial hypoplasia, micrognathia) or disorders associated with abnormal muscle tone are at risk.

C. **What is patient's clinical status?** Initial evaluation and management includes rapid assessment of airway, breathing, and circulation (ABCs).

D. **What is patient's sleep pattern?** OSAS, which occurs only during sleep, is associated with snoring, pauses in or labored breathing, abnormal movements or head positioning, and excessive sweating during sleep.

E. **Who was with patient when ALTE occurred?** May raise suspicion of abuse or Munchausen syndrome by proxy.

F. **What are characteristics of patient's sleep position and environment?** Supine sleep position and presence of gas-trapping objects in cribs (eg, stuffed animals, pillows) place young infants at risk of SIDS. Tobacco, alcohol, or other substance exposures increase the risk of SIDS and child abuse.

G. **Are other problems associated with event?** Fever and symptoms of upper respiratory infection suggest an underlying infectious process. Abnormal eye or body movements suggest seizures. Associated feeding problems may suggest dysphagia, gastroesophageal reflux, or cardiac abnormalities.

H. **Is there a family history of ALTEs or SIDS?** SIDS can run in families, but may suggest child abuse and certain metabolic conditions.

I. **Is there a history of prematurity or an underlying condition?** Infants and children with underlying medical conditions are at risk of apneic events. OSAS is associated with adenotonsillar hypertrophy, allergic rhinitis, obesity, trisomy 21, craniofacial syndromes, skeletal dysplasia syndromes, neuromuscular disorders, cerebral palsy, and sickle cell disease.

III. **Differential Diagnosis.** ALTE is a heterogeneous disorder with a broad differential diagnosis. The more common causes are listed below.

A. **Idiopathic.**

B. **Gastroesophageal Reflux Disease (GERD) or Dysphagia.** GERD can be associated with obstructive apnea, esophagitis, bronchospasms, and growth failure. Stimulation of chemoreceptors in the upper airway and lower esophagus can lead to obstructive apnea.

C. Seizure or Other Neurologic Abnormality. Usually associated with behavioral changes and daytime symptoms.

D. Sepsis or Infection (Bacterial, Viral). Respiratory syncytial virus (RSV), pertussis, and serious underlying infections can often present with central apnea.

E. Cardiac Disease. History and physical exam usually provide clues to these disorders.

F. Anemia. Consider, particularly in a young infant with a history of prematurity.

G. Breath-holding Spell. Associated with emotional outbursts or stressful situations.

H. Upper Airway Obstruction (eg, laryngomalacia). See Chapter 84, Stridor, p. 393.

I. Metabolic Disorder. Inborn errors of metabolism can present as ALTE in young infants. Metabolic disorders often present with metabolic acidosis.

J. Traumatic Child Abuse. See Chapter 14, Child Abuse: Physical, p. 70.

K. Munchausen Syndrome by Proxy.

IV. Database

A. Physical Exam Key Points

1. **Vital signs.** Is heart rate normal for age and regular? Is there an absence of breathing movements? Are there pauses or irregularities in respiration? Is respiratory effort effective? What is the oxygen saturation, and is it maintained in the normal range?

2. **General appearance.** Is patient alert and vigorous or lethargic? Any obvious deformities?

3. **Growth parameters.** Rarely, in severe cases of OSAS, failure to thrive may be evident. Obesity, however, is much more common.

4. **HEENT.** Evaluate for rhinitis, adenotonsillar hypertrophy, and polyposis. Check for retinal hemorrhages.

5. **Cardiopulmonary findings.** Check perfusion and abnormal sounds (eg, murmurs, rales, wheezing). Pectus excavatum suggests prolonged or severe upper airway obstruction, or both. Cor pulmonale is rarely associated with OSAS.

6. **Neuromuscular exam.** Assess tone, cranial nerves, and deep tendon reflexes.

7. **Skin.** Any signs of trauma or poor perfusion?

B. Laboratory Data. Laboratory investigation should be guided by findings from history and physical exam. Bedside observation of snoring, labored breathing, or obstructed breaths with or without oxyhemoglobin desaturation can be highly suggestive of OSAS.

1. **CBC.** Evidence of infection or anemia?

2. **Serum electrolytes.** Evidence of acidosis or electrolyte imbalance?

   3. **Cultures as indicated.** ALTE may be a manifestation of bacterial or viral infection, particularly RSV.
   4. **Metabolic studies.** See Chapter 66, Metabolic Diseases, p. 301.
C. **Radiographic and Other Studies**
   1. **Chest x-ray.** Can provide evidence of infection, congenital heart disease or aspiration.
   2. **Anteroposterior (AP) and lateral neck x-rays.** Assess patency of airway.
   3. **Barium swallow.** Useful in patients with dysphagia or GERD.
   4. **ECG.** Can identify congenital heart disease.
   5. **EEG.** Can identify seizure disorders.
   6. **Multichannel pneumocardiogram and polysomnogram.** Assesses respiratory control and adequacy of gas exchange.
   7. **pH probe.** Used to evaluate for GERD. Often useful when performed with multichannel pneumocardiogram.

V. **Plan**
   A. **Initial Management.** Assess ABCs and correct any problems. Intervene for any life-threatening conditions (eg, meningitis).
   B. **Monitoring.** A period of hospital monitoring is often recommended for infants with ALTE. Selected infants, in whom ALTE can be well characterized as an observer's overreaction to a normal episode, may be discharged home with good follow-up.
   C. **Medical and Nonmedical Therapies.** Medical therapy for any newly diagnosed condition should be established and explained, as well as any nonmedical therapies (eg, reflux precautions). In OSAS resulting from adenotonsillar hypertrophy, adenotonsillectomy is usually curative; weight loss is recommended if child is obese.
   D. **Discharge Planning.** Parents and other caregivers of infants with ALTE should undergo CPR training. Review safe infant sleep practices, most importantly supine sleep in a safe crib environment.
   E. **Home Cardiorespiratory (Apnea) Monitors.** Use of home apnea monitors for infants with ALTE is recommended by some centers, but this remains an area of controversy. If prescribed, the monitor should have an event recorder, so that any further episodes at home can be correlated with data recorded on the monitor. It should be emphasized, however, that apnea monitors have never been shown to prevent SIDS and that prospective identification of SIDS is not possible. Monitor should be prescribed only as long as is necessary and should be discontinued if no further episodes occur or after any episodes have resolved. Continued episodes in otherwise healthy or treated infants are uncommon and warrant reevaluation.
   F. **Airway Support.** For patients with OSAS, airway support can be provided by continuous or bilevel positive airway pressure (CPAP

or BiPAP) administered with a nasal mask. Supplemental oxygen therapy should be used with care, however, because blunting of the hypoxic drive to breathe in a child with CO_2 retention due to OSAS can theoretically worsen obstructive hypoventilation.

VI. Problem Case Diagnoses
  A. The initial diagnosis of GERD in the 3-month-old male infant was confirmed by pH probe.
  B. AP and lateral neck x-rays supported a diagnosis of adenotonsillar hypertrophy in the 3-year-old boy. During sleep, persistent oxyhemoglobin desaturation was treated with repositioning and supplemental oxygen therapy, maintaining oxyhemoglobin saturation levels in the 90–92% range. Clinical improvement occurred after urgent adenotonsillectomy.

VII. Teaching Pearl: Question. What is the most common cause of severe apnea associated with viral infection?

VIII. Teaching Pearl: Answer. RSV; it can cause bronchiolitis and sometimes pneumonia in affected infants.

REFERENCES

Brooks JG. Apparent life-threatening events and apnea of infancy. *Clin Perinatol* 1992;19:809–838.

Committee on Fetus and Newborn. Apnea, sudden infant death syndrome, and home monitoring. *Pediatrics* 2003;111:914–917.

Marcus CL, Ward SL, Mallory GB, et al. Use of nasal continuous positive airway pressure as treatment of childhood obstructive sleep apnea. *J Pediatr* 1995;127:88–94.

Ramanathan R, Corwin MJ, Hunt CE, et al. Cardiorespiratory events recorded on home monitors: Comparison of healthy infants with those at increased risk for SIDS. *JAMA* 2001;285:2199–2207.

Sterni LM, Tunkel DE. Obstructive sleep apnea in children: An update. *Pediatr Clin North Am* 2003;50:427–443.

10. BACK PAIN

  I. Problem. A 6-year-old girl has back pain of several weeks' duration and now refuses to walk.

  II. Immediate Questions
    A. Is there evidence of neurologic disability? Back pain in children, as opposed to adults, is more likely to have a serious organic cause. Although "adult-type" low back pain is now recognized in children, a careful evaluation for structural or organic causes is warranted in children. Of utmost importance is a history and physical exam directed toward any potential evidence of spinal cord involvement, which would mandate urgent radiologic and neurosurgical involvement.
    B. When and how did pain begin? It is important to recognize acute or more chronic onset. Trauma is a common cause, especially in athletes. Repetitive trauma (eg, in gymnasts) may have a more indolent onset.

C. **Are there constitutional symptoms?** Fever, weight loss, and malaise may be signs of infectious, inflammatory, or malignant processes. Patients with trauma generally are otherwise well.

D. **Is there a history of prior episodes or a congenital problem with the spine?** Patients with visible evidence over the spine (hair tufts, vascular malformations) are predisposed to spinal cord entrapment and may have prior or even progressive gait disturbances.

E. **Any change in spinal curvature?** Chronic juvenile scoliosis is usually not painful, but acute, painful scoliosis is a clue to a new structural cause.

F. **Is pain worse at night?** Trauma, overuse, spondylolisthesis, and muscle strain disorders usually improve with rest. Worsening of symptoms at night suggests inflammatory, infectious, or malignant processes.

III. **Differential Diagnosis**
   A. **Infectious Diseases.** Bacterial osteomyelitis, rarely including tuberculosis; diskitis, either infectious or noninfectious; epidural abscess; or psoas abscess, which may present with limp and back pain.

   B. **Parainfectious Diseases.** Includes transverse myelitis, demyelinating disorders, and radiculopathies that occasionally start with pain.

   C. **Trauma or Structural Causes.** Spondylolysis, spondylolisthesis, Scheuermann disease, intervertebral disk herniation, compression fractures, or diastematomyelia (tethered cord).

   D. **Mass Lesions.** Primary bone tumors (osteoid osteoma, aneurysmal bone cyst, eosinophilic granuloma, Ewing sarcoma, neuroblastoma); intraspinal tumors (lipoma, cysts, neurofibroma).

   E. **Inflammatory Conditions.** Ankylosing spondylitis, Reiter syndrome, or disk calcification (usually cervical).

   F. **Referred Pain.** Usually from the abdomen (appendicitis, pyelonephritis, gallbladder disease, endometriosis).

   G. **Metabolic Alterations.** Hemolytic anemia, storage disease (Gaucher disease), or osteoporosis.

   H. **Conversion or Psychogenic Disorders.** Less common in children, but gait disturbance, headache, abdominal pain, and fatigue may accompany back pain in patients with these disorders.

IV. **Database**
   A. **Physical Exam Key Points**
      1. **Vital signs and general appearance.** Evidence of systemic disorders is key: fever, weight loss, hypertension, adenopathy.
      2. **Spine.** Check for congenital lesions, such as hair tufts. Observe flexion, extension, and lateral bending. Paraspinous muscle spasm is often seen with structural disorders. Does patient have scoliosis, either new onset or preexisting? Is there loss or

accentuation of the lumbar curve? Search for a palpable ridge or "step," which may be seen with spondylolisthesis. Is there a localized tender area? Palpation and percussion of vertebrae is helpful.

3. **Maneuvers**
   a. **Prone-supine to sitting-standing.** Observe as patient changes position. Guarding of spine is present with serious disorders.
   b. **Gait and standing.** Painful or weak?
   c. **Forward bending and then hyperextension of spine.** Aids in a search for deformities and location of pain.
   d. **Straight leg raising.** Patient lifts leg slowly with knee extended; pain at 30–60 degrees is positive.
   e. **FABERE.** Mnemonic for **F**lexion (knee, with lateral malleolus on the opposite knee), **AB**duction, **E**xternal **R**otation, and **E**xtension (hip). Downward pressure on the leg causes pain in patients with sacroiliac disease.
4. **Neurologic exam.** Critical in identifying conditions that require emergency treatment of potential spinal cord involvement. Evaluate tendon reflexes, strength, sensation, and bowel and bladder function.

B. **Laboratory Data**
   1. **CBC, differential, platelet count.**
   2. **ESR, C-reactive protein.** Inflammatory markers.
   3. **Cultures.** Blood and, on occasion, direct bone aspirate may be indicated.
   4. **Other workup.** HLA-B27, ANA, and other specialized testing may be required.

C. **Radiographic and Other Studies**
   1. **Plain x-rays.** Initial spinal films may be helpful in patients with structural disorders (eg, spondylolisthesis).
   2. **Radionucleotide bone scan.** Helpful in acute infectious processes (osteomyelitis, diskitis), but may also be useful in defining more chronic processes such as repetitive trauma. Single-photon emission computed tomography (SPECT) links CT with radioisotope scanning and may increase sensitivity, especially when looking for fractures of the lumbar spine.
   3. **CT scan.** Useful in evaluating structural processes and can be used with myelography to define the spinal cord area.
   4. **MRI scan.** Allows the most complete look at all structures, including nerve roots in inflammatory or demyelinating disorders. Very helpful in viewing extent of paraspinous processes, such as osteomyelitis.

V. **Plan.** Initial evaluation should center on establishing whether there is any evidence of spinal cord involvement. Follow with emergency radiographic and neurosurgical consultation. Next, decide whether a systemic disorder is present, and whether this primarily involves the spine or is referred pain. A detailed history will help in this situation. Search for any structural process involving the spine by examination and radiography.

  A. Infection. In patients with osteomyelitis, diskitis, or paraspinous infection, obtain a culture of infected material, usually by CT-guided biopsy or aspiration. Then immobilize the spine and administer long-term antibiotic therapy. Orthopedic consultation is indicated.

  B. Trauma. Often these patients are athletes with repetitive injury. Once the diagnosis is suspected (eg, spondylolysis, spondylolisthesis), a comprehensive rehabilitation program is needed, supervised by a specialist in orthopaedic or sports medicine.

  C. Mass Lesions or Neurologic Condition. A planned approach involving multiple disciplines is necessary. Maximum care must be taken to protect the spinal cord from any injury or progression of disease. Biopsy may be indicated after careful radiographic studies are completed.

VI. Problem Case Diagnosis. The 6-year-old girl had low back pain for several months that became acutely worse after she underwent chiropractic manipulation. Later that night, she refused to walk. Examination revealed markedly decreased deep tendon reflexes and sensation in the legs. Plain films were normal, but CT scan revealed a hemorrhagic, cystic lesion in the upper lumbar spine that was later confirmed to be an aneurysmal bone cyst. Neurosurgical intervention led to slow but complete return of neurologic function.

VII. Teaching Pearl: Question. What is a typical history for a school-aged child with an osteoid osteoma of the lumbar spine?

VIII. Teaching Pearl: Answer. Osteoid osteoma often produces pain that is worse at night and awakens child from sleep. Pain, described as "boring," is dramatically relieved by aspirin or other NSAIDs. Plain films are often normal initially, but the lesion may be seen by other imaging modalities.

REFERENCES

King HA. Back pain in children. *Pediatr Clin North Am* 1999;30:467–474.
McIntire SC. Back pain. In: Gartner JC, Zitelli BJ, eds. *Common and Chronic Symptoms in Pediatrics.* Mosby, 1997:15–31.

11. BRADYCARDIA

  I. Problem. A 9-month-old infant is brought to the emergency department with acute bronchiolitis. The infant's heart rate has decreased to 58 beats/min.

II. Immediate Questions

A. Is the heart rate abnormal? Heart rate varies with age and is greatly influenced by factors such as crying, anxiety, fever, and activity. Table I–7 lists normal heart rate ranges in infants and children. See Appendix H, p. 768, for other age-specific heart rate values.

B. Is patient hemodynamically compromised? Assess the following:
  1. **Level of consciousness.** Remember the mnemonic **AVPU: A**lert, responsive to **V**oice, responsive to **P**ain, **U**nresponsive.
  2. **Peripheral pulses.** Normal, thready, or absent?
  3. **Skin perfusion**
     a. **Color.** Pink, mottled, gray, or blue?
     b. **Temperature.** Warm, cool, or cold?
     c. **Capillary refill.** Normal (< 2 seconds) or delayed (> 2 seconds)?
  4. **BP.** Differentiates extent of shock. (See Table I–12 in Chapter 52, Hypotension … for estimates of the lower limit [fifth percentile] of systolic BP based on age. For other age-specific BP values, refer to Appendix B, p. 759).
     a. **Compensated (early) shock.** Normal BP, poor systemic perfusion.
     b. **Decompensated (late) shock.** Hypotension, weak central pulses, decreased level of consciousness.
  5. *Clinically significant bradycardia is defined as heart rate < 60 beats/min associated with hemodynamic compromise and shock.*

C. Does patient have a history of cardiac anomaly or disease? If so, prompt cardiac consultation is required.

III. Differential Diagnosis.
As a mnemonic remember the **6 H's and a T: H**ypoxemia, **H**igh (metabolic) acid, (intracranial) **H**ypertension, **H**ypothyroidism, **H**ypothermia, **H**eart condition, and **T**oxins.

A. Hypoxemia.

B. High Acid (Metabolic Acidosis). Any condition causing shock and lactic acidosis can result in bradycardia. This often precedes asystole and needs to be treated emergently.

TABLE I–7. NORMAL HEART RATE RANGES FOR INFANTS AND CHILDREN

Age	Heart Rate (beats/min)
Newborn	80–180
1 wk–3 mo	80–180
3 mo–2 y	80–160
2–10 y	65–130
10 y–adult	55–90

C. Intracranial Hypertension

1. Bradycardia is part of Cushing triad, along with hypertension and irregular respirations.

2. Head injury, CNS space-occupying lesion (tumor; abscess; epidural, subdural, or intracranial hemorrhage), hydrocephalus, malfunctioning ventricular shunt, meningitis, cerebrovascular event, or diabetic ketoacidosis.

D. Hypothyroidism.

E. Hypothermia.

F. Primary Heart Conditions

1. **Complete heart block.** The most common cause of significant primarily cardiac bradycardia in infants and children. May be asymptomatic or cause shock and congestive heart failure (CHF). Usually does not respond to normal resuscitative measures such as ventilation, oxygenation, treatment of acidosis, and catecholamine support.

   a. Congenital
   - i. Idiopathic.
   - ii. Associated with congenital heart defects such as corrected transposition of the great arteries or left atrial isomerism and polysplenia syndromes (heterotaxy).
   - iii. Associated with collagen disease in mother.

   b. Acquired, nonsurgical heart block
   - i. Idiopathic.
   - ii. Associated with congenital heart defects.
   - iii. Infectious diseases: myocarditis (viral or Lyme) or endocarditis.
   - iv. Connective tissue diseases: lupus, rheumatic fever.
   - v. Kawasaki disease.
   - vi. Muscle disease.
   - vii. Cardiac tumor.
   - viii. Cardiac sclerosis.

   c. Postsurgical. Incidence < 1% because of improved operative technique.
   - i. **Transient.** Resolves within 8 days.
   - ii. **Permanent.** Usually develops immediately after surgery but may occur many years later.

2. **Sick sinus syndrome.** Depressed sinus node function.

   a. Presentation. Sinus bradycardia or slow junctional rhythm alternating with episodes of tachycardia. May present with syncope.

   b. Causes. Surgery to correct atrial septal defect, Mustard procedure for d-transposition of the great vessels, Fontan repair for single ventricle complexes, viral myocarditis, idiopathic.

G. Toxins. Common drugs and toxins that can cause bradycardia include:

1. Antidysrhythmics.
2. α-Adrenergic agonists.
3. β-Adrenergic agonists.
4. Calcium channel blockers.
5. Ciguatera.
6. Clonidine.
7. Digitalis glycosides.
8. Opioids.
9. Organophosphates and carbamates.

IV. Database
A. Physical Exam Key Points
1. **Vital signs and general appearance.** Assess vital signs; airway, breathing, and circulation (respiratory rate, BP, temperature, and pulse oximetry); level of consciousness; peripheral pulses; and skin perfusion.
2. **Chest and lungs**
   a. Observe for old surgical scars suggesting past cardiac surgery.
   b. Rales and wheezing may indicate CHF or infection.
3. **Heart.** Rhythm, murmurs?
4. **Abdomen.** Hepatomegaly may indicate CHF.
5. **Skin.** Perfusion, rashes (eg, meningococcemia, lupus, endocarditis, rheumatic fever)?

B. Laboratory Data
1. **ECG.** Will differentiate sinus bradycardia from complete heart block.
2. **Blood gas analysis.** Will confirm hypoxemia or acidosis.

C. Radiographic and Other Studies. Chest x-ray may reveal cardiomegaly, congenital heart defect, or CHF.

V. Plan. Figure I–3 depicts an approach to the patient with bradycardia.
A. **Support ABCs.** Secure airway, administer 100% oxygen, and obtain IV access.
B. Attach patient to a cardiorespiratory monitor or defibrillator.
C. If patient remains hemodynamically compromised despite adequate ventilation and oxygenation, begin chest compressions.
D. Identify and treat possible causes of bradycardia (**6 H's and a T;** see III, earlier). Refer to Figure I–3.
E. If patient does not improve, administer epinephrine or atropine, or both.
F. If patient remains bradycardic or has a history of cardiac disease, consult a cardiologist emergently. For complete heart block, consider isoproterenol, epinephrine infusion, or transcutaneous or transthoracic cardiac pacing.

VI. Problem Case Diagnosis. The 9-month-old infant was in respiratory distress and hemodynamically compromised when admitted to the emergency department. Endotracheal intubation was performed and

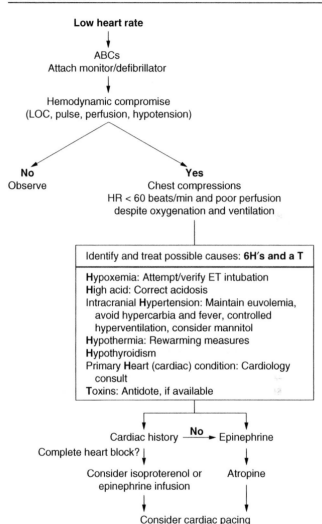

Figure I–3. Management algorithm for bradycardia. (ABCs = airway, breathing, circulation; ET = endotracheal; HR = heart rate; LOC = level of consciousness.)

ventilation with 100% oxygen was provided. Patient's heart rate immediately improved to 120 beats/min.

VII. Teaching Pearl: Question. What is the most common cause of clinically significant bradycardic rhythms in infants and children?

VIII. Teaching Pearl: Answer. Hypoxemia; therefore, immediate support of airway, ventilation, and oxygenation is warranted.

REFERENCES

Gewitz MH, Vetter VL. Cardiac emergencies. In Fleisher GR, ed. *Textbook of Pediatric Emergency Medicine.* Lippincott Williams & Wilkins, 2000:659–700.
Hazinski MF, Zartsky AL, eds. *Pediatric Advanced Life Support Provider Manual.* American Heart Association Publication, 2002.

12. CARDIOPULMONARY ARREST

I. Problem. A 4-month-old boy is brought to the emergency department by his parents, who found him lifeless, apneic, and pulseless this morning.

II. Immediate Questions

A. Is patient unresponsive? Establish unresponsiveness using vocal or physical stimulation.

B. Is airway patent? Open airway using the head tilt–chin lift maneuver.

C. Is there a history or suspicion of injury to head or neck? If injury is present or suspected, immobilize cervical spine and perform the jaw-thrust maneuver to open the airway. If airway remains obstructed, patient should be repositioned and maneuvers for relieving airway obstruction attempted.

D. Is patient breathing? If patient does not have spontaneous respirations, assist ventilation using a bag-valve-mask device, while delivering 100% oxygen (rate of 1 breath every 5 seconds in infants).

E. Does patient have a pulse? Recommended sites to assess presence of a pulse in infants are brachial and femoral. If patient is pulseless, start chest compressions (rate of 100 per minute or ratio of 5 compressions to 1 ventilation in infants). Establish IV access rapidly. If attempt at peripheral IV access is unsuccessful, place an intraosseous (IO) line immediately. Administer epinephrine by endotracheal (ET), IV, or IO route every 3–5 minutes. Reassess pulse between dosages of epinephrine.

F. Is patient in shock? If patient is in shock, secure the airway, provide 100% oxygen, and obtain IV access. Provide fluid boluses of 20 mL/kg of isotonic (NS or Ringer lactate) solution at least twice. Reassess patient after each fluid bolus. Consider an inotropic agent drip if there is no or minimal improvement in BP or perfusion after second fluid bolus. Some patients will require additional fluid boluses.

G. Are there treatable causes of cardiopulmonary arrest? Consider the **5 H's and 4 T's:** **H**ypoxemia; **H**ypovolemia; **H**ypothermia; **H**yperkalemia or hypokalemia and metabolic disorders; intracranial **H**ypertension; cardiac **T**amponade; **T**ension pneumothorax; **T**oxins, poisons, and drugs; and **T**hromboembolism.

III. Differential Diagnosis

A. Upper Respiratory Conditions. Airway obstruction, croup, epiglottitis, retropharyngeal abscess, suffocation, strangulation, trauma, or tracheitis.

B. Lower Respiratory Conditions. Pneumonia, asthma, bronchiolitis, foreign body aspiration, drowning, smoke inhalation, or pulmonary edema.

C. Infection. Sepsis or meningitis.

D. Cardiac Disorders. Congenital heart disease, pericarditis, or rhythm disturbances.

E. Shock. Hypovolemic shock from dehydration or hemorrhage, cardiogenic shock from myocardial dysfunction, or distributive shock from sepsis or anaphylaxis.

F. Neurologic Disorders. CNS infection, meningitis or encephalitis, head injury, or cerebrovascular event.

G. Trauma or Environmental Causes. Hypovolemia, hypothermia, hyperthermia, or submersion injury.

H. Metabolic Disorders. Hypoglycemia, hypocalcemia, or hyperkalemia.

I. Sudden Infant Death Syndrome.

IV. Database

A. Physical Exam Key Points

1. General assessment and vital signs. Assess responsiveness and obtain vital signs.

a. Respiratory rate. Fast rate can indicate a toxic or metabolic abnormality. Slow rate is often an ominous sign that is suggestive of impending respiratory arrest, a toxin, or intracranial hypertension. Assess oxygenation by pulse oximetry.

b. Heart rate and rhythm. Is heart rate absent or is a collapse rhythm present? Identify asystole, pulseless electrical activity, ventricular fibrillation, and pulseless ventricular tachycardia. Is rate slow (sinus bradycardia, complete heart block) or rapid (sinus tachycardia, supraventricular tachycardia, or ventricular tachycardia)? Evaluate rate and rhythm, and listen for murmurs suggestive of congenital heart defect or acquired heart disease.

c. BP. Is BP high (intracranial hypertension, toxin, or hypertensive emergency) or low (decompensated shock)?

d. Temperature. High or low temperature suggests an infection or toxin. Hypothermia may be indicative of the environment.

2. **CNS.** Low Glasgow Coma Scale score may indicate head injury. Examine head and fontanelle; bulging fontanelle can occur with intracranial hypertension or meningitis, whereas sunken fontanelle indicates hypovolemia and dehydration. Look for boggy swelling, palpable fracture, or other signs of trauma. Note presence of a ventricular shunt.

3. **Eyes.** Examine for signs of trauma (raccoon's eyes) or hypovolemia and dehydration (sunken). Assess pupil size and reaction. Pupillary size can give clues to the presence of a toxin. Depressed or absent reaction may indicate structural CNS lesion, herniation or impending herniation, or cardiopulmonary arrest. Asymmetry can indicate structural CNS lesion. Papilledema of the optic disk may occur with intracranial hypertension; however, absence of papilledema does not rule it out. Hemorrhages of the disk suggest intracranial injury.

4. **Neck and trachea.** Palpate for injury to the cervical spine or tracheal deviation. Look for venous distention that may indicate tension pneumothorax.

5. **Thorax.** Observe for old surgical scars or signs of rib fractures.

6. **Lungs.** Auscultate lungs and assess effectiveness of ventilation. Listen for decreased breath sounds (consolidation, pneumonia, pleural effusion, or pneumothorax), rales (pneumonia, bronchiolitis, or pulmonary edema), and wheezing (asthma, bronchiolitis, foreign body aspiration, pulmonary edema), which are suggestive of lower airway disease, or stridor (foreign body, croup, tracheitis, epiglottitis, retropharyngeal abscess), suggestive of upper airway disease.

7. **Abdomen.** Palpate for signs of injury, tenderness, and hepatomegaly.

8. **Skin and extremities.** Look for any signs of injury or bruising, perfusion, and rash.

B. **Laboratory Data**
   1. **Blood gas analysis.** Hypoxemia, acidosis.
   2. **CBC.**
      a. **WBC count.** Infection, sepsis.
      b. **Hemoglobin and hematocrit.** Hemorrhage.
   3. **Bedside dextrose determination.** Hypoglycemia.
   4. **Basic metabolic panel.** Electrolyte abnormalities, acidosis.
   5. **Blood and urine cultures.** Sepsis.
   6. **CSF cell count, chemistry, Gram stain, and culture.** CNS infection. Perform lumbar puncture only if patient is stable.
   7. **Serum or urine drug screening.** Toxin.

C. **Radiographic and Other Studies**
   1. **Chest x-ray.** ET tube placement, pneumonia, foreign body aspiration, pneumothorax, rib fractures, congenital heart defect, congestive heart failure.
   2. **ECG.** Rhythm abnormalities, congenital heart defect.

   3. Trauma series. Cervical spine series, chest, and pelvis.
   4. CT scan of head. Head injury (epidural, subdural, or intracranial hemorrhage), CNS infection (abscess), tumor, cerebral edema, cerebrovascular event.
   5. Abdominal CT scan. Abdominal injury.
   6. Skeletal survey. Suspected inflicted injury or child abuse among children younger than 3 years of age.

V. Plan

A. Responsiveness. Establish using vocal or physical stimulation.

B. Airway
   1. Open airway using the head tilt–chin lift maneuver.
   2. If head or neck injury is present or suspected, immobilize cervical spine and perform jaw-thrust maneuver to open airway.
   3. If airway remains obstructed, reposition patient and attempt maneuvers to relieve airway obstruction.

C. Breathing. If patient does not have spontaneous respirations, assist ventilation using a bag-valve-mask device, while delivering 100% oxygen. If patient continues to have ineffective or no respirations, perform ET intubation and ventilate through the ET tube.

D. Circulation
   1. Palpate brachial or femoral pulse.
   2. Attach patient to cardiorespiratory monitor or defibrillator.
   3. Establish IV access rapidly. If attempt at peripheral IV access is unsuccessful, place an IO line immediately.
      a. Patient is pulseless
         i. Monitor shows **asystole** or **pulseless electrical activity:** Start chest compressions. Administer epinephrine via ET, IV, or IO route every 3–5 minutes.
         ii. Monitor shows **ventricular fibrillation** or pulseless **ventricular tachycardia:** Defibrillate immediately (time should not be spent on ET intubation or IV or IO access), up to 3 times as needed. Start with 2 joules/kg, then 4 joules/kg, then 4 joules/kg. If no response, administer epinephrine via ET, IV, or IO route. Perform CPR. Defibrillate. If no response, administer antiarrhythmics (amiodarone, lidocaine, or magnesium) ET, IV, or IO. Perform CPR. Defibrillate.
      b. Patient has slow pulse (< 60 beats/min) and shows severe cardiorespiratory compromise despite adequate oxygenation and ventilation.
         i. Start chest compressions. Administer epinephrine via ET, IV, or IO route every 3–5 minutes.
         ii. Consider atropine if primary AV block or increased vagal tone is suspected.
         iii. Consider cardiac pacing.

       c. Patient has rapid pulse and shows severe cardiorespiratory compromise despite adequate oxygenation and ventilation.

         i. Monitor shows narrow complexes (probable **supraventricular tachycardia**): Perform cardioversion immediately with 0.5 joules/kg. Increase dose to 2 joules/kg if initial dose is ineffective, **or** administer adenosine IV or IO if immediately available.

         ii. Monitor shows wide complexes (probable **ventricular tachycardia**): Perform cardioversion immediately with 0.5 joules/kg. Increase dose to 2 joules/kg if initial dose is ineffective. Consider antiarrhythmics (amiodarone, procainamide, lidocaine).

    4. If patient is in **shock,** provide fluid boluses of 20 mL/kg of isotonic (NS or Ringer lactate) solution at least twice. Reassess patient after each fluid bolus. Consider infusion of inotrope if there is no or minimal improvement after second fluid bolus.

    5. Consider the **5 H's and 4 T's** (see II, G, earlier).

    6. Involve consultants promptly for the following conditions: congenital or acquired heart disease, arrhythmias (cardiologist); injuries (trauma surgeon); head injury, and intracranial hypertension (neurosurgeon).

    7. Other actions

       a. Administer antidote when available for suspected toxins.

       b. Provide empiric antimicrobial therapy for suspected sepsis or meningitis.

VI. Problem Case Diagnosis. The 4-month-old boy was unresponsive and apneic on arrival in the emergency department. He underwent ET intubation and received 100% oxygen but remained pulseless and asystolic. Cardiac compressions were initiated. IO access was obtained, and epinephrine was given every 3 minutes for a total of three times. Patient remained pulseless. Postmortem examination was consistent with sudden infant death syndrome.

VII. Teaching Pearl: Question. Among industrialized nations, what is the leading cause of death from the age of 6 months through young adulthood?

VIII. Teaching Pearl: Answer. Injury; therefore, injury prevention is the first link in the so-called pediatric chain of survival.

REFERENCES

Hazinski MF, Zartsky AL, eds. *Pediatric Advanced Life Support Provider Manual.* American Heart Association Publication, 2002.

Seidel JS. Cardiopulmonary resuscitation. In Barkin RM, ed. *Pediatric Emergency Medicine.* Mosby, 1997:104–117.

13. CHEST PAIN

I. **Problem.** A 15-year-old boy complains of chest pain 1 week after experiencing minor trauma. For the past 3 days he has had low-grade fever and achy, stabbing chest pain that is worse with exertion or walking, as well as mild dizziness with standing and nocturnal shortness of breath.

II. **Immediate Questions.** Most children with chest pain have a benign, noncardiac cause of pain. However, the complaint should be taken seriously because of patient and parental concerns, and because underlying heart disease or other serious pathology can sometimes exist. Thorough history and careful physical exam can guide diagnosis and determine when laboratory studies should be ordered.

A. **When did pain begin?** Children with sudden onset of pain (within 48 hours of presentation) are more likely to have an organic cause (pneumonia, asthma, trauma, pneumothorax) of pain. Chronic, undiagnosed pain is more likely to be idiopathic or have a psychogenic cause.

B. **What precipitates pain? Are there associated symptoms?** Chest pain precipitated by exercise should be taken seriously (suggesting cardiac disease or, more commonly, exercise-induced asthma). History of trauma, rough play, or choking on a foreign body may be relevant. Chest pain associated with syncope or palpitations is more significant and may also relate to cardiac disease. History of fever suggests an infectious process (eg, pneumonia, myocarditis).

C. **What is patient's past medical and family history?** Past medical history may reveal asthma that places patient at risk for more serious causes of pain. Previous heart disease or conditions such as diabetes mellitus (hyperlipidemia) or Kawasaki disease (coronary artery aneurysms) may increase risk of cardiac pathology. Obtain family history, because cardiac disorders can be familial. Patients with hypertrophic cardiomyopathy may relate a family history of chest pain or sudden death.

D. **How severe is pain?** Determine if pain is frequent, severe, or interrupts child's daily activity. Pain that awakens child from sleep is more likely to have an organic etiology.

E. **How is pain characterized (location, quality)?** Young children may be imprecise in language and description, which can decrease usefulness of the history. Suspect esophagitis if burning sternal pain is present; pericarditis if there is sharp pain that is relieved by sitting up and leaning forward and associated with fever.

F. **How old is patient?** Young children are more likely to have a cardiorespiratory cause for their pain (eg, cough, asthma, pneumonia, or heart disease); adolescents are more likely to have pain associated with stress or a psychogenic disturbance.

III. Differential Diagnosis

A. Cardiac Causes. Previously undiagnosed cardiac disease is a rare cause of chest pain in children (< 5%).

1. **Myocardial ischemia or infarction.** Conditions that place children at risk of angina or myocardial infarction include anomalous coronary arteries, long-standing diabetes mellitus, past medical history of Kawasaki disease, chronic anemia (eg, sickle cell disease), and cocaine use. In many cases, exercise induces chest pain with these disorders because coronary blood flow is limited. Therefore, pain with exertion or syncope, or both, especially in these children should always be carefully evaluated.

2. **Arrhythmia.** Associated with palpitations or abnormal cardiac exam. Supraventricular tachycardia is the most common of these arrhythmias, but premature ventricular contractions can also lead to brief, sharp chest pain.

3. **Structural cardiac abnormalities.** Hypertrophic obstructive cardiomyopathy has an autosomal dominant pattern of inheritance; therefore, a family history may exist. These children are at risk for ischemic chest pain, especially when exercising, and have a murmur that is best heard with standing or Valsalva maneuver. Most other cardiac structural disorders rarely cause chest pain; however, severe pulmonic stenosis with associated cyanosis and aortic valve stenosis can lead to ischemia. In these latter conditions, pain is described as squeezing, choking, or a pressure sensation in the sternal area. These conditions are almost always diagnosed before child presents with pain, and associated murmurs are found on physical exam. Mitral valve prolapse may cause chest pain by papillary muscle or left ventricular endocardial ischemia. Midsystolic click and late systolic murmur are found in many cases. However, studies show that mitral valve prolapse is no more common in children with chest pain than in the general population.

4. **Cardiac infections.** Uncommon cause of pediatric chest pain. Pericarditis presents with sharp stabbing pain that improves when patient sits up and leans forward. Child is usually febrile and has respiratory distress, friction rub, distant heart sounds, neck vein distention, and pulsus paradoxus. Myocarditis is somewhat more common and can present in more subtle fashion. After a few days of fever and other systemic symptoms such as vomiting and lightheadedness, patient may develop pain with exertion and shortness of breath. Exam may reveal muffled heart sounds, fever, gallop rhythm, or tachycardia that is out of proportion to degree of fever present. Patient also may have orthostatic changes in pulse or BP. This is often misinterpreted as volume depletion, because child with this infection may not be taking oral fluids well and may indeed have mild dehydration. However, if orthostatic vital signs do not improve

with fluid resuscitation, cardiogenic causes such as myocarditis should be suspected.

B. Musculoskeletal Disorders. One of the most common diagnoses in children with chest discomfort.

1. **Muscle strain.** Active children frequently strain chest wall muscles while wrestling, carrying heavy books, or exercising. Pain is generally reproducible by palpation or with movement of the torso and upper extremities.

2. **Costochondritis.** A related disorder that is common in children. Diagnosis is made by eliciting tenderness (reproducible pain) over costochondral junctions with palpation. Pain may be sharp, bilateral, and exaggerated by physical activity or breathing, and may persist for several months.

3. **Direct chest wall trauma.** Some children suffer direct trauma to the chest, resulting in mild contusion of the chest wall or, with more significant force, rib fracture, hemothorax, or pneumothorax. In most cases there is a straightforward history of trauma, and diagnosis is clear. Careful physical exam reveals chest tenderness or pain with movement of torso or upper extremities.

C. Respiratory Causes

1. **Asthma.** When associated with severe, persistent cough or wheezing, may lead to chest pain due to overuse of chest wall muscles. Diagnosis is made by history or findings of wheezes, tachypnea, or decreased breath sounds. Chest pain with exercise secondary to exercise-induced asthma can be confirmed with a treadmill test.

2. **Pneumonia.** Suspect in febrile children with chest pain. Most such patients have a history of cough and physical findings of rales, tachypnea, or decreased breath sounds. Pleural effusion may develop and may cause pain that is worsened by deep inspiration. Although x-rays are helpful in confirming presence of effusion, tachypnea and auscultation of decreased breath sounds should raise suspicion about this condition.

3. **Spontaneous pneumothorax or pneumomediastinum.** Causes chest pain with respiratory distress, decreased breath sounds on affected side (if pneumothorax is significant), and possibly palpable subcutaneous air. Children with asthma, cystic fibrosis, and Marfan syndrome are at high risk for these conditions, although in previously healthy children an unrecognized subpleural bleb may rupture with minimal precipitating factors. Adolescents who snort cocaine are at risk for similar barotrauma and may complain of severe, sudden chest pain with associated anxiety, hypertension, and tachycardia.

4. **Pulmonary embolism.** Extremely rare in pediatric patients but should be considered in adolescent girls with dyspnea, fever, pleuritic pain, cough, and hemoptysis. Likelihood of this diagnosis is increased in the presence of birth control pill use or

recent abortion. Young boys with recent leg trauma are also at risk.

D. Psychogenic Disturbances. Stress precipitates chest pain in both boys and girls at equal rates; often anxiety and stress are not easily apparent. Not all such children present with hyperventilation or an anxious appearance. However, if child has had a recent major stressful event (eg, separation from friends, divorce in family, or school failure) that correlates temporally with the onset of chest pain, it is reasonable to conclude that symptoms are related to the underlying stress.

E. GI Disorders
  1. **Reflux esophagitis.** Causes chest pain in young children and adolescents. Classically described as burning, substernal in location, and worsened by reclining or eating spicy foods. Therapeutic trial of antacids can aid diagnosis.
  2. **Foreign body ingestion.** Significant pain, along with drooling, dysphagia, or both, occurs if a coin or other foreign body is trapped in the upper esophagus. Child or parents often give a clear history of recent foreign body ingestion and a plain-film x-ray can confirm diagnosis.
  3. **Pill-induced esophagitis.** Can develop in teenagers who take pill medications (eg, tetracycline or doxycycline), especially with minimal water, and then lie down. Prior history of esophageal dysmotility or stricture will make pain more likely. Doxycycline produces an acidic solution or gel as it dissolves and thus is caustic when it remains in the esophagus. Symptoms may be noted several days after beginning medication, but frequently pain occurs after taking the first dose. Diagnosis relies on a careful history because physical exam is usually unremarkable. Because these medications are chronically used by adolescents for treatment of acne, teenage patients may not reveal they take them unless specifically asked.

F. Miscellaneous Causes: Pain Related to Underlying Diseases
  1. **Sickle cell disease.** Children with vasoocclusive crisis may have pain that localizes to the chest or produces acute chest syndrome.
  2. **Marfan syndrome.** May result in chest pain and fatal dissection of an abdominal aortic aneurysm.
  3. **Herpes zoster infection.** Shingles may produce severe chest pain that precedes the classic vesicular rash by several days or occurs simultaneously.
  4. **Coxsackievirus infection.** This common viral infection may lead, rarely, to pleurodynia with paroxysms of sharp pain in chest or abdomen ("devil's grip").
  5. **Breast tenderness.** Teenagers or preteens may complain of chest pain from physiologic changes of puberty or from early changes of pregnancy.

6. **Thoracic tumor.** Hodgkin disease or non-Hodgkin lymphoma may present with chest pain but undoubtedly there will be other signs and symptoms of disease.

7. **Precordial catch syndrome.** Texidor twinge or "stitch in the side" is thought to cause unilateral chest pain that lasts a few seconds or minutes and is associated with bending or a slouched posture. It is believed the pain arises from parietal pleura or from pressure on an intercostal nerve, but etiology is unclear. Straightening up and taking shallow breaths or one deep breath relieves the pain, which may recur often or remain absent for months.

8. **Slipping rib syndrome.** This is a rare "sprain disorder" caused by trauma to costal cartilages of the 8th, 9th, and 10th ribs that do not attach to the sternum. Children with slipping rib syndrome complain of pain under the ribs or in upper abdominal quadrants. They also hear a clicking or popping sound when lifting objects, flexing the trunk, or even with walking. It is believed that the pain is caused by one of the ribs hooking under the rib above and irritating intercostal nerves. Pain can be duplicated and syndrome confirmed by performing the "hooking maneuver," whereby the affected rib margin is grasped and then pulled anteriorly. Surgery is thought to be the only definitive management, although most patients are treated satisfactorily with nonopioid analgesics.

9. **Idiopathic chest pain.** Diagnosed in 20–45% of patients with pediatric chest pain, when no other diagnosis can be determined with certainty.

IV. Database
A. Physical Exam Key Points
1. **Vital signs**
   a. **Hypotension.** May be present in cases of tension pneumothorax, myocarditis, or myocardial infarction. All of these diagnoses are quite rare in children.
   b. **Hypertension.** May be due to pain or an underlying medical condition related to chest pain (eg, systemic lupus erythematosus).
   c. **Fever.** May be a sign of infection (eg, pneumonia, myocarditis, or pericarditis).
   d. **Tachycardia.** May be related to pain or could indicate an arrhythmia such as supraventricular tachycardia or ventricular tachycardia (less common).

2. **General assessment.** Differentiate child in severe distress who needs immediate treatment for life-threatening conditions (eg, pneumothorax). Hyperventilation can be distinguished from respiratory distress by absence of cyanosis or nasal flaring. Next, look for signs of chronic disease (pallor,

poor growth), which may suggest that chest pain is one symptom of a more complex problem (eg, tumor or collagen vascular disease). Consider Marfan syndrome if patient is tall and thin with an upper extremity span that exceeds his or her height. Note any signs of anxiety that could indicate emotional stress.

   3. Skin. Examine child for rashes or other skin lesions. Bruises on parts distant from the chest may indicate unrecognized trauma to the chest.

   4. Abdomen. This area deserves careful evaluation because it may be a source of pain that is referred to the chest.

   5. Chest. Exam may reveal rales, wheezes, or decreased breath sounds if there is pulmonary pathology. Murmurs, rubs, muffled heart sounds, or arrhythmias may be noted if there is cardiac pathology. A murmur that intensifies with Valsalva maneuver and the standing position is the hallmark of hypertrophic cardiomyopathy. Evaluate the chest wall for signs of trauma, tenderness (suggesting musculoskeletal pain), or subcutaneous air (suggesting pneumothorax or pneumomediastinum).

B. Laboratory Data. If history and physical exam do not lead to a specific diagnosis for chest pain, it is unlikely that laboratory tests will be helpful. Laboratory studies usually confirm previously known disorders or abnormal findings that are suspected clinically. These studies are probably unnecessary in children with chronic pain, normal physical exam, and no history to indicate cardiac or pulmonary disease (Table I–8).

   1. Blood counts and ESR. Of limited value unless sickle cell disease, collagen vascular disease, infection, or malignancy is suspected.

   2. Drug screening for cocaine. May be indicated in older children with acute pain associated with anxiety, tachycardia, hypertension, or shortness of breath.

   3. Cardiac enzymes. Rarely of value unless there are specific concerns from history or exam.

C. Radiographic and Other Studies. Chest x-rays and ECGs should not be routinely ordered unless indicated by history and physical exam.

   1. Chest x-ray. Helpful if patient has fever, respiratory distress, decreased or abnormal breath sounds, or other pulmonary disease. Fever with chest pain is highly correlated with pneumonia. Chest film may lead to diagnoses of pericarditis or myocarditis if cardiomegaly is found in a febrile child with chest pain. Children with asthma and chest pain may have pneumothorax or pneumomediastinum.

   2. ECG. Warranted if patient has an abnormal cardiac exam, including unexplained tachycardia, arrhythmia, murmur, rub, or click.

   3. Chest x-ray plus ECG. Both studies are indicated if history reveals pain that is acute in onset (ie, began in past 2 or 3 days)

TABLE I–8. INDICATIONS FOR LABORATORY STUDIES IN CHILDREN WITH CHEST PAIN

- **WORRISOME HISTORY**
  Acute onset of pain
  Pain on exertion
  History of heart disease
  Serious associated medical problems (eg, diabetes mellitus, asthma, Marfan syndrome,
    Kawasaki disease, sickle cell anemia, systemic lupus erythematosus)
  Use of drugs (cocaine, oral contraceptives)
  Associated complaints (syncope dizziness, palpitations)
  Significant trauma
  Foreign body ingestion or aspiration
  Fever

- **ABNORMAL PHYSICAL EXAM**
  Respiratory distress
  Palpation of subcutaneous air
  Decreased breath sounds
  Cardiac findings (eg, murmurs, rubs, arrhythmias)
  Fever
  Trauma

---

or is otherwise concerning for cardiac disease. If there is pain with exertion, be particularly concerned about cardiac disease or asthma and obtain an ECG and chest x-ray. If patient has a history of heart disease, chest x-ray or ECG may also be desirable.

4. **Echocardiogram.** It may be wise to refer child for this study if structural heart disease is suspected. It is not necessary to obtain an echocardiogram on all children with ill-defined chest pain to look for mitral valve prolapse.

V. Plan

A. **Initial Management.** Assess vital signs and general appearance to determine if immediate treatment is needed. Check for thoracic trauma. Assess degree of pain and impact of pain on child's life. Determine if chest pain is part of a chronic underlying condition. Consider serious associated conditions (eg, asthma, lupus, sickle cell disease, Marfan syndrome). Consider serious organic pathology if child has fever or pain induced by exercise. Consider laboratory studies if history is of concern or physical exam findings are abnormal. In most cases of pediatric chest pain (musculoskeletal, psychogenic, or idiopathic pain), child will respond to reassurance, acetaminophen or NSAIDs, and rest. Heat and relaxation techniques may also be useful to manage pain.

1. **Severe distress or abnormal vital signs.** Admit child to the hospital for monitoring, further diagnostic studies, and extended treatment.

2. **Pain with exertion.** Refer for exercise stress tests or pulmonary function tests.
3. **Suspected esophageal foreign body.** Refer to a specialist for rapid removal of foreign object.
4. **Emotional problems.** Consider referral to a psychiatrist if serious problem cannot be managed by pediatrician.
5. **Known or suspected heart disease.** Consider referral to a cardiologist, even if pain proves to be unrelated.
6. **Chest pain associated with exercise, syncope, dizziness, or palpitations.** Refer for further evaluation. Consider Holter monitor or echocardiogram, or both, to look for an arrhythmia or structural heart disease.

B. **Specific Etiologies**
1. **Pneumonia.** Treat with oral antibiotics (eg, amoxicillin or erythromycin). Consider IV antibiotics and hospital admission if child is in respiratory distress, hypoxic, unable to take oral medications, or having an inadequate response to initial treatment.
2. **Asthma.** Treat with bronchodilators and consider oral steroids.
3. **Esophagitis.** A trial of antacids may be beneficial. When pill-induced esophagitis is suspected, discontinue medication and treat with sucralfate or proceed directly to endoscopic evaluation.
4. **Pneumothorax.** Immediate decompression of tension pneumothorax can be lifesaving (see Chapter 73, Pneumothorax, p. 336).
5. **Myocarditis.** Establish vascular access; give oxygen by mask or nasal canula. Consider IV inotropic or vasopressor medications and admit.

C. **Follow-up.** Appropriate follow-up should be arranged in all cases, because many children with ill-defined chest pain have persistent symptoms for many months. Serious organic pathology is unlikely to be found in the future, but some patients are kept from participating in their usual activities because of pain, and some manifest psychoemotional problems or symptoms of exercise-induced asthma that were not recognized at the initial visit. Have patient and family keep a pain diary listing occurrences, characteristics, and associated signs and symptoms.

VI. **Problem Case Diagnosis.** The 15-year-old boy was diagnosed with myocarditis. He presented with typical features (mild, progressive pain for 1 week, associated with shortness of breath) and had a worrisome history of pain with exertion and fever (suggesting an infectious etiology). He was dizzy with standing, suggesting hypovolemia or cardiac insufficiency. Minor trauma is sometimes misleading.

VII. **Teaching Pearl: Question.** Why is chest pain that is associated with exercise cause for concern?

VIII. Teaching Pearl: Answer. Although rare, sudden death that occurs in young children is often preceded by chest pain with exercise. Pain related to serious conditions such as myocarditis, coronary artery disease, and hypertrophic cardiomyopathy is worsened by exertion. Such patients should be referred to a cardiologist for further testing, including an echocardiogram, Holter monitoring, or exercise stress tests. Exercise-induced asthma is another condition in which chest pain is precipitated or worsened by exercise.

REFERENCES

Brumund MR, Strong WB. Murmurs, fainting, chest pain: Time for a cardiology referral? *Contemp Pediatr* 2002;19:155–166.

Selbst SM, Ruddy RM, Clark BJ, et al. Pediatric chest pain; a prospective study. *Pediatrics* 1988;82:319–323.

Selbst SM. Chest pain in children; consultation with the specialist. *Pediatr Rev* 1997;18:169–173.

Swenson JM, Fischer DR, Miller SA. Are chest radiographs and electrocardiograms still valuable in evaluating new pediatric patients with heart murmurs and or chest pain? *Pediatrics* 1997;99:1–3.

Washington RL. Sudden deaths in adolescent athletes caused by cardiac conditions. *Pediatr Ann* 2003;32:751–756.

14. CHILD ABUSE: PHYSICAL

I. Problem. During a diaper change, the mother of a 3-week-old girl notices that the infant has a painful, swollen left thigh. X-rays show a spiral fracture of the femur.

II. Immediate Questions

A. How long have symptoms been present? Recent onset of pain and swelling, particularly if severe, suggests an acute process. Pain or other symptoms from injury are exacerbated by diaper changes, feeding, dressing, and bathing.

B. Any history of trauma? Noninflicted, unintentional ("accidental") injury is common in infants and children. Unexplained or spontaneous injuries, explanations that are implausible or inconsistent with degree or mechanism of injury or child's developmental abilities, or changing explanations should raise concerns of inflicted injuries. Discrepancies between history and physical findings are common in abuse.

C. What other symptoms are present? History of perinatal infection exposure, immunizations, and recent fever or systemic symptoms is important in considering an infectious cause of leg swelling and pain. Additional symptoms may be associated with the cause of injury or the result of additional occult injury. Although irritability, colic, frequent crying, and difficulty feeding may be sources of frustration leading to abuse, they may also be due to prior skeletal, head, or abdominal trauma. Lethargy, apnea, and respiratory difficulty may also suggest occult head or abdominal injury.

D. Who is involved in care of child? Who are primary caretakers, and does child spend time with substitute caretakers, relatives, baby-sitters, or at daycare? An infant's mother is more likely to know about or be responsible for injuries if she reports that she has been the exclusive caretaker for several days than if she has just returned from a several-day business trip and discovered the injury. Who was with child when symptoms began and who else has had access to child? The individual who brings child for medical care may be the abuser, may be covering up for the abuser, or may have no knowledge of what caused the injury.

E. Are other risk factors present? Child abuse occurs in families from all socioeconomic, ethnic, and cultural backgrounds. Factors increasing risk of abuse include family issues of poverty, isolation, domestic violence, alcohol or drug abuse, and parents being abused as children. Maternal depression is also a significant risk factor, particularly for infants. Children are at increased risk if they were premature, have physical or developmental disabilities, or have perceived or actual behavioral problems. Abuse may be precipitated by a family crisis or triggering behavior such as a family argument, child's misbehavior, toilet training, or crying infant.

III. Differential Diagnosis

A. Child Abuse. Child abuse should always be considered, however briefly, in any child who presents with trauma. Significant injury, including fractures in an infant, has a higher risk of being inflicted.

B. Birth Trauma. Linear skull fractures (sometimes seen with cephalohematomas) and clavicle fractures can occur, and, less frequently, long bone fractures. Long bone fractures from birth trauma should be symptomatic within minutes to days of delivery.

C. Unintentional, Noninflicted Injury. Child abuse is most commonly confused with unintentional, noninflicted injury. Many inflicted injuries in children are indistinguishable from "accidental" trauma on clinical or radiologic grounds. The most important factor in deciding whether the injury is inflicted is a detailed description of the "accidental" event.

D. Metabolic, Genetic, and Infectious Bone Disorders. Abnormalities suggesting fractures or bone injury can be seen in several metabolic and genetic disorders that include abnormal or easily fractured bones. These disorders are often easily differentiated from abuse by presence of a family history, associated symptoms or physical findings, and specific abnormal-appearing bone configuration and density. Osteomyelitis may produce similar clinical signs in the extremities and radiologic changes in bone that mimic injury (eg, periosteal reaction), but fever, systemic symptoms, and elevated WBC counts, ESR, and C-reactive protein are typical of osteomyelitis.

E. **Coagulation Disorders.** Bruises are common in inflicted injury. Genetic diseases, including hemophilia and von Willebrand disease, and acquired disorders, including idiopathic thrombocytopenia and leukemia, may present with unusual bruising.

F. **Dermatologic Conditions.** Burns are a common form of inflicted injury. Impetigo, toxic epidermal necrolysis, pemphigus, and staphylococcal scalded skin syndrome can produce burnlike lesions.

G. **Other Conditions.** Henoch-Schönlein purpura can present with leg swelling and bruiselike lesions. Sickle cell crisis can present with extremity pain and swelling.

IV. **Database**

A. **Physical Exam Key Points**

1. **General features.** Child abuse can present with a single injury, but presence of multiple injuries, particularly involving multiple body surfaces or planes, in different stages of healing, caused by different mechanisms or agents, showing inflicted patterns, or found "by surprise" on examination are hallmarks of inflicted injury.

2. **Measurements.** Below-average weight, length (height) and head circumference, particularly infants and toddlers with measurements below the fifth percentile, suggest growth delay or failure to thrive (see Appendix G, Growth Charts, p. 766). Psychosocial factors or neglect are responsible for many cases of failure to thrive. It is important to compare current measurements with prior measurements.

3. **Vital signs.** Fever is typically absent, except in some cases of inflicted abdominal injury. Hypotension can occur with significant bleeding into an extremity, but shock or unusual respiratory patterns raise concerns about intracranial, thoracic, or intra-abdominal injury.

4. **Skin.** Inflicted bone, head, and abdominal trauma can occur without any cutaneous findings; however, skin findings are the most common manifestation of inflicted injury. All body surfaces should be inspected.

   a. **Bruises.** Normally occurring bruises are found over bony prominences (knees, shins, elbow, forehead, and chin); they are typically oval or rounded with indistinct borders. Inflicted bruises are often found over soft tissue areas and show patterns and shapes with distinct borders suggestive of the striking implement. Bruises in noncruising and nonambulatory infants are unusual.

   b. **Burns.** Noninflicted scald burns show a pattern of cooling liquids, following gravity down a surface, and splash marks. Inflicted scald burns are often circumferential on extremities or involve buttocks and show clear lines of demarcation between normal and burned skin with no splash marks.

Noninflicted contact burns typically involve palmar surface of the hand and show no distinct shapes. Inflicted contact burns often show distinct shapes with distinct margins.

5. **HEENT.** Scalp bruises and swelling are associated with impact injury. Large head circumference and full or bulging fontanel may be evidence of intracranial injury. Bilateral retinal hemorrhages are suggestive of, but not specific for, inflicted head injury. Oral lacerations or injury to the frenulum may result from forced feeding or forcing objects into the mouth to stop crying. Blood in the ear canal or behind the tympanic membrane may be associated with head trauma.

6. **Extremities.** Inspect, palpate, and test range of motion of all joints of all extremities for signs of tenderness, pain, or deformity.

7. **Abdomen.** Abdominal distention and tenderness should raise concerns about intra-abdominal injury. Bruising over abdomen is unusual, but should raise concerns about blunt injury to abdominal organs when present.

8. **Neurologic exam.** An infant with an isolated cutaneous injury or fracture should have normal findings on neurologic exam. Lethargy, decreased responses, increased or decreased tone, cranial nerve signs, or focal neurologic findings suggest intracranial injury.

B. **Laboratory Data**

1. **CBC.** Low hemoglobin and hematocrit should raise concerns about significant blood loss with severe injury such as intra-abdominal trauma. In children with excessive bruising, screen for leukemia and thrombocytopenia.

2. **Coagulation studies.** Platelet count, PT, and PTT can serve as a minimal screen for coagulopathies in children presenting with bruises.

3. **Liver function tests, pancreatic enzymes.** Elevated liver function tests or elevated amylase and lipase may indicate blunt abdominal trauma. When enzyme levels are elevated, consider abdominal CT scan.

C. **Radiographic and Other Studies**

1. **Skeletal survey.** Radiographs of the entire skeleton, including views of chest, skull, spine, pelvis, and extremities, should be obtained to look for occult fractures in all children younger than 2 years of age with suspected physical abuse. A single x-ray of the entire body ("babygram") is not adequate. X-rays should be the primary screening test for skeletal trauma. Routine skeletal x-rays in children older than 2 years are considered on a case-to-case basis.

   a. Fractures highly associated with abuse include rib fractures, metaphyseal "corner" or bucket-handle fractures, and fractures of sternum, scapula, or vertebral spinous processes.

    b. Suspicious fractures include multiple fractures, especially when bilateral or at different stages of healing, and complex skull fractures.

    c. Any fracture in a nonambulatory infant and all fractures when there is no history of trauma or the history is inconsistent with the injury should raise concerns of abuse.

    d. Repeat skeletal survey is often recommended 2 weeks after initial x-rays to help identify healing fractures that may not have been seen on initial films.

2. Nuclear medicine bone scan. Can pick up minor fractures before they are seen on x-rays and may remain positive after complete healing is seen on x-rays. Not useful for diagnosis of acute skull fractures or acute metaphyseal fractures of long bones. Should not be primary screening test for skeletal trauma.

3. CT scan of head. The primary screening test for acute inflicted head trauma. Essential for evaluation of children with suspected head trauma but should be considered in all young infants with any signs of inflicted injury.

    a. Subdural hematomas with or without skull fractures and associated with bilateral retinal hemorrhages are classic findings for inflicted head trauma.

    b. Subarachnoid hemorrhages, brain contusions, and focal or diffuse brain edema may be seen in some cases of inflicted head injury.

4. MRI scan of head. Useful in delineating small subdural hematomas and lesions of brain parenchyma.

V. Plan

A. Report Suspected Abuse. All 50 states have laws that require heath care providers to report suspected child abuse to child protective service (CPS) agencies or police. Generally the threshold for reporting should be when physician has a reasonable suspicion that child's condition may have been caused by abuse. Physician's job is to report suspected abuse, not to investigate abuse. Physician should not accuse the individual who brought child for medical care, but should explain why report is being made. Explanation should include statements such as child's injuries are too severe for or otherwise do not fit description of how injuries occurred and that physician is concerned that someone may be hurting child. Physician can add that he or she is required by law to report these types of injuries for further investigation. Reporting laws typically require a telephone report immediately to report suspected abuse and discuss immediate concerns about child's safety, followed by a written report.

B. Manage Acute Injuries. Most abusive injuries require only outpatient therapy. Consider hospitalization of young infants and more severely injured children for observation and management of their injuries, as well as for child whose home is unsafe, if CPS worker cannot obtain emergency placement for child.

   C. Follow-up. Medical follow-up will depend on type and severity of injuries. Although obtaining signed releases is appropriate, state laws pertaining to criminal investigation and investigation of suspected child abuse take precedence over HIPAA regulations, allowing physicians to discuss otherwise protected health information with CPS workers and police.

VI. Problem Case Diagnosis. The 3-week-old infant has an acute spiral fracture of the left femur, with no explanation given for this injury. Infant was a healthy term neonate, with an uncomplicated prenatal and perinatal course. The spiral nature of this fracture suggests a twisting force applied to the leg. A skeletal survey showed no additional fracture and otherwise normal-appearing bones. CT scan of the head was negative. During the CPS and police investigation, the mother's boyfriend admitted that he might have hurt the infant when he became frustrated while trying to change the diaper. A follow-up skeletal survey 2 weeks later showed multiple healing posterior rib fractures.

VII. Teaching Pearl: Question. How can you be certain the femur fracture in the infant described in the opening problem was not caused by birth trauma?

VIII. Teaching Pearl: Answer. A femur fracture occurring at birth would be expected to cause decreased mobility or "pseudoparesis" of the leg and signs of tenderness shortly after birth, not 3 weeks later. The x-rays themselves show an acute injury with no signs of healing of the fracture. Fractures, except for skull fractures, typically show radiographic signs of healing within 7–14 days of injury. A fracture showing no early signs of healing could not have occurred more than 14 days prior to x-ray. An acute nonhealing fracture in a 3-week-old infant could not have occurred at birth. The healing rib fractures, not seen initially, but seen in follow-up x-rays further emphasize this point.

REFERENCES

American Academy of Pediatrics. *Visual Diagnosis of Child Abuse on CD-ROM,* 2nd ed. AAP, 2003.

Kleinman P. *Diagnostic Imaging of Child Abuse,* 2nd ed. Mosby, 1998.

Reece R, Ludwig S, eds. *Child Abuse: Medical Diagnosis and Management,* 2nd ed. Lippincott Williams & Wilkins, 2001.

15. CHILD ABUSE: SEXUAL

   I. Problem. A 6-year-old girl is brought to the physician after telling her mother that her uncle touches her "privates" with his hand and his "privates."

II. Immediate Questions

A. **Does hospital, county, or state have specific protocols or evaluation centers for suspected sexual abuse or sexual assault?** Multidisciplinary evaluation programs for suspected chronic sexual abuse and acute sexual assault best serve many child and adolescent victims.

B. **How should the history be obtained?** It is essential to understand what happened, when it happened, and what symptoms are present. Initial history should be obtained from adults who accompany child, preferably without child present, including past medical history, review of systems, and content and context of child's disclosure. Some direct history from child is appropriate and should be obtained in a relaxed manner, preferably with child's caretaker out of the room. Questioning should be open-ended and nonleading. A general inquiry such as "why are you here to see the doctor?" or "has anything happened to you that hurt, scared, or confused you?" or instruction to "tell me what happened" is a good place to start. Use phrases such as "tell me more," or "how did that happen," or "what happened next" to continue the interview. *Do not* start by saying "your mother told me your uncle touched your privates—is that true?" Document the history carefully, indicating which portion is from caretaker and which from child. Indicate direct quotations by using quotation marks.

C. **When did last sexual contact occur?** Disclosure of abuse is often a social and emotional, but not a medical, emergency. If sexual abuse occurred within the last 72 hours and type of sexual contact suggests body fluids from abuser might be recovered, perform immediate evaluation at a facility capable of forensic evidence collection. Most cases of child sexual abuse do not fit these criteria.

D. **What symptoms are present?** Does child have genital pain, discharge, bleeding, sores, or itching? Urinary burning or frequency? Anal pain, bleeding, or itching? Although these symptoms are nonspecific, prompt evaluation is indicated when acute symptoms are present. Were anogenital symptoms present at time of abuse incident or at any other time in the past? Have there been other physical symptoms or changes in child's behavior?

III. Differential Diagnosis.
Sexually abused children present for medical care in three ways: disclosure of sexual abuse, behavioral symptoms, and signs and symptoms of anogenital problems.

A. **Child Sexual Abuse.** Most common presentation is a complaint or disclosure of sexual contact. Abuse is primary reason that child makes a disclosure. History of sexual abuse provided by child is also the most important and frequently present evidence.

B. **Behavioral Conditions.** Presenting symptoms of sexual abuse may be very general in nature and include changes in child's behavior, emotional responses, and activity. These behaviors are nonspecific and may be indicators of physical, emotional, or other nonabuse-related stresses. Sexually "acting out" behavior should raise concern about abuse but is not diagnostic.

C. **Dermatologic Conditions.** Genital signs and symptoms are commonly associated with improper hygiene, irritant or contact dermatitis, atopic dermatitis, or seborrhea. Lichen sclerosus et atrophicus may present with hemorrhagic, bruised, or abraded appearance in anogenital area.

D. **Congenital Conditions.** Congenital variations of anal and genital structures are common. Midline fusion abnormalities suggesting injury may involve either genital or anal openings.

E. **Urethral Disorders.** Painless genital spotting or bleeding is associated with urethral prolapse, most often found in prepubertal African-American girls.

F. **Anal Conditions.** Midline perianal tags are common normal variations. Anal fissures and bleeding may be associated with constipation. Perianal lesions may accompany inflammatory bowel disease.

G. **Nonsexual Trauma.** Straddle injuries can be associated with pain, bruising, bleeding, and lacerations. Injuries are often anterior, typically involve the external genitalia (not the hymen), and are asymmetric.

H. **Infectious Conditions.** Perianal streptococcal infection can produce painful defecation and intense redness with fissuring and bleeding of perianal tissues. Streptococcal vaginitis may produce intense genital pain and redness with purulent or bloody discharge. Other nasopharyngeal or respiratory pathogens can produce purulent vaginitis. *Shigella* infection may produce bloody vaginal discharge. Genital lesions can be associated with varicella and molluscum contagiosum. Pinworms are associated with either genital or anal pain, itching, and excoriation.

I. **Other Conditions.** Intravaginal foreign bodies are associated with purulent or bloody discharge. Normal physiologic leukorrhea in pubertal girls may be misinterpreted as infections. Labial adhesions or agglutination often result from an irritant or infectious process.

IV. Database
A. Physical Exam Key Points
1. General features of exam
a. Purpose.
Most important purpose of exam is to reassure child that he or she is or will be physically all right. Other purposes are to document physical or forensic findings produced by sexual contact, screen for sexually transmitted infections, and look for physical findings indicative of other medical conditions. Most physical exams of sexually abused

children will not yield any specific physical findings for sexual contact.

b. **Preparation.** Exam should not require physical force. It is essential to describe steps of exam in advance and reassure child that it will not be painful. A general physical exam should be conducted before the anogenital exam.

c. **Documentation.** Photograph significant or suspicious findings (or draw a detailed diagram if camera is unavailable).

2. **Behavior.** Document child's behavior and demeanor during exam, although no specific behavior proves abuse did or did not occur.

3. **Skin.** Skin findings (eg, bruising, abrasions, or ligature marks) are occasionally seen in support of history of use of physical force. Findings are typically absent in younger children because use of physical force is uncommon.

4. **HEENT.** Palatal bruising and lip injury are occasionally seen in forced oral penetration.

5. **Genital exam.** Anogenital exam should be done with child in multiple positions, including supine frog-leg, supine knee-chest, and prone knee-chest positions. Specific genital findings are uncommon. Erythema is a common nonspecific finding, often associated with hygiene problems. Warts, vesicular or ulcerative rashes, or purulent discharges raise concerns about STDs. Genital bruises, abrasions, and lacerations can be seen in sexual abuse or accidental injury. Hymenal lacerations or scars, or missing portions of the posterior hymeneal margin, are specific for penetrating trauma.

6. **Anal exam.** Specific anal findings are rare. Erythema is a common nonspecific finding, often associated with hygiene problems. Anal fissures, perianal abrasions, midline anal tags, and anal dilation are common nonspecific findings. Anal tears or scars that extend through the anal sphincter are diagnostic for anal penetration.

B. **Laboratory Data**

1. **Testing for STDs**

a. **Prepubertal children.** Routine testing for STDs is not needed, but STD testing should be considered in children with specific risk factors, including known or clinically suspected STD, sibling of a child with known STD, genital discharge or anal or genital injury present on exam, or perpetrator with known or suspected STD.

b. **Pubertal and postpubertal adolescents.** Adolescents who describe sexual contact that could transmit an STD should be tested routinely, with culturing for *Neisseria gonorrhea* and *Chlamydia,* wet mount of secretions for trichomonas (in girls), and rapid plasmin reagin (RPR). Consider hepatitis B virus and HIV testing.

   2. Drug screening. Routine testing is not recommended. Consider if history or exam suggest drug or alcohol use.
   3. Forensic evidence collection ("rape kit"). Attempt to collect and preserve physical evidence of seminal fluid, blood, saliva, or pubic hair from perpetrator. Typically, collection is guided by specific protocols using prepackaged collection "kits."
      a. Prepubertal children. Collection of forensic evidence is often limited in prepubertal children by types of sexual contacts typically experienced and interval between sexual contact and evaluation. A selective approach is warranted based on history and physical findings. Higher yields of positive forensic evidence come from clothing and bedclothes than from child's body.
      b. Pubertal and postpubertal adolescents. Forensic evidence should be collected if adolescents present for evaluation within 72 hours (some protocols specify within 96 hours) of sexual contact that is likely to transfer secretions from perpetrator.
   C. Radiographic and Other Studies
   1. Imaging studies. May be of benefit in selected patients with suspected sexual abuse *and* other signs of physical injury.
   2. Pregnancy testing. Urine or blood pregnancy test should be performed on all menarcheal adolescents at risk of pregnancy, particularly those being considered for emergency contraception.

V. Plan
   A. Report Suspected Abuse. All 50 states have laws that require heath care providers to report suspected child abuse including suspected sexual abuse (see also Chapter 14, Child Abuse: Physical, p. 73). State laws vary as to when reports need to be made to child protective service (CPS) agency or police, or both.
   B. Manage Acute Injuries. Most sexually abused children will have no injuries or minor injuries not requiring surgical repairs. Treatment includes maintaining good perineal hygiene, sitz baths, and topical lubricant ointments or topical antibiotics.
   C. Sexually Transmitted Disease Prophylaxis
   1. Prepubertal children. Prophylactic antibiotics are not routinely administered.
   2. Pubertal and postpubertal adolescents. Adolescents should be offered antibiotic prophylaxis for gonorrhea, chlamydia, bacterial vaginosis, and trichomoniasis. Current recommendations include:
      a. Cefixime, 400 mg IM or IV for 1 dose, or ceftriaxone, 125 mg IM or IV for 1 dose; **or**
      b. Spectinomycin, 40 mg/kg IM for 1 dose (maximum 2 g) for children allergic to penicillin; **and** azithromycin, 1 g PO, or

doxycycline, 100 mg PO twice daily for 7 days (if older than 8 years); **and** metronidazole, 2 g PO for 1 dose.

3. **Other.** Some protocols recommend hepatitis B vaccine administration to previously unimmunized children and consideration of HIV prophylaxis in high-risk cases.

D. **Emergency Contraception.** Offer pregnancy prophylaxis to postmenarcheal girls with a history of sexual contact that places them at risk for pregnancy and who present within 72 hours (perhaps up to 96 hours) of sexual assault. Treatment is two Ovral tablets orally initially, followed by two Ovral tablets 12 hours after first dose. Nausea is a common side effect.

E. **Follow-up.** Medical follow-up depends on type and severity of injuries and presence of STDs. Consider referral for psychological screening or counseling. Physicians should be willing to discuss medical findings and answer questions raised by CPS workers and police during their investigations. State laws pertaining to criminal investigation and investigation of suspected sexual abuse take precedence over HIPAA regulations, allowing physicians to discuss otherwise protected health information with CPS workers and police.

VI. **Problem Case Diagnosis.** The 6-year-old girl described being sexually abused by a teenaged uncle over several months. He bribed her to keep the abuse "secret." The most recent episode occurred about 1 week ago. Patient has had intermittent complaints of genital pain and dysuria but no history of bleeding or discharge. She has no current symptoms, and exam was normal. The uncle had a history of a prior incident with a young cousin that the family "dealt with themselves."

VII. **Teaching Pearl: Question.** When sexual contact occurs between children, how does one differentiate abuse from sexual experimentation?

VIII. **Teaching Pearl: Answer.** Normal sexual experimentation involves age-appropriate activities between children of similar age or developmental stage. Motivation for the activity is mutual curiosity and pleasure and involves mutual "consent." Sexual abuse involves manipulation, pressure, coercion, threat, or force to involve child in developmentally inappropriate sexual activity and maintain secrecy. Episodes that are very frequent, very intense, or compulsive should also raise concerns.

REFERENCES

American Academy of Pediatrics, Committee on Child Abuse and Neglect. Guidelines for the evaluation of sexual abuse of children: A subject review. *Pediatrics* 1999;103:186–191.

American Academy of Pediatrics, Committee on Adolescence. Care of the adolescent sexual assault victim. *Pediatrics* 2001;107:1476–1479.

American Academy of Pediatrics. *Visual Diagnosis of Child Abuse on CD-ROM,* 2nd ed. AAP, 2003

Reece R, Ludwig S, eds. *Child Abuse: Medical Diagnosis and Management,* 2nd ed. Lippincott Williams & Wilkins, 2001.

16. COAGULAPATHY

I. Problem. A 14-month-old boy is admitted to the general pediatric service with dehydration attributed to viral gastroenteritis. He is noted to have multiple bruises. After venipuncture, he develops a hematoma.

II. Immediate Questions

   A. Are there any identifiable factors that predispose patient to bleeding? For example, an underlying infection causing disseminated intravascular coagulation (DIC)?

   B. Pertinent Past Medical History: Is there a history of liver disease? Any previous history of bleeding? A previous history of easy bruising in the first year of life raises suspicion of a bleeding disorder. Inquire about nutritional status. Vitamin K deficiency can result from malabsorption syndromes or malnutrition.

   C. Pertinent Past Surgical History: Has patient had bleeding with past procedures? Approximately 30% of male infants with hemophilia bleed during circumcision.

   D. Pertinent Family History. Attempt to characterize bleeding in relatives. Most patients with a family history of hemophilia are diagnosed at birth. However, one third of hemophiliacs represent new mutations.

   E. What medication(s) does patient take? Aspirin and NSAIDs affect platelet function but typically do not cause bleeding unless patient has an underlying defect in hemostasis.

III. Differential Diagnosis

   A. Blood Draw Technique. Bleeding from venipuncture sites from lack of pressure should be brief and minimal.

   B. Thrombocytopenia. Patients with thrombocytopenia, platelet dysfunction, and von Willebrand disease (vWD) usually present with mucocutaneous hemorrhage, including ecchymoses, petechiae, epistaxis, gingival bleeding, GI hemorrhage, and menorrhagia (see Chapter 87, Thrombocytopenia, p. 408).

   C. Platelet Dysfunction

      1. Congenital

         a. Defects in platelet-vessel wall interaction (disorders of adhesion). VWD, Bernard-Soulier syndrome.

      b. Defects in platelet-platelet interaction (disorders of aggregation). Congenital afibrinogenemia, Glanzmann thrombasthenia.

      c. Defects in platelet secretion. Storage pool disease (deficiencies of dense granules; ie, May-Hegglin anomaly, Hermansky-Pudlak syndrome, Chédiak-Higashi syndrome, thrombocytopenia–absent radius [TAR] syndrome).

   2. Acquired

      a. Drug-induced. Aspirin, NSAIDs.

      b. Uremia. Precise cause of platelet dysfunction in uremia is unknown.

D. Coagulation Defects

   1. Congenital

      a. Hemophilia A. X-linked recessive bleeding disorder attributable to deficiency of factor VIII.

      b. Hemophilia B. X-linked recessive disorder caused by deficiency of factor IX.

   2. Acquired

      a. Vitamin K deficiency. Vitamin K–dependent factors include II, VII, IX, and X. Malabsorption of vitamin K can follow administration of broad-spectrum antibiotics that alter normal intestinal flora. Deficiency can also follow ingestion of drugs that interfere with vitamin K absorption (ie, cholestyramine, megadoses of vitamin E or A, salicylate overdose). Other causes of vitamin K deficiency include cystic fibrosis, biliary atresia, obstructive jaundice, and short bowel syndrome.

      b. Liver disease. Virtually all coagulation factors are synthesized by the liver.

      c. DIC. Hemorrhagic disorder associated with activation of procoagulant, anticoagulant, and fibrinolytic mechanisms predisposing host to microvascular hemorrhage as well as thrombosis. Causes include gram-negative sepsis, hypotensive shock, massive trauma, and malignancy.

      d. Acquired inhibitory antibodies of hemostasis. Antibodies to coagulation factors, including vWF and factors II, V, and X, may arise spontaneously in a variety of clinical conditions.

E. Child Abuse. Should be suspected when:

   1. Child has an injury with no history of trauma.

   2. History is inconsistent with severity of injury.

   3. There is a delay in seeking medical care for significant injury.

   4. There is a history of poorly explained, recurrent injuries.

IV. Database

  A. Physical Exam Key Points

1. **Vital signs.** Significant blood loss may results in increased tachycardia and hypotension.
2. **Skin and mucous membranes.** Examine for petechiae, purpura, ecchymoses, hemangiomas, oozing from venipuncture sites, and jaundice. Examine mucous membranes for gingival oozing of blood, mucosal purpura, or oropharyngeal petechiae.
3. **Abdomen.** Examine for hepatosplenomegaly.
4. **Musculoskeletal system.** Examine muscles for hematoma and atrophy; joints for decreased range of motion and degeneration.
5. **Neurologic exam.** Assess for signs of CNS bleeding.

B. **Laboratory Data**
   1. **CBC.** Monitor hemoglobin to assess for blood loss. Platelet counts > 50,000/mm^3 are adequate to maintain hemostasis if function is normal. Petechiae may appear when platelet count drops below 50,000/mm^3 but do not tend to be generalized unless count is < 20,000/mm^3.
   2. **Peripheral blood smear.** Normally, there are 10–20 platelets per oil-immersion field, about 10% of which are larger than average. RBC fragments may suggest DIC.
   3. **PT.**
      a. Prolonged whenever plasma levels of one or more of the factors in the extrinsic pathway (V, VII, X, prothrombin, or fibrinogen) fall to levels below ~30% of normal. PT measures thrombin generation following activation of factor X by factor VIIa.
      b. PT can be expressed as an international normalized ratio (INR), calculated as patient PT/control PT to the power of the international sensitivity index (ISI). The ISI is a measure of the sensitivity of each individual laboratory's thromboplastin reagent to coagulation factor deficiencies. The INR allows for uniform monitoring of the degree of anticoagulation in different laboratories.
      c. PT is prolonged at birth. Causes of prolonged PT include vitamin K deficiency, DIC, liver disease, congenital factor deficiencies, and oral anticoagulant therapy.
   4. **APTT.** Becomes prolonged whenever plasma levels of one or more coagulation factors other than factor VII drop below ~30% of normal. Reflects plasma concentration of the four contact factors (XI, XII, prekallikrein, and high-molecular-weight kininogen [HMWK]) and factors II, V, VIII, IX, and X. APTT is prolonged in healthy newborns and reaches adult values by ~6 months of age. The most common cause of prolonged APTT is heparin contamination in samples obtained from indwelling catheters. Other causes of prolonged APTT are congenital factor deficiencies, DIC, liver disease, and lupus anticoagulant.

5. **Thrombin time.** Measures conversion of fibrinogen to fibrin. It is prolonged by heparin, hypofibrinogenemia, and dysfibrinogenemias.
6. **Platelet aggregation testing.** Requires platelet count > 100,000/mm^3 and relatively large volume of blood (> 10 mL). Patterns of aggregation to ADP, epinephrine (EPI), collagen, arachidonic acid, and ristocetin are measured. Patients with vWD show decreased aggregation with ristocetin as do those with Bernard-Soulier syndrome. In platelet storage pool disease, abnormal aggregation to ADP, EPI, and collagen is seen. Patients with Glanzmann thrombasthenia show abnormal aggregation to ADP, EPI, collagen, and arachidonic acid.
7. **Plasma fibrinogen concentrations.** Decreased in patients with significant DIC.
8. **Fibrin split products and D-dimer.** Increased levels are consistent with DIC.
9. **Bone marrow aspiration and biopsy.** Indicated in bleeding patients when malignancy or aplasia is suspected.

C. **Radiographic and Other Studies**
1. **Skeletal survey.** Indicated in cases of suspected child abuse.
2. **CT scan.** Should be considered for patients with known or suspected bleeding disorders who suffer trauma, especially to the head or abdomen.

V. Plan

A. **Suspected Child Abuse.** Consult child protective services (see Chapter 14, Child Abuse: Physical, p. 73). If bleeding is significant enough to warrant immediate treatment, draw one or two tubes to hold for future diagnostic tests, and treat appropriately.
B. **Thrombocytopenia or Platelet Dysfunction.** To correct or prevent bleeding due to thrombocytopenia from lack of platelet production or due to platelet dysfunction, transfuse single donor pheresis platelets at a dose of 10 mL/kg to raise platelet count by 50,000/mm^3.
C. **Thrombocytopenia**
1. **Due to immune destruction (ie, idiopathic thrombocytopenic purpura [ITP]).** Can be treated with IV immune globulin at a dose of 1 g/kg/day for up to three doses or Rho(D) immune globulin, 50 mcg/kg as a single dose. Alternative therapy for ITP includes prednisone, 2 mg/kg/day, or high-dose methylprednisolone, 30 mg/kg/day for up to 3 days. Patients should avoid use of NSAIDs and aspirin products.
2. **From drug reaction.** Discontinue drug and transfuse platelets as necessary.
D. **vWD.** Treatment of patients with type 1 vWD (the most common form) is as follows.
1. **Minimal bleeding or minor surgical procedures.** Give desmopressin acetate (DDAVP), which promotes release of vWF from endothelial cells.

      a. Intranasal dose. Administer 150 mcg for patients < 50 kg and 300 mcg for patients > 50 kg (use 1.5 mg/mL concentration).

      b. IV dose. Administer 0.3 mcg/kg.

  2. Major surgery or significant bleeding. Administer a factor VIII concentrate containing high levels of vWF (ie, Humate P); vWF 1 unit/kg will raise plasma level 2 units/dL.

 E. Hemophilia. Recombinant factor products are the preferred treatment for deficiencies of factors VIII and IX. Treatment depends on severity of disease, presence of an inhibitor, and medical circumstances.

  1. Factor VIII. Dose of factor VIII = unit/dL(%) desired rise in plasma factor VIII × body weight (kg) × 0.5; $T_{1/2}$ of factor VIII is 12 hours.

  2. Factor IX. A 1 unit/kg dose of factor IX results in 1 unit/dL rise in plasma factor IX level; $T_{1/2}$ of factor IX is 18–24 hours.

 F. DIC. Treat the underlying disease and support patient with appropriate blood products, including RBCs, platelets, plasma, and cryoprecipitate. Dose guidelines are packed RBCs, 10–15 mL/kg; fresh frozen plasma, 10–20 mL/kg; and cryoprecipitate, 1 bag (unit)/5 kg up to 10 bags.

 G. Vitamin K deficiency. SQ route is preferred due to hypersensitivity to IV and IM injections. Dose is 1–2 mg SQ as a single dose. Oral dose is 2.5–5 mg daily.

VI. Problem Case Diagnosis. The 14-month-old boy was diagnosed with moderate factor VIII deficiency (factor VIII level of 1–5%). The APTT was also noted to be prolonged. Patient improved with factor VIII replacement and IV fluids.

VII. Teaching Pearl: Question. A patient with severe hemophilia A is treated for bleeding with 25 units/kg recombinant factor VIII concentrate. What is the expected postinfusion factor VIII level?

VIII. Teaching Pearl: Answer. The expected factor VIII level is 50%.

REFERENCES

Lusher JM. Clinical and laboratory approach to the patient with bleeding. In: Nathan DG, Orkin SH, Look T, Ginsburg D, eds. *Hematology of Infancy and Childhood.* Saunders, 2003:1515–1526.

Montgomery RR, Gill JC, Scott JP. Hemophilia and von Willebrand disease. In: Nathan DG, Orkin SH, Look T, Ginsburg D, eds. *Hematology of Infancy and Childhood.* Saunders, 2003:1547–1576.

Pruth RK, Bleeding disorders: An overview and clinical practice. In: Tefferi A, ed. *Primary Hematology.* Humana Press, 2001:303–316.

17. COMA

 I. Problem. An unresponsive 18-month-old boy is brought to the emergency department for evaluation.

II. Immediate Questions

A. Is patient breathing spontaneously? What are the other vital signs? As in all emergencies, rapid evaluation and support of airway, breathing, and circulation (ABCs) are initial management priorities. All patients should receive 100% oxygen via face mask. Comatose patients may not have effective spontaneous respirations or may have lost their protective airway reflexes and therefore may require assisted ventilation with a bag-valve-mask device or endotracheal intubation.

B. Is patient's condition the result of head injury? If head injury is suspected, immediately immobilize the cervical spine using in-line manual stabilization or placement of a cervical spine collar. Maintain cervical spine immobilization during airway management, especially during endotracheal intubation. Obtain rapid IV access.

C. What is patient's Glasgow Coma Scale (GCS) score? Although it was originally proposed for patients with head injury, the GCS is helpful in assessing the depth of nontraumatic coma (see Appendix F, p. 765). Patients with a GCS score ≤ 8 should be intubated.

D. Does patient have signs of herniation (dilated nonreactive pupil, papilledema, posturing) or intracranial hypertension (Cushing triad: hypertension, bradycardia, irregular respirations)? These patients should be intubated and given controlled mild hyperventilation. IV administration of mannitol or normal saline should be considered. They will require emergent CT scan of the head and neurosurgical consultation.

E. What is patient's dextrose level? Hypoglycemia is a common cause of coma and is readily detected by bedside determination. Timely glucose administration to hypoglycemic patients can be lifesaving.

F. Is drug overdose suspected? Does patient have small pupils? Consider administering IV naloxone for opiate overdose.

G. Pertinent Historical Information
1. Is there a history of witnessed or suspected trauma?
2. Does patient have fever?
3. What is the probability of poisoning, ingestion, or overdose?
4. What are the associated symptoms (eg, headache, seizures, diplopia, weakness, vomiting, bloody diarrhea)?
5. Is there a contributing past medical history (eg, seizure disorder, brain tumor, ventricular shunt, sickle cell disease, metabolic disorder, diabetes, liver disease, renal failure)?

III. Differential Diagnosis.
Etiologies of coma may be divided into structural or medical causes (Table I–9) and are similar to those for altered mental status, discussed in Chapter 6 (see pp. 27–31).

A. Structural Causes. Tend to result in asymmetric or focal neurologic findings, particularly affecting pupillary response, extraocular

TABLE I-9. COMMON DIAGNOSES OF COMA BY AGE

Infant	Child	Adolescent
Abuse	Abuse/Trauma	Psychiatric
Inborn error	Infection	Seizure
Infection	Seizure	Toxin
Metabolic	Toxin	Trauma
Seizure		

movements, and motor response to pain. (For additional discussion of these causes, see Chapter 6, Altered Mental Status, III, A, 1–4, p. 27.)

    1. Trauma (eg, from shearing forces). When mechanism of injury does not fit the extent of child's injuries, always consider inflicted trauma or child abuse.

    2. Tumor.

    3. Cerebrovascular event (hemorrhagic and ischemic strokes occur with same frequency in children).

    4. Hydrocephalus (communicating or noncommunicating).

    5. Infection (eg, epidural abscess, usually in older children and adolescents from contiguous spread of middle ear or sinus infection).

B. Medical Causes. Include any process that decreases delivery of substrate to the brain. Pupils are generally equal and reactive and neurologic exam is nonfocal. (See Chapter 6, Altered Mental Status, III, B, p. 28, for additional discussion.)

    1. Infection (eg, meningitis, encephalitis, subdural empyema, sepsis).

    2. Poisoning or overdose. See Table I–3, p. 29, for examples of common drugs that may cause coma. Because many drugs and toxins are not detectable on serum and urine screening tests, a high index of suspicion should be maintained. Some ingested substances cause a specific constellation of signs (toxidrome), which aids in diagnosis and management (see Table I–4, p. 30).

    3. Metabolic alterations (eg, hyperglycemia or hypoglycemia, electrolyte abnormalities, buildup of waste or metabolic products due to renal or hepatic failure, or inborn errors of metabolism).

    4. Hemolytic uremic syndrome (eg, secondary to infection with *E coli* O157:H7).

IV. Database

    A. Physical Exam Key Points

        1. Depth of coma. Assess using GCS.

2. **Ocular and motor responses.** Assess the following to help determine whether etiology is structural or medical. Asymmetry points to a structural lesion.
   a. **Pupillary size.** Normal or asymmetric?
   b. **Pupillary reflex.** Fixed or reactive?
   c. **Extraocular movements.** Normal, asymmetric, or absent?
   d. **Motor response to pain.** Decorticate, decerebrate, or flaccid?
3. **Respiratory pattern.** Identification of abnormal patterns of respiration can help differentiate a structural from a medical cause of coma (see Figure I–1, p. 33).
   a. **Cheyne-Stokes respiration.** Implies dysfunction of structures deep in both cerebral hemispheres or diencephalon; usually seen in metabolic encephalopathy.
   b. **Central neurogenic hyperventilation.** May occur with lesions of midbrain and pons.
   c. **Cluster breathing.** May result from primary or secondary brainstem lesions.
   d. **Ataxic breathing.** May result from primary disruption of medullary respiratory centers.
4. **Toxidromes** (see Table I–3, p. 29).
5. **Neurologic findings.** Perform a thorough neurologic exam.
6. **Smell of patient's breath.** May reveal alcohol intoxication or diabetic ketoacidosis.
7. **Signs of trauma.** Boggy scalp swelling, Battle sign, raccoon eyes, retinal hemorrhages, hemotympanum, bruises, hematomas.

B. **Laboratory Data**
   1. **Glucose.** Rapid bedside serum glucose determination immediately identifies hypoglycemia or hyperglycemia.
   2. **Serum electrolytes.** Identify electrolyte abnormalities that could cause seizures (Na^+ and Ca^{2+}), as well as acidosis (bicarbonate) or uremia (BUN and creatinine).
   3. **Liver function tests.** Reveal presence of hepatic failure.
   4. **Serum ammonia.** Elevated level is associated with common inborn errors of metabolism or liver failure.
   5. **Serum or urine drug screening.** Although limited, can identify potential toxins.
   6. **Anticonvulsant drug levels.** Obtain in patients with known seizure disorders.
   7. **CBC, differential, blood and urine cultures.** Obtain in febrile patients or whenever sepsis or CNS infection is likely. CBC is also helpful in evaluation of patients who have sickle cell disease or who may have hemolytic uremic syndrome.
   8. **Cerebrospinal fluid evaluation (cell count, chemistry, and culture).** Obtain whenever CNS infection or sepsis is suspected. To avoid the risk of cerebral herniation, consider obtaining CT scan of the head before performing lumbar puncture in

patients with suspected structural CNS lesions or increased intracranial pressure.

9. **ABGs.** Helps tailor degree of hyperventilation.

C. Radiographic and Other Studies

1. **CT scan of head.** Obtain emergently whenever increased intracranial pressure or presence of a structural lesion is suspected. Obtain in all comatose patients with coma of unclear etiology.

2. **Skeletal survey.** Obtain in children younger than 3 years of age who may have suffered inflicted injuries or child abuse.

3. **ECG.** May be helpful in management of certain ingested substances or toxins.

V. Plan.
Management is similar to that of a patient with altered mental status, discussed in Chapter 6. See Figure I–1 on p. 33, which depicts a systematic approach to patient care.

A. Initial Management

1. Support ABCs. Secure airway, administer 100% oxygen, and obtain IV access.

2. Immobilize cervical spine for known history of or suspected head trauma.

3. Assess GCS and perform endotracheal intubation if ≤ 8.

4. Assess for signs of herniation (dilated nonreactive pupil, papilledema, posturing) or increased intracranial pressure (Cushing triad). If present, provide controlled mild hyperventilation, consider administration of mannitol or normal saline, and obtain emergent CT scan of the head and neurosurgical consultation.

5. Perform rapid bedside glucose determination; if glucose ≤ 40, administer IV dextrose.

B. Specific Plans

1. **Narcotic overdose.** If suspected and patient has small pupils, administer IV naloxone to reverse opiate toxicity.

2. **Head injury or focal neurologic finding.** If suspected or present, or if there is a focal neurologic finding, obtain CT scan of the head and neurosurgical consultation.

3. **Inflicted injury or suspected child abuse.** If suspected in a child younger than 3 years of age, obtain a skeletal survey.

4. **Metabolic alterations.** Correct metabolic and electrolyte abnormalities and acidosis.

5. **Poisoning or overdose.** If suspected, administer charcoal (if ingestion occurred within 1 hour) and antidote if available.

6. **Fever, CNS infection, or sepsis.** Perform a lumbar puncture if patient is stable and does not have signs of increased intracranial pressure. Administer appropriate antibiotics.

7. **Hyperammonemia.** Consider workup for metabolic disorder.

VI. Problem Case Diagnosis.
The 18-month-old patient had slow, irregular respirations and a GCS score of 8. Physical exam showed

boggy swelling on the right temporal area. The cervical spine was immobilized, patient was intubated, and IV access obtained. Rapid blood glucose determination showed a glucose level of 98. Emergent CT scan of the head showed a subdural hemorrhage on the right side. Patient was admitted to the ICU with neurosurgical consultation. Subsequent evaluation revealed multiple rib fractures in different stages of healing and metaphyseal long bone fractures, all consistent with child abuse.

VII. Teaching Pearl: Question. What is the most important sign that differentiates structural from medical etiologies of coma?

VIII. Teaching Pearls: Answer. Pupillary response; it is usually preserved when coma is secondary to toxic and metabolic causes. Although pupils may be small, they are usually symmetric and reactive.

REFERENCES

King D, Avner JR. Altered mental status. In: Isaacman DJ, ed. Neurologic Emergencies. *Clin Pediatr Emerg Med* 2003;4:171–178.

Nelson DS. Coma and altered level of consciousness. In: Fleisher GR, ed. *Textbook of Pediatric Emergency Medicine.* Lippincott Williams & Wilkins, 2000:165–176.

18. CONSTIPATION

I. Problem. A 4-year-old boy has infrequent and painful bowel movements.

II. Immediate Questions

  A. What is patient's usual pattern of stooling? Normal frequency varies from 4 times daily in infants to once every 3 days in children.

  B. Age at onset of symptoms? Consider congenital anomalies, obstruction, or chronic diseases if constipation has been present since infancy. Functional constipation starts in toddler or preschool years.

  C. Consistency and size of stool? Hard, large stool that is painful to pass is consistent with the diagnosis of constipation regardless of stool frequency.

  D. Symptoms when having a bowel movement? Pain may be due to large or hard stool, anal fissure, or, less commonly, perianal streptococcal infection. Functional constipation results in recurrent cycle: pain with passing stool → withhold stool → increased stool volume in rectum → dilated rectum, decreasing sensory function → increased stool volume → pain with passing stool, and so on.

  E. Any associated symptoms (eg, abdominal pain, bloating, distention)? Patients with severe constipation have decreased appetite and weight loss. Approximately 30% of patients have day or night enuresis, or both, and ~60% have recurrent abdominal pain.

F. Difficulties with toilet training? Coercive training or resistance may lead toddlers to withhold stool, starting a recurrent cycle of functional constipation.

G. What is patient's usual diet? Diets low in fiber, high in complex carbohydrates, and high in dairy products contribute to slowed bowel elimination.

H. Any associated fecal soiling? Most encopresis occurs in association with chronic constipation (eg, retentive encopresis). The full, distended rectum loses the ability to signal the urge to pass stool, which, in turn, leads to stool leakage.

I. What medication(s) does patient take? Constipation is a common side effect of many prescribed, over-the-counter, and alternative remedies.

J. Pertinent past or present medical history? Acute injury, illness, or hospitalization is a common precipitator; reasons may include decreased activity, medications, or electrolyte disturbance. Underlying endocrine, neuromuscular, or chronic disease may alter bowel habits.

K. Any stressful events in home or school environment? Stress may affect diet, sleep, and activity level and thus produce changes in bowel habits.

III. Differential Diagnosis

A. Functional Constipation. The most common type in patients showing no evidence of structural, endocrine, or metabolic disease.

B. Congenital Anomalies of Neuromuscular Function. Consider when constipation is evident in infancy. Includes congenital aganglionic megacolon or Hirschsprung disease, intestinal neuronal dysplasia, and chronic intestinal pseudoobstruction.

C. Structural Anomalies. Often evident on inspection (eg, imperforate or ectopic anus, anal stenosis, anteriorly displaced anus in girls). Intestinal defects include intestinal bands, intestinal stenosis, and strictures secondary to inflammatory bowel disease. Consider spinal cord defects (eg, tethered cord, spina bifida, spinal cord injury).

D. Metabolic Disorders. Hypokalemia, hypercalcemia, hypothyroidism.

E. Abdominopelvic Mass. Direct external pressure on GI tract.

F. Lead Poisoning. Causes constipation, microcytic anemia, and abdominal pain.

G. Infant Botulism. Progressive symptoms, including constipation, weak cry, and ascending paralysis.

H. Medication Side Effect. In particular, calcium supplements, opiates, and tricyclic antidepressants.

IV. Database
  A. Physical Exam Key Points
   1. General appearance
      a. Evidence of systemic or chronic illness (eg, growth parameters).
      b. Features consistent with hypothyroidism.
   2. Abdomen. Distention, fecal masses, quality and presence of bowel sounds.
   3. Rectal exam
      a. Inspection. Size and position of anus, presence of soiling, anal fissures, streptococcal perianal cellulitis, skin tags.
      b. Digital exam. Anal tone is decreased in functional constipation and spinal cord defects. Presence of increased volume of stool in large distended rectum is consistent with functional constipation. Small, empty rectum is consistent with Hirschsprung disease.
   4. Neurologic exam. Absence of anal wink and decreased lower extremity reflexes suggests neurologic condition.
  B. Laboratory Data. Laboratory investigation should be guided by the findings from history and physical exam. Additional studies are unnecessary if history and exam are consistent with functional constipation. Obtain appropriate studies if metabolic or endocrine abnormality is suspected. Test stool for heme if digital exam is performed.
  C. Radiographic and Other Studies
   1. Abdominal x-ray. To detect dilated rectum or megacolon, evidence of obstruction, or stool impaction. It is normal to see some stool in colon.
   2. Barium enema. Unprepped is useful in Hirschsprung disease; prepped, for intestinal structural defects; but not commonly used.
   3. Rectal biopsy. To rule out Hirschsprung disease and other neuromuscular disorders.
   4. Anal manometry. Unnecessary for diagnosis of most cases.

V. Plan. Goals include relieving impaction, softening stool, and retraining patient to have regular, painless bowel movements.
  A. Parental Education. Imperative for successful treatment of functional constipation. Long-term treatment is often required, and relapse is common. Discuss social and emotional impact of encopresis.
  B. Dietary Changes. These changes alone are not successful in most cases. Increase fiber and fluids, and limit milk intake to 8–16 oz/day in patients older than 1 year of age.
  C. Cleansing and Maintenance Therapies
   1. Enema. Consider for patients with large volume of stool in rectum or colon. Produces rapid results. Use adult-sized enema in children older than 3 years of age.

2. **Nonstimulant laxative or stool softener.** Relieves pain associated with passing stool.
   a. **Maltsupex (1 tsp in 8 oz of formula) or Dark Kayro syrup.** Consider for young infants.
   b. **Milk of magnesia.** Effective, but many children have issues with lack of palatability. Causes increased magnesium in renal-impaired patients.
   c. **Mineral oil.** Effective but disliked due to consistency and potential leakage onto clothing. There is an aspiration risk in young children and those who are developmentally impaired.
   d. **Nonabsorbable sugar (eg, lactulose and sorbitol).** Work by osmotic effect. Product can be diluted in drink of choice. May produce bloating, cramping, or diarrhea.
   e. **Polyethylene glycol 3350 (MiraLax).** Effective in stool-impacted children without initial enema.
   f. **For slower cleansing.** Use MiraLax daily over 2 weeks; a 3–6-month regimen may be necessary before resumption of normal bowel pattern is seen.
3. **Stimulant laxative.** Acceptable for short-term use until rectum returns to normal size and function.

VI. Problem Case Diagnosis. Findings of palpable stool on abdominal exam and large, hard stool in the rectum of this well-appearing, age-appropriate child led to the diagnosis of functional constipation.

VII. Teaching Pearl: Question. How should parents be counseled when they express concerns because their infant cries and strains for several minutes just prior to passing a soft stool?

VIII. Teaching Pearl: Answer. It is common for infants younger than 6 months of age to cry, strain, and appear to have pain with passing stool. If stool is soft, infant is not constipated but rather exhibiting what is known as infant dyschezia. Reassure parents that these symptoms will resolve over time.

REFERENCES

Baker SS, Liptak GS, Colletti RB, et al. Constipation in infants and children: Evaluation and treatment. A medical position statement of the NASPGHAN. *J Pediatr Gastroenterol Nutr* 1999;29:612–626.

Behrman RE, Kliegman RM, Jenson HB, eds. *Nelson Textbook of Pediatrics,* 17th ed. Saunders, 2004.

Bishop W, DiLorenzo C, Loening-Baucke V, et al. New paradigm in the diagnosis and management of constipation. *Pediatr News* (Suppl) 2004.

19. COUGH

I. Problem. An 18-month-old patient is admitted with persistent, paroxysmal cough associated with posttussive vomiting, inability to sleep, and poor intake.

II. Immediate Questions

A. What are key characteristics of the cough?

1. How long has child had cough (ie, acute or chronic)? Has cough lasted more than 3 weeks?
2. Did cough come on suddenly, as with choking, or gradually with signs and symptoms of upper respiratory tract infection?
3. What were circumstances at onset of cough?
4. Do any of the following situations aggravate cough: cold air, deep inspiration, exercise, feeding, position, time of day, time of year (ie, seasonal, spring or fall)?
5. Is cough paroxysmal, as in cystic fibrosis, asthma, pertussis, or foreign body aspiration?
6. Does cough produce mucus?
7. Is mucus clear (indicating asthma) or yellow or green (indicating suppurative lung disease)? Is blood present in mucus, as in cystic fibrosis, foreign body aspiration, tuberculosis, or bronchiectasis?
8. Does cough disappear completely during sleep, suggestive of psychogenic cough?

B. What are accompanying symptoms?

1. Chest pain or heartburn suggests gastroesophageal reflux of cardiac origin.
2. Dyspnea or tachypnea suggests pneumonia, atelectasis, edema, pneumothorax, or pulmonary embolism.
3. Sore throat, earache, or headache, with upper respiratory infection.

C. Pertinent Past Medical History

1. Birth history, including prematurity or respiratory distress syndrome.
2. Respiratory syncytial virus in infancy.
3. Growth velocity.
4. Previous episodes of coughing spells and response to bronchodilators, antihistamine, or antacids.
5. Recurrent upper or lower respiratory infections.

III. Differential Diagnosis.
Cough receptors are present throughout respiratory tract from upper airway (nose, pharynx) to terminal bronchioles. Stimulation of these receptors can occur from an array of sites, including ear, diaphragm, pericardium, and stomach.

A. Ear.
Foreign body or impacted cerumen.

B. Oropharynx or Nasopharynx.
Postnasal drip from allergic or infectious rhinosinusitis is a common cause of cough.

C. Larynx.
Congenital abnormalities (eg, laryngotracheal cleft) or viral infections cause croupy cough.

D. Tracheobronchial Tree.
Irritation of mucosal receptors or retention of secretions can result in cough.

1. **Bronchospasm.** Asthma is a frequent cause of cough that can be productive and paroxysmal.

  2. **Congenital abnormalities.** Includes tracheoesophageal fistula, cysts, and vascular rings.
  3. **Bronchitis.** Includes infectious or inflammatory irritation of mucosal receptors, as in asthma and cystic fibrosis.
  4. **Pneumonia.** Includes viral, bacterial, and atypical pneumonia as well as typical and atypical mycobacteria. *Pneumocystis* pneumonia occurs in immunocompromised patients with respiratory distress, patients receiving chemotherapy, and those with severe combined immunodeficiency syndrome or ciliary dyskinesia syndrome.
  5. **Aspiration syndromes.** Patients with either swallowing dysfunction or gastroesophageal reflux can present with cough. Cough is minimal after the cough receptors are desensitized.
  6. **Inhaled irritants** (eg, passive smoking).
  E. **Other Causes**
   1. Slow recovery from viral lower respiratory tract infection or recurrent lower respiratory infection.
   2. Congestive heart failure.
   3. Pericardial effusion.
   4. Interstitial lung disease: nonproductive cough with infectious (tuberculosis, histiocytosis, coccidioidomycosis) or inflammatory etiology (sarcoidosis).
  F. **Cause of Cough in Neonatal Period.** As a mnemonic remember **CRADLE: C**ystic fibrosis; **R**espiratory infection; **A**spiration from tracheoesophageal fistula swallowing dysfunction, gastroesophageal reflux; **D**yskinesia of cilia; **L**ung, airway, vascular malformation; **E**dema, heart failure.

IV. **Database**
  A. **Physical Exam Key Points**
   1. **Vital signs and general appearance.** Check vital signs, including height and weight percentiles, oxygen saturation, temperature, respiratory rate, and use of accessory muscles.
   2. **Ear.** Is there inflammation or foreign body?
   3. **Mouth.** Postnasal drip or cobblestoning of posterior pharynx, indicating lymphoid hyperplasia?
   4. **Sinuses.** Tenderness, swelling, or opacification?
   5. **Neck.** Tracheal shift, indicating pneumothorax or parapneumonic effusion?
   6. **Lungs**
    a. **Stridor?** Infection, crouplike viral illness.
    b. **Epiglottitis?** Rare after *Haemophilus influenza* type b vaccine.
    c. **Congenital abnormality?** Subglottic hemangioma laryngeal cysts, vocal cord paralysis.
    d. **Rhonchi?** Inflammation in proximal airway with infections or irritants.

      e. Crackles? Pneumonia, pulmonary edema, interstitial lung disease, congestive heart failure.

      f. Wheezing?

         i. Generalized polyphonic. Asthma, generalized monophonic-tracheobronchomalacia.

         ii. Localized. Foreign body, lymph node, tuberculosis, Hodgkin or non-Hodgkin lymphoma, sarcoidosis, histoplasmosis, or coccidioidomycosis.

7. Heart. Check rate and rhythm. Is there increased jugular venous pressure, third heart sound, or gallop, as in congestive heart failure?

8. Extremities. Is there clubbing (bronchiectasis, cystic fibrosis, or hypogammaglobulinemia) or cyanosis (congestive heart failure)?

B. Laboratory Data. Obtain CBC with differential. Check WBCs for leukocytosis with left shift (infectious diseases), lymphocytosis (pertussis), or lymphopenia (immunodeficiency diseases). Low hemoglobin and hematocrit may indicate pulmonary hemosiderosis or chronic infection.

C. Radiographic and Other Studies. Obtain as directed by history and physical exam.

1. Chest x-ray. To study airway, parenchyma, lung volume, diaphragm, and cardiovascular structure. Use lateral film to assess retrocardiac region behind diaphragm.

2. Inspiratory, expiratory, or decubitus films. To rule out foreign body and air trapping.

3. Barium swallow study. To detect swallowing dysfunction, gastroesophageal reflux, congenital anomalies or masses (slings).

4. Sinus film or CT scan of sinuses.

5. Milk scan. To evaluate for aspiration.

6. Pulmonary tests. Pulmonary function tests, bronchodilator response, bronchial challenge test.

7. Bronchoscopy. To evaluate unexplained cough, wheeze, and persistent air-space disease, including bronchoalveolar lavage in immunocompromised patients with pneumonia.

8. Sweat test. If cystic fibrosis is suspected.

9. Purified protein derivative (PPD) skin test.

10. Immunoglobulins.

11. α_1-Antitrypsin level.

12. *Mycoplasma* serology.

13. Biopsy of lung and bronchoalveolar lavage. In immunocompromised patients to rule out opportunistic infection and pneumocystitis.

V. Plan. Management is tailored to the specific diagnosis.

A. Antibacterial Treatment. Has little effect on cough in patients with *Mycoplasma* or pertussis.

B. Bronchodilators.

C. Anti-inflammatory Agents.

D. Antihistamine. For patients with postnasal drip.

E. Cough Suppressants. Act by depressing the central component of the cough reflex. Anticipate CNS and respiratory depression.

    1. Contraindicated in very young children, suppurative lung disease, or other conditions with increased sputum production.

    2. May be indicated for dry, irritative cough with posttussive emesis, exhaustion, or insomnia.

    3. Codeine, 1 mg/kg/day for a total of < 60 mg/day. *Lethal dose is 7–14 mg/kg.* Codeine should *not* be given to infants younger than 6 months of age because primary route of inactivation is glucuronization (histamine releaser).

    4. Effectiveness of over-the-counter cough suppressants is controversial.

    5. Antihistamine (eg, diphenhydramine) is an effective cough suppressant but causes drowsiness.

F. Mucolytics.

G. Chest Physical Therapy.

VI. Problem Case Diagnosis. The 18-month-old patient had viral, lower respiratory infection–induced airway hyperreactivity and cough, which promoted gastroesophageal reflux.

VII. Teaching Pearl: Question. Are cough suppressants indicated in all situations of cough in children?

VIII. Teaching Pearl: Answer. Cough is a very primitive protective reflex. Always seek to identify the cause before prescribing treatment. Cough suppressants are contraindicated in patients with suppurative lung disease.

REFERENCES

Guilbert TW, Taussig LM. "Doctor, he's been coughing for a month. Is it serious?" *Contemp Pediatr* 1998;15:155, 159, 161–167, 169–172.

Irwin RS, Madison JM. The persistently troublesome cough. *Am J Respir Crit Care Med* 2002;165:1469–1474.

Kamei RK. Chronic cough in children. *Pediatr Clin North Am* 1991;38:593–605.

Newson T, McKenzie S. Cough and asthma in children. *Pediatr Ann* 1996;25:156–161.

20. CYANOSIS

    I. Problem. A 1-week-old female infant is brought to the emergency department because she has turned blue.

    II. Immediate Questions

        A. What are the vital signs? Respiratory rate and respiratory effort are important indicators of the severity of illness in an infant. Increased respiratory rate with retractions, nasal flaring, and grunting indicates significant respiratory disease. An infant who has cyanosis with increased respiratory rate but no increased effort (so-called comfortable tachypnea) is more likely to have congenital heart disease. Oxygen saturation, obtained by peripheral pulse oximetry, may help establish a differential diagnosis, especially if saturations are different in upper versus lower extremities (differential saturations). Significant tachycardia or bradycardia is an indicator of severe physiologic derangement requiring immediate attention.

B. **How easily does air move into and out of lungs?** Wheezing or stridor indicates airway obstruction. Poor air movement, prolonged expiration, or other lung sounds (rales, wheezes, rhonchi) assist in the differential diagnosis. Poor aeration on only one side may indicate pneumothorax or pneumonia.

C. **Is there a murmur?** A murmur is present in some types of cyanotic congenital heart disease (eg, significant right ventricular outflow obstruction seen in critical pulmonary stenosis or tetralogy of Fallot) but may not be present in others (eg, transposition of the great arteries, atrioventricular canal defect, total anomalous pulmonary venous connection, and hypoplastic left heart syndrome). An infant with a hypercyanotic episode (so-called tet spell) may not have a murmur if the episode is severe, because there is not enough pulmonary blood flow to create a murmur.

D. **Is cyanosis peripheral, central, or differential?** Cyanosis that affects skin and lips but spares oral mucosa, tongue, and conjunctivae is termed *peripheral cyanosis*. It occurs in the presence of normal arterial saturation. Cyanosis that affects mucosa of the mouth and conjunctivae in addition to skin and lips is termed *central cyanosis* and suggests arterial desaturation or abnormal hemoglobin. *Differential cyanosis*, blueness of the upper or lower portion of the body, only, is an indicator of heart disease. Cyanosis of the lower extremities is seen in infants with critical aortic coarctation or interrupted aortic arch. The lower portion of the body is supplied by systemic venous blood coursing right to left across a patent ductus arteriosus (PDA). This differential cyanosis may also be seen in a newborn with persistent pulmonary hypertension. Transposition of the great arteries with PDA may produce differential cyanosis of the upper extremities (oxygenated blood courses right to left across ductus arteriosus, supplying the lower body).

E. **When does cyanosis occur?** Cyanosis that occurs intermittently is associated with apnea, cold exposure (acrocyanosis), or intermittent airway obstruction. Intermittent cyanosis that occurs with feeding is seen with choanal atresia, esophageal atresia (especially with coughing, sputtering), or severe gastroesophageal reflux. Cyanosis as a result of cardiac disease, respiratory disease, or abnormal hemoglobin usually is present continuously.

F. How old is patient? Differential diagnosis for a child or an adolescent with cyanosis can be quite different from that of a newborn. In-depth prenatal and birth history and past medical history may supply important information for diagnosis. For example, patients presenting outside of infancy generally do not have a cardiac cause for cyanosis without a known history of cardiac disease or illness predisposing them to cardiac disease.

G. Pertinent Historical Information
  1. Is there a relevant family history?
  2. Any recent illnesses or surgeries?
  3. What is the possibility of exposures or ingestions?

III. Differential Diagnosis. Cyanosis refers to the bluish skin color attributable most often to the presence of desaturated hemoglobin (5 g/dL). Primary etiologies include respiratory, cardiac, circulatory, and nervous system disorders, as well as abnormal hemoglobin.

A. Respiratory Diseases
  1. Lung disease
    a. Newborn. Lung hypoplasia (diaphragmatic hernia), respiratory distress syndrome, transient tachypnea of the newborn, bronchopulmonary dysplasia, pulmonary interstitial emphysema, congenital adenomatoid malformation, meconium aspiration.
    b. Infectious. Pneumonia, pneumonitis, bronchiolitis.
    c. Asthma.
    d. Cystic fibrosis.
    e. Infiltrative disease. Pulmonary hemosiderosis, sarcoidosis.
  2. Airway abnormalities or obstruction
    a. Congenital. Choanal atresia, macroglossia, micrognathia (Pierre Robin sequence), laryngeal web, tracheal stenosis, vascular ring, tracheoesophageal fistula.
    b. Infectious. Acute epiglottitis, croup, retropharyngeal abscess, laryngospasm.
    c. Traumatic. Vocal cord injury, pneumothorax, pneumomediastinum.
    d. Other. Lymphoma, cystic hygroma, goiter, laryngeal hemangioma or neoplasm, foreign body, obesity.
  3. Trauma. Pneumothorax, pneumomediastinum, vocal cord injury.

B. Pulmonary Vascular Diseases
  1. Primary pulmonary hypertension. Cyanosis requires a right-to-left shunt at the atrial or ductal level unless lung disease is present.
  2. Pulmonary arteriovenous malformation. Idiopathic or associated with congenital heart, hepatic, or portal disease.

C. Cardiac Diseases
  1. Cyanotic congenital heart disease

        a. As a mnemonic, remember the **6 T's: T**ransposition of the great arteries (most common neonatal cyanotic congenital heart defect), hypoplastic left heart syndrome (**T**richamber), **T**etralogy of Fallot (most common cyanotic congenital heart defect in children), **T**runcus arteriosus, **T**ricuspid atresia, **T**otal anomalous pulmonary venous connection.

        b. Atrioventricular canal defect, Ebstein malformation of the tricuspid valve, critical pulmonary stenosis, pulmonary atresia, Eisenmenger syndrome.

    2. Persistent pulmonary hypertension of the newborn.

    3. Severe congestive heart failure. As a result of congenital heart disease or acquired heart disease, sustained tachycardia or bradycardia, or infection (myocarditis).

D. Circulatory Disorders. Cyanosis is the result of increased venous desaturation due to increased extraction of oxygen in peripheral tissues from diminished supply of blood to (hypoperfusion) or venous blood return from (venous stasis) those tissues.

    1. Shock.

    2. Sepsis.

    3. Hypoglycemia.

    4. Cardiomyopathy.

    5. Vena cava obstruction. Inferior or superior obstruction as a result of cardiac or hepatic disease.

    6. Hypotension. May be associated with autonomic dysfunction or vasovagal syncope.

    7. Peripheral cyanosis. Acrocyanosis related to cold exposure, Raynaud disease.

E. Neurologic Problems

    1. Apnea. Prematurity, cerebral anomalies, intracranial hemorrhage, meningitis or encephalitis.

    2. Breath-holding spells.

    3. Respiratory muscle weakness (neuromuscular). Myotonic or muscular dystrophy, Guillain-Barré syndrome, Werdnig-Hoffman disease, myasthenia gravis, infant botulism.

    4. Seizures.

F. Hemoglobin Abnormalities

    1. Methemoglobinemia. Familial, nitrate exposure, aniline dye ingestion.

    2. Low-oxygen-affinity hemoglobin.

    3. Polycythemia or hyperviscosity syndrome.

IV. Database

A. Physical Exam Key Points

    1. Extent of cyanosis. Constant or intermittent? Peripheral or central? Is differential cyanosis present?

    2. Airway and breathing. Is patient apneic? Any airway noises audible? Is patient breathing comfortably or with increased effort? Is there weakness or asymmetry to chest movement?

Is patient able to speak or cry? What is the character of speech or crying?

3. **Lungs.** Listen for symmetry of breath sounds and quality of air movement. Any abnormal lungs sounds (eg, wheezing)?
4. **Heart.** Assess heart rate and BP. Listen to heart sounds and examine for murmur, gallop, or rub.
5. **Pulses.** Simultaneously assess pulses for quality in upper and lower extremities. Use right arm and either femoral area. Left arm may be distal to an aortic coarctation and misleading in the assessment. Evaluate for equality of pulsation and presence of femoral delay.
6. **Abdomen.** Assess for liver size, presence of ascites, or spider veins across the abdomen (indicators of congestive heart failure or liver disease).
7. **Neurologic exam.** Assess muscular tone and symmetry of movement. Is there gross seizure activity? Check pupil size and symmetry. Assess for sunset sign.

B. Laboratory Data

1. **ABGs on room air.** Significant hypoxemia suggests cardiac or pulmonary etiology. Relatively normal PaO_2 suggests other causes (eg, methemoglobinemia, neurologic disorder, polycythemia). If cardiac cause is suspected, check response to 100% oxygen (hyperoxia test).
2. **Hyperoxia test.** Administer 100% oxygen to patient for 10–15 minutes, then obtain ABGs and compare to values previously obtained on room air.
   a. In patients with cardiac disease, PaO_2 will change little with 100% oxygen. PaO_2 will remain < 125 mm Hg in cardiac disease.
   b. Patients with pulmonary disease will respond to 100% oxygen with an increase in PaO_2 to > 150 mm Hg.
   c. In those with severe pulmonary disease or persistent pulmonary hypertension, PaO_2 may not increase significantly.
3. **CBC with differential.** May demonstrate polycythemia (hematocrit > 65%), anemia, or evidence of infection.
4. **Glucose.**
5. **Cultures.** Obtain if infection is suspected.
6. **Methemoglobin level.** When exposed to air, a drop of arterial blood has a chocolate-brown color. Patient with methemoglobin level > 40% deserves treatment, as does patient with neurologic changes or chest pain.

C. Radiographic and Other Studies

1. **Chest x-ray.** Examine for abnormal cardiac size (decreased in hypovolemic shock; increased in cardiac shock), presence or absence of pulmonary vasculature (increased or decreased blood flow to lungs), signs of interstitial lung disease, evidence of mediastinal mass, pneumothorax, foreign body ingestion, or bony abnormalities.

     2. ECG. Abnormalities suggest presence of cardiac disease or abnormal cardiac rhythm.

     3. Echocardiogram. Use to confirm cardiac disease when suspected or determine presence of cardiac disease in cases less certain.

     4. Imaging studies of head. Consider CT scan, MRI scan, or ultrasonography of the head if neurologic disease is suspected.

V. Plan

A. Initial Management

1. Assess and maintain airway, breathing, and circulation (ABCs). Tracheal intubation and mechanical ventilation may be necessary, as might inotropic support. Investigate airway if foreign body aspiration is suspected.

2. Perform appropriate testing rapidly. Select studies that will give the most diagnostic information in the shortest amount of time. In some situations, an echocardiogram may be obtained more quickly than the hyperoxia test.

B. Prostaglandin Therapy.
Cyanotic heart disease in a newborn is likely to be dependent on the ductus arteriosus for pulmonary or systemic blood flow. In a severely ill infant, prostaglandin E_1 infusion (0.01–0.05 mcg/kg/min initially) should be started until diagnosis can be confirmed by echocardiogram. Lower infusion rates may avoid prostaglandin-induced apnea.

C. Treatment of Underlying Cause of Cyanosis.
After diagnosis is determined, treat emergently as necessary or obtain specialist consultation.

D. Specific Therapies

1. **Methemoglobinemia.** Infuse 1–2 mg/kg of methylene blue as a 1% solution in normal saline over 5 minutes.

2. **Tet spell.** In an infant with known or suspected tetralogy of Fallot, hypercyanotic episodes (tet spells) should be managed by increasing preload and systemic vascular resistance to overcome right ventricular outflow obstruction and increase pulmonary blood flow. Treatment typically consists of IV fluid bolus, knee-to-chest positioning, and oxygen (may or may not be useful). In addition, sodium bicarbonate (0.5–1.0 mEq/kg IV) should be administered for metabolic acidosis and morphine sulfate (0.05–0.1 mg/kg IV or SQ) for sedation. Phenylephrine (5–10 mcg/kg) can be administered IV to increase systemic vascular resistance and increase pulmonary blood flow.

VI. Problem Case Diagnosis.
Results of the hyperoxia test in the 1-week-old infant suggested a diagnosis of cyanotic congenital heart disease, which became symptomatic after PDA closed. Prostaglandin E was infused to reopen the ductus. An echocardiogram confirmed transposition of the great arteries.

VII. Teaching Pearl: Question. Why is cyanosis not apparent in a new-born at the same arterial oxygen saturation that causes cyanosis in a 1-year-old child?

VIII. Teaching Pearl: Answer. Fetal hemoglobin has a higher affinity for oxygen than does hemoglobin A.

REFERENCES

Grifka RG. Cyanotic congenital heart disease with increased pulmonary blood flow. *Pediatr Clin North Am* 1999;46:405–425.

Tingelstrad J. Consultations with the specialist: Nonrespiratory cyanosis. *Pediatr Rev* 1999;20:350–352.

Waldman JD, Wernly JA. Cyanotic congenital heart disease with decreased pulmonary blood flow in children. *Pediatr Clin North Am* 1999;46:385–404.

Zorx JJ, Kanic Z. A cyanotic infant: True blue or otherwise? *Pediatr Ann* 2001;30:597–601.

21. DIARRHEA

I. Problem. A 9-month-old boy has a 2-day history of watery diarrhea, vomiting, and decreased urine output. He is afebrile but irritable, with sunken eyes, thick tenacious saliva, and poor skin turgor.

II. Immediate Questions

A. How old is patient? In a young infant, the intestinal mucosa tends to be more permeable to water than in an older child or adult. This can result in greater net fluid and electrolyte losses. Diarrhea in the first few months of life requires more immediate attention.

B. What are the vital signs? Tachycardia suggests volume depletion. Hypotension suggests hypovolemic or septic shock. Fever implies an infectious etiology. Diarrhea with associated tachycardia, hypotension, or fever should be evaluated immediately.

C. Is diarrhea grossly bloody? Bloody diarrhea is seen with invasive bacterial infections, ischemic bowel or infarction, allergic phenomenon or inflammatory bowel disease (IBD). It requires more active and immediate intervention.

D. Is this an acute or chronic problem?

1. Acute diarrhea. Usually a self-limited disease, which can often be treated symptomatically. The most common cause is infection. Other common causes include drugs (eg, antibiotics) as well as excessive intake of high-carbohydrate fluids or non-absorbable fillers (eg, sorbitol).

2. Chronic diarrhea. Defined as diarrhea that lasts longer than 4 weeks. Common causes include chronic, nonspecific diarrhea (toddler's diarrhea), lactose intolerance, milk-protein allergy, encopresis, irritable bowel syndrome, various infections, drugs, and IBD. It can present with an acute exacerbation.

E. **Are there risk factors that suggest a specific cause?** Risk factors include day care, winter season, ill contacts, drugs, travel, animal exposure, constipation, excessive juice intake, poorly prepared or stored poultry or salads, untreated water sources, prior abdominal surgery, immunodeficiency, and prematurity.

F. **Is there associated vomiting?** Small bowel processes, most commonly associated with viral agents, cause delayed gastric emptying and luminal distention, often leading to vomiting before the onset of diarrhea. Vomiting increases risk of significant dehydration.

G. **Associated abdominal pain?** Absence of pain makes inflammatory causes such as ulcerative colitis less likely. Malabsorption presents with diarrhea, abdominal pain, flatulence, and greasy stools without concurrent fever.

H. **What is the volume of stool?** Small bowel conditions tend to produce large-volume, watery stools that are relatively infrequent. Conversely, large bowel involvement, usually due to a bacterial-induced inflammatory process, tends to produce frequent, less watery stools.

I. **Has patient participated in any recreational water activities?** Infectious causes have been associated with recreational water activities (eg, swimming pools, water parks, lakes, rivers, hot tubs); includes *Shigella sonnei* and *Cryptosporidium parvum*.

J. **Is there a reason to suspect laxative abuse (eg, adolescent girl with history of bulimia)?** Testing stool for laxatives may secure the diagnosis without an extensive workup.

III. **Differential Diagnosis**
   A. **Infection**
      1. **Viral.** Usually resolves in a few days and can be treated symptomatically. Rotavirus, adenovirus, and Norwalk virus are more common.
      2. **Bacterial.** *Shigella dysenteriae, S sonnei, Salmonella* spp, *Campylobacter jejuni, Yersinia* spp, and enterohemorrhagic *Escherichia coli* cause diarrhea by enteroinvasion. *Staphylococcus aureus, E coli, Vibrio cholerae, Vibrio parahaemolyticus, Clostridium perfringens, Clostridium difficile,* and some *Shigella* species cause diarrhea by producing enterotoxins. Spectrum of illness may range from asymptomatic to life threatening. *S aureus* and *C perfringens* are often associated with food poisoning. Enterohemorrhagic *E coli* causes bloody diarrhea and may be associated with hemolytic uremic syndrome.
      3. **Parasitic.** *Giardia lamblia* is often contracted by drinking contaminated water and can cause abdominal distention, diarrhea and, at times, failure to thrive. *Giardia* is easily passed by the fecal-oral route and is particularly troublesome in day-care centers and

schools. *Entamoeba histolytica* produces severe colitis; however, it is generally acquired only by travel to developing countries. *Cryptosporidium* can cause a self-limited diarrhea in
immunocompetent individuals or severe, unremitting diarrhea
in patients with an immune deficiency.

B. Postinfectious State. Several viruses can cause severe enteritis
resulting in prolonged intestinal mucosal damage, acquired carbohydrate intolerance, and malabsorption in infants. Patients
present initially with fever and diarrhea, followed by intractable
watery diarrhea that may resolve in as short a time as 2 weeks or
last as long as several months.

C. Drugs
  1. **Antibiotics.** Can alter bowel flora and cause loose, watery
     stools. Broad-spectrum antibiotics (eg, clindamycin and some
     cephalosporins) can lead to induction of *C difficile* overgrowth
     and toxin production, resulting in pseudomembranous colitis,
     which can occur as long as 4 months after antibiotic use.
  2. **Laxatives.**
  3. **Antacids.** Magnesium-containing antacids can cause osmotic
     diarrhea.
  4. **Cholinergic agents.** Metoclopramide and bethanechol are
     frequently used in children with gastroesophageal reflux dis-
     ease and may cause significant diarrhea.
  5. **Chemotherapy.** Mucositis and enteritis can follow radiation
     and chemotherapy.

D. Diet
  1. **Overfeeding.**
  2. **Adverse response to an ingested food or food additive.**
     Common offenders include cabbage, chocolate, peppers, soy-
     beans, chickpeas, carrots, licorice, spinach, celery, fava beans,
     rhubarb, mushrooms, turnips, radishes, monosodium gluta-
     mate, nitrates or nitrites, sulfites, and parabens.
  3. **Excessive intake of high-carbohydrate fluids or nonab-
     sorbable fillers (eg, sorbitol).**
  4. **Malnutrition.**

E. Chronic Nonspecific Diarrhea (Toddler's Diarrhea). Typically
occurs in children aged 1–3 years. Children appear healthy and
continue to grow and develop normally. Excessive fluid intake
and an unbalanced diet that consists mostly of low-residue, high-
carbohydrate, and low-fat foods may play a role.

F. Lactose Intolerance. Frequent cause of chronic diarrhea in
pediatric patients. Often associated with bloating and flatulence.
Milk or milk products exacerbate the diarrhea. Congenital lactase
deficiency is an autosomal-recessive disorder that presents in
infancy and is extremely rare. Late-onset lactose intolerance is
due to a progressive loss of enzyme activity in the brush border

of the small bowel mucosa; this can begin as early as 5 or 6 years of age in some ethnic groups. Acquired lactose intolerance occurs after any illness that causes damage to the small bowel mucosa.

G. Encopresis or Fecal Impaction. In the toddler or older child, encopresis often presents as diarrhea and is almost always caused by severe constipation. Any apparently healthy child who has a history of uncontrollable diarrhea should be evaluated for constipation or encopresis.

H. Inflammatory Diseases

1. **IBD.** Presentation of IBD (Crohn disease and ulcerative colitis) is quite variable and depends on the site and severity of inflamed bowel and chronicity of the disease. Most commonly, children present with growth failure, diarrhea, abdominal pain, mucous or bloody stools, or weight loss.

2. **Milk-protein allergy.** Milk-protein allergy is a pathologic immune reaction induced by milk-protein antigens. Up to 50% of children with milk-protein allergy can have a concomitant soy-protein allergy. Usually present with heme-positive or bloody diarrhea and poor growth.

3. **Necrotizing enterocolitis.** Occurs almost exclusively in premature infants.

I. Malabsorption

1. **Pancreatic dysfunction.** Leads to fat malabsorption and steatorrhea, with large, greasy, foul-smelling stools; growth failure; and deficiencies of fat-soluble vitamins. Causes include cystic fibrosis, Schwachman syndrome, and chronic pancreatitis.

2. **Bacterial overgrowth.** Consider in postsurgical patients. Leads to bile salt deconjugation, which typically promotes watery diarrhea.

3. **Celiac disease.** Allergic response to gluten, characterized by proximal small bowel mucosal damage and subsequent malabsorption. Can occur at any time after gluten is introduced into the diet, from about 6 months to adulthood. Symptoms include diarrhea, abdominal distention and discomfort, lactose intolerance, poor growth, vitamin deficiencies, and iron-deficiency anemia.

4. **Eosinophilic gastroenteritis.** Typically presents with signs and symptoms of malabsorption, hypoalbuminemia, and anemia.

J. Irritable Bowel Syndrome. Intermittent diarrhea may alternate with constipation. Abdominal pain and flatulence may be present. Symptoms are aggravated by stress. Physical exam and routine laboratory tests are normal.

K. Anatomic Abnormalities. Short-bowel syndrome or intestinal lymphangiectasia.

    L. Endocrine Disorders. Hyperthyroidism, diabetes, or Addison disease.

    M. Immunodeficiency. HIV infection, isolated IgA deficiency, combined immune deficiency.

    N. Tumor. Familial polyposis coli, functional tumors (eg, VIPoma, somatostatinoma, gastrinoma), or lymphoma involving the bowel.

    O. Inborn Metabolic Errors. Familial chloride diarrhea, Wolman disease, abetalipoproteinemia, or hypobetalipoproteinemia.

IV. Database

A. Physical Exam Key Points

1. **General appearance.** Child's mental status as evident during interaction with clinician and parents can be used as a measure of the seriousness of illness and dehydration. All children should be weighed unclothed for comparison with previous weights and to provide a baseline for monitoring subsequent weights.

2. **Vital signs.** Elevated temperature increases insensible water losses and may lead to more rapid dehydration. Decreased BP, elevated pulse, or decreased peripheral perfusion may indicate intravascular volume depletion due to dehydration or sepsis. Tachypnea may indicate fever, anxiety, pain, sepsis, or compensation for metabolic acidosis.

3. **HEENT.** Assess anterior fontanelle and eyes for sunken presentation. Evaluate mucous membranes (more than the lips) for moistness. Aphthous ulcers are associated with IBD.

4. **Abdomen.** Distended abdomen may be associated with an ileus, as seen in enteritis or gaseous dilation due to malabsorption. Auscultation may reveal high-pitched sounds of peristaltic rushes found in enteritic and secretory diarrheas. Dysenteric diarrheas tend to be associated with a quieter abdomen. Carefully assess signs of peritonitis, which may cause diarrhea due to inflammation and local enteric irritation.

5. **Rectum.** Look for fissures (seen with fecal impaction) and skin tags (suggesting IBD).

6. **Musculoskeletal system.** Arthritis is associated with IBD and infection by *Yersinia enterocolitica*.

7. **Skin.** Skin turgor may give a sense of the degree of dehydration. Doughy, tented skin suggests hypernatremic dehydration. Hyperpigmentation can be seen in Addison disease. Erythema nodosum and pyoderma gangrenosum point to IBD.

B. Laboratory Data

1. **Serum electrolytes.** Assess, particularly Na^+ and bicarbonate, in any child considered significantly dehydrated. Knowing the serum Na^+ concentration is crucial when determining composition of the fluids and rate of rehydration to be used in a child who is dehydrated.

    2. **CBC with differential.** Anemia may be associated with IBD, hemolytic uremic syndrome, malabsorption, tumor, or HIV infection.

    3. **ESR, C-reactive protein.** Elevated in IBD and systemic infections.

    4. **Stool analysis**
        a. **Occult blood.** Suggests inflammation, ischemia, tumor, or various infections.
        b. **Leukocytes.** Fecal leukocytes have a high positive predictive value for bacterial diarrhea.
        c. **Cultures.** Indicated if history (eg, blood, travel) or stool exam (> 5 fecal leukocytes per high power field) strongly suggest a bacterial cause or if diarrhea is prolonged.
        d. **Ova and parasites (O&P).** Fresh stool for O&P should be examined, especially when *G lamblia* or *Cryptosporidium* is suspected (eg, day-care setting).
        e. **pH and reducing substances.** Presence of reducing substances and a low pH are indicative of malabsorption.

    5. **Rapid antigen tests.** Enzyme-linked immunoassays for rotavirus (Rotazyme) and *Giardia* can be done on appropriate stool samples if clinically indicated.

    6. ***C difficile* toxin.** Indicated if diarrhea is prolonged or severe and antibiotics have been given in the past 4 months (usually 4–14 days); decreased specificity in young infants

    7. **Fecal fat.** Twenty-four– to 72-hour collection of stool for fecal fat is essential for workup of fat malabsorption.

C. Radiographic and Other Studies
    1. **Proctosigmoidoscopy or colonoscopy.** Indicated if patient remains ill with negative stool cultures. Useful in determining presence of mucosal inflammation (suggesting IBD), obtaining biopsies, and examining for masses.

    2. **Upper GI series with small bowel follow-through.** May suggest Crohn disease, celiac disease, or lymphoma.

    3. **Breath hydrogen lactose tolerance test.** Increase in breath hydrogen approximately 2 hours after administration of a standard oral lactose dose indicates lactose intolerance.

    4. **D-xylose test.** Abnormal in diseases involving small bowel mucosa (eg, Crohn disease, celiac disease, small bowel bacterial overgrowth, and regional enteritis). Reserve for workup of chronic or recurring diarrhea.

V. Plan
  A. General Management. Dehydration is most common complication of acute diarrhea. Initial treatment should focus on correcting dehydration and any associated electrolyte disturbances. Antidiarrheal agents in the pediatric population, particularly in younger patients, should be used with caution and are not

indicated in most acute diarrheal episodes. Antibiotic therapy should be avoided and implemented only in specific situations, guided by stool culture results. Many causes of diarrhea resolve by addressing the underlying cause (eg, discontinuation of a drug).

B. Fluid Replacement. Management of dehydration due to diarrhea requires initial rapid rehydration, replacement of ongoing losses, and provision of maintenance fluid during recovery.

   1. Intravenous. Indicated if patient is markedly volume depleted or has accompanying nausea and vomiting. First stage consists of rapid infusion of isotonic saline to expand intravascular volume (eg, 20 mL/kg over 20–60 minutes). Subsequent IV hydration is a combination of replacement of estimated fluid deficit added to regular maintenance needs. This should occur over 24 hours unless child has hypernatremic dehydration, in which case rehydration should occur over 48 hours.

   2. Oral. Indicated for patients who are mildly to moderately dehydrated. Ideal oral hydration solutions are high in Na^+ (40–90 mEq/L) with appropriate concentrations of glucose (~2%) to facilitate uptake of Na^+ and water without causing osmotic diuresis. Initial fluid resuscitation consists of administration of oral hydration solution in a volume equal to estimated fluid deficit (usually 50–100 mL/kg) given over ~4 hours. This is followed by continual administration of oral hydration solution in volumes calculated to satisfy maintenance requirements and ongoing losses. Patients who present with vomiting as well as diarrhea should be given small, frequent sips of oral hydration solution. Despite vomiting, more than 90% of infants will tolerate oral rehydration given in a gradual manner.

C. Diet. Early refeeding is recommended in managing acute gastroenteritis because luminal contents are a known growth factor for enterocytes and help facilitate mucosal repair following injury. Introducing a regular diet within a few hours of rehydration or continuing the diet during diarrhea without dehydration has been shown to shorten duration of disease. Infants and children with more severe diarrhea may require lactose restriction to prevent exacerbating the diarrhea because of transient lactase deficiency resulting from acute gastroenteritis. Avoid heavily sweetened juices and encourage intake of complex carbohydrates such as rice and potatoes.

D. Antimicrobial Therapy

   1. *Salmonella*. Antibiotic treatment is associated with prolonged excretion of the organism and does not appear to change the natural course of the disease. Antibiotics are indicated only for ill-appearing children, patients at risk of *Salmonella* bacteremia (including young infants and immunocompromised patients), and secondary infections (eg, osteomyelitis, meningitis).

Antibiotic sensitivity is crucial because resistance is common. Treatment is ampicillin, trimethoprim-sulfamethoxazole (TMP-SMX), or a third-generation cephalosporin.

2. **Shigella.** Antibiotics are recommended to decrease duration of illness and fecal shedding. Antibiotic sensitivity is crucial because resistance is common. Treatment is TMP-SMX or ciprofloxacin.

3. **Campylobacter.** Most cases are self-limited and do not require antibiotic therapy. More severe cases can be treated with erythromycin or ciprofloxacin. Treatment generally improves clinical course of disease.

4. **Yersinia.** Most cases are self-limited. Antibiotics are of questionable value because no clear relationship exists between antibiotic administration and clinical improvement.

5. **E coli.** Most illnesses caused by these organisms are acute and self-limited and do not require antibiotic therapy.

6. **C difficile.** Often associated with previous or ongoing antibiotic treatment; therefore, discontinue offending antibiotic. Documented enterocolitis is treated with oral or IV metronidazole or oral vancomycin.

7. **G lamblia.** Metronidazole is drug of choice for treating symptomatic giardiasis. Furazolidone is an alternative that is supplied in a liquid form.

E. **Other Specific Therapies**

1. **Postinfectious gastroenteritis.** Elemental formulas (ie, lactose-free with hydrolyzed amino acids and medium-chain triglycerides) usually improve absorption across damaged intestinal epithelium. Severe cases may require continuous nasogastric feeding or TPN.

2. **Chronic, nonspecific diarrhea.** Often responds to high-fat diet and reduction in clear fluid intake.

3. **Lactose intolerance.** Dietary exclusion of lactose-containing foods. In infants, a lactose-free formula can be used temporarily during acute illness. In older children, use of LactAid tablets and products can be used on a more permanent basis.

4. **Encopresis.** Therapy relies on initial, aggressive bowel cleansing using enemas, followed by long-term maintenance therapy with stool softeners or laxatives (see Chapter 18, Constipation, p. 91).

5. **Milk-protein allergy.** Because of the high cross-reactivity between milk and soy protein, switching to a soy formula is usually ineffective. Most patients respond to an elemental formula (ie, protein hydrolysate formula) and should be maintained on this for 1 year before performing a challenge. Prognosis is excellent, with most infants tolerating milk-containing products by 1–2 years of age.

6. **Irritable bowel syndrome.** Therapy consists of high-fiber diet, fiber supplements, antispasmodic agents, and behavioral modification (eg, relaxation techniques).
7. **IBD.** Treatment depends on location and severity of the inflamed bowel and should be determined by a pediatric gastroenterologist.
8. **Celiac disease, fat malabsorption, and pancreatic disorders.** If suspected, referral to a pediatric gastroenterologist is indicated.

VI. **Problem Case Diagnosis.** The 9-month-old boy had acute viral gastroenteritis complicated by dehydration. Physical exam was unremarkable except for dry mucous membranes, absence of tears, and poor skin turgor. He responded well to two boluses of IV fluids before tolerating adequate oral fluids.

VII. **Teaching Pearl: Question.** What clinical and simple laboratory findings are useful in differentiating between viral and bacterial enteritis?

VIII. **Teaching Pearl: Answer.** Vomiting before the onset of diarrhea and large, watery, and relatively infrequent stools suggest viral gastroenteritis. Fever, abdominal pain, and frequent, small-volume, and often bloody stools containing mucus and leukocytes are more commonly seen in bacterial enteritis.

REFERENCES

Baldassano RN, Liacouras CA. Chronic diarrhea: A practical approach for the pediatrician. *Pediatr Clin North Am* 1991;38:667–686.
Berman J. Heading off the dangers of acute gastroenteritis. *Contemp Pediatr* 2003;20:57–74.
Reis EC, Goepp JG, Katz S, Santosham M. Barriers to the use of oral rehydration therapy. *Pediatrics* 1994;93:708–711.

22. DYSURIA

I. **Problem.** A mother tells the pediatrician that her 4-year-old daughter has pain with urination.

II. **Immediate Questions**
   A. **When did painful urination begin?** Trauma to the urinary tract must be ruled out if pain develops after an injury. Bicycle and straddle injuries commonly cause damage to the kidneys or urethra, leading to hematuria or dysuria, or both. Consider behavioral problems, including attention seeking, if symptoms occur only at a particular time of day (ie, during school).
   B. **Where is the pain located? In the urethra? In the pelvis or abdomen? Is there back pain?** Pain originating from another organ system may be referred to the urethra. An intra-abdominal abscess or a low-lying inflamed appendix may produce complaints

of dysuria. Dysuria associated with back pain is a common presentation of pyelonephritis. Renal stones in the pelvis, calyx, or ureter can cause abdominal or flank pain with radiation into the scrotum or vulva. Stones in the urethra or distal ureter cause dysuria. Stones in the bladder are not associated with pain.

C. Are there associated complaints (eg, fever, drainage or discharge between urinations, abnormal urine odor or color, or changes in volume or frequency of urination)? Fever, dark and foul-smelling urine, frequency, and urgency are all symptoms associated with UTIs. If patient is sexually active and experiencing discharge or dyspareunia, consider STDs (eg, gonorrhea, chlamydia).

D. What is the quality and strength of the urinary stream? Patients with obstructive processes (eg, posterior urethral valves) have small, frequent voidings. Patients with urethral strictures or meatal stenosis have a decrease in the force of their urine stream.

E. Has there been any bleeding? Bleeding may be present after trauma or associated with infection or congenital anomalies. Excess calcium excretion and renal stones cause dysuria as well as hematuria.

F. What medication(s) does patient take? Some medications (eg, cyclophosphamide) may cause irritation to the urethra and painful urination.

G. Has there been any change in brand of soap, detergent, or fabric softener? Does patient take showers or baths? Certain soaps or cleansers can be associated with urethral irritation and pruritus. Bubble baths, for example, remove protective lipids from the urethra, causing irritation.

III. Differential Diagnosis

A. UTI. Cystitis is a bacterial infection of the bladder; pyelonephritis is an infection of the kidneys (see Chapter 91, Urinary Tract Infection, p. 424).

B. Urethritis. Predominantly an infection of sexually active individuals, usually observed in boys. Signs and symptoms include painful or burning urination and discharge from the urethral meatus. Causes may be gonococcal (*Neisseria gonorrhea*) and nongonococcal urethritis (NGU), which is now more frequent in the United States. NGU may be due to *Chlamydia trachomatis, Ureaplasma urealyticum,* and, less commonly, *Trichomonas vaginalis* or herpesvirus infection.

C. Vaginitis or Vulvitis

1. Group A streptococci. Common cause of vaginitis in prepubertal girls. Presents with serous discharge, marked erythema and irritation of the vulvar area, and discomfort on walking and urination.

2. *Candida*. Can also cause vaginitis but typically causes intense pruritus. Labia may be pale or erythematous with satellite lesions. Vaginal discharge, if present, is usually thick and adherent, with white curds.

3. **Other causes.** In sexually active adolescents, the most common causes include bacterial vaginosis ("fishy," foul-smelling discharge), candidal vulvovaginitis (white, "cottage-cheese"–appearing discharge), and trichomoniasis (malodorous yellow, frothy discharge).

D. **Contact or Candidal Dermatitis.** Frequently seen in infants wearing diapers because the diaper area is warm, often moist, and frequently contaminated by feces laden with organisms. Failure to change diapers frequently is a major predisposing factor. Harsh soaps, irritating chemicals, and detergents contribute to the process.

1. **Irritant or contact dermatitis.** Usually confined to convex surfaces of the perineum, lower abdomen, buttocks, and proximal thighs; spares the intertriginous areas.

2. **Candidal dermatitis.** Appears as a bright red eruption, with sharp borders and pinpoint satellite papules and pustules; tends to involve the intertriginous areas.

E. **Urethral Stricture and Meatal Stenosis.** Usually result from urethral trauma, either iatrogenic (catheterization or endoscopic procedures) or accidental (straddle injuries). Symptoms include decrease in force of the urine, bladder instability, hematuria, and dysuria.

F. **Urinary Lithiasis.** Most children with renal stones have an underlying metabolic abnormality. Exceptions include those with a neuropathic bladder and those who have urinary tract reconstruction with intestine. Pain from stones varies depending on location (see II, B, earlier).

G. **Posterior Urethral Valves.** Most common cause of bladder outlet obstruction in boys. In the presence of a persistent valve, the prostatic urethra becomes dilated, vesicoureteral reflux may be present, and a small bladder with hypertrophied walls develops. Infants may present with poor voiding stream, bilateral flank masses, or UTI and dysuria.

IV. **Database**

A. **Physical Exam Key Points**

1. **Vital signs.** Evaluate for fever, tachycardia, or hypotension, which suggest upper tract involvement and, in the case of hypotension, urosepsis.

2. **Abdomen and back.** Examine for abdominal or flank masses, suprapubic tenderness, or costovertebral angle tenderness.

3. **Genitalia.** Inspect skin and perineum for evidence of rashes, redness, or irritation. Look for evidence of discharge. Perform pelvic exam in sexually active adolescent girls who present with dysuria and discharge to rule out vaginitis, cervicitis, and pelvic inflammatory disease.

B. **Laboratory Data**
   1. **Urinalysis, urine culture.** Obtain both studies if UTI is suspected (see Chapter 91, Urinary Tract Infection, p. 425). Presence of leukocytes, leukocyte esterase, nitrites, erythrocytes, or bacteria on urinalysis is highly indicative of UTI. Erythrocytes alone can be seen with renal calculi. Bacteria or yeast alone may be detected in urine specimens due contamination by normal flora of vagina and urethra.
   2. **CBC with differential and blood culture.** Order in all patients who are ill-appearing and are admitted (see also Chapter 91, Urinary Tract Infection, p. 426).
   3. **Urethral discharge.** Obtain Gram stain and culture on Thayer-Martin medium. Presence of intracellular, gram-negative diplococci on Gram stain requires empiric treatment for gonorrhea. Always evaluate for the possibility of coinfection with *Chlamydia.* Giemsa stain will show cytoplasmic inclusion within epithelial cells if infection is present. Alternatively, discharges can be sent for DNA probe for *C trachomatis* and *Gonococcus.*
   4. **Urine test for *N gonorrhea* and *Chlamydia.*** Less-invasive method of diagnosing these organisms. Involves a ligase chain reaction. Test looks for the presence of both organisms and amplifies their DNA if present.
   5. **Vaginal discharge.** Use wet mount to look for *T vaginalis,* which has flagella and moves rapidly and erratically. Clue cells (activated squamous cells coated with bacteria) indicate bacterial vaginosis. Presence of hyphae indicates infection with *C albicans.*

C. **Radiographic and Other Studies**
   1. **Ultrasound and voiding cystourethrogram.** See Chapter 91, Urinary Tract Infection, p. 427. Order ultrasound if congenital anomaly is suspected. Voiding film obtained during IV urography or retrograde urethrography is diagnostic of urethral strictures or stenosis. Diagnosis of posterior urethral valves is made by a voiding cystourethrogram.
   2. **X-ray of abdomen and pelvis.** May diagnose renal calculi. Approximately 90% of stones are calcified, and diagnosis can be made by plain abdominal film alone.
   3. **CT scan of abdomen and pelvis.** Stones that are small or radiolucent are often seen using a nonenhanced spiral CT scan of the abdomen and pelvis.

V. **Plan**
   A. **UTI or Pyelonephritis.** See Chapter 91, Urinary Tract Infection, p. 427.
   B. **Urethritis**
      1. **Chlamydial urethritis.** Suspect when dysuria, pyuria, but no bacteriuria, is present. Treatment with azithromycin, 1 g in a single dose, or doxycycline, 100 mg twice daily for 7 days, is

effective. Alternative treatments: erythromycin, 500 mg 4 times daily for 7 days, or ofloxacin, 300 mg twice daily for 7 days. Patient's sexual partner should also be evaluated and treated. Doxycycline should *not* be used in children younger than 9 years of age. Ofloxacin should be used *with caution* in those younger than 18.

   2. Gonococcal urethritis. With the emergence of penicillin resistance, cefixime, 400 mg in a single dose, or ceftriaxone, 125 mg IM in a single dose, should be given. Alternative treatments: ciprofloxacin, 500 mg, or ofloxacin, 400 mg, in single doses. Because of frequent coexistence of chlamydial urethritis, appropriate antichlamydial treatment should also be given (see preceding paragraph). Patient's sexual partner should also be evaluated and treated. Use ciprofloxacin and ofloxacin *with caution* in children younger than 18 years.

C. Vaginitis. Therapy is directed at specific cause.

   1. Bacterial vaginitis (group A streptococci). Treatment consists of topical antibiotic ointment (mupirocin).

   2. Candidal vaginitis. Topical antifungal (miconazole, butoconazole, or clotrimazole) for 3–7 days. Alternative treatment for older adolescent: 150-mg single oral dose of fluconazole.

   3. Bacterial vaginosis or trichomonal vaginitis. Metronidazole, 2 g as a single dose, is effective.

   4. Atrophic vaginitis or labial adhesions. Topical Premarin cream is effective. It should be applied daily for 1 week, then 2–3 times per week thereafter.

D. Dermatitis. Management is tailored to the cause.

   1. Contact dermatitis. Frequent diaper changes; gentle, thorough cleansing of area; and application of lubricants and barrier pastes is usually all that is needed. Occasionally a short course of low-potency steroids hastens resolution.

   2. Candidal dermatitis. Most cases respond well to topical antifungal therapy and worsen with steroids.

E. Urethral Strictures and Meatal Stenosis. Treatment involves dilation if mild stenosis; urethroplasty if stenosis is more severe.

F. Urinary Stones. Treatment depends on size and type of stone and ranges from fluid hydration (to help pass the stone) to lithotripsy with or without extracorporeal shock, to surgical removal. In children with urolithiasis, treatment of the underlying metabolic disorder should be addressed.

G. Posterior Urethral Valves. Treatment consists of surgical valve ablation.

VI. Problem Case Diagnosis. The 4-year-old patient had complained of pain with urination for 3 days. Her urine was reportedly of normal color and smell, and she had neither frequency nor urgency. Review of systems was negative for fever or symptoms of upper respiratory infection, but significant for pruritus in the perineum. Physical exam showed a well-appearing girl in no acute distress. There was no back pain and no abdominal tenderness. Significant erythema of the labia minora and vulva was noted. There was no appreciable discharge. Urinalysis was normal. Patient was diagnosed with contact dermatitis and started on lubricant ointment 4 times a day. Her symptoms resolved in 5 days.

VII. Teaching Pearl: Question. Is dysuria the most common presentation in patients with *C trachomatis* infection?

VIII. Teaching Pearl: Answer. Although dysuria is a more common presenting feature of chlamydial infection in children, up to 50% of patients are asymptomatic. Girls often present with mucopurulent cervical discharge; boys, with urethral discharge.

REFERENCES

Behrman RE, Kliegman RM, Jenson HB, eds. *Nelson Textbook of Pediatrics*, 17th ed. Saunders, 2004.
Friedman S, Nelson N, Seidel H. *Primary Pediatric Care*. Mosby, 1992.
Garfunkel L, Kaczorowski J, Christy C. *Pediatric Clinical Advisor*. Mosby, 2002.
Schwartz W, ed. *The 5 Minute Pediatric Consult*. Lippincott Williams & Wilkins, 2000.

23. EPISTAXIS

I. Problem. A 3-year-old boy has a history of periodic nosebleeds of increasing frequency (several times this week).

II. Immediate Questions
  A. How old is patient? Nosebleeds are unusual in very young children. In adolescent boys, juvenile nasopharyngeal angiofibroma (JNA) is a rare, benign, highly vascular neoplasm of the nasopharynx that can cause significant bleeding.
  B. Was there trauma to the nose? Allergic rhinitis can cause itching and subsequent rubbing of the nose, traumatizing mucosa. Prior trauma from a direct blow on the nose may cause septal injury and bleeding. A dry environment causes crusting, and young children may be prone to picking the nose, irritating septal mucosa. Unilateral foul or purulent nasal discharge suggests a foreign body. In hospitalized patients, indwelling nasal tubes or suction trauma may injure mucosa and promote bleeding.
  C. What medication(s) has patient taken? Use of NSAIDs promotes bleeding, particularly in children with undiagnosed coagulopathy. Antihistamines may thicken secretions and cause drying and cracking of mucosa. Nasal sprays, particularly those not in an aqueous vehicle or that rely on propellants, can traumatize mucosa. Patient should be instructed on proper way to spray nasal medications, directing stream away from septum. Herbal or

alternative medications (eg, ginseng) may be associated with bleeding.

D. Is there a history of recent surgeries? Procedures requiring nasal intubation can injure mucosa. Adenoidectomy, sinus surgery, and repair of nasal fracture, among other procedures, all carry a small risk of postoperative bleeding, as does use of a nasal tube with a pH probe or nasogastric (NG) tube after an abdominal procedure.

E. History of bleeding problems? Many children have never been surgically challenged; therefore, seek information suggesting coagulopathy (eg, unusual or prolonged bleeding with circumcision, umbilical cord separation, or dental extractions; unusual bruising with play or immunizations; history of unusual or large bruises in muscles or joints; unusually heavy menstrual flow in adolescent girls; history of blood transfusion; family history of bleeding problems).

F. Any systemic illnesses? Renal and hepatic diseases are associated with bleeding problems. Does child have a hematologic malignancy?

G. What therapy has been offered to prevent or stop nose-bleeds? Measures to moisten mucosa and humidify the nasal cavity are most effective in preventing bleeding. With active bleeding, using ice, pinching nasal bones, or having child lie down are not effective. Lying down may cause blood to enter the posterior pharynx, causing child to choke and gag.

H. Is bleeding unilateral? Is there blood in the mouth? Most bleeding occurs from anterior septal vessels and may be unilateral or switch from side to side. Consider posterior epistaxis if blood is seen entering the posterior oropharynx when child has not been lying down.

III. Differential Diagnosis

A. Anterior Epistaxis. The most common source of bleeding in children is at the confluence of anterior ethmoidal, sphenopalatine, and nasopalatine arteries and veins in the anterior septum (Kiesselbach plexus or Little area). Bleeding may be unilateral or switch from one side to the other. Dry ambient environment contributes to bleeding, as does nose picking. Bleeding may recur on frequent basis.

B. Posterior Epistaxis. Unusual in children. Bleeding can be brisk and appear to be bilateral. Blood often pours down back of nose and into oropharynx.

C. Neoplasms. JNA in adolescent boys is associated with prior self-limited bleeding before a more brisk event occurs. May cause nasal obstruction, initially unilateral. Nasopharyngeal carcinoma (NPC) is seen in teenage African-American boys in the United States. Nasal obstruction and ipsilateral serous otitis media or firm cervical lymph nodes are noted on exam.

  D. Coagulopathies. Bleeding history serves as guide to possibility of coagulopathy. Obtain laboratory tests as indicated.

  E. Foreign Body. Small children may present with a long-standing history of unilateral purulent or foul nasal discharge. Diagnosis is by examination; treatment is removal.

  F. Trauma. History of overt injury is usually easily obtained. Fractures will have physical signs of displaced nasal bones or septum. Picking or rubbing nose may be a response to allergic itching.

  G. Systemic Illness. History and physical exam should provide clues to presence of systemic disease causing nosebleed.

IV. Database

 A. Physical Exam Key Points. Diagnosis of epistaxis is usually readily made based on history or physical exam.

  1. General appearance. Pallor, toxicity, and signs of shock or malignancy may be present, but pediatric epistaxis is rarely severe enough to cause hemodynamic instability or chronic anemia. Most children appear healthy and active; patients with malignancy or severe systemic disease are exceptions.

  2. Vital signs. Tachycardia and hypotension are not expected without unusual brisk hemorrhage.

  3. EENT. Unilateral serous otitis media with a firm ipsilateral cervical lymph node suggests NPC. Hypoesthesia over V2 or abnormalities of extraocular muscles suggests invasion of inferior orbital fissure, seen with advanced JNA. Blood pouring into the posterior oropharynx is suggestive of posterior bleeding. Excoriation of the nares on one side with foul odor suggests a foreign body. Evaluate for signs of atopy (eg, allergic shiners, Denny crease, mouth breathing).

  4. Anterior rhinoscopy. Keys to locating an active source of anterior bleeding or intranasal foreign body are adequate light, appropriate instruments, cooperative patient, and skilled assistance. Assess color and texture of mucosa. Clear secretions, boggy turbinates, and bluish mucosa are seen in patients with allergic rhinitis.

  5. Nasopharyngoscopy. Used to define presence of a nasopharyngeal mass and carried out, in the absence of active bleeding, after topical decongestion and analgesia of nasal mucosa.

 B. Laboratory Data. Routine laboratory studies, including PT and PTT, are not needed in healthy children with negative personal and family bleeding histories and diagnosis suggestive of common anterior epistaxis.

  1. CBC with platelet count and differential. Warranted with history of significant blood loss, suspicion of bleeding disorder in patient or family, or with long-standing, recurrent bleeding.

  2. Von Willebrand evaluation. Useful when medical or family history suggests coagulopathy.

C. **Radiographic and Other Studies**
   1. **CT scan.** Has advantage of showing bony erosion when JNA with cranial neuropathies is suspected. Contrast enhancement demonstrates vascular extent of the lesion. Sinus disease is demonstrated well, particularly on coronal views.
   2. **MRI scan.** Specifically defines soft tissues and is useful in patients with NPC and JNA.
   3. **Magnetic resonance angiography (MRA).** Demonstrates vascularity of JNA.
   4. **Angiography.** Necessary to define feeding vessels and for embolization of JNA before resection.

V. **Plan**
   A. **Anterior Epistaxis**
      1. **Minor active bleeding.** Have child sit up, lean forward over a basin or towel, and gently blow nose to rid nasal cavity of clots. Nostrils should be pinched, applying direct pressure to anterior septum, for a full 5 minutes. Should this fail, nasal cautery is indicated.
      2. **Active bleeding.** Reassurance to calm all involved and allow for orderly treatment is important. Adequate support personnel, good lighting, and appropriate instruments must be available. To cauterize the anterior nasal septum, topical decongestion or analgesia is achieved using 4% lidocaine mixed with oxymetazoline. If bleeding site is located, silver nitrate sticks can be applied to the spot. Apply silver nitrate only to the area to be cauterized. Scar formation between lateral and medial nasal walls may result if both areas are cauterized. A small pledget of absorbable topical hemostatic agent soaked in oxymetazoline can be placed against the bleeding point and left in place if needed. Antibiotic ointment is instilled at the end of cautery. Use acetaminophen for analgesia. **Given the risk of inhaling or choking on blood, conscious sedation should be avoided for control of active bleeding. In uncooperative children, general anesthesia allows effective management of bleeding in a controlled environment.**
      3. **Packing.** Rarely needed. Oral antibiotics are warranted when packing is used. In general, packs need to be removed in 48 hours.
      4. **Therapy to prevent bleeding.** Directed at keeping mucosa moist. Frequent use of saline nose spray (at least 3–4 times daily) and twice-daily use of petroleum jelly prevents cracking and crusts and enhances healing of mucosa. If ambient environment is dry, an ultrasonic humidifier in bedroom is beneficial.
   B. **Posterior Epistaxis**
      1. **Packing**

    a. Posterior bleeding can cause significant loss of blood. Because posterior packs can interfere with oxygenation, consider admission to an ICU or stepdown unit to monitor oxygenation.

    b. Posterior packs are painful. Although adequate analgesia is mandatory for patient comfort, injudicious use of narcotics can increase the risk of hypoventilation and hypoxia. Supplemental oxygen can be given when indicated, but not at the risk of depressing respiratory drive in patients with CO_2 retention.

  2. Antibiotics. Administer antistaphylococcal antibiotics to prevent sinusitis associated with packing.

  3. Consult. Consultation with an otolaryngologist may be the most effective and expedient way to effect control of bleeding.

  4. Other actions. Obtain CBC with differential, platelet count, PT, and PTT. Transfusion may be warranted. After discharge, consider iron replacement.

C. Neoplasms

  1. Imaging with CT, MRI, MRA, or angiography will help define extent of nasopharyngeal neoplasms. Because of the highly vascular nature of JNA, biopsy should never be performed. NPC does, however, require tissue diagnosis. Workup to define extent of disease is necessary prior to chemotherapy and radiation therapy.

  2. Treat patients with JNA using embolization 24–48 hours prior to surgical resection. Extent of tumor determines approach. Significant blood loss can occur with resection.

  3. Rule out hematologic malignancies by appropriate blood work and bone marrow biopsy.

D. Coagulopathies. Hematologic malignancies or systemic illnesses associated with epistaxis should be sought by history and physical exam and confirmed by appropriate laboratory tests. Management of bleeding is directed toward correction of clotting abnormalities. Packing should be avoided; it can traumatize mucosa, creating a larger surface that rebleeds when packing is removed. In the event of active bleeding, a temporary packing of oxymetazoline is useful. Head elevation and measures to moisten mucosa, as discussed earlier (see V, A, 4), can be used to help prevent rebleeding.

E. Foreign Body. Anterior rhinoscopy is performed using appropriate lighting and instrumentation with skilled assistance to hold child. Consider using a papoose board. Frazier suction is used to rid nose of purulent exudate and confirm presence of a foreign body. Various instruments (eg, appropriately sized nasal forceps or an angled ear hook) can then be used to extract foreign material. If bleeding is not active, refer to otolaryngologist for outpatient extraction. After removal, child and parents should be given instructions to use saline nose spray to rid nose of purulent discharge. Prescribe an oral antibiotic to combat concomitant sinusitis.

F. Trauma. Avoidance of further trauma to mucosa and moisturizing therapy will allow healing and prevent rebleeding. With facial fractures, refer child to specialist for reduction.

G. Systemic Illness. Correction of hematologic abnormalities associated with systemic disease is the mainstay of treatment.

VI. Problem Case Diagnosis. The 3-year-old boy was treated with a 2-week trial of aggressive measures to keep nasal mucosa moist. Nosebleeds persisted, and he was referred to an otolaryngologist. Nasal exam and cautery were performed in the operating room. Minimal manipulation of the septum caused brisk oozing from a small branch of the nasopalatine vessels. Silver nitrate failed to control bleeding, and electrocautery was applied. Patient was discharged the same day and did well on therapy of daily saline and petroleum jelly.

VII. Teaching Pearl: Question. What is the anatomic basis of direct pressure to the anterior septum to control epistaxis?

VIII. Teaching Pearl: Answer. The nasal mucosa has a rich blood supply from the anterior ethmoidal, sphenopalatine, and nasopalatine vessels. These vessels converge on the anterior septum. This area is easily traumatized from rubbing and picking. Turbulent airflow from septal deformities causes eddy currents and drying and cracking of mucosa, making this site the most common source of bleeding. Direct pressure on the area by pinching the nostrils for 5 minutes will control most uncomplicated nosebleeds.

REFERENCES

Emanuel JM. Epistaxis. In: Cummings CW, Fredrickson JM, Harker LA, et al, eds. *Cummings Otolaryngology: Head and Neck Surgery,* 3rd ed. Mosby, 1998:852–865.

Goldman, JL, Winstead W, Ganzel TM. Embolization as the definitive treatment of epistaxis in the pediatric patient. *Ear Nose Throat J* 1995;74:490-492.

Makura ZG, Porter GC, McCormick MS. Paediatric epistaxis: Alder Hey experience. *J Laryngol Otol* 2002;116:903-906.

Sandoval C, Dong S, Visintainerer P, et al. Clinical and laboratory features of 178 children with recurrent epistaxis. *J Pediatr Hematol Oncol* 2002;24:47–49.

24. EYE DISCHARGE (CONJUNCTIVITIS) AND SWELLING

I. Problem. A 10-year-old girl has eye redness and discharge, which started 2 days ago.

II. Immediate Questions

A. How old is patient? Age of child is important in determining the etiology of conjunctivitis. In newborns, typical cause is chemical, chlamydial, or bacterial (including gonococcal). Chemical conjunctivitis is related to irritation from eye drops (silver nitrate) administered at birth. Gonococcal and chlamydial conjunctivitis are infections acquired by passage through the birth canal of an infected mother. In older children, bacteria, viruses, and allergies are more likely causes. Large outbreaks may occur in day-care settings or schools. Bacterial etiologies include *Haemophilus influenzae* (most common bacterial cause), *Streptococcus pneumoniae, Moraxella catarrhalis,* staphylococci, and *Pseudomonas.* Viruses include adenovirus (most common viral cause), enteroviruses (coxsackievirus), herpes simplex virus (HSV), Epstein-Barr virus, rubeola, rubella, and mumps. Allergic conjunctivitis is typically seasonal (pollen) and may also be caused by mold, fungus, dust, and food.

B. When did symptoms appear? Time of onset is especially important in the neonatal period. With chemical conjunctivitis, inflammation begins a few hours after drops have been placed and usually lasts 24–36 hours. Gonococcal conjunctivitis develops between 2 and 5 days of life (later if prophylaxis was given). Chlamydial conjunctivitis occurs between 5 and 23 days of life.

C. Is discharge unilateral or bilateral? Although this finding is not useful to differentiate among viral and bacterial causes (one or both eyes involved), occasionally it can help in distinguishing an allergic cause (typically bilateral).

D. Characteristics of discharge? Viral conjunctivitis typically causes watery or serous discharge. Bacteria cause purulent or mucopurulent discharges. Allergies produce serous or mucoid discharge, often very stringy.

E. Associated symptoms? Viral conjunctivitis is often associated with upper respiratory symptoms or other systemic complaints (pharyngitis and conjunctivitis with adenovirus). Preauricular adenopathy or rashes may be present. With vesicles or corneal ulcerations, HSV must be ruled out. Bacterial conjunctivitis may have associated infections (eg, ipsilateral otitis media with conjunctivitis suggests *H influenzae*). Allergic conjunctivitis is associated with intensely itchy eyes, runny nose, and sneezing. Pain with movement of the eye is never normal; orbital cellulitis must be ruled out (see III, G, later).

III. Differential Diagnosis

A. Keratitis. Inflammation of the cornea caused by infection, trauma (contact lens use), or UV light radiation. Symptoms include severe pain as well as clouding and swelling of the cornea. Infectious etiologies include HSV, adenovirus, *S pneumoniae, Staphylococcus* *aureus,* and *Pseudomonas.* Treatment involves specific antibiotics for bacterial infections or acyclovir for HSV.

B. Uveitis (Iritis, Iridocyclitis). Inflammation of the iris and ciliary muscle typically caused by an autoimmune response (ie, juvenile rheumatoid arthritis, Reiter syndrome, sarcoidosis). Causes unilateral or bilateral, painful, associated photophobia; small or irregular pupil; and poor vision. Treatment includes topical steroids and therapy of underlying disease.

C. Scleritis. Focal or diffuse scleral inflammation due to idiopathic autoimmune disease. Causes unilateral, intense erythema and localized pain. May cause globe perforation. Topical steroids provide relief of symptoms.

D. Episcleritis. Focal inflammation of the deep subconjunctival tissues, similar to scleritis. Unilateral pain is caused by an autoimmune response. Typically self-limited. Topical steroids provide fast relief.

E. Foreign Body. Causes unilateral, red eye, with "gritty" feeling in the eye. There is a positive history of exposure, and object may be visible. Treat by irrigation and removal of object, and check for corneal ulceration.

F. Periorbital (Preseptal) Cellulitis. Infection of the anterior eye and eyelid caused by *S aureus,* streptococci, or *H influenzae.* Causes skin redness, swelling, and warmth. Patients retain normal vision, and there is minimal involvement of the orbit. Associated with fever, ill appearance, and an elevated WBC count. Treatment includes systemic antibiotics if patient appears ill, is very young, or is unresponsive to outpatient therapy.

G. Orbital (Septal) Cellulitis. Caused by the same organisms responsible for sinusitis (often contiguous extension of ethmoid sinusitis) but involves the back of the eye (postseptal area). Associated with vision loss, limitation or pain with eye movement, and proptosis. Significant lid edema may be present. Child often appears ill, with fever and elevated WBC count. Treatment includes systemic antibiotics and drainage of orbital abscesses when indicated.

IV. Database

A. Physical Exam Key Points

1. **Ophthalmic exam.** Check both eyes for swelling of eyelids, redness of conjunctiva, movement, and associated pain. Inspect for gross anatomic defects (proptosis). Note any discharge (color and consistency). Vision, pupils, and motility should be normal.

2. **Complete physical exam.** Should always be done to rule out signs of systemic infection. Pay particular attention to oropharynx and ears.

B. Laboratory Data. Studies in older children are usually not warranted; diagnosis typically is based on history and physical exam.

Gram stain and culture are obtained in neonates to rule out gonococcal and chlamydial disease.

1. **Gram-stained smear of discharge.** Can be done quite rapidly. Check for WBCs and presence of bacteria.
   a. *Neisseria gonorrhea.* Gram-negative intracellular diplococci.
   b. *S aureus.* Gram-positive cocci in clusters.
   c. *Pseudomonas aeruginosa.* Gram-negative bacilli.
   d. **Streptococci.** Gram-positive spherical cocci.
   e. **Enterococci.** Gram-positive, lancet-shape, encapsulated diplococci.
   f. *H influenzae.* Gram-negative coccoid rods.
   g. *Chlamydia trachomatis,* **HSV (or other viruses), chemical, or allergic conjunctivitis.** Gram-negative.
2. **Culture and sensitivity testing of discharge.** Identifies specific organism, but results are not available for several days. Special transport media are required for viral specimens (eg, Thayer-Martin for gonococcal).
3. **Giemsa stain.** Obtain if chlamydial infection is suspected to check for cytoplasmic inclusion bodies within epithelial cells. Presence of many eosinophils may indicate an allergic cause.

C. **Radiographic and Other Studies.** Usually are not required. CT scan with thin orbital slices may be useful for patients in whom orbital cellulitis is suspected.

V. **Plan**
A. **Nonpharmacologic Management.** Apply warm or cool compresses to eye for comfort.
B. **Pharmacologic Management**
   1. **Antibiotic therapy.** Necessary to prevent sight-threatening complications of gonococcal, chlamydial, and herpes conjunctivitis in neonates.
      a. **Gonococcal.** Aqueous penicillin G or ceftriaxone for 1–7 days and ocular irrigation.
      b. **Chlamydial.** Oral erythromycin for 14 days.
      c. **Herpes simplex.** Topical trifluorothymidine 9 times a day for at least 14 days with or without systemic acyclovir.
   2. **Topical antibiotic treatment.** Erythromycin, tetracycline, or polymyxin B solution qid for bacterial conjunctivitis hastens resolution of symptoms but may not be necessary when oral medications are administered.
   3. **Antiviral therapy.** Except for HSV, no specific treatment is available.
   4. **Topical antihistamine or mast cell stabilizer.** For allergic conjunctivitis.
C. **Preventive Therapy**
   1. Good hand washing to decrease transmission.

    2. Avoidance of allergen or irritant if allergic.
    3. Neonatal prophylaxis with 1% silver nitrate, 0.5% erythromycin, or 1% tetracycline.

VI. Problem Case Diagnosis. On examination, the 10-year-old girl had clear drainage involving both eyes, but no pruritus or pain. She complained of sore throat. Conjunctivae were injected in both eyes. No foreign body was visible. Eyelids were not edematous, and extraocular muscles and vision were intact. Preauricular adenopathy was noted bilaterally, and the oropharynx was injected without exudate. Clinical diagnosis is viral conjunctivitis (probably adenovirus). Patient's mother was counseled about use of cool compresses for comfort and importance of washing hands to prevent transmission. Family was asked to follow up in 3 days, and to call back sooner if worrisome features develop or symptoms worsen.

VII. Teaching Pearl: Question. What is a common cause of mucopurulent eye discharge in neonates that is noninfectious in etiology?

VIII. Teaching Pearl: Answer. Neonates with malformation or incomplete canalization of a nasolacrimal tear duct can present with excessive tearing or mucopurulent discharge days or weeks after birth. The condition usually resolves with conservative treatment by 1 year of age.

REFERENCES

Behrman RE, Kliegman RM, Jenson HB, eds. *Nelson Textbook of Pediatrics,* 17th ed. Saunders, 2004.
Garfunkel L, Kaczorowski J, Christy C. *Pediatric Clinical Advisor.* Mosby, 2002.
Schwartz W, ed. *The 5 Minute Pediatric Consult.* Lippincott Williams & Wilkins, 2000.

25. FAILURE TO THRIVE

  I. Problem. At a well-child visit, a 4-month-old infant is noted to have fallen below the third percentile for weight.

  II. Immediate Questions
    A. What is patient's height (recumbent length in infant) and head circumference? Failure to thrive (FTT) is growth failure confined to weight, unless the deprivation is of long duration. Low weight for height suggests a short-term problem. Low weight and height, or head circumference, or all three, suggests long-term deprivation or organic disease rather than familial disease.
    B. What are past growth parameters? Evaluate the growth trend. Values that consistently fall below the 3rd percentile support an etiology of prematurity, familial, or chronic disease. FTT is often defined as a 2-standard–deviation decline in weight velocity (two major percentile lines on growth curve).

C. What is patient's feeding history? FTT is undernutrition, regardless of etiology. Decreased caloric intake is the most common cause, but FTT may also result from increased caloric requirements or decreased absorption of calories. Ask about appetite, routine meals, and fluid intake (what is offered and when). Specific questions include:

1. Is formula mixed properly? Overly dilute formula results in decreased caloric intake.
2. How much formula does infant actually ingest from each bottle?
3. Is there evidence of effective breast feeding (eg, latching on, milk production, time at breast)?
4. Are other foods and fluids being offered?

D. Any feeding difficulties? In an infant, choking, slow feeding, tiring with feeding, poor suck, vomiting, or regurgitation suggests GI, cardiac, or neurologic disorder. In a toddler or older child with decreased appetite, consider dental disease, constipation, chronic illness, or apathy.

E. What is the prenatal history and birth history? Relevant information includes maternal nutrition, prenatal laboratory values, perinatal infections, illnesses, medications, delivery complications, extended nursery or NICU stay, and newborn screening tests.

F. Has patient achieved normal developmental milestones? Developmental delays may provide clues to the cause of FTT. FTT itself can cause delay.

G. What is the past medical history? Hospitalizations, recurrent infections, and chronic diarrhea suggest chronic disease.

H. What medication(s) does patient take? Ask about prescribed, over-the-counter, and alternative remedies.

I. What is the social history? Specific questions include:

1. Who is primary caregiver?
2. Who lives at home?
3. Who cares for patient if caregiver is away?
4. Any changes in family dynamics?

J. Family history? Relevant information includes siblings or parents with chronic disease or recurrent infection, chromosomal or metabolic abnormality, fetal or infant deaths, and stature and growth trends, including FTT.

K. Interaction among patient, caregiver, and family? FTT usually involves environmental or psychosocial factors, or both. Child maltreatment and neglect take many forms, from overt physical and emotional abuse to nonintentional neglect.

III. Differential Diagnosis. FTT is a sign, not a diagnosis. The cause of the undernutrition must be determined. Most patients are younger than 3 years of age. Often FTT may involve a combination of organic (ie, major disease process or single organ dysfunction) and environmental or psychosocial factors (ie, no distinct pathophysiologic abnormality but, rather, insufficient emotional-physical nurturing). Presence of one factor does not preclude a search for others.

A. Environmental, Psychosocial, or Nonorganic FTT. Most common type in the United States. Includes neglect (intentional, nonintentional), feeding issues (decreased amount, improper mixing of formula, poor technique), poverty (food unavailable), and parental incompetence (maternal depression, substance abuse, diminished mental capacity).

B. Congenital or Anatomic Anomalies. Chromosomal defect, congenital anomalies, cardiac defect, infection, cystic fibrosis, in utero exposure to toxins.

C. GI Abnormalities. Gastroesophageal reflux disease, milk-protein intolerance, celiac disease, Hirschsprung disease, irritable bowel disease, malabsorption, malrotation.

D. Renal Disorders. Occult UTI, renal tubular acidosis, chronic renal insufficiency.

E. Cardiac Disorders. Persistent patent ductus arteriosus, acquired heart disease, congestive heart failure.

F. Pulmonary Disorders. Bronchopulmonary dysplasia, poorly controlled asthma, chronic aspiration.

G. Infectious Diseases. HIV, tuberculosis, parasitic infestations, dental disease.

H. Metabolic Alterations. Inborn errors, galactosemia, amino or organic acidurias, storage diseases, hypercalcemia.

I. Endocrine Disorders. Thyroid, parathyroid, adrenal, pituitary, or growth hormone disorders; diabetes mellitus type 1.

J. Neurologic Disorders. Degenerative disorders, cerebral palsy, oral motor dysfunction, structural defects.

K. Medications. Prescribed, over-the-counter, and alternative remedies.

L. Other Causes. Malignancy, sickle cell disease, environmental toxins (lead).

IV. Database. Further evaluation (laboratory and other studies) is rarely useful unless suggested by history or physical exam findings.

A. Physical Exam Key Points

1. Growth parameters. Plot height (if age > 2 years) or recumbent length (if < 2 years), weight, and head circumference on a standard growth chart (see Appendix G, p. 766).

2. Overall appearance and behavior. Assess for eye contact, interaction, inappropriate behaviors, dysmorphic features, signs of endocrine or metabolic disease, psychosocial neglect, or emotional abuse.

3. Signs of malnutrition. Loss of subcutaneous fat, muscle wasting, sparse hair or alopecia, cheilosis, hydration.

4. Signs of maltreatment or neglect. Cutaneous injuries (eg, bruises, burns, unusual marks) or poor hygiene.

5. **HEENT.** Fontanelle, funduscopic exam, neck masses, dental disease, tonsillar or sinus disease, cleft palate or lip.
6. **Cardiopulmonary system.** Abnormal chest wall, evidence of reactive airway disease, atypical murmur or abnormal heart sounds, digital clubbing.
7. **Abdomen.** Protuberance, organomegaly.
8. **Neurologic exam.** Abnormal muscle tone and strength, coordination, deep tendon reflexes.
B. **Laboratory Data.** Initial laboratory tests to consider in severe cases include CBC, electrolytes, BUN and creatinine, total CO_2 or HCO_3, urine culture, HIV, and PPD. Order other tests as dictated by history and exam findings.
C. **Radiographic and Other Studies.** These tests have minimal yield if not suggested by history or exam findings. Perform skeletal survey, if maltreatment is suspected.

V. **Plan**
A. **Hospitalization.** Admit patients with severe malnutrition or when infant or child is at risk for harm, follow-up is not reliable, caregiver is neither competent nor compliant, or outpatient management fails.
B. **Parental Education and Training.** Key component of treatment, regardless of cause. Avoid placing blame. Parents may require referral to nutritional, occupational therapy, physical therapy, psychiatric, and social services.
C. **Psychosocial Causes.** Ensure that home environment is safe, caregiver is competent and compliant, and follow-up is reliable.
   1. **Infants.** Observe feeding techniques.
   2. **Toddlers.** Institute routine mealtimes, offer solids before liquids, and limit juice or water.
D. **Organic Causes.** Treat underlying condition. Institute slow introduction of high-calorie foods, with close monitoring.
E. **Caloric Supplementation.** Depends on specific diagnoses and severity. Patients often require 50% increase in caloric requirements.
F. **Follow-up.** Frequent follow-up and close monitoring of growth and development are important because patients are at risk for cognitive and developmental delays.

VI. **Problem Case Diagnosis.** Exam findings in the 4-month-old infant were normal except for loss of subcutaneous fat, and interaction with family was appropriate. Mother reported that she had been mixing 2 cans of water to every can of formula concentrate, "trying to make ends meet." This provided two thirds of infant's required caloric intake per day (13.3 cal/oz rather than 20 cal/oz). Diagnosis is FTT caused by environmental factors.

VII. **Teaching Pearl: Question.** If a healthy thriving infant shows a decline over two or more major percentiles late in infancy, is this cause for concern?

VIII. Teaching Pearl: Answer. Normal changes in linear growth occur in infants. Studies show that healthy thriving infants channel to higher or lower percentiles over the first 18 months of life, at times crossing over two or more major percentiles, then staying within that new channel of growth.

REFERENCES

Behrman RE, Kliegman RM, Jenson HB, eds. *Nelson Textbook of Pediatrics,* 17th ed. Saunders, 2004.

Gahagan S, Holmes R. A stepwise approach to evaluation of undernutrition and failure to thrive. *Pediatr Clin North Am* 1998;45:169–187.

Schwartz ID. Failure to thrive: An old nemesis in the new millennium. *Pediatr Rev* 2000;21:257–264.

Zenel J Jr. Failure to thrive: A general pediatrician's perspective. *Pediatr Rev* 1997;18:371–378.

26. FEEDING PROBLEMS

I. Problem. A 2-year-old child who has exhibited decreased appetite and frank food refusal over the past several days is brought to the pediatrician for evaluation.

II. Immediate Questions

  A. How long have symptoms been present? Has patient been acutely ill with fever, vomiting or diarrhea, or symptoms of upper respiratory infection? Or have symptoms existed chronically with recent flare-up? Children commonly decrease food intake prior to and immediately following acute, self-limited illness. The situation is urgent only if symptoms of dehydration (dry mucous membranes, decreased urine output, poorly perfused skin) or change in mental status (lethargy, excessive irritability, inconsolable crying) are noted.

  B. Does patient have underlying medical conditions that are associated with poor oral intake? Conditions that predispose to disordered passage of food from the mouth to the stomach - (dysphagia) include central and peripheral nervous system disorders, diseases of muscle, and structural abnormalities of the oral cavity, pharynx, and esophagus. Decreased food intake having a behavioral basis or resulting from developmental delay is more likely to be associated with disruptive mealtime behavior and food selectivity than acute cessation of liquids and solids. Development of or exacerbation of known reflux esophagitis can lead to refusal to feed, especially if retching during or post-feeding is present.

  C. Is choking, gagging, or respiratory distress present? Choking, gagging, and ultimate respiratory distress with feeding should prompt assessment for aspiration and pulmonary sequelae (see IV, C, later). Food refusal having a behavioral basis is less likely to present with acute choking and is never associated with increased work of breathing or true respiratory distress.

D. Is patient taking any new medication(s) or herbal supplement(s)? Has there been any exposure to toxins? Food refusal can be secondary to acute ingestion of poisons that ulcerate or scar the mucosal lining of the mouth. Some decrease in appetite may be seen with medications or herbal supplements that directly cause disordered taste sensations or exacerbation of GI upset.

III. Differential Diagnosis

A. Acute Viral or Bacterial Illness. Infectious processes can directly affect the GI tract, with resultant vomiting or diarrhea that decreases oral intake. Likewise, symptoms of upper respiratory tract infection, streptococcal pharyngitis, or pneumonia can affect child's oral intake.

B. Reflux Esophagitis. Acute presentation of reflux esophagitis, especially in infants, can diminish oral intake. Pain associated with feeding efforts (secondary to acid reflux) may initially present post-prandially or generalize to food refusal and selectivity. Children taking antireflux medications can experience flare-up of dysphagia if the medication dose is subtherapeutic or intercurrent illness exacerbates acid production in the stomach.

C. Developmental or Behavioral Food Refusal. Children with developmental disabilities (including mental retardation and autistic spectrum disorder) may "shut down" feeding efforts as a behavioral response to their environment. Typically, developing children (especially around age 2 years and in summer) can also go on "hunger strikes," but rarely will they cease all oral intake for more than a day if mealtime structure is maintained.

D. Airway or Foodway Anomalies. Children with congenital defects of the nasopharynx, oral cavity, and laryngeal region are predisposed to disordered passage of food from mouth to stomach. With growth and introduction of more highly textured food, decompensation of feeding may occur, with possible aspiration risk. Acquired anatomic defects secondary to tumor, trauma, or post-surgical manipulations can also disorganize feeding.

E. Neurologic Deficits. CNS disease affecting the signals to swallow safely may underlie decreased feeding efforts. In peripheral nerve disorders and neuromuscular diseases, acute decline of oral intake may be associated with decompensation in neurologic status.

F. Ingestion. See II, D, earlier.

IV. Database

A. Physical Exam Key Points

1. **Vital signs.** Check for fever, tachypnea, or poor perfusion associated with respiratory distress, dehydration, or infection.

Decreased weight-for-height percentiles may indicate chronic poor oral intake (see Chapter 25, Failure to Thrive, p. 126).

2. **Mouth.** Inspect oral mucosa for lesions consistent with infection or ingestion.

3. **Lungs.** Auscultate for symmetric breath sounds, rales, rhonchi, or wheezes. Decreased breath sounds, especially in right lung fields, may be consistent with aspiration pneumonia.

4. **Abdomen.** Reproducible midline or epigastric pain may be present with reflux esophagitis (but is often absent in chronic conditions).

B. **Laboratory Data.** Generally not indicated in feeding disorders. CBC with differential may be obtained in patients with infectious processes (high WBC count) or chronic reflux (anemia secondary to mucosal erosion and blood loss).

C. **Radiographic and Other Studies**

1. **Modified barium swallow (MBS).** The gold standard study used to delineate oral, pharyngeal, and esophageal phases of swallowing, but rarely indicated acutely unless anatomic considerations or persistent aspiration are suspected.

2. **Plain film, chest X-ray.** Warranted if pneumonia, ingestion pneumonitis, or anatomic abnormalities are suspected.

3. **Routine neuroimaging.** Not done to work up feeding disorders. Rare, direct CNS etiologies, such as mass effects from tumor or trauma, or pressure phenomena from congenital lesions such as Chiari malformations, warrant CT or MRI scan.

V. **Plan.** Evaluation of feeding problems in young children aims to assess acute impact on wellness. Life-threatening presentations secondary to feeding difficulties are rare. Aspiration, as well as unrecognized reflux, can result in nutritional inadequacy, failure to thrive, and immunologic compromise.

A. **Acute Viral or Bacterial Illness**

1. Acetaminophen or NSAIDs for symptomatic relief for fever and discomfort.

2. Rapid strep and throat cultures, and chest X-ray, as clinically warranted.

3. Antibiotics, if infectious pneumonia is suspected; but generally not indicated if aspiration is the proven cause.

B. **Reflux Esophagitis.** Often under-recognized as a cause of food refusal; it can "reactivate" after intercurrent illness.

1. Thicken formula with rice cereal (using 1 tsp/oz initially). Use of upright positioning post-prandially may provide symptomatic relief.

2. Pharmacologic therapy is aimed at neutralizing acid production and promoting GI motility.

3. Assess concomitant constipation that may increase abdominal pressure and exacerbate reflux. Stool softeners, prokinetic agents, and laxatives by mouth are preferable initially.

    C. Developmental or Behavioral Food Refusal

       1. Assess aspiration risk. Chest x-ray or MBS, or both, may be indicated, especially in nonverbal children.

       2. Counsel caregivers to provide structure to mealtime.

       3. Use 3-day diet diary to assess nutritional repleteness. Supplemental products (drinks, protein, or carbohydrate powders) can provide calorie boosters.

    D. Airway or Foodway Anomalies

       1. Look for clinical signs of other congenital defects that may affect midline structures, thereby causing disorganized swallowing.

       2. MBS study is often necessary to delineate swallowing safety.

    E. Neurologic Deficits

       1. Careful physical exam is imperative to rule out decompensation in baseline status underlying swallowing dysfunction.

       2. MBS study, as noted in D, 2, earlier.

       3. Thickening of feedings, modification of textures presented, and upright positioning may decrease aspiration potential.

  VI. Problem Case Diagnosis. The 2-year-old child had had a recent febrile illness with GI symptoms, leading to decreased appetite and food refusal over several days. In most children, such presentations are self-limiting. If declining appetite and frank food refusal were to persist, however, clinician should begin to suspect other processes. Unmasked reflux esophagitis with pain during and immediately following feeding may present as dysphagia. Suspicion for this should be higher in children with developmental disabilities, in whom chronic reflux can present atypically with poor weight gain in the setting of intercurrent irritability, nighttime restlessness, or disruptive mealtime behavior.

  VII. Teaching Pearl: Question. If the safety of feeding integrity is in doubt, what is the most definitive examination that can be obtained to assess swallowing safety?

  VIII. Teaching Pearl: Answer. With acute food refusal, a history of infectious process, reflux symptoms, or ingestion will determine workup and clinical management. Suspicion of chronic dysphagia, neurologic decompensation, or underlying developmental disabilities should prompt an MBS study to delineate aspiration risks.

REFERENCE

Tuchman D, Walter R. *Disorders of Feeding and Swallowing in Infants and Young Children.* Singular Publishing, 1994.

27. FEVER

  I. Problem. A 9-month-old boy is brought to the pediatrician for evaluation. He has a 24-hour history of fever, ranging from 101.3°F to 103.6°F, that is associated with fussiness and lethargy.

II. **Immediate Questions**

A. **Has patient been afebrile either spontaneously or as response to antipyretic therapy since onset of the fever? If so, how did patient seem when afebrile?** It is important to clarify whether ill behavior (lethargy and irritability) is a result of fever or of the underlying illness.

B. **What signs and symptoms are associated with the fever?** Most infants have self-limited viral syndromes, primarily from respiratory viruses. GI symptoms or cutaneous manifestations (rash) are also frequently caused by viruses. Although these findings provide useful insight, their presence should not foreshorten an evaluation. Recent data suggest that presence of some viral diseases (eg, respiratory syncytial virus) reduces the risk of another more serious infection in a febrile child; however, other studies have shown that viral diseases and an established focus of infection do not protect infants from a concurrent serious, deep infection.

C. **Are there any known sick contacts?** Does a sibling or caregiver have a similar illness? Does a contact have a serious infectious or contagious illness (ie, meningococcemia) that demands immediate diagnostic consideration?

D. **Are there any known or possible immune deficiencies that need to be considered?** Fever may be the primary presentation of a child with severe combined immunodeficiency syndrome or indicate a first instance of bacteremia from an encapsulated organism (eg, *Pneumococcus*) in a child with a sickling syndrome.

E. **Does patient have bacterial meningitis?** This is the most important question confronting the clinician when a child presents with fever. Meningitis must be considered and ruled out by history, physical exam, and, if necessary, diagnostic testing.

III. **Differential Diagnosis.** Dependent on age of child.

A. **Infection**

1. **Bacterial.** Most common pathogen varies, depending on age (Table I–10).

TABLE I–10. MOST COMMON BACTERIAL PATHOGENS IN FEBRILE CHILDREN AGED 1–24 MONTHS

< 1 Month	1–3 Months	3–24 Months (and Older)
Group B streptococci	*S pneumoniae*	*S pneumoniae*
E coli and other enteric pathogens	Group B streptococci	*N meningitides*
Listeria monocytogenes	*N meningitides*	*Salmonella species*
Salmonella species	*Salmonella species*	
*Staphylococcus aureus**	*L monocytogenes*	

*Epidemic setting.

    2. **Viral**
      a. **Newborn.** TORCH infection.
      b. **Infant and young child.** Enterovirus and respiratory viruses.
      c. **Older child and adolescent.** Respiratory viruses and Epstein-Barr virus (EBV).
    3. **Fungal.** Newborn or immune-compromised host.
    4. **Mycobacterial.** In exposed populations.
    5. **Rickettsial.** In appropriate geographic locations.
    6. **Other vector-transmitted infection** (eg, Lyme disease).
  B. Rheumatologic Disorders. Includes Kawasaki disease, Still disease, acute rheumatic fever, juvenile rheumatoid arthritis, systemic lupus erythematosus (SLE), vasculitic syndrome, onset of periodic fever syndrome, and inflammatory bowel disease.
  C. Neoplasia. Includes leukemia, neuroblastoma, Wilms tumor, non-Hodgkin lymphoma, Hodgkin lymphoma, histiocytosis, osteogenic sarcoma, and Ewing sarcoma. Onset is usually insidious but sudden onset of fever may indicate a solid neoplasm that has undergone internal bleeding (eg, neuroblastoma) or is complicated by infection due to immune suppression or obstruction.
  D. Fictitious Disease. Falsified symptoms of fever (eg, Munchausen syndrome).
  E. Thermoregulatory Disorders. Dysautonomia, diabetes insipidus, anhydrosis.
  F. Miscellaneous. Drug-induced, hypermetabolic, or malignant neuroleptic states.

IV. Database
  A. Physical Exam Key Points
    1. **General appearance.** Very important, especially in younger children. Recognition of the "toxic infant" with fever should trigger medical urgency.
    2. **Vital signs.** High degree of fever and its association with other risk indicators in a young child increases the likelihood of bacteremia. Hypotension should raise concern about hypovolemia, sepsis-induced loss of peripheral vascular resistance, or myocardial dysfunction. Hypotension in the absence of tachycardia raises concern about disturbance of cardiac function or rhythm. Absence of tachycardia with fever is a feature of *Salmonella typhi*. Tachycardia in the absence of hypotension may be related to fever (10–20 beats/min increase for each degree above normal temperature), incipient vascular collapse (particularly in the setting of narrowed pulse pressure), depressed cardiac function, or an associated rhythm disturbance (eg, supraventricular tachycardia). Elevated respiratory rate, which also may be a response to fever, may signal a pulmonary source of the fever when the rate is elevated disproportionately to heart rate and BP. Alternatively, increased

respiratory rate may be respiratory compensation for metabolic acidosis resulting from the underlying etiology of the fever.

3. **Skin.** Rashes frequently accompany viral syndromes (viral exanthemas). The critical distinction in assessing rash in a febrile child is whether or not the rash blanches with pressure. Nonblanching rash may indicate a vasculitic injury with extravasation of blood into the surrounding dermis. It should raise suspicion of infecting organisms that are tropic to vascular structures, which includes enteroviruses, *Neisseria meningitides* (meningococcemia), and *Rickettsia rickettsiae* (Rocky Mountain spotted fever [RMSF]). Distribution of rash can be useful in distinguishing source of infection. Varicella starts centrally (truncal) and moves out, whereas variola begins peripherally. Palms are more often involved in RMSF.

4. **HEENT.** Acute otitis media is the most frequent diagnosis in children presenting with fever. Diagnosis in a screaming child requires diagnostic skill beyond mere assessment of tympanic membrane erythema. Drum appearance and membrane mobility are important signs. Conjunctival suffusion may be one of the diagnostic clues to Kawasaki disease. It is important to evaluate for pharyngitis (eg, group A streptococcus, EBV), peritonsillar abscess, retropharyngeal abscess, and rhinosinusitis (eg, upper respiratory allergic diathesis). Drooling may suggest upper airway obstruction, including retropharyngeal abscess.

5. **Neck.** Assess for nuchal rigidity, including Brudzinski and Kernig signs. Note that these signs become progressively less reliable in children younger than 15 months of age. Tilted head due to torticollis may indicate an inflamed node in contact with the sternocleidomastoid (eg, peritonsillar abscess).

6. **Lymph nodes.** Suppurative nodes are usually caused by either *Staphylococcus aureus* or group A streptococcus. Catscratch fever usually is associated with a cold lymphadenitis. Often an entry punctum can be found on skin in the anatomic area associated with the abnormal node. Generalized adenopathy directs clinician away from focal infections with considerations of certain viral, rheumatologic, or malignant processes.

7. **Lungs.** Respiratory tract is the most frequent site of infection in children with fever. Altered pattern of normal breath sounds is a clue (especially tachypnea). Rales may direct clinician to a pulmonary infiltrate. Diffuse wheezes can be heard in bronchospastic processes and lower airway infection (bronchiolitis). Unilateral or segmental wheezes suggest foreign body aspiration.

8. **Heart.** New murmur, particularly mitral or aortic regurgitant, should raise suspicion of acute rheumatic fever. Occasionally

this will only be heard on serial exams, because it may not be present at onset of fever. Muffled or distant heart sounds may be a clue to pericardial effusion as part of viral pancarditis or due to septic pericardial effusion.

9. **Abdomen.** Examination often requires diversionary tactics. Exam findings such as localized tenderness often need to be repeated from different approaches to validate finding. Rupture of the appendix before operative treatment is the rule in infants and young toddlers. Tenderness at McBurney point, if elicited, is reliable as a sign of appendicitis. Liver size, as measured by distance of the edge below the right costal margin at the mid-clavicular line (MCL), requires knowledge of changing anatomic ratios with growth. A liver edge 3 cm below the right costal margin at the MCL may be normal in a newborn but marks hepatomegaly in a 10-year-old child. Tenderness of the costovertebral angle (CVA) in older toddlers and children points to a renal source of infection.

10. **GU system.** Perform a GU exam to evaluate for pelvic inflammatory disease in a sexually active febrile adolescent. Consider UTI in a febrile girl without other evidence of an infectious focus. Physical findings (eg, CVA tenderness) are less reliable in younger children. Male adolescents must be assessed for testicular tenderness of epididymitis.

11. **Extremities.** Trauma from childhood play can be noted on the extremities, and evidence of infecting cellulitis should be sought. The punctum of cat-scratch disease is most often seen on extremities (upper > lower) as this is the site of most human contact with cats. Extremity findings can be seen in Kawasaki disease, dermatomyositis, SLE, and vasculitic syndromes (eg, septic vasculitis).

B. **Laboratory Data**

1. **CBC with differential.** Often overutilized in well-appearing febrile children. Total WBC is a risk factor for bacteremia in highly febrile child. Low total WBC is not a reliable predictor of meningitis because low WBC counts are seen in viral infection, overwhelming infection (including meningitis), and immune deficiency states.

2. **Lumbar puncture.** Remains the gold standard for diagnosis of meningitis and must be performed, if not contraindicated, when history and physical exam cannot convincingly rule out bacterial meningitis.

3. **Blood culture.** Has little practical value to assess for occult bacteremia (bacteremia unexpected on clinical grounds). Most of these episodes are benign and resolve without treatment. Children who develop serious deep infections often present for medical care before positive testing of the blood culture. Multiple (three or four) blood cultures are warranted when

certain diseases (eg, osteomyelitis, endocarditis) are suspected to increase their yield. Blood cultures should be obtained through central lines if present.

4. **Urinalysis.** A useful test in female children without other evidence of infectious foci; it has a significantly lesser yield in male children but should be considered in uncircumcised boys during infancy if fever is not self-limited. Urine nitrites, leukocyte esterase, Gram stains, and direct cell visualization add to the immediate diagnostic value of urinalysis.

5. **Urine culture.** The gold standard for diagnosing UTI.

6. **Other cultures.** Throat culture and rapid antigen tests can be useful in diagnosing streptococcal pharyngitis; occasional culture from the maximum area of induration of a cellulitis yields an infecting organism. Stool culture in selected patients may lead to a diagnosis of enteric infection (bloody diarrhea, elevated fecal leukocytes, or protracted diarrhea).

7. **Miscellaneous tests.** Consider cultures of central lines, if present. Hepatic transaminases may suggest viral disease and lead to more specific hepatitis studies. C-reactive protein and ESR, although nonspecific, can occasionally help direct diagnoses or assess progress of treatment in some infectious diseases.

C. **Radiographic and Other Studies**

1. **Chest x-ray.** Useful in patients who have fever without localizing signs, particularly if physical exam findings raise suspicion of pulmonary involvement (especially tachypnea).

2. **Abdominal imaging.** "Blind" abdominal imaging for clues to an abdominal source of fever seldom is useful. Abdominal imaging, as well as imaging in general, should be guided by clinical suspicion.

3. **Ultrasound.** By virtue of its rapid availability, often a useful study if clinical signs or symptoms direct an evaluation to a given area. May reveal abscesses or other fluid collections.

4. **Bone scan or MRI.** Particularly useful if bone infection is suspected.

5. **Thoracentesis, arthrocentesis, bone aspirate.** As a general rule, obtaining material for culture from locations of fluid collections has a high yield and is warranted whenever possible. Perform whenever possible prior to antimicrobial treatment, because it can direct treatment.

6. **Echocardiogram.** Can be useful to assess for myocardial dysfunction, as seen in viral myocarditis, acute rheumatic fever, and Kawasaki disease. May also implicate valvular disease of acute rheumatic fever, infective endocarditis, and coronary dilation or aneurysm of Kawasaki disease.

V. **Plan.** Age of the involved child is a critical ingredient in the clinical decision tree. Any ill-appearing child requires thorough evaluation.

A. Young Infants. Approach each febrile infant with the goal of first ruling out meningitis or overwhelming sepsis. Neonates must be considered functionally "immunocompromised" as they not only often fail to localize infection but also have a limited repertoire of clinical responses.

   1. Infants, especially those who are younger than 1 month or who appear ill, require thorough evaluation with blood culture, urine evaluation and culture, and cerebrospinal fluid (CSF) evaluation with culture and appropriate CSF polymerase chain reaction (eg, herpes, enterovirus).

   2. Admission and empiric treatment to cover group B *Streptococcus, Listeria monocytogenes,* and gram-negative enteric organisms is warranted, as well as consideration of empiric treatment of herpesvirus with acyclovir. A third-generation parenteral cephalosporin or an aminoglycoside (usually gentamicin) coupled with ampicillin is the current treatment of choice in most settings. Clinician must still rule out meningitis in this patient.

B. Children One Month to 2 Years of Age

   1. Treatment approach. Evaluation and management of this age group requires the most consideration. First, a compulsive search for the source of the fever must be performed. If found, treatment can proceed by clinical diagnosis as long as clinician recognizes that the diagnosed clinical syndrome does not necessarily eliminate more worrisome diagnoses.

   2. Fever Without Localizing Signs (FWLS). If no source of infection is found, child fits into the diagnostic group of FWLS. Although most infants with FWLS have self-limited viral disease, a rare but real number of such patients are early in the course of a serious infection. Choices for therapeutic management include:

   a. "Sepsis workup" on all such patients, with subsequent hospitalization and empiric antibiotic treatment. This aggressive approach will treat hundreds perhaps even a thousand such patients to avoid missing the single patient at the early stage of an illness, either viral or occult bacteremia, that is destined to go on to bacterial meningitis. This option is fraught with problems, including issues of medical complications (eg, phlebitis, medication errors) and the psychosocial disruption of hospitalization.

   b. Evaluation and empiric treatment of all infants who are "toxic," while assuring close follow-up in FWLS infants who look well despite fever. Clinician may choose to perform acute phase testing, CBC and differential, C-reactive protein, and urine studies to add diagnostic comfort to the choice to follow patient expectantly. Follow-up in this instance requires that infant's parents or caregiver realize they are assuming a small risk in not hospitalizing child. Parents must be given appropriate information to enable them to recognize progression of the illness (irritability, lethargy, loss of interest in feeding, petechiae or purpura, seizures or neurologic alteration) and respond to those changes (return immediately for care). Follow-up when these elements cannot be put in place may require hospitalization for observation without empiric treatment.

C. Children Older Than 2 Years of Age. Manage as for an older child. In this age group, child's response to serious illnesses is sufficiently developed to be recognized (eg, nuchal rigidity is a reliable finding of meningeal irritation).

D. Infant With Otitis Media. In an infant with otitis media, meningitis must be ruled out. The finding of a source of infection (eg, acute otitis media) in a highly febrile infant does not remove the onus on clinician to rule out serious deep infection. Although data suggest that a patient with one focus of infection is unlikely to have a second source of infection, the first diagnosis source does not protect patient from a second, more serious, source.

VI. Problem Case Diagnosis. Evaluation in the emergency department showed a febrile infant (103.1°F) who was irritable but consolable by his parents. Physical findings were negative for an infectious focus. Lumbar puncture was deferred in favor of antipyretic treatment with acetaminophen to clarify role of fever in infant's altered behavior. Upon reevaluation 1 hour later, infant was laughing and actively engaged in play with his father. Information was provided to parents regarding risks and findings that warrant return and reevaluation, and infant was sent home. Phone follow-up found that fever persisted for the next 3 days but occasional antipyretic therapy confirmed infant's well-being. On the third day, infant developed a diffuse, blanching, erythematous macular rash. Fever and other symptoms simultaneously resolved. Diagnosis is roseola (herpesvirus 6).

VII. Teaching Pearl: Question. What are the key considerations when assessing an infant with high fever?

VIII. Teaching Pearl: Answer. Assessment is dependent on child's age. Most neonates require a sepsis workup, with admission and empiric antibiotic treatment. Patients beyond the neonatal period, but younger than 2 years, require concise review of the history to assess for altered risk indicators (immune compromise) and infectious contacts, and thorough physical exam to search for an infectious focus. Management is then based on the clinical syndrome (pneumonia, cellulitis, meningitis, FWLS) or degree of toxicity. Fever itself, rather then the source of the fever, may cause irritability and lethargy. Antipyretic therapy may have its most substantive role in the ill but nontoxic infant in which defervescence allows a more effective assessment of infant's status. Patients older than 2 years of age can be managed based on their clinical syndrome and degree of toxicity as one would older children.

REFERENCES

Malatack JJ, Consolini DM. Fever without localizing signs and occult bacteremia. In: Klein JD, Zaoutis TE, eds. *Pediatric Infectious Disease Secrets.* Hanley & Belfus, 2003:211–220.

Shapiro ED. Fever without localizing signs. In: Long SS, Pickering LK, Prober CG, eds. *Pediatric Infectious Disease.* Churchill Livingstone, 1997:110–114.

28. FEVER OF UNKNOWN ORIGIN

I. **Problem.** A 7-year-old boy who has had daily fever for 2 weeks is brought to the clinic for evaluation.

II. **Immediate Questions**
   A. **What is the degree of fever and who has documented it?** Normal body temperature is highest in children who are preschool aged. Several studies have documented that peak temperature tends to be in the afternoon and is highest at about 18–24 months of age when many normal children will have a temperature of 101°F. It is important to document fever (usually in an office setting) prior to beginning extensive testing.
   B. **Is this truly fever of unknown origin (FUO)?** Definition in adults is 2 weeks of outpatient fever and 1 week in hospital without a diagnosis. In children, variable definitions have been used. Generally, most clinicians would accept fever documented for more than 1 week in which initial cultures and other investigations fail to yield a diagnosis. This is quite different from **fever without localizing signs (FWLS),** which is a more common and acute disorder in pediatrics, often involving risks and outcomes of bacteremia (for further discussion, see Chapter 27, Fever, p. 132). Another key question is whether this is a **"periodic" fever interspersed with wellness,** pointing to additional possible diagnoses.
   C. **What symptoms does patient have now? At onset?** Clues to diagnosis of FUO are often obtained from the history, including meticulous review of systems (eg, rashes, skin breaks, and GI complaints).
   D. **What testing has been done?** Initial effort should be to ensure complete data collection (ie, cultures, laboratory work, x-rays, antibody titers).
   E. **Are there known exposures?** In difficult cases patients and families may, with careful questioning, recall exposures (eg, insect or tick bites, animal contact, other children or adults with illness).
   F. **What treatment has been initiated previously?** At times, prior treatment may mask the fever history, make cultures negative, suppress bacterial growth (eg, urine or throat), or be the source of fever in the form of a drug reaction.
   G. **Has patient traveled outside the country or to an endemic area?** Certain areas are far more likely to be sources of individual

illnesses (eg, Lyme disease, *Salmonella* infection), and a history of travel to these areas may provide valuable clues.

III. **Differential Diagnosis.** The list of potential etiologies of FUO is enormous, but with care, a systematic approach using key major screening tests and categories will prove useful.

   A. **Infection.** In almost all reviews of FUO in pediatric patients, infection is the largest category, with a figure of at least 50% of all final diagnoses. It is important to recognize *uncommon manifestations* of common disorders (infectious mononucleosis with hepatitis or pneumonia) rather than unusual or *uncommon infections,* such as tularemia. About half of the *localized* infections involve the **respiratory tract,** and a careful history and x-rays may confirm this diagnosis. Other locations that are sources of prolonged fever include **urinary tract, bone,** and **CNS.** A random search for abscesses may not be warranted, but if patient has abdominal symptoms with FUO, a CT scan may be useful. Look for clues to more generalized infections (Epstein-Barr virus, enteric infection, cat-scratch disease, tuberculosis, and cytomegalovirus) in which there may be evidence of multiple organ involvement.

   B. **Collagen or Connective Tissue Disease.** Juvenile rheumatoid arthritis may present with a long duration of fever before a diagnosis is established (ie, fever precedes evidence of joint or skin involvement). Additional causes include Kawasaki disease, systemic lupus erythematosus, rheumatic fever, and other vasculitic syndromes, such as Wegener granulomatosis. Most of these conditions produce additional physical findings, but patients with Kawasaki disease who are younger than 1 year of age may have "incomplete" or atypical presentations with only a few manifestations of the disorder.

   C. **Neoplasia.** Most common in this group are lymphoreticular malignancies (eg, lymphoma, leukemia). If there are joint symptoms, these may, at times, be confused with juvenile rheumatoid arthritis. Neuroblastoma and occasionally other sarcomas may present with fever as the major symptom.

   D. **Inflammatory Bowel Disease.** This is an unusual cause of isolated FUO because other symptoms (eg, diarrhea, weight loss, poor growth) are usually present.

   E. **Miscellaneous.** There are always rare causes not evident on an initial search. Examples are ectodermal dysplasia with poor thermal regulation, diabetes insipidus with dehydration and fever in infancy, and central fever in patients with disordered thermoregulation. Another rare cause is so-called inflammatory pseudotumor, usually found in the abdomen.

   F. **Pseudo FUO.** This entity is likely much more common than true FUO because frequent, minor, viral illness may be overinterpreted. A careful recording of illnesses and overall function of child and family is necessary, including school attendance.

    G. Periodic Fever. This is a separate entity in which fever is truly episodic, followed by "normal" times. This category includes periodic fever with aphthous stomatitis, pharyngitis (PFAPA) and familial Mediterranean fever and variants. Many of these latter disorders are being delineated using newer genetic techniques as well as by studying pathways of inflammation.

IV. Database

A. Physical Exam Key Points

1. **Vital signs and growth parameters.** Fever should be confirmed and weight loss or growth failure recorded. Hypertension may be a clue to renal involvement. Respiratory rate may be elevated in patients with chest disorders.

2. **Skin.** Examination should be meticulous, evaluating for skin breaks, nodules, and rashes, which may be clues to the diagnosis. Petechiae may be another clue.

3. **EENT.** Conjunctivae may demonstrate injection or even splinter hemorrhages in endocarditis. Fundi and disk margins should be examined. EENT exam should include pneumatic otoscopy (otitis media is overdiagnosed) and clinical exam of the sinuses.

4. **Lymph nodes, organomegaly.** Generalized disorders often include generalized adenopathy and enlargement of liver spleen, or both. Regional lymph node enlargement may be a clue to disorders such as cat-scratch disease.

5. **Chest and lungs.** Changes in breath sounds or adventitious sounds may confirm a localized process.

6. **Heart.** A new murmur may be a result of infection or a disorder such as rheumatic fever.

7. **Abdomen and perianal area.** Assess for pain, masses, and bowel sounds. Patients with a previously ruptured, walled-off appendix may present with prolonged fever and diarrhea. Regional enteritis commonly involves the anus; skin tags and fissures may be clues.

8. **Extremities, bones, back.** A search for localized tenderness may be critical to making a correct diagnosis. Be certain to examine the spine for flexibility and paraspinous muscle spasm.

B. Laboratory Data

1. **Cultures.** Be certain that key cultures (usually blood, urine, throat, and occasionally stool or local lesions) have been taken for analysis.

2. **Screening tests.** Several studies have documented that inflammatory markers are strong evidence of more serious causes of prolonged fever: **increased ESR, elevated C-reactive protein,** and **low albumin with reversal of the albumin–globulin ratio.** These tend to be sensitive but not specific for serious disorders. Patients without markers of chronic inflammation

may warrant observation rather than intense investigation. Although a specific diagnosis is usually not made, **CBC with platelets and comprehensive metabolic profile** should be ordered for most patients, especially to screen renal and hepatic function.

3. **Titers.** Several disorders are best diagnosed with antibody titers (eg, Lyme disease, Epstein-Barr infection, tularemia, cat-scratch disease). If these are likely diagnoses, titers should be sent rapidly because paired titers may be necessary.

4. **Bone marrow exam.** Should not be routine, except perhaps in immunocompromised patients. If there are reductions in at least two cell lines from a CBC, marrow exam may be useful to look for malignancy.

C. **Radiographic and Other Studies.** Radiology consultation is extremely useful when making decisions about the best imaging test.

1. **Chest x-ray.**
2. **Bone scan.** Useful with localized tenderness.
3. **CT scan.** May be useful, especially when there are localized findings in areas such as chest, abdomen, bones, and CNS. Routine use of CT scan in all patients without localizing findings is not useful and may give misleading information.
4. **Leukocyte tagged scans.** Occasionally useful to localize infection, but there are reports of false-negative results.
5. **MRI scan.** Rapidly becoming the most useful test to evaluate certain areas (eg, bone, spine, and CNS).

V. **Plan.** Treatment is based on whether or not patient has an identifiable condition. Inflammatory markers help clinician to decide whether further extensive testing is necessary. Even when present, at times there must be a period of watchful waiting and repeat examination, seeking additional information from history or physical exam.

A. **Pursue Clues, Only.** Most clinicians approach patients with FUO by random testing (x-rays, CT scans, etc) without any clear information as to a possible diagnosis.

B. **Seek Additional Information From History and Exam.** This is clinician's strength: New data may lead to the correct diagnosis. Examples may be new exposures, hearing a new murmur, a new skin rash.

C. **Use Laboratory Wisely.** Repeat cultures may be helpful. Blood may be sent for additional titers or for "vasculitis" screens (eg, ANCA).

VI. **Problem Case Diagnosis.** Patient had an increased ESR, low albumin, and negative throat, blood, urine, and stool cultures as an outpatient. He had mild abdominal pain at onset, which was improving. Additional history revealed exposure to a neighbor's new kitten. Physical exam uncovered several resolving old papules on the right arm where he had been scratched, as well as axillary adenopathy. Sonogram and abdominal CT scan, performed because of initial abdominal pain, showed typical granulomatous lesions in the liver. Titers for *Bartonella henselae* were strongly positive, confirming a diagnosis of systemic cat-scratch disease.

VII. Teaching Pearl: Question. A patient presents with generalized adenopathy and fever of 8 days' duration. The patient had periorbital edema early in the illness and now has splenomegaly and mild hepatitis. What diagnosis should be considered?

VIII. Teaching Pearl: Answer. Periorbital edema is seen occasionally in infectious mononucleosis and is known as Hoagland sign. Mild hepatitis is seen almost universally in the 2nd week of illness.

REFERENCES

Gartner JC Jr. Fever of unknown origin. *Adv Pediatr Infect Dis* 1992;7:1–4.
Miller M, Szer I, Yogev, R, Bernstein B. Fever of unknown origin. *Pediatr Clin North Am* 1999;42:999–1015.

29. FOREIGN BODY: GASTROINTESTINAL TRACT

I. Problem. A 2-year-old boy old is brought to the physician's office 1 hour after a gagging episode. His mother states that he has had some difficulty swallowing, has been acting normally, but is not interested in drinking or eating. The boy is unwilling to open his mouth for his mother.

II. Immediate Questions

A. Is there a history of gagging, drooling, vomiting, sore throat, or dysphagia? Many of these symptoms indicate the presence of a foreign body in the GI tract.

B. Is patient refusing food? All of these symptoms could point to an esophageal foreign body.

C. Is there a history of midepigastric or chest pain? Lodging of a foreign body in the esophagus can lead to abdominal and chest pain.

D. Does patient have shortness of breath, coughing, or wheezing? If the object is compressing the trachea, these respiratory symptoms would be expected.

E. Were symptoms sudden in onset? The timing can be helpful in identifying a discrete event.

F. Is fever associated with the pain? These symptoms may indicate perforation, which is a very rare complication of foreign body ingestion.

G. Was the foreign body ingestion witnessed? Some patients with known foreign body ingestion are *asymptomatic*. In 30–40% of cases, patients with esophageal foreign bodies present without symptoms.

   H. What is the foreign body? Common foreign bodies in children are coins, bones, pins, pencils, crayons, batteries, buttons, marbles, and paper clips. Food impactions occur most often with meat. Coins account for the majority of esophageal foreign bodies.

   I. Does patient have a history of GI dysmotility? Dysmotility disorder can mimic or be caused by foreign body ingestions.

   J. Is there a history of esophageal strictures? Strictures could be due to a caustic ingestion or follow repair of esophageal atresia or tracheoesophageal fistula.

III. Differential Diagnosis
   A. Pharyngitis. Causes sore throat, dysphagia, and drooling in some cases. Often the pharynx is injected with exudates.
   B. Gastroenteritis. May present with abdominal cramping and vomiting.
   C. Gingivostomatitis. Usually presents with oral pain, drooling, and anorexia.
   D. Airway foreign body. May compress the esophagus, leading to painful swallowing and dysphagia.

IV. Database
   A. Physical Exam Key Points
      1. ABCs. Assess airway, breathing, and circulation first.
      2. General appearance and vital signs. Often normal if the foreign body has passed beyond the proximal esophagus.
      3. Oropharynx. May reveal excoriations or bloody streaks resulting from the ingested foreign body.
      4. Neck. Swelling, redness, or crepitus of the neck may be present if there is esophageal perforation.
      5. Lungs. If the foreign body is compressing the trachea, stridor or wheezing may be present. Asymmetric breath sounds may be auscultated.
      6. Abdomen. Evaluate for tenderness and signs of peritonitis.
   B. Laboratory Data. Not useful when considering a foreign body in the GI tract.
   C. Radiographic and Other Studies. The most important goal in treatment of any foreign body in the GI tract is *locating* the object.
      1. Plain chest x-ray. Obtain AP and lateral views; include the upper airway and upper stomach. These views usually indicate the location of the foreign body. Note that esophageal foreign bodies usually become lodged in one of three places in the esophagus: the thoracic inlet (60–80%), the level of the aortic arch (5–20%), and the gastroesophageal junction (10–20%). Coins are usually seen on edge on lateral films. Coins in the esophagus are seen in the coronal orientation, and coins in the

airway appear in the sagittal orientation. X-ray films will also determine the *number* of foreign bodies ingested.

2. **Abdominal x-ray.** Foreign bodies that have traversed the esophagus and are present in the stomach or intestines will be visualized on these views.

3. **Thin barium esophagogram.** Perform when a *radiolucent* foreign body is suspected (eg, plastic toys, glass, aluminum, pieces of wood).

4. **Hand-held metal detectors.** May be used as adjunctive tests in an initial screening to locate the foreign body. These devices should be operated by persons experienced in their use.

V. Plan

A. Support ABCs.

B. Determine Whether Foreign Body Should Be Removed

1. **Esophageal foreign body.** Foreign bodies located in the upper third of the esophagus should be removed within 12 hours. For objects located in the middle third of the esophagus, an x-ray should be repeated within 12–24 hours. A sharp object in the esophagus raises the risk of perforation and becomes a medical emergency.

   a. **Techniques for removal.** These techniques vary, depending on the nature of the foreign body. Coins may be removed by rigid endoscopy, Foley removal, or bougienage.

      i. **Rigid endoscopy.** Long the method of choice; usually occurs in the operating room under general anesthesia and is performed most often by an ENT surgeon or a gastroenterologist. It allows direct inspection of the esophagus to identify esophageal injury or unsuspected additional foreign bodies.

      ii. **Foley catheter method.** Usually performed under fluoroscopic guidance by a radiologist. The uninflated balloon end of the Foley catheter is inserted until it is located beyond the coin. The balloon is then inflated with contrast material and the coin is pulled upward into patient's mouth. This technique works best for round, smooth objects. It does not permit inspection of the esophagus and should be reserved for use in healthy children who have had uncomplicated coin ingestion. A concern about the balloon-tipped catheter technique is the lack of airway control.

      iii. **Bougienage.** The least commonly used procedure for coin removal. A lubricated esophageal dilator is passed into the esophagus, dislodging the coin and causing it to pass into the stomach. This technique should be reserved for use in healthy children who were seen ingesting a single foreign body.

2. **Nonesophageal foreign body**

    a. Stomach. Foreign bodies in the stomach should be removed immediately when they are causing symptoms of abdominal pain, obstruction, or vomiting. Sewing needles have a propensity to perforate, and removal is usually recommended. Long foreign bodies (> 5 cm) should also be removed from the stomach. Foreign bodies that remain in the stomach usually require no acute intervention. Parents can be reassured that 98% of stomach foreign bodies are expelled per rectum. If a sharp object is found in the stomach, vigilance may be all that is required if the child is asymptomatic.

    b. Intestine. If at the time of evaluation, a long foreign body has passed into the small intestine, serial abdominal x-rays may be indicated. Smooth, round foreign bodies usually pass through the GI tract within 1 week. Asking parents to search child's stools for evidence of the foreign body is a controversial approach, as parents may discontinue the task before the foreign body is retrieved.

  3. Disc batteries. Disc button batteries, such as those found in watches, calculators, toys, and hearing aids, are a relatively new cause of GI ingestion. Disc batteries can be distinguished from coins radiographically. In the AP projection, a battery appears as a double-density shadow and in the lateral projection, the edges are rounded and reveal a step-off at the junction of the anode and cathode. Several types of disc batteries may cause corrosive injury to the mucosa; however, most ingestions of disc batteries are benign. A disc battery located in the esophagus should be removed immediately. Once the battery reaches the stomach; however, it is likely to pass through the remainder of the GI tract without complication, thus requiring no intervention.

 C. Medications. Historically, it had been suggested that medications such as glucagon and diazepam could be used to enhance motility or to relax the lower esophageal sphincter. Guidelines about the use of these medications are lacking due to limited investigation.

VI. Problem Case Diagnosis. Plain chest x-ray confirmed the diagnosis of an esophageal foreign body, revealing a coin at the level of the thoracic outlet in this 2-year-old boy. Because of the symptoms produced and the location of the foreign body, the coin was removed.

VII. Teaching Pearl: Question. Do clinical features of stridor, wheezing, and dysphagia indicate a foreign body in an airway rather than in the GI tract?

VIII. Teaching Pearl: Answer. Upper esophageal foreign bodies can present with stridor, wheezing, and dysphagia.

REFERENCES

Chen MK, Beierle EA. Gastrointestinal foreign bodies. *Pediatr Ann* 2001;30:736–742.

Connors GP. A literature-based comparison of three methods of pediatric esophageal coins removal. *Pediatr Emerg Care* 1997;13:154–157.

Ruben CW, Liacouras CA. Evaluation and Management of foreign bodies in the upper gastrointestinal tract. *Pediatr Case Rev* 2003;3:150–156.

Wyllie R. Foreign bodies and bezoars. In: Behrman RE, Kliegman RM, Jenson HB, eds. *Nelson Textbook of Pediatrics,* 17th ed. Saunders, 2004:1244.

30. FOREIGN BODY: RESPIRATORY TRACT

I. **Problem.** A 2-year-old girl has had a cough for the past 3 weeks. Her mother recalls an episode of "choking" several weeks ago, but her daughter seemed fine right after the episode and she has noticed no drooling since. There is no history of fever.

II. **Immediate Questions**
   A. **Did patient eat anything before or during the choking episode?** Food items are the most commonly aspirated foreign bodies in the pediatric population. The foods most often responsible for choking in this age group are hot dogs, grapes, peanuts, and popcorn.
   B. **Did patient play with any small toys prior to the choking episode?** Nonfood items that are aspirated include balloons, toys, and coins. Balloons comprise one third of the foreign bodies that are not food. Many nonfood foreign bodies are nonradiopaque.
   C. **Does patient have dysphagia?** If the foreign body is lodged in the larynx, there could be associated laryngeal swelling compressing the esophagus and leading to dysphagia.
   D. **Is there a cough?** Cough is present in > 90% of cases. It is usually abrupt in onset but can become quiescent after the initial choking episode. Cough can recur if the foreign body is mobile. Persistent cough and fever may indicate a long-standing retained bronchial foreign body.
   E. **Is stridor present?** Stridor suggests upper airway obstruction due to inflammation, infection, or foreign body aspiration.
   F. **What is the character of the cough?** Often if the foreign body is retained in the larynx, there will be a croupy cough and hoarseness. The cough may also be paroxysmal.
   G. **Does patient have a history of upper airway stenosis?** Stenotic lesions from previous intubations or tracheal surgery predispose to specific areas of lodging of the foreign bodies.

III. **Differential Diagnosis**
   A. **Upper Respiratory Infection.** May cause significant upper airway congestion and cough. Etiology is usually viral, and chest exam, normal.

   B. Esophageal Foreign Body Ingestion. May be associated with
      hoarseness or dysphagia, or both, as well as drooling. Lung exam
      is normal.
   C. Retropharyngeal Cellulitis or Abscess. May present with fever,
      cough, and drooling. Lung exam is normal, but there may be stri-
      dor.
   D. Croup. Presents with a barking cough and stridor. Lung fields are
      clear.
   E. Reactive Airway Disease. May present with diffuse or focal
      wheezing.
   F. Bronchiolitis. Presents with diffuse or unilateral wheezing in
      association with preceding symptoms of an upper respiratory
      infection.
   G. Pneumonia. Often presents with a persistent cough and fever.
      Exam may reveal decreased breath sounds or focal rales.

IV. Database
   A. Physical Exam Key Points
      1. ABCs. Assess airway, breathing, and circulation immediately.
         In children, foreign bodies are much more often located in a
         bronchus than in the trachea.
      2. General appearance and vital signs. Crucial when assess-
         ing child who may have aspirated a foreign body. Patients with
         foreign bodies in the upper airway may present with acute res-
         piratory failure and cyanosis if there is total obstruction of the
         larynx.
      3. Upper airway. If there is a partial obstruction of the upper
         airway, patient may demonstrate respiratory distress, including
         stridor.
      4. Lungs. Look for retractions and an increased respiratory rate.
         Foreign bodies in the lower airway generally present with
         wheezing that is localized in the early phases. Wheezing may
         become bilateral as time elapses. Lung exam may demonstrate
         rales, rhonchi, and retractions. There may only be subtle differ-
         ences in air entry heard with the stethoscope.
   B. Laboratory Data. There is no role for laboratory studies when
      considering a foreign body in the respiratory tract.
   C. Radiographic and Other Studies
      1. Plain chest x-ray. In suspected lower airway foreign body
         aspirations, this should be the first x-ray ordered. It frequently
         reveals unilateral aeration disturbance such as air trapping
         ("ball-valve" phenomenon), atelectasis (complete obstruction),
         or consolidation. Many foreign bodies are not visualized on
         plain x-rays because they are nonradiopaque, but the afore-
         mentioned findings will suggest aspiration.
      2. Inspiratory and expiratory films. May be required if plain film
         is not revealing. Often these additional films show unilateral air

trapping. In young children who cannot cooperate for these views, **lateral decubitus films** are a helpful adjunct. With an obstructed lung, the air that is trapped prevents the lung from collapsing and it does not become smaller in the dependent decubitus position.

3. **Fluoroscopic airway exam.** Rarely required, but if so, it can be diagnostic if differential ventilation of the lungs causes mediastinal shifting during respiration.

4. **Soft tissue lateral neck x-ray.** Indicated if an upper airway foreign body is suspected. Radiopaque objects are readily seen. Complications of nonradiopaque foreign bodies may be visualized.

5. **Endoscopy (laryngoscope, bronchoscopy).** Useful for diagnosis and treatment. Ideally should be performed during the day with pediatric airway specialists present.

V. **Plan**

A. **Support ABCs.** If complete airway obstruction is suspected, basic life support (BLS) measures should be started.

B. **Complete Airway Obstruction**

1. Begin bag-valve-mask ventilation immediately after airway positioning. If patient cannot be adequately ventilated, immediately initiate the Heimlich maneuver in children older than 1 year or age or use back blows and chest thrusts in infants.

2. If these measures fail to dislodge the foreign body, it may be necessary to visualize the foreign body and extract it. If appropriate equipment is available, attempt direct visualization of the oropharynx with a laryngoscope. Use caution to avoid pushing the foreign body further into the airway, leading to complete obstruction. Most foreign bodies are located at the base of the tongue. If the foreign body is visualized, a Magill forceps should be used to extract it.

C. **Lower Airway Foreign Body.** If suspected, the radiographic workup should begin promptly. If a foreign body is discovered peripherally, bronchoscopy must be performed to remove it. Child should have nothing by mouth in preparation for the procedure. If there is an associated pneumonia, appropriate antibiotics are indicated.

VI. **Problem Case Diagnosis.** The 2-year-old patient had aspirated a Barbie doll shoe. A chest x-ray revealed right middle lobe air trapping without pneumonia. The object was removed from the right mainstem bronchus using bronchoscopy.

VII. **Teaching Pearl: Question.** Is it true that most respiratory foreign bodies in children are located in the right mainstem bronchus?

VIII. **Teaching Pearl: Answer.** There is only a slight preponderance of right bronchial foreign bodies in young children.

REFERENCES

Holinger LD. Foreign bodies of the airway. In: Behrman RE, Kliegman RM, Jenson HB, eds. *Nelson Textbook of Pediatrics,* 17th ed. Saunders, 2004:1410–1411.

Poirer MP, Ruddy RM. Acute upper airway foreign body removal: The choking child. In: Henretig FM, King C, eds. *Textbook of Pediatric Emergency Procedures.* Williams & Wilkins, 1997:621–627.

Stenklyft PH, Cataletto ME, Lee BS. The pediatric airway in health and disease. In: Gausche-Hill M, Fuch S, Yamamoto L, eds. *APLS: The Pediatric Emergency Resource,* 4th ed. Jones & Bartlett, 2004:64–66.

Swischuck LE, ed. Foreign bodies in the lower airway. In: *Emergency Imaging of the Acutely Ill or Injured Child,* 4th ed. Lippincott Williams & Wilkins, 2000:88–94.

31. GASTROINTESTINAL BLEEDING: LOWER TRACT

I. **Problem.** A 1-month-old infant is brought to the emergency department because his parents have noticed blood in the diaper.

II. **Immediate Questions**

A. **What are the current vital signs and appearance of patient?** Vital signs and appearance provide an indication of patient's hemodynamic stability. Age-adjusted tachycardia is the most sensitive indicator of severe bleeding. Are parents able to quantify and describe the blood seen in the diaper? Has this been an acute or chronic process?

B. **Are there symptoms of an acute abdominal process (eg, pain, distention, vomiting, lethargy)?** Painful rectal bleeding is often seen in patients with infectious, inflammatory, or ischemic causes. Pain, vomiting, and small amounts of blood in stool should raise suspicion of bowel obstruction. Intussusception, intestinal volvulus and malrotation, and necrotizing enterocolitis are important diagnoses to consider early in evaluation.

C. **Is there a history of recent diarrheal illness? What is patient's normal bowel pattern?** Rectal fissures can be caused by either diarrhea or constipation.

D. **What is patient's current dietary history?** Brief dietary history should include information about weight loss, feeding intolerance, or multiple formula changes. All may be suggestive of allergic colitis.

E. **If school-aged, has patient had any extraintestinal manifestations?** Symptoms such as rash, arthralgias, anorexia, and weight loss are all indicative of inflammatory bowel disease, although this condition is rarely diagnosed before age 5 years.

F. **Any recent medications or ingestions?** Recent antibiotic exposure raises the possibility of *Clostridium difficile*–associated colitis.

G. **Does patient have any underlying medical conditions?** Brief past medical history should include information about previous bleeding, liver disease, or coagulation disorder. Also ask about family history of bleeding diathesis, familial polyposis, or inflammatory bowel disease.

III. Differential Diagnosis

A. **Necrotizing Enterocolitis.** It is important to exclude this diagnosis in infants. Condition is most commonly seen in preterm infants with rectal bleeding, feeding intolerance, and systemic instability, but 10% of cases occur in full-term infants. Antenatal exposure to maternal cocaine and formula feeding are risk factors.

B. **Obstructive Lesions.** Include Hirschsprung disease, intestinal volvulus and malrotation, and ileocolic intussusception. Pain or irritability can indicate ischemia. Children with Hirschsprung disease present with abdominal distention and difficulty stooling and are occasionally septic looking. Patients with intestinal volvulus and malrotation may have a history of bilious emesis, irritability, and blood streaks in stool. Ileocolic intussusception classically presents with cyclic abdominal pain, lethargy, and current-jelly stools, but patient may have only altered mental status (ie, withdrawal, disinterestedness) and occult blood in the stool.

C. **Milk-Protein Allergy.** Affects approximately 2% of infants younger than 2 years of age. Clinical spectrum ranges from immediate-type reactions, including urticaria and angioedema, to intermediate and late-onset reactions, such as atopic dermatitis, gastroesophageal reflux, enterocolitis, and proctitis.

D. **Anorectal Fissure.** The most common proctologic disorder during infancy and childhood. Most cases occur in infants younger than 1 year of age. May be associated with diarrhea, causing perineal irritation, but more commonly is associated with constipation. Recurrent fissures or perianal excoriation are associated with perianal β-hemolytic *Streptococcus* and pinworm infections.

E. **Infectious Enterocolitis.** Bacterial causes include *Salmonella, Shigella, Campylobacter, Yersinia enterocolitica, C difficile,* and *Escherichia coli. Entamoeba histolytica* and *Giardia* are important parasitic pathogens. Opportunistic infections in immune-compromised hosts include cytomegalovirus, *Mycobacterium avium* complex, and disseminated aspergillosis.

F. **Vasculitis.** Henoch-Schönlein purpura (HSP) and hemolytic uremic syndrome (HUS) are common vasculitides in children. HSP typically consists of purpuric rash of buttocks and lower extremities, arthralgias, angioedema, and acute abdominal pain. GI symptoms, including abdominal pain, occult bleeding, massive bleeding, and intussusception, may precede dermatologic findings. Hematuria also can be present. HUS classically presents with a triad of microangiopathic hemolytic anemia, thrombocytopenia, and oliguric renal failure. One of the many complications of HUS is colitis causing melena and possibly perforation. The cause is unknown.

G. Inflammatory Bowel Disease. Ulcerative colitis or Crohn disease must be considered in older children or adolescents who present with rectal bleeding. Search for extraintestinal manifestations, as noted earlier.

H. Structural Anomaly, Intestinal Duplication, or Meckel Diverticulum. Often presents with painless rectal bleeding. Occasionally can be lead point of intussusception.

I. Vascular Lesions. Include angiodysplasia, hemorrhoids, hemangiomas, and arteriovenous malformations. Such lesions are rare causes of bleeding in children.

J. Polyps. The most common forms are hamartomatous and adenomatous polyps. Hamartomatous polyps are benign and are associated with juvenile polyps, juvenile polyposis coli, and Peutz-Jeghers syndrome. Adenomatous polyps are potentially premalignant and are associated with familial adenomatous polyposis and Gardner syndrome.

K. Coagulopathy. Consider hemorrhagic disease of newborn, a coagulation defect, or disseminated intravascular coagulation as a possible cause of bleeding. Bleeding caused by a coagulopathy is not limited to the GI tract.

L. Tumors. Occur rarely in children, although leiomyoma and histiocytosis have been described.

M. Ingestions. Foreign body ingestions are common in toddlers; considerations include glass or rectal thermometers. Ingested medications (antibiotics, bismuth, or iron) and foods (commercial dyes and certain vegetables) can mimic the appearance of blood.

IV. Database
A. Physical Exam Key Points
1. **General appearance.** Does child appear acutely ill? Does child demonstrate pallor and lethargy, indicating significant blood loss?
2. **Vital signs.** Tachycardia is the most sensitive indicator of severe bleeding. A positive orthostatic change is a decrease in systolic BP of 10 mm Hg or an increase of 20 beats/min in pulse, indicating a 10–20% loss of intravascular fluid volume. Hypotension is a late finding and demands immediate resuscitation with fluids (compatible blood if available).
3. **Abdomen.** This is a critical component of physical exam. Assess for signs of obstruction or ischemia, as evidenced by tenderness, distention, peritoneal signs, or mass. Always consider age of patient in relation to physical findings. A mass in the right lower quadrant in a toddler suggests intussusception but in an older child is more likely to indicate inflammatory bowel disease.
4. **Rectum.** Rectal exam is important in the evaluation of rectal bleeding. Eversion of anal mucosa may reveal a rectal fissure

or polyp. Perianal skin tags suggest Crohn disease. Rectal polyps may be palpated on digital exam. Stool in the rectal vault should be tested for occult blood.

5. **Skin.** Eczema is seen in association with milk-protein allergy. Cutaneous hemangioma or telangiectasia suggests internal vascular anomalies. Petechia or bruising may suggest liver disease or coagulopathy. Purpura is seen with the vasculitis of HSP. Erythema nodosum frequently is found with inflammatory bowel disease.

6. **Extremities.** Examine for joint swelling or erythema, which can be seen with inflammatory bowel disease.

B. Laboratory Data

1. **Type and crossmatch.** Indicated for significant blood loss.

2. **Guaiac test for occult blood.** Is patient really bleeding? Many substances ingested by children, including red food coloring and iron supplements, look like blood.

3. **CBC.** Stable hematocrit can give clinician a false sense of security. Hematocrit declines only after extravascular fluid enters the intravascular space. A significant drop may not occur for hours.

4. **PT and PTT.** The first steps in evaluation of a primary coagulopathy or disseminated intravascular coagulation.

5. **Liver transaminases.** Indicated if clinician suspects liver failure as the cause of a clotting abnormality.

6. **Serum electrolytes, BUN, creatinine.** Obtain, along with urinalysis, if HUS is strongly suspected.

7. **Stool studies.** Include bacterial culture, *C difficile* toxin assay, and Wright stain (to demonstrate eosinophils seen in allergic colitis), if suggested clinically.

C. Radiographic and Other Studies

1. **Colonoscopy.** The preferred study for significant rectal bleeding.

2. **Abdominal x-ray.** May provide useful information if pain or vomiting is present. Include supine and upright (or lateral decubitus) views to check for air fluid levels indicative of obstruction. Pneumoperitoneum or focal bowel wall thickening are indicative of colitis. A distorted bowel gas pattern may suggest a mass effect.

3. **Air contrast or barium enema.** Necessary in the evaluation and treatment of intussusception.

4. **CT or MRI scan.** Usually indicated for evaluation of a mass lesion or vascular lesion.

5. **Angiography or scintigraphy.** May be used to locate obscure sites of bleeding or Meckel diverticulum.

V. Plan

A. Initial Management

1. In the face of hemodynamic instability, aggressive fluid resuscitation is started with initial evaluation. If patient demonstrates tachycardia or orthostatic changes, infuse 20 mL/kg of normal saline or Ringer lactate solution (or compatible blood when available) and reassess.

2. Verify that substance is actually blood using guaiac test. In patients with significant bleeding, perform gastric lavage to rule out upper GI bleeding. Infants have rapid gastric emptying time, so upper GI bleeding can present as blood in the diaper. A negative aspirate does not rule out upper tract bleeding; up to 10% of patients with duodenal ulcers can have a negative gastric aspirate.

3. Obtain samples for laboratory analysis based on clinical presentation. In a healthy infant with a few streaks of blood, stool culture and observation is acceptable. If suspicious of significant GI bleeding, immediately obtain type and cross-match, CBC, PT, and PTT.

4. If suspicious of an obstructive lesion, order flat and upright abdominal films. Proceed as needed to additional imaging studies and surgical consultation.

5. Patients who have undergone significant volume loss with vital sign changes should undergo endoscopy as soon as bleeding is controlled. Avoid use of contrast if endoscopy is planned because it may obscure mucosal lesions.

B. **Specific Therapies**
   1. Treatment is directed at underlying problem. Allergic colitis is managed with hydrolyzed formula. Necrotizing enterocolitis is managed with supportive care. Appropriate antibiotics, most notably metronidazole, are used in treatment of *C difficile* colitis. Immunosuppressive agents are used in management of inflammatory bowel disease; they have also been successful in patients with rapidly proliferating hemangiomas.
   2. **Endoscopic Therapy.** Most common indication for this therapy is polypectomy; it is also used for sclerotherapy, electrocautery, and elastic band ligation.
   3. **Surgery.** Reserved for nonreducible intussusception, vascular anomaly, and structural lesions.

VI. **Problem Case Diagnosis.** The 1-month-old patient appeared well, with normal vital signs. Parents described streaks of bright red blood on formed stool with each diaper change. Child was consuming cow's milk formula without any evidence of intolerance or emesis. Physical exam was completely benign. Presence of blood was confirmed with guaiac test. CBC was normal, but stool was positive for eosinophils. Diagnosis is allergic colitis; a hydrolyzed formula is recommended.

VII. Teaching Pearl: Question. What is the most common cause of lower GI bleeding in children younger than 1 year of age compared with those older than 1 year?

VIII. Teaching Pearl: Answer. Allergic colitis and anorectal fissure are frequent diagnoses in children younger than 1 year of age. Infectious gastroenteritis and anorectal fissures are common diagnoses in children older than 1 year. Painless rectal bleeding is more common with vascular malformation, polyp, or Meckel diverticulum. Painful rectal bleeding is seen with infectious, inflammatory, or ischemic lesions. Inflammatory bowel disease is rarely diagnosed before the age of 5 years.

REFERENCES

Fleisher GR, Ludwig S. *Textbook of Pediatric Emergency Medicine,* 4th ed. Lippincott Williams & Wilkins, 2000.

Fox VL. High risk, underappreciated, obscure, or preventable causes of gastrointestinal bleeding: Gastrointestinal bleeding in infancy and childhood. *Gastroenterol Clin* 2000;29:37–66.

Lawrence WW, Lawrence W, Wright JL, Cheng TL. Causes of rectal bleeding in children. *Pediatr Rev* 2001;22:394–395.

Squires RH. Gastrointestinal bleeding. *Pediatr Rev* 1999;20:95–111.

32. GASTROINTESTINAL BLEEDING: UPPER TRACT

I. Problem. A 2-month-old infant is brought to the emergency department by his parents, who state that he "just spit up blood."

II. Immediate Questions

A. Are parents able to quantify amount of bleeding? Would parents estimate blood loss as a spoonful, cupful, or more? Were there blood streaks or coffee-ground material in emesis? Was there frank bright red blood? Estimated volume of blood loss should be correlated with child's clinical condition. If required, initiate fluid resuscitation immediately.

B. Does patient appear to be in pain? Pain suggests an inflammatory or ischemic lesion. Causes needing urgent care include an obstructive lesion or abdominal trauma resulting in ischemia or massive hemorrhage. Bleeding into the biliary tract after abdominal trauma can also produce right upper quadrant pain and jaundice.

C. Was the substance truly blood? Was it the patient's blood? Many foods ingested by children mimic the appearance of blood. Food coloring is contained in fruit juices and gelatins. Breast-feeding infants may swallow maternal blood from cracked nipples.

D. Is bleeding coming from GI system? Does patient have any history of nasopharyngeal trauma, chronic nasal congestion, or epistaxis? Swallowed nasopharyngeal bleeding from trauma or mucosal ulceration can cause hematemesis.

E. Was there a possible ingestion? Does patient regularly take medication(s)? Possible ingestions resulting in mucosal irritation include NSAIDs, aspirin, theophylline, steroids, batteries, and alcohol. In toddlers or mentally handicapped patients, consider the possibility of a foreign body.

F. Are there any other concurrent sites of bleeding (rectal, oral mucous, urinary tract, bruising)? Rule out a systemic problem such as coagulopathy or disseminated intravascular coagulation.

G. What is the past medical history? Is there any history of umbilical artery catheterization, sepsis, previous episodes of bleeding from the GI tract or other sites; any past hematologic disorders or liver disease?

III. Differential Diagnosis. Always consider patient's age.

    A. Swallowed Maternal Blood. Relatively common occurrence in infants during delivery or after breast-feeding from mother's irritated nipple. Common presentation is a well-appearing infant with hematemesis.

    B. Gastritis or Ulcer. Causes in children are multifactorial and not completely understood. Can occur in a stressed preterm or a healthy term infant. May be related to maternal medications (eg, tolazoline, α-adrenergic agonists, or NSAIDs). Maternal cocaine use also can be a risk factor. Ingesting certain medications, including aspirin, NSAIDs, and steroids, is a risk factor. Hemodynamically significant GI bleeding can result from standard dosing of NSAIDs. Parents may not consider these as "medications," so ask specifically about their use. Stresses, including surgery, burns, increased intracranial pressure, or sepsis, can cause gastritis or ulceration. Other causes include mucosal irritation from milk-protein allergy, a lodged foreign body, gastrostomy tubes, or infection (*Haemophilus pylori*).

    C. Esophagitis. Can result from gastroesophageal reflux disease (GERD). Children with bleeding esophagitis as a result of GERD are more likely to have a neuromuscular disease or hiatal hernia. Other causes of esophagitis include mechanical injury by a foreign body, chemical injury from caustic ingestion, medication (pill esophagitis), or infection (*Candida albicans, Aspergillus,* herpes simplex virus, cytomegalovirus).

    D. Coagulation Disorders. Hemorrhagic disease of the newborn is rarely seen today because vitamin K administration at birth has become routine. Risk factors include altered bowel flora as a result of antibiotics or fat malabsorption (ie, cystic fibrosis). A coagulopathy can occur as a primary defect of the coagulation cascade (ie, hemophilia) or secondary to liver disease or disseminated intravascular coagulation as a result of overwhelming infection.

E. Varices. Variceal bleeding is rare in infancy, although gastroesophageal varices associated with portal hypertension are the most common cause of significant GI bleeding in older children. Gastroesophageal varices form in children with intrahepatic or extrahepatic causes of portal hypertension; rarely in association with congenital heart disease or vascular malformations. Portal vein thrombosis is a common cause of extrahepatic obstruction. Risk factors include omphalitis, history of umbilical vein cannulation, and dehydration. Intrahepatic portal hypertension is caused by hepatic parenchymal disorders. More common associated diagnoses include biliary cirrhosis with biliary atresia, hepatitis, congenital hepatic fibrosis, α_1-antitrypsin deficiency, and cystic fibrosis.

F. Structural Anomalies. Include hypertrophic pyloric stenosis, duodenal web, and antral web. These anomalies usually present with emesis but may be associated with bleeding. GI duplication can occur anywhere in the intestinal tract, but it is most commonly found in the small bowel. These patients usually present with signs of GI tract obstruction and abdominal mass.

G. Vascular Anomalies. A rare cause of GI bleeding. These anomalies include focal lesions (hemangiomas or Dieulafoy lesion) or more diffuse lesions (hereditary hemorrhagic telangiectasia or Kasabach-Merritt syndrome).

H. Oropharyngeal Causes. Include epistaxis, facial trauma, and tooth extraction, resulting in swallowed blood.

I. Mallory-Weiss Tears. These mucosal lacerations of gastric mucosa are caused by significant vomiting.

IV. Database

A. Physical Exam Key Points

1. **Vital signs and general appearance.** Used to assess patient's hemodynamic condition. A child may lose up to 15% of body fluid volume without significant hemodynamic change. Tachycardia is the first cardiovascular change seen.

2. **Head and neck.** Visualize posterior nose and pharynx to exclude epistaxis. Examine for scleral icterus for possible liver disease. Periorbital petechiae suggest vigorous vomiting associated with Mallory-Weiss tear.

3. **Abdomen.** Presence of distention, absence of bowel sounds, or peritoneal findings are associated with ischemic or obstructive lesions. Hepatosplenomegaly and ascites suggest chronic liver disease or failure. Epigastric tenderness may be elicited with gastroesophageal ulcerations.

4. **Skin.** Prominent abdominal venous pattern or spider nevi suggest liver disease; cutaneous hemangiomas may suggest an underlying vascular malformation.

B. Laboratory Data

1. **Fecal occult blood test (Gastroccult).** Will determine whether substance is actually blood.
2. **Apt-Downey test.** Differentiates fetal hemoglobin from maternal hemoglobin, identifying whether blood comes from infant or mother.
3. **Type and cross-match.** Indicated with significant hemorrhage.
4. **CBC.** Hematocrit is an unreliable indicator in acute blood loss, declining only after extravascular fluid enters the intravascular space. Low WBC and platelet counts may be seen in hypersplenism from portal hypertension and cancer. Microcytic anemia suggests chronic mucosal bleeding.
5. **Liver function panel.** Evaluates liver function and ability to produce coagulation factors.
6. **PT and PTT.** Used to evaluate coagulation cascade and liver function.
7. **Basic metabolic panel.** A BUN:creatinine ratio > 30 suggests blood resorption from the GI tract. Electrolyte abnormalities may be seen with hemolysis.

C. Radiographic and Other Studies

1. **Abdominal x-ray.** Useful if foreign body, bowel perforation, or bowel obstruction is suspected.
2. **Ultrasonography.** Helpful when liver disease, portal hypertension, or vascular anomalies are strong possibilities in differential diagnosis.
3. **Barium contrast.** Too insensitive to detect superficial mucosal lesions; may delay diagnosis because presence of contrast material in stomach and duodenum at the time of endoscopy can obscure the bleeding source.
4. **CT or MRI scan.** Useful for evaluation of mass lesions and vascular malformations.
5. **Upper GI endoscopy.** Diagnostic test of choice for significant bleeding because it has a high degree of sensitivity and allows for therapeutic intervention. Patients who have had significant volume loss with vital sign changes should undergo endoscopy as soon as bleeding is controlled. If endoscopy is planned, avoid use of contrast radiology.
6. **Angiography.** Consider when bleeding is so massive that it obscures the view via endoscopy; can be both diagnostic and therapeutic.
7. **Scintigraphy.** Rarely indicated except in cases of suspected enteric duplications or obscure bleeding sites.

V. Plan. Upper GI tract bleeding is defined as bleeding above the ligament of Treitz. Approximately 20% of all GI tract bleeding in children arises from this area. Children typically present with hematemesis, melena, or both. Children can also present with hematochezia because of their accelerated intestinal transit times, and because blood acts as a cathartic.

A. Initial Management. The primary focus should be stabilization of patient. Always address resuscitative efforts first in a child who shows hemodynamic compromise.

  1. First determine that vomited or excreted material actually contains blood. Many foods ingested by children may give the appearance of blood in stool or emesis, including many food colorings. This question can simply be answered with a fecal occult blood test. The Apt-Downey test can identify infants who may have swallowed maternal blood

  2. Obtain vital signs, including orthostatics and clinical condition of patient. Tachycardia is indicative of acute blood loss. A child with hemodynamic instability requires placement of a large-bore IV line and administration of normal saline or lactated Ringer solution in boluses of 20 mL/kg until compatible blood products are available or patient is stable.

  3. Patients with severe or significant GI bleeding

    a. Order immediate blood studies, including type and cross-match, CBC, PT and PTT, and electrolyte panel with liver function studies.

    b. Insert a nasogastric tube. Nasogastric aspirate that is positive for occult blood will differentiate upper GI from lower GI bleeding. If gastric contents clear following initial lavage, gastric irrigation can be performed every 15 minutes for 1 hour, and than every 2–3 hours to assess continued bleeding.

  4. Medications. Early use of antacid therapy and an H_2 antagonist is recommended because of the prevalence of peptic disease.

B. Recurrent Hemorrhage. Patients with significant and recurrent hemorrhage should undergo endoscopy. Medications, including vasopressin and octreotide, may be indicated to control active bleeding. Arteriographic embolization can be used in treatment of vascular anomalies.

VI. Problem Case Diagnosis. On arrival in the emergency department, infant appeared happy, playful, and in no apparent distress. Vital signs were within normal limits except for mild tachypnea. Upon questioning, parents indicated that infant had coughed up blood-tinged secretions earlier in the day, and they had been aggressively suctioning copious nasal secretions, which were also blood tinged. Infant had no history of feeding intolerance or previous bleeding. Physical exam was significant only for nasal mucosal inflammation and excoriation. Clinician suspects that this minimal amount of bleeding is secondary to swallowed epistaxis. As in this case, good history-taking and clinical exam can avert unnecessary workup in patients with minimal, self-limited bleeding.

VII. Teaching Pearl: Question. What are the five most common causes of upper GI bleeding in children?

VIII. Teaching Pearl: Answer. The most common causes of GI bleeding in children are (1) duodenal ulcer, (2) gastric ulcer, (3) esophagitis, (4) gastritis, and (5) varices.

REFERENCES

Fleisher GR, Ludwig S. *Textbook of Pediatric Emergency Medicine,* 4th ed. Lippincott Williams & Wilkins, 2000.

Fox VL. High-risk, underappreciated, obscure, or preventable causes of gastrointestinal bleeding: Gastrointestinal bleeding in infancy and childhood. *Gastroenterol Clin* 2000;29:37–66.

Rodgers BM. Upper gastrointestinal hemorrhage. *Pediatr Rev* 1999;20:171–176.

Squires RH. Gastrointestinal bleeding. *Pediatr Rev* 1999;20:95–111.

33. HEADACHE

I. Problem. A 12-year-old girl complains of severe headaches.

II. Immediate Questions

A. Is this an emergency, urgent, or routine clinical condition? Determine if care needs to be administered emergently. An emergency case requires the same attention to detail as does a routine case; however, the pace and order in which actions are completed differs. Remember the ABCs (airway, breathing, circulation).

B. Has patient had similar episodes before? If patient has a history of prior, similar events, it is much less likely this is an urgent medical or surgical condition.

C. How is headache described? Obtain a thorough description of the headache, related symptoms, and exacerbating and relieving factors, as well as symptoms prior to, during, and after episode(s). Obtain descriptions from child, parent, and a witness, if possible. Specific questions include:

1. If a recurrent problem, what is the usual duration of headache? When does it occur?

2. Are there any complaints associated with headache(s)? Any associated activities, such as involuntary motor movements, falling, or stiffening, with headache(s)?

3. What was patient doing before and after episode(s)?

4. Are there any precipitants to headache(s)? Any alleviating factors for headache(s)?

D. Pertinent Historical Information

1. What was the prenatal and neonatal course? May identify risks for long-term neurologic sequelae.

2. Were developmental milestones achieved at appropriate ages?
3. Any significant medical or surgical history, including head trauma?
4. Is there any family history of neurologic disorders? Current medical disorders?
5. Does patient take any medication(s)?

III. **Differential Diagnosis.** Differential diagnosis is broad. Many conditions can present with headaches, including intoxications, intracranial mass lesions, medical disorders, behavioral disorders, sleep disorders, and neurologic disorders.

A. **Migraines.** Migraines are the first group of disorders that most people think of when a child has recurrent headaches with photophobia, phonophobia, and nausea and or vomiting. Defined as recurrent headaches that vary widely in their intensity, frequency, and duration, migraines may be associated with typical features (aura, unilaterality, nausea, vomiting, and family history) in addition to a transient alteration of neurologic function (motor, sensory, or mood). Migraines are presumed to be related to vasospasm; however, they are most likely related to the effects of intracranial neurochemical release. There are two basic types: with and without aura (ie, a symptom perceived prior to onset of headache, often visual [scotoma]). Depending on the intracranial location of the migrainous event, patient may experience GI symptoms (anorexia, nausea, and vomiting), fear, unusual sensations (hallucinations), localized weakness (involving extremities or eyes), sensory changes, dizziness, or visual loss. Other forms of migraine include complicated (associated with neurologic deficit) and migraine variants with cyclic vomiting and benign paroxysmal vertigo.

B. **Headaches (Nonmigraine).** Idiopathic headaches have no identifiable etiology. Other headaches may be caused by intracranial mass lesions (neoplasm, abscess, stroke, vascular anomalies), subarachnoid hemorrhage (ruptured aneurysm), head trauma, infections (sinusitis, meningitis, or encephalitis), toxicity, or ingestion (antibiotics, steroids, carbon monoxide, cocaine, amphetamines, alcohol). Withdrawal of certain medications (barbiturates, caffeine, acetaminophen, ibuprofen, narcotics, SSRIs, indomethacin) can also cause headaches. Headaches can occur after a seizure, as a result of pseudotumor cerebri, or a cerebral or vertebral artery dissection.

C. **Tension-Type Headache.** The probable cause of common headache. Results from muscle tension in scalp muscles, which produces a bilateral "bandlike" squeezing sensation around the head. Pain is located in regions of the head with muscles—frontal, temporal, and occipital—and can last from minutes to days.

D. Chronic Daily Headache. Extremely frequent form of tension-type headache. Occurs at least 20 days per month. Patients can often recall the exact date of onset of these frequent and bothersome headaches.

E. Cluster Headaches. Severe, unilateral headaches classically associated with ipsilateral nasal congestion, conjunctival injection, and lacrimation. Pain is severe but limited to less than 2 hours' duration. Can be treated with inhaled oxygen.

F. Associated Oral and Facial Disorders. Includes trigeminal neuralgia, sometimes caused by dental abscesses; sinus disease; temporomandibular joint dysfunction or malocclusion; glaucoma; and uveitis.

G. Sleep Disorders. Insufficient or inefficient sleep may result in headaches, excessive daytime sleepiness, and cognitive and behavioral phenomena. Can be an isolated diagnosis or a complication of other medical conditions, including obstructive sleep apnea, adverse effects of medications, behavior disorders, and nocturnal seizures.

H. Behavior Disorders. Complaint of headache may be a sign of a mood or conversion disorder (eg, depression). Conversion disorder or psychogenic headache is a diagnosis of exclusion.

I. Medical Disorders. Common febrile illness, CNS infections (meningitis and encephalitis), diabetes, severe respiratory conditions with hypoxia, vasculitic disorders, and toxic effects on the CNS of severe liver, kidney, metabolic, or neurodegenerative disorders can all present as headache.

IV. Database
  A. Physical Exam Key Points. A complete physical exam is important to identify a systemic disorder. When evaluating any patient, assess ABCs to avoid missing an emergency condition.
    1. Vital signs. Heart rate and BP changes may reflect systemic infection, cardiac disease, or intoxication. Alteration of temperature may reflect infection or effects of intoxication.
    2. General appearance and affect. Growth and development problems may reflect an underlying medical or neurologic disorder. Is patient cooperative, interactive, or in distress?
    3. Skin. Inspect skin for signs of trauma, birthmarks (erythematous, hypopigmented or hyperpigmented lesions), and rash that suggests infectious or vasculitic disorder.
    4. Head and neck. Check for microcephaly and macrocephaly, reflecting alteration in brain parenchyma or hydrocephalus. Scalp tenderness may suggest tension headache, migraine, or temporal arteritis. Inspect for signs of head trauma. Perform funduscopic exam to check for papilledema (intracranial mass lesion or pseudotumor cerebri). The constellation of unilateral conjunctival injection, nasal congestion, and lacrimation

suggests cluster headache. Examine teeth and temporo-mandibular joint for pain, crepitus, or limited range of motion. Neck stiffness (meningismus) may indicate meningitis or sub-arachnoid hemorrhage.

5. **Neurologic findings.** Detailed neurologic exam allows clinician to localize the condition to specific regions of central and peripheral nervous systems. Disorders of the cerebral cortex will affect cognition, whereas lesions in the brainstem will affect specific cranial nerves. Spinal cord lesions demonstrate motor or sensory levels on examination, or both.

   a. **Mental status.** Exam must be carried out at an age-appropriate level.

   b. **Cranial nerves.** Pupil size and reactivity in addition to eye movements reflect function of portions of the upper brainstem. Symmetric movement of face, soft palate, and tongue demonstrates integrity of the lower brainstem.

   c. **Motor system.** Muscle bulk, tone, and strength demonstrate function of the motor pathways. Fine motor skills may suggest developmental abilities. Note any involuntary movements. Weakness and gait problems may be seen in "functional" disorders.

   d. **Sensory system.** Localized sensory deficits may reflect dysfunction of central or peripheral nervous system; they are also seen in functional disorders.

   e. **Deep tendon reflexes.** Demonstrate integrity of specific reflex pathways from peripheral muscle through the levels of the spinal cord.

   f. **Cerebellar exam.** Cerebellar dysfunction may be a sign of localized space-occupying lesion, destructive process, or degenerative disorder.

B. **Laboratory Data**

   1. **Basic metabolic panel, glucose, calcium.** Electrolyte abnormalities (hypernatremia, hyponatremia, hypocalcemia) and hypoglycemia or hyperglycemia can present with headache. Metabolic acidosis may be seen with underlying metabolic disorder or intoxication; respiratory acidosis is seen in other intoxications (alcohol, benzodiazepines, and barbiturates).

   2. **Renal and hepatic profile.** Can indicate acute or chronic end-organ dysfunction.

   3. **CBC with differential.** Elevated WBC count may indicate active infection.

   4. **Toxicology screening or drug levels.** Based on patient's history; blood levels of prescription medications, ingested medications, or substances of abuse may point to cause of headache.

   5. **ABGs.** Obtain if hypoxia or acid-base problems are suggested by history or physical exam.

C. Radiographic and Other Studies
  1. Lumbar puncture. If history or physical exam suggests an intracranial infection (meningitis or encephalitis) or pseudotumor cerebri. Also confirms subarachnoid hemorrhage. *Do not* perform in the presence of increased intracranial pressure or mass-occupying lesions because of risk of herniation.
  2. Ancillary testing
    a. Neuroimaging (CT or MRI scan). Consider for all patients with headache. If patient has normal findings on exam and has only a history of headache, neuroimaging study is not needed emergently. MRI scan is more sensitive than CT but requires that patient remain still for a prolonged period of time, and therefore often requires sedation.
    b. Sinus x-ray or CT imaging. If clinically indicated.
    c. EEG. The gold standard for seizures; can demonstrate cerebral cortical dysfunction due to generalized encephalopathy or localized destructive or space-occupying lesion.
    d. ECG. If a cardiac disorder is suspected.

V. Plan. ABCs must be assessed in any clinical setting. A next, crucial step is to determine if a specific clinical condition requires emergency intervention, urgent management, or routine care.
  A. Emergency Management. If patient was having active vomiting with signs of dehydration or increased intracranial pressure, emergent medical or surgical management may be required. Migraine can progress to status migrainosus. IV medication may be required for this condition.
    1. During status migrainosus, establish IV access and obtain appropriate blood tests.
    2. Administer medications. Possible agents include:
      a. Prochlorperazine, 5–10 mg, or metoclopramide, 10 mg IV.
      b. DHE, 0.5–1 mg IV. If headache persists for 30 minutes, repeat 0.5 mg IV; can be repeated q8h until headache clears. DHE should *not* be used in patients with peripheral vascular or coronary artery disease, hypertension, renal or hepatic failure, hyperthyroidism-complicated migraines, or pregnancy.
      c. Ketorolac, 30–60 mg IM.
      d. Dexamethasone, 4 mg IV.
      e. Depacon, 15–25 mg/kg IV.
  B. Migraine Management
    1. Infrequent migraines. Can be managed with symptomatic medication use (ie, "when headache occurs, take an analgesic medication"). These medications include acetaminophen, aspirin, NSAIDs, and a variety of combination medications (containing butalbital, caffeine, and codeine), such as Midrin and Fioricet. Triptans (eg, sumatriptan, rizatriptan, zolmitriptan,

and naratriptan) can be used for infrequent headaches occurring less than once per week. Triptan medications are effective in treating migraine headache along with accompanying symptoms of nausea and vomiting. Dose can usually be repeated in 2 hours.

2. **Prophylactic treatment.** Various agents from many medication classes have been used to treat headaches prophylactically. Choose medications based on efficacy in various headache types. Symptomatic medications are used to treat rare or occasional headaches. Most patients will not start a prophylactic headache medicine until they regularly have at least three or four headaches per month (ie, weekly).

   a. The first-line prophylactic agent is often a β-blocker; these agents should *not* be used in patients with asthma.

   b. Anticonvulsant medications (eg, carbamazepine, sodium valproate, lamotrigine, and topiramate) are often used for migraines.

3. **Other useful agents.** Tricyclic antidepressants (also used for chronic daily headache and post-traumatic headache) and calcium channel blockers. Recent evidence demonstrates headache improvement with botulinum toxin type A.

4. **Adverse medication effects.** All medications have potential adverse effects. Triptan medications are contraindicated in patients with ischemic heart disease, hypertension, peripheral vascular disease, hemiplegic or basilar migraine, recent MAOI or ergotamine medication use, or liver failure. Routine blood testing can identify some adverse effects, but blood tests are not predictive of impending adverse effects.

5. **Nonmedical interventions for recurrent headaches.** These interventions include local application of heat or massage, biofeedback, relaxation techniques (meditation or yoga), psychotherapy, and acupuncture.

6. **Rebound headache.** Some patients have recurrent headaches because of overuse of analgesic medications, usually referred to as rebound headache. Once analgesic medications are used more than 4 days per week, for several weeks, there may be a rebound effect in which headache occurs when patient does not take analgesic medication. This is essentially a chronic, recurrent withdrawal syndrome. Patients often compensate for this by increasing the dose and frequency of their analgesic medication. This disorder is treated by withdrawal from the analgesic medication.

C. **Follow-up.** It is important to be able to quantify frequency and severity of headaches to determine the appropriate treatment, as well as efficacy of treatment. Patients taking prophylactic headache medications are typically followed regularly until headache-free for at least 6–12 months.

VI. Problem Case Diagnosis. The 12-year-old girl reported headache episodes that lasted between 2 and 10 hours. Episodes had occurred for 2 years, both at home and at school, with a frequency of one to three per month. Headaches occurred at various times of the day and were associated with nausea, photophobia, and phonophobia, but not involuntary motor activity. Episodes began without warning and interrupted activities because of previously described symptoms. Patient's prenatal, developmental, and past medical histories were unremarkable; however, her mother and older sister had had similar symptoms when they were her age. Physical exam was unremarkable, and neurologic exam, normal. Diagnosis is migraine without aura. This disorder typically presents between the ages of 5 and 11 years (peak onset between 10 and 13 years of age). Patient's condition is not a medical emergency because the headaches have been noted for at least 2 years.

VII. Teaching Pearl: Question. How are migraines categorized?

VIII. Teaching Pearl: Answer. There are three subsets of complicated migraine: (1) *basilar,* with symptoms of vertigo, tinnitus, blurred or double vision, and scotoma secondary to vasoconstriction of basilar and posterior cerebral arteries; (2) *ophthalmoplegic,* which present with 3rd nerve palsy ipsilateral to the side of the headache; and (3) *hemiplegic,* in which unilateral sensory or motor signs develop during headache, including numbness, weakness, and aphasia. Although these forms of migraine are not common, keep them in mind because their presentation suggests the presence of an underlying structural lesion, thus requiring more urgent management than common migraine.

REFERENCES

Lipton RB, Diamond S, Reed M, et al. Migraine diagnosis and treatment: Results from the American Migraine Study II. *Headache* 2001;41:638–645.

Silberstein SD, Lipton RB, Goadsby PJ. *Headache in Clinical Practice,* 2nd ed. Martin Dunitz, 2002.

Winner P, Rothner AD. *Headaches in Children and Adolescents.* BC Decker, 2001.

34. HEART MURMURS AND HEART SOUND ABNORMALITIES

I. Problem. A 6-week-old infant admitted with respiratory distress is noted to have a heart murmur.

II. Immediate Questions
   A. Is there cyanosis? Congenital heart disease with right-to-left shunting or single-ventricle physiology produces cyanosis that persists despite administration of supplemental oxygen.
   B. Are there signs and symptoms of heart failure? Symptoms of heart failure in infants include slow feeding, tiring with feeding, or

diaphoresis associated with feeding. Signs of heart failure in this age group are resting tachycardia and tachypnea.

C. Has this murmur been noted previously? A murmur from a left-to-right shunting lesion, such a ventricular septal defect, presents as the pulmonary vascular resistance falls and a gradient develops between the systemic and pulmonary circulations (usually in the first week of life). Murmurs due to valve stenosis typically are present from birth. A murmur attributed to carditis (associated with Kawasaki disease, rheumatic fever, endocarditis, or myocarditis) would be a new finding, in association with other systemic signs.

D. Are there other systemic signs or symptoms? Persistent fever, conjunctivitis, rash, extremity changes, and lymphadenopathy are seen in Kawasaki disease. Joint swelling and pain in association with a new murmur in an older patient could be indicative of acute rheumatic fever. Evidence of bacteremia with persistent fever and a new or changing murmur may suggest infective endocarditis. Failure to thrive may be associated with chronic volume overload, heart failure, or pulmonary hypertension.

E. Is there a history of prematurity? Premature infants, especially those with low birth weight, are more likely to have persistent patent ductus arteriosus.

F. Has there been a prior cardiac evaluation? Many patients with congenital heart disease are identified prenatally by fetal echocardiography and have had subsequent postnatal evaluations. Information from any prior cardiac evaluations, including findings of diagnostic tests, should be reviewed.

III. Differential Diagnosis

A. Innocent Murmurs. Refers to murmurs that are not associated with any underlying structural heard disease (ie, heart is anatomically normal). These sounds are considered nonpathologic and physiologic. Patients with innocent murmurs do not require bacterial endocarditis precautions.

1. **Peripheral pulmonic stenosis.** Common systolic murmur of neonates, typically heard over pulmonic area (left second intercostal space), with wide radiation to back and into axillae bilaterally. Reflects the more acute angle of origin of branch pulmonary arteries from the main pulmonary artery. Rarely persists beyond 3–6 months of age.

2. **Still's murmur.** Common systolic murmur of childhood, rare in neonates. Typically grade 2–3/6, heard over the left lower sternal border and cardiac apex, and louder in supine posture. Distinguished by characteristic vibratory, honking, or twanging-quality overtone. This murmur, as with other innocent murmurs, may be accentuated with fever or increased cardiac output.

3. **Venous hum.** The only innocent continuous murmur; reflects the sound of normal systemic venous return through jugular

veins. Diastolic component is louder, distinguishing it from arterial continuous murmurs. Heard at the right infraclavicular area in children in the sitting position; changes with head turning maneuvers, and eliminated by compression over jugular vein.

4. **Pulmonary flow murmur.** A systolic ejection murmur, heard over the pulmonic area. There is no click, as would be heard in valvar pulmonic stenosis, and the second heart sound (S2) is normally split. Exaggerated in older patients with absent thoracic kyphosis (straight back syndrome), which brings the pulmonary trunk closer to the anterior chest wall.

B. **Murmurs From Left-to-Right Shunts**

1. **Ventricular septal defect (VSD).** Typically holosystolic (same frequency and intensity throughout systole) and may obscure S2. May have a harsh or blowing character and be associated with a thrill.

2. **Atrial septal defect.** Classic auscultatory findings are persistently and widely split second heart sound (reflecting delayed closure of the pulmonary valve), pulmonary flow murmur, and middiastolic rumble caused by increased flow across the tricuspid valve.

3. **Patent ductus arteriosus (PDA).** Represents failure of the vessel connecting the aorta and the pulmonary artery to close after birth. Flow is throughout the cardiac cycle, because aortic pressure is higher than pulmonary pressure, except if there is pulmonary hypertension. Typically produces a continuous murmur, peaking at S2.

C. **Valvular Heart Disease.** Valvular pulmonic or aortic stenosis presents as a systolic ejection murmur and may be associated with a thrill. A systolic click may precede the murmur, which reflects a referred sound of the stenotic valve opening.

D. **Outflow Tract Obstruction.** Obstruction to flow across the outflow tracts from each ventricle causes a systolic murmur. Intensity of murmur will increase with degree of obstruction. Left ventricular outflow obstruction can be caused by a subaortic membrane or occur in association with hypertrophic cardiomyopathy. The most common cause of right ventricular outflow obstruction in cyanotic patients is infundibular obstruction in tetralogy of Fallot.

IV. **Database**

A. **Physical Exam Key Points**

1. **Vital signs and general appearance**

a. **Height and weight.** Slow weight gain, or crossing growth percentiles, can be seen in left-to-right shunting lesions associated with volume overload.

b. **Pulse oximetry.** Cyanosis that persists despite supplemental oxygen suggests intracardiac mixing, or right-to-left shunting from a cyanotic form of congenital heart disease.

    c. **Heart rate.** Neonates cannot increase stroke volume and thus rely on increased heart rate to maintain cardiac output.

    d. **BP.** A wide pulse pressure can be seen in diastolic run-off lesions, such as PDA, aortic insufficiency, coronary fistula, aortopulmonary window, or arteriovenous malformation. Discrepancy between upper and lower extremity BP is seen in coarctation of the aorta and interrupted aortic arch.

2. **Chest.** Extreme ventricular hypertrophy can cause chest asymmetry. Single-ventricle lesions or ventricular hypertrophy causes a ventricular lift or heave.

3. **Heart.** Auscultation is the most important aspect of the cardiac physical exam. Listen for the first and second heart sounds (S1 and S2), and for normal splitting of S2 with inspiration. Decide if murmur is systolic, diastolic, or continuous. Listen for extra heart sounds, such as systolic clicks or a rub. A third heart sound (S3), or diastolic rumble, in an infant is most often attributable to increased flow across atrioventricular valves in left-to-right shunting lesions. A fourth heart sound (S4) is not common in pediatric patients, but may be heard in cardiomyopathies.

    a. **Holosystolic murmur.** A murmur that is the same frequency and intensity throughout systole and may obscure S2. VSD causes a holosystolic murmur because there is shunting between the higher-pressure left ventricle and lower-pressure right ventricle throughout systole. Intensity of the murmur diminishes as right ventricular pressure increases in association with development of pulmonary hypertension, or if the defect is large enough to not be pressure restrictive. Tricuspid or mitral regurgitation also causes a holosystolic murmur.

    b. **Systolic ejection murmur.** Sometimes referred to as a "crescendo-decrescendo" murmur, it begins after S1, increases in midsystole, and decreases before S2; both heart sounds will be audible. This type of murmur is heard in semilunar (aortic or pulmonary) stenosis but may be innocent as well. Pulmonary valve stenosis is heard at the pulmonic area (left second intercostal space), with radiation to lung fields and back. Valvular aortic stenosis is best heard at the left midsternal border, radiating toward the right base and neck. An ejection click, or high-pitched opening sound, often precedes the systolic ejection murmur in aortic or pulmonic stenosis, distinguishing it from an innocent flow murmur

    c. **Diastolic murmur.** The murmur of semilunar valve insufficiency (eg, pulmonary or aortic regurgitation) begins immediately after S2 and has a blowing, decrescendo quality. A middiastolic sound of relative tricuspid valve stenosis is heard at the left lower sternal border in atrial septal defect. Left heart volume overload (eg, from VSD or large PDA) causes a diastolic rumble of relative mitral stenosis, heard at the apex and left fifth intercostal space.

    d. Continuous murmur. A murmur that is systolic and continues into or throughout diastole. Lesions associated with continuous murmurs include PDA, less commonly arteriovenous malformation, aortopulmonary window, and coronary artery fistula. Also includes venous hums.

  4. Pulses. Examine distal pulses, and palpate brachial and femoral pulses simultaneously. Absent or delayed femoral pulses, associated with higher arm BP, are indicative of coarctation of the aorta. Wide pulse pressure is associated with sharp upstroke, and rapid fall-off (water-hammer pulse), with aortic run-off lesions.

  5. Skin. Examine for the characteristic rash of erythema marginatum, seen in rheumatic fever, as well as rare cutaneous manifestations of bacterial endocarditis (Janeway lesions, Olser nodules).

B. Laboratory Data

  1. CBC. Anemia can cause a systolic flow murmur associated with high-output heart failure. Physiologic nadir of hemoglobin, which occurs at about 6 weeks in neonates, may be associated with a murmur or accentuation of the murmur from underlying valvular stenosis. Elevated WBC count can be seen in infective endocarditis. Platelet count elevation is seen in Kawasaki disease.

  2. Serial blood cultures. Useful when infective endocarditis is suspected.

  3. ESR, C-reactive protein, antistreptolysin O titers. Useful if rheumatic fever is suspected.

C. Radiographic and Other Studies

  1. ECG. Interpretation gives indirect information on ventricular hypertrophy, atrial enlargement, and ventricular strain. Note that left axis deviation (QRS axis –30 to –120) is abnormal in neonates, associated with tricuspid atresia or complete common atrioventricular canal.

  2. Chest X-Ray. Gives cardiac and visceral situs, which is helpful in patients with dextrocardia or heterotaxy syndrome. Cardiothymic silhouette can be used to detect enlargement of cardiac structures (eg, enlargement of pulmonary artery segment in pulmonic stenosis, or left atrial enlargement in VSD). Cardiothoracic ratio generally is less than 0.55 but may appear larger in neonates because of prominent thymic tissue. Increased pulmonary vascular markings are associated with left-to-right shunting lesions and pulmonary overcirculation.

3. **Echocardiogram.** Two-dimensional imaging provides complete anatomic information. Physiologic information can be inferred by assessment of ventricular performance and cardiac chamber size. Septal defects can be diagnosed. Doppler exam of cardiac valves detects stenosis or regurgitation.

V. Plan. Management of patients with murmur is determined by the etiology of the murmur. Following complete cardiac exam, ECG, chest x-ray, pulse oximetry, and four-extremity BP provide useful information. Pediatric cardiology consultation is appropriate if patient is symptomatic from the murmur, or if management of patient's primary clinical problem would be influenced by an underlying cardiac diagnosis.

   A. Cyanosis. If cyanosis and hypoxemia are not corrected with administration of supplemental oxygen, then cyanotic heart disease should be suspected. Consult pediatric cardiology.

   B. Innocent Murmurs. Provide reassurance. In the absence of structural heart disease, these sounds may be accentuated by anemia or circumstances that increase cardiac output (fever, hyperthyroidism).

   C. Left-to-Right Shunts. If there is pulmonary overcirculation and evidence of congestive heart failure, decongestive therapy with diuretics and digoxin may be appropriate. Fluid restriction may be appropriate, because volume boluses may exacerbate congestive heart failure.

   D. Valvular Disease. Patients with stenotic or regurgitant valves, as well as those with VSD or outflow tract gradients, require antibiotic prophylaxis for invasive procedures that are associated with bacteremia (eg, GI or GU instrumentation, dental work).

   E. Outflow Tract Obstruction. Dynamic gradients across left or right ventricular outflow tracts are improved by correcting dehydration, anemia, and tachycardia. In tetralogy of Fallot, severe infundibular obstruction is associated with progressive cyanosis and loss of the systolic murmur. *This is a cardiac emergency.*

VI. Problem Case Diagnosis. An asymptomatic murmur, auscultated at the 2-week visit, was clinically monitored because newborn was doing well. At 6 weeks, infant presented with a 1-week history of difficulty feeding. Chest x-ray showed an enlarged heart and signs of congestive heart failure. Echocardiography confirmed the diagnosis of VSD.

VII. Teaching Pearl: Question. What clinical features suggest the presence of an underlying cardiac disease and preclude the diagnosis of an innocent murmur?

VIII. Teaching Pearl: Answer. Underlying cardiac disease should be suspected if patient has associated clinical features (tiring with feeding, diaphoresis, poor weight gain), cyanosis, diastolic murmur, a widely transmitted loud murmur (> grade 3), abnormal pulses, abnormal heart sounds (S2, rub, click, gallop), abnormal ECG, and abnormal chest x-ray.

REFERENCES

Gidding SS. Heart murmurs. In: Stockman JA III, ed. *Difficult Diagnoses in Pediatrics.* Saunders, 1990:91–98.
Pelech AN. Evaluation of the pediatric patient with a cardiac murmur. *Pediatr Clin North Am* 1999;46:167–188.
Perloff JK. *The Clinical Recognition of Congenital Heart Disease,* 4th ed. Saunders, 1994.

35. HEMATURIA

I. **Problem.** A screening urinalysis shows hematuria in a 10-year-old girl admitted for a planned course of chemotherapy. This finding has not been noted before.

II. **Immediate Questions**
A. **Are RBCs present on microscopic evaluation?** The reagent strip reacts to hemoglobin and myoglobin. It can also be cross-contaminated by other chemicals on the strip.
B. **Is patient having menses or was urine collected by catheter?** Both would be expected reasons for hematuria.
C. **Is there a known bleeding disorder or is patient receiving anticoagulation therapy?** Patients who have coagulation abnormalities usually have other sites of bleeding.
D. **Has patient had recent abdominal surgery or trauma?** Although gross hematuria is usually present in such patients, sometimes microscopic hematuria persists.
E. **What medication(s) does patient take?** Patient may have been receiving an antineoplastic agent, such as cyclophosphamide, which is associated with hemorrhagic cystitis or urinary tract tumors (very rare in children).
F. **Does patient have a history of urologic or renal abnormalities?** Many of these abnormalities are associated with hematuria.
G. **Any symptoms of UTI?** The most common cause of hematuria in a child, UTI is usually associated with pain, urgency, and frequency. WBCs are also present in urine.
H. **Is gross hematuria present, or is there a history of gross hematuria?** Gross hematuria is more likely to have been noticed by patient or family and to have a cause, such as infection, trauma (including local perineal irritation), stones, nephritis, or cystic kidney disease.
I. **If hematuria is microscopic, how is it characterized?**

1. **Microscopic with symptoms**
   a. **General.** Fever, abdominal pain, hypertension, and edema may point toward a cause.
   b. **Non-UTI.** Rash, purpura, arthritis, GI symptoms, and respiratory symptoms all may point to other diseases that may have renal involvement (systemic lupus erythematosus, hemolytic uremic syndrome, Henoch-Schönlein purpura).
   c. **Urinary tract–specific symptoms.** Dysuria and frequency often point to hypercalciuria, stones, or infections as a cause.
2. **Asymptomatic microscopic hematuria with proteinuria.** Urine protein is usually ≥ 2+ on dipstick; or, urine protein-to-creatinine ratio is > 0.2. Presence of proteinuria is more likely to be associated with glomerular disease but could be benign.
3. **Asymptomatic microscopic hematuria without proteinuria.** The cause for this group is almost always (> 90%) benign and may not require immediate evaluation, especially if the RBC count is low (≤ 5–10/HPF).

III. **Differential Diagnosis.** Categorized as either (1) outside of or (2) from the urinary tract. If from the urinary tract, it can either be from the upper tract (kidneys) or from the lower tract (ureter, bladder, or urethra). If from the kidneys, it can be either glomerular or nonglomerular in nature.
   A. **Hematuria Unrelated to Urinary System**
   1. **Coagulopathy (primary or medication related).** Usually associated with other signs of bleeding.
   2. **False hematuria.** Rectal or vaginal bleeding; myoglobin or hemoglobin.
   3. **Factitious hematuria.** Contamination of dipstick by other chemicals (microscopic normal).
   B. **Hematuria That Is Glomerular in Nature**
   1. **Postinfectious nephritis (streptococcal or other causes).** Low C3.
   2. **IgA nephropathy.** Normal C3; occurs with viral upper respiratory infection.
   3. **Henoch-Schönlein nephritis.** Systemic findings include rash, abdominal pain, and joint problems.
   4. **Chronic nephritis.** Focal segmental, membranous, or membranoproliferative disease usually causes significant proteinuria.
   5. **Lupus nephritis.** Low C3; other systems may be affected.
   6. **Vasculitis.** Scleroderma, Wegener granulomatosis, or polyarteritis nodosa.
   7. **Hemolytic uremic syndrome (HUS).**
   8. **Hereditary nephritis.** Alport syndrome (hearing loss); thin membrane disease (little proteinuria).

C. **Hematuria From Kidneys That Is Not Glomerular**
   1. **Interstitial disease (usually with proteinuria).** Analgesic nephropathy, toxins (heavy metal, drugs); eosinophils may be present in urine.
   2. **Infections (pyelonephritis, tuberculosis).** Always associated with pyuria.
   3. **Malformations.** Cystic disease (family history); obstructive disease (can occur with minimal trauma); vascular problem (hemangioma, arteriovenous fistula).
   4. **Tumors.** Rare in children.
   5. Ischemia related; emboli (post–cardiac catheterization or surgery); thrombosis (coagulation disorder, nephrotic syndrome).
   6. Trauma.
D. **Hematuria From Lower Urinary Tract (Ureter, Bladder, Urethra)**
   1. Mechanical (stones, usually associated with pain).
   2. Obstruction (posterior urethral values).
   3. **Infection or inflammation**
      a. **Cystitis.** Bacterial, viral (adenovirus), or chemical (cyclophosphamide).
      b. **Urethritis.** Sexually transmitted.
      c. **Prostatitis, periurethritis, vaginitis.** Pelvic inflammatory disease; STDs.
   4. **Hypercalciuria.** In children, commonly presents without stones but often with dysuria; few WBCs in urine; urine calcium-to-creatinine ratio is > 0.2.
E. **Miscellaneous**
   1. Exercise-related hematuria or myoglobinuria.
   2. **Benign recurrent hematuria.** Diagnosis of exclusion; patient may have positive family history.

IV. **Database.** The effort involved in the search for a cause of hematuria is expensive and time-consuming. Remember that *isolated* hematuria *without or with minimal proteinuria* is almost always a *benign* condition and *workup can be deferred.* On the other hand, *gross* hematuria, *symptomatic* hematuria, and hematuria *with heavy proteinuria* need an *aggressive and early evaluation.*
   A. **Physical Exam Key Points**
      1. **BP.** Often elevated with nephritis.
      2. **Abdomen.** Examine for mass effect (tumor, obstruction, cystic disease), pain, and tenderness (infection, infarction, obstruction, stone).
      3. **Genitalia.** Examine urethral meatus (discharge, blood), vagina (discharge, blood), and rectum (blood, fissure, hemorrhoids).
      4. **Skin and joints.** Observe for rashes, petechiae, purpura, ecchymosis, and swelling suggestive of vasculitis or systemic disease.

B. **Laboratory Data**
   1. **Urinalysis**
      a. **RBC casts (sometimes), proteinuria (usually).** Think nephritis.
      b. **WBCs (> 10/HPF), bacteria (unspun urine).** Think infection.
      c. **Crystals with pain.** Think stones or hypercalciuria.
      d. **Positive urine dipstick for blood with few or no RBCs.** Think myoglobin or hemoglobinuria (check LDH, CPK, blood smear).
   2. **Urine for calcium and creatinine.** Think hypercalciuria if ratio is > 0.2.
   3. **CBC**
      a. **Increased WBC count with left shift.** Think infection and inflammation.
      b. **Elevated ESR (C-reactive protein).** Think infection (pyelonephritis).
      c. **Abnormal smear (low platelets, abnormal RBCs).** Think HUS.
      d. **Anemia.** Hemoglobinopathies, HUS.
   4. **Sickle cell screen.** Obtain, if not known, in African-American children.
   5. **Metabolic panel**
      a. **Elevated BUN and creatinine, abnormal electrolytes.** Think primary renal disease.
      b. **Low total protein and albumin.** Think nephritis and nephrotic syndrome.
   6. **Immunologic screening tests.** If significant proteinuria accompanies hematuria, obtain C3, C4, ANA, antistreptolysin O, ANCA, IgA, hepatitis panel, HIV.
   7. **Cultures**
      a. **Urine.** For bacterial, viral (in special cases; many RBCs and few WBCs); acid-fast bacilli.
      b. **Blood.** When patient has significant fever or systemic symptoms.
      c. **Stool.** Bloody diarrhea fits picture of HUS.
   8. **Coagulation studies.** When CBC is abnormal or other sites of bleeding are present.
C. **Radiographic and Other Studies**
   1. **Ultrasound.** Simple, noninvasive, and useful in patients with microscopic hematuria; will show anatomy (cysts, obstruction), possible stone, evidence of renal parenchymal disease if tissue is echodense, and loss of cortical-medullary junction.
   2. **CT scan.** First choice in patients with gross, painful hematuria; post-traumatic hematuria; or possible stone. Before contrast is given, renal function (serum creatinine) must be evaluated.

   3. **KUB.** Simple, and easy to obtain; 80% of stones are radio-
      dense. May also reveal GI abnormality.
   4. **Special studies.** Cystogram, nuclear renal scan, and angiog-
      raphy are second-line studies that should be obtained only
      after urology or nephrology consultation.

V. Plan. Treatment depends on etiology. Cause of hematuria is rarely
   an emergency except for gross hematuria (with or without clots), for
   which the cause could be trauma, severe coagulation abnormality, or
   cyclophosphamide-induced cystitis.

   A. UTI. Begin treatment before culture results are known if patient is
      ill with symptoms and there are > 10 WBCs/HPF (infection is very
      likely) or if evidence of sepsis or pyelonephritis is present
      (increased C-reactive protein, ESR, high WBC count with left
      shift).

   B. Urolithiasis. Stones ≤ 5 mm are usually passed by patient
      (manage with hydration and analgesics). Obtain urology consul-
      tation if stones are large or associated with obstruction or infec-
      tions.

   C. Obstruction or Other Urologic Abnormalities. Consult urology
      colleagues; arrange nephrology consultation if renal impairment
      is present.

   D. Neoplasm. Consult oncology, urology, or surgery colleagues.

   E. Glomerulonephritis. Obtain nephrology consultation for consid-
      eration of renal biopsy, further evaluation, and treatment.

   F. Coagulopathy. Attempt to correct the clotting abnormality, and
      consult hematology colleagues.

   G. Hemorrhagic Cystitis. Consult urology colleagues. Treatment of
      a patient with hemorrhagic cystitis consists of saline irrigation, but
      primary treatment is prevention with hydration and mesna.

VI. Problem Case Diagnosis. The 10-year-old patient had hemorrhagic
   cystitis. On further investigation, the inciting agent for the bladder
   injury was found to be cyclophosphamide therapy.

VII. Teaching Pearl: Question. What are clues that a UTI involves the
   kidney (upper tract infection)?

VIII. Teaching Pearl: Answer. Flank or back pain, vomiting, elevated C-
   reactive protein, WBC or RBC casts, loss of urine concentrating ability,
   abnormal DMSA scan.

REFERENCES

Ahn JH, Morey AF, McAninch JW. Workup and management of traumatic hematuria.
   Emerg Med Clin North Am 1998;16:145–164.
Cohen RA, Brown RS. Microscopic hematuria. *N Engl J Med* 2003;348:2330–2338.
Diven SC, Travis LB. A practical primary care approach to hematuria in children.
   Pediatr Nephrol 2000;14:65–72.

Patel HP, Bissler JJ. Hematuria in children. *Pediatr Clin North Am* 2001;48:
1519–1537.

36. HEMOPTYSIS

I. Problem. A 10-year-old boy who is seen in the emergency department has a 3-day history of cough. Yesterday he heard a gurgling noise and then began coughing up bright red sputum. A similar episode occurred this morning.

II. Immediate Questions

  A. Is it hemoptysis? Blood from a nasal, oral, or gastric source may be aspirated to the larynx and expectorated. Look for bright red or rust color, frothiness, or a mixture with purulent sputum. May be preceded by a gurgling noise in the large airway.

  B. What is volume of blood loss? May be blood-tinged to massive.
   1. Mild. Blood loss is < 15–20 mL/24 h.
   2. Moderate. Blood loss is 20–200 mL/24 h.
   3. Massive. Blood loss is > 8 mL/kg/24 h, or 200–600 mL/24 h. *This is a life-threatening problem* that demands ICU admission and rapid diagnostic evaluation.

  C. Are there associated respiratory symptoms? Chronic cough suggests infection, cystic fibrosis (CF), bronchiectasis, or foreign body. Dyspnea suggests pulmonary hypertension or idiopathic pulmonary hemorrhage (IPH). Wheezing suggests foreign body or IPH.

  D. Does patient have chest pain? Chest pain can occur with acute lower respiratory infection, trauma, or pulmonary embolism.

III. Differential Diagnosis

  A. Infection. Acute lower respiratory tract infection is the single most common cause of hemoptysis; may be tracheobronchitis, pneumonia (bacterial, fungal, parasitic, but rarely tuberculous), or lung abscess. If bronchiectasis is present, think CF, immunodeficiency, chronic aspiration, foreign body, allergic bronchopulmonary aspergillosis (ABPA), or ciliary dyskinesia syndrome.

  B. Foreign Body. Must always be considered, even in the absence of a positive history.

  C. Pulmonary Arteriovenous Malformation. Presents with dyspnea on exertion, palpitations, and chest pains. When large, may produce neurologic symptoms (headaches, confusion, dizziness, syncope, cerebral vascular accidents).

  D. Alveolar Hemorrhage Syndrome. Idiopathic, associated with renal disease, or with rheumatologic disease.

  E. Trauma. Can be blunt, penetrating, or iatrogenic trauma (especially with tracheostomy).

F. Pulmonary Thromboembolism. Prolonged inactivity; calf pain or leg edema.

G. Tumor. Rare, but must be considered (bronchial adenoma, carcinoid, mediastinal teratoma, bronchogenic carcinoma, metastatic lesions).

H. Cardiac Disease. Pulmonary vascular obstructive disease and enlarged collateral bronchial circulation.

I. Coagulopathy. Drugs, thrombocytopenia, disseminated intravascular coagulation, liver disease.

J. Factitious. Consider when medical history or patient's behavior is unusual.

IV. Database

A. Physical Exam Key Points

1. **Vital signs.** Look for fever, signs of impending respiratory failure, orthostatic changes, or hypotension.
2. **HEENT.** Look for signs of nasal or oropharyngeal sources of bleeding and for evidence of head or neck trauma.
3. **Chest.** Examine for signs of trauma. Listen for pleural rub, localized crackles, bruits, or signs of consolidation.
4. **Heart.** Listen at apex with bell for a low diastolic rumble of mitral stenosis. Gallop rhythm and jugular venous distention suggest congestive heart failure.
5. **Extremities.** Look for cyanosis, clubbing, edema, or calf pain.
6. **Skin.** Look for petechiae, telangiectasia, ecchymoses, angiomata, or rashes.

B. Laboratory Data

1. **CBC with differential.** Look for signs of chronic anemia or acute blood loss. Is WBC count elevated? Eosinophilia suggests parasites or allergy.
2. **Coagulation studies (PT, PTT, platelets, bleeding time).** Coagulation problems are uncommon in children but need to be ruled out.
3. **Urinalysis, BUN, creatinine.** Evaluate for pulmonary-renal syndromes.
4. **ABGs.** Evaluate for impending respiratory failure.
5. **Sputum.** Obtain for bacterial, mycobacterial, and fungal cultures; cytology.
6. **Other workup.** Consider IgE level (ABPA, allergies, parasitic infection), hemosiderin-laden macrophages (alveolar hemorrhage syndromes), milk precipitins (Heiner syndrome), antiglomerular basement membrane antibodies (Goodpasture syndrome), ANCAs (Wegener granulomatosis).

C. Radiographic and Other Studies

1. **Chest x-ray.** Order PA and lateral views. Up to one third are normal. When abnormal, the most common findings are atelectasis and alveolar, and interstitial parenchymal infiltrates.

Look for tram-track appearance characteristic of bronchiectasis. Obtain inspiratory and expiratory films if foreign body aspiration is a possibility.

2. **High-resolution CT scan.** Ideal for following up chest x-ray abnormalities. Use contrast to evaluate for vascular lesions.
3. **Ventilation-perfusion (V/Q) scan.** Obtain if pulmonary embolism is suspected; can be performed in almost all age groups.
4. **Bronchoscopy.** Consider when bleeding persists or in absence of diagnosis from other studies. Rigid scope is preferred for massive hemoptysis. Obtain lavage specimen for bacteriologic cultures, cytology, and histopathologic studies.
5. **Angiography.** To evaluate for possible arteriovenous malformation (AVM) and to rule out pulmonary embolus when V/Q scan is equivocal.
6. **ECG or echocardiogram.** Obtain in patients with suspected cardiac disease.

V. Plan
A. Initial Management
1. Arrange ICU admission for patients with massive hemoptysis or impending respiratory failure.
2. Protect airway; this may require early intubation. Death occurs from asphyxia rather than hemorrhage.
3. Establish IV access for fluid resuscitation and medications.
4. Correct any underlying coagulopathy.
5. Order bed rest, with partial cough suppression using narcotics.

B. Bronchoscopy.
Arrange early if diagnosis is in doubt or hemoptysis continues. Bleeding may be controlled with topical therapy, bronchoscopic pressure, or endobronchial tamponade.

C. Pulmonary Medicine Consultation.
Consider ENT, general surgery, or thoracic surgery consultation for massive or continuous hemoptysis. May require laser therapy, endoscopic tumor resection, or lobectomy. Pneumonectomy is rarely required in children.

D. Treatment of Underlying Cause
1. **Infection.** Treat with antibiotics as dictated by clinical picture.
2. **Pulmonary emboli.** Treat acutely with low-molecular-weight heparin.
3. **Diffuse alveolar hemorrhage or pulmonary-renal syndrome.** Administer IV steroids.
4. **Nonsurgical patient with localized bleeding.** Perform bronchial arteriography followed by embolization.

E. Surgery.
Consider when embolization has failed or is not feasible.

VI. Problem Case Diagnosis.
Physical exam of the 10-year-old boy was unremarkable except for a soft murmur over the left chest. ECG was normal, but a chest CT scan revealed a pulmonary AVM that

was confirmed and further defined by selective arteriogram. Patient underwent an uncomplicated resection of the AVM.

VII. Teaching Pearl: Question. What does the presence of pallor suggest when seen in conjunction with hemoptysis?

VIII. Teaching Pearl: Answer. Pallor in conjunction with hemoptysis indicates that massive bleeding has occurred.

REFERENCES

Batra PS, Holinger LD. Etiology and management of pediatric hemoptysis. *Arch Otolaryngol Head Neck Surg* 2001;127:377–382.

Pianosi P, Al-saddon H. Hemoptysis in children. *Pediatr Rev* 1996;17:344–348.

Sheikh S, Sisson B, Senler SO, Eid N. Moderate hemoptysis of unknown etiology. *Pediatr Pulmonol* 1999;27:351–355.

Sidman JD, Wheeler WB, Cabalka AK, et al. Management of acute pulmonary hemorrhage in children. *Laryngoscope* 2001;111:33–35.

37. HYPERBILIRUBINEMIA, DIRECT (CONJUGATED)

I. Problem. A 6-week-old male infant who was born at full term is brought to the pediatrician's office with a 1-week history of jaundice.

II. Immediate Questions
   A. How has infant been acting and feeding? A toxic-appearing child needs to be evaluated for sepsis or acute infection. Irritability and poor feeding may be a sign of neurologic effects of metabolic disorders, severe hepatic decompensation, or infection.
   B. Has infant been growing and developing as expected? Many metabolic conditions cause developmental delays. Significant liver disease often results in poor weight gain and growth.
   C. Has infant had fever? Sepsis, UTI, and cholangitis may present with fever. Bacterial peritonitis must also be considered in a patient with ascites and fever.
   D. Is abdomen distended? Abdominal distention often represents organomegaly or ascites, both seen with progressive liver dysfunction.
   E. What is the color of stool and urine? Acholic (clay-colored or pale) stool and dark urine suggest biliary obstruction (eg, biliary atresia), which requires urgent evaluation for timely surgical referral.

III. Differential Diagnosis
   A. Anatomic Causes
      1. Extrahepatic biliary atresia. The most common cause of neonatal cholestasis; more common in females. Underlying process is progressive destruction of the biliary tree lumen, resulting in complete obliteration by 3 months of age. Although

injury seems to begin in the extrahepatic biliary tree, it progresses to include intrahepatic biliary radicals as well. Etiology is undetermined. Approximately 10% of patients have the embryonic form of disease with associated anomalies, including polysplenia or asplenia, preduodenal portal vein, situs inversus, and malrotation. Most patients present with jaundice and acholic stools between the 2nd and 4th weeks of life.

2. **Gallstone disease.** Seen in patients with hemolytic disease, hypothyroidism, cystic fibrosis, or those receiving prolonged diuretic or parenteral nutrition therapy.

3. **Choledochal cyst.** Essentially a cystic outpouching of the biliary tree; there are five different types.

4. **Other.** Sclerosing cholangitis, infectious cholangitis, inspissated bile plugs, spontaneous bile duct perforation, biliary hypoplasia, Caroli disease, extrinsic compression of bile ducts, congenital hepatic fibrosis.

B. **Infectious Causes.** Include cytomegalovirus (CMV), rubella, hepatitis A though G, herpesviruses (simplex, zoster, HHV 6), adenovirus, enteroviruses, Epstein-Barr virus (EBV), reovirus 3, parvovirus B19, HIV, bacterial sepsis, *E coli* UTI, cholangitis, syphilis, listeriosis, tuberculosis, toxoplasmosis. Most of these patients present with other signs of infection. Laboratory evaluation usually reveals evidence of hepatocellular injury with elevated ALT and AST in addition to cholestasis.

C. **Metabolic Causes**
   1. Disorders of metabolism of amino acids (tyrosinemia).
   2. Disorders of lipid metabolism (Niemann-Pick, Gaucher, and Wolman diseases).
   3. Disorders of carbohydrate metabolism (galactosemia, fructosemia, type IV glycogenesis).
   4. Endocrinopathies (hypopituitarism, hypothyroidism).
   5. Urea cycle defects.
   6. Neonatal hemochromatosis; characterized by acute hepatic failure in newborn period. Antioxidant therapy may ameliorate symptoms, but process is essentially fatal without liver transplantation. Etiology is unclear, but subsequent pregnancies may be affected.
   7. Ultrastructural abnormalities, such as peroxisomal (or Zellweger syndrome) and mitochondrial disorders.
   8. Bile acid disorders.

D. **Inherited or Familial Causes**
   1. α_1-**Antitrypsin deficiency.** The most common inherited disease resulting in pediatric liver transplantation. Patients may present with transient cholestasis in infancy. Family history of early emphysema in nonsmokers should be a red flag. Has autosomal-recessive inheritance. Liver disease affects children; pulmonary disease typically occurs in adulthood, but pulmonary

function tests should be obtained in any symptomatic child or by 10 years of age as baseline.

2. **Cystic fibrosis (CF).** Cholestasis or gallstone formation can be seen. Liver disease associated with CF can progress to cirrhosis. About one quarter of patients with CF have liver involvement; therefore, all patients need screening laboratory evaluations. Treatment with ursodeoxycholic acid seems to improve cholestasis but may not influence natural progression of disease.

3. **Alagille syndrome.** Also known as arteriohepatic dysplasia. Liver lesion is intrahepatic bile duct hypoplasia. Has autosomal-dominant inheritance with variable penetrance. Mutations are seen in *Jagged1* gene on chromosome 20. Patient has associated cardiac disease (usually peripheral pulmonic stenosis but can be any cardiac anomaly, including tetralogy of Fallot or coarctation of the aorta), vertebral anomalies (most commonly butterfly vertebrae), and retention of posterior embryotoxon on slit-lamp eye exam. Classic facial features may not be well-defined in infants but are often apparent in adult family members.

4. **Wilson disease (hepatolenticular degeneration).** Has autosomal-recessive inheritance with mutations on chromosome 13. Most patients present in second decade of life with hepatic involvement. Neuropsychiatric disease is apparent by third and fourth decades of life. Associated abnormalities include hematologic, endocrine, ocular (Kayser-Fleischer ring), and renal anomalies, with copper accumulation in these tissues.

5. Progressive familial intrahepatic cholestasis (Byler syndrome).

6. Benign recurrent cholestasis.

7. Familial cholestasis of North American Indians.

E. **Toxic Causes.** Drugs (acetaminophen, amiodarone, estrogens, isoniazid, ketoconazole, phenytoin, valproic acid, halothane, L-asparaginase, among others), toxins (eg, mushroom poisoning, some herbs), or parenteral nutrition.

F. **Other Causes**

1. **Idiopathic neonatal hepatitis.** Also known as giant cell hepatitis. Second most common "diagnosis" in neonatal cholestasis, after biliary atresia. However, with improved ability to diagnose some metabolic and genetic disorders, the number of patients who fall into this category has been decreasing over the past 10–20 years. In general, presentation of infants with this condition is similar to that of infants with biliary atresia (ie, acholic stools and jaundice by 3 months of age). There is a slight male preponderance, and 10–20% of cases are familial (these patients have a worse clinical outcome).

2. Shock.

3. Histiocytosis X.

    4. Neonatal lupus.
    5. Extracorporeal membrane oxygenation.
    6. Graft-versus-host disease.
    7. Venoocclusive disease.
    8. Autosomal trisomies.
    9. Erythroblastosis fetalis.

IV. Database

A. Physical Exam Key Points

1. **Vital signs.** Fever may indicate infectious cholangitis or viral hepatitis

2. **Growth parameters.** Poor weight gain and linear growth stunting can occur with chronic liver disease, endocrine abnormalities, and malabsorptive conditions. Weight may be falsely elevated due to ascites or edema, and organomegaly. Consider anthropometric measurements in that setting.

3. **Physical findings.** Jaundice, scleral icterus, hepatosplenomegaly, ascites, peripheral edema, caput medusa, xanthomas, palmar erythema, telangiectasia, male gynecomastia, peripheral wasting, hemorrhoids or occult blood in stool, clubbing, changes on neurologic exam (includes mental status, pupillary size, asterixis, hyperreflexia or hyporeflexia, clonus, Babinski sign).

B. Laboratory Data. Evaluation is guided by clinical presentation.

1. **Blood.** CBC with platelets and reticulocyte count, electrolytes, glucose, BUN, creatinine, liver enzymes (ALT, AST, alkaline phosphatase, GGTP, 5′-nucleotidase), direct and total bilirubin, PT and PTT, albumin, ammonia, cholesterol, TORCH titers, EBV, CMV, hepatitis B and C, α_1-antitrypsin level and phenotype, ceruloplasmin, serum ferritin and iron, RBC galactose-1-phosphate uridyl transferase, and thyroid function tests. Consider blood culture, serum amino acids, and serum bile acids.

2. **Urine.** Urinalysis, including reducing substances. Consider urine culture, urine amino acids, urine organic acids, urine bile acids. Suspect galactosemia if urinalysis has reducing substance without glucosuria.

3. **Other workup.** Sweat chloride analysis to evaluate for CF.

C. Radiographic and Other Studies

1. **Radiologic studies.** Long bone films for possible congenital infection; abdominal ultrasound with Doppler flows of hepatic and portal vessels; hepatobiliary scintigraphy (HIDA, DiSIDA) to evaluate hepatobiliary flow; MRCP/ERCP.

2. **Other.** Liver biopsy; exploratory laparotomy with intraoperative cholangiogram; bone marrow for suspected storage diseases.

V. Plan. A few of the previously listed disorders are amenable to medical or surgical treatment. For most, however, management is directed toward identifying and treating the complications of cholestasis.

A. **Malnutrition.** Secondary to malabsorption or steatorrhea and decreased intake.
   1. Provide age-appropriate nutritional supplements that are relatively high in medium-chain triglycerides (about 40–60% of fat calories).
   2. If oral intake is inadequate, patient may require nasogastric tube feedings.
   3. Fat-soluble vitamin replacement. Follow levels of vitamin A, 25-hydroxyvitamin D, and vitamin E, as well as PT.
   4. Closely monitor weight, anthropometrics, and linear growth.
   5. Follow serum calcium, phosphorus, magnesium, zinc, and iron levels; may need replacement.

B. **Pruritus.** Various medications can be tried, including bile-acid binding agents (cholestyramine, colestipol, antacids), phenobarbital, rifampin, ursodeoxycholic acid, antihistamines, and carbamazepine. Efficacy is not uniform. Biliary diversion surgery is occasionally used in severe pruritus. Intractable pruritus may be an indication for transplantation.

C. **Hyperlipidemia and Xanthomas.** More common with intrahepatic cholestasis than extrahepatic disease. Severe hyperlipidemia in Alagille disease is associated with atherosclerosis and renal lipidosis. Treat with bile-acid binding resins such as cholestyramine or ursodeoxycholic acid. No significant effect is seen with dietary saturated fat or cholesterol restriction, or with cholesterol-lowering agents.

D. **Disease Progression.** Monitor closely for progression of liver dysfunction with laboratory studies (CBC, electrolytes, glucose, BUN, creatinine, ALT, AST, alkaline phosphatase, GGTP, total and direct bilirubin, albumin, PT, ammonia levels, lipid profile, prealbumin) and physical exams.

E. **Complications.** Manage expectantly for complications such as ascites, infections, bleeding, and encephalopathy.

F. **General Care.** Support patient and family, and promote maintenance of general pediatric care, especially immunization. All live viral vaccines should be given, in an accelerated schedule if needed, prior to transplantation.

G. **Referral.** Provide early referral to a pediatric liver transplantation center if patient's diagnosis suggests chronic liver disease. Surgical referral for portoenterostomy in patients with presumed extrahepatic biliary atresia should occur before 6–8 weeks of age for optimal results.

VI. **Problem Case Diagnosis.** The 6-week-old male infant had cholestasis, hepatosplenomegaly, and recent onset of poor feeding with slow weight gain. Abdominal ultrasound confirmed organomegaly but did not detect a gallbladder. HIDA scan revealed no excretion after 24 hours. Liver biopsy and subsequent intraoperative cholangiogram showed biliary atresia. Kasai procedure was performed before 8 weeks of age, and infant had good bile drainage postoperatively.

VII. Teaching Pearl: Question. Until what age is cholestatic jaundice considered physiologic?

VIII. Teaching Pearl: Answer. Although a moderate, indirect hyperbilirubinemia may be normal in neonates (so-called physiologic jaundice), direct hyperbilirubinemia (cholestasis) is always pathologic.

REFERENCES

Diwakar V, Pearson L, Breath S. Liver disease in children with cystic fibrosis. *Paediatr Respir Rev* 2001;2:340–349.

Feranchak AP, Ramirez RO, Sokol RJ. Medical and nutritional management of cholestasis. In: Suchy FJ, Sokol RJ, Balistreri WF, eds. *Liver Disease in Children,* 2nd ed. Lippincott Williams & Wilkins, 2001:195–238.

Piccoli DA. Alagille syndrome. In Sokol RJ, Balistreri WF, eds. *Liver Disease in Children,* 2nd ed. Lippincott Williams & Wilkins, 2001:327-342.

Primhak RA, Tanner MS. Alpha-1-antitrypsin deficiency. *Arch Dis Child* 2001;85:2–5.

Sokol RJ. Approach to the infant with cholestasis. In: Sokol RJ, Balistreri WF, eds. *Liver Disease in Children,* 2nd ed. Lippincott Williams & Wilkins, 2001:187–194.

Sokol RJ, Mack C, Narkewicz MR, Karrer FM. Pathogenesis and outcome of biliary atresia: Current concepts. *J Pediatr Gastroenterol Nutr* 2003;37:4–21.

38. HYPERBILIRUBINEMIA, INDIRECT (UNCONJUGATED)

I. Problem. A 3-day-old male infant who was born at 37 weeks' gestation is being evaluated in the emergency department for jaundice. His indirect bilirubin level is elevated.

II. Immediate Questions

A. How has infant been acting lately? Irritability, high-pitched cry, and seizures may be seen with bilirubin encephalopathy or kernicterus.

B. Has infant had fever? Always consider the diagnosis of infection or sepsis in an infant presenting with jaundice, particularly if jaundice appears in the first 24 hours of life or develops after 3 days of life. Other signs suggestive of infection include temperature instability, poor color or perfusion, tachypnea, lethargy, apnea, and poor feeding.

C. How has infant been feeding? Infants with poor feeding are at risk for dehydration and jaundice. In the first week of life, many infants and mothers have difficulty with breast-feeding, especially when infants are born before 38 weeks' gestation. Inadequate feeding may result in delayed stooling, which, in turn, may contribute to increased enterohepatic circulation of bilirubin.

D. What is mother's blood type? Are isoimmune antibodies present in mother's serum? Infants born to mothers with O-type blood are at highest risk for ABO incompatibility. Antibodies to other minor group antigens also may uncommonly contribute to jaundice.

E. Infant's birthweight? Weight loss in the first few days of life is expected, but excessive weight loss may occur in the setting of dehydration and poor caloric intake. It is important to recognize dehydration in young infants to avoid life-threatening acidosis.

III. Differential Diagnosis. Indirect hyperbilirubinemia is much more common in neonates than in older children. When seen in an older infant or child, consider diagnoses of hemolytic anemia and hepatic disease.

A. Physiologic Jaundice. Jaundice that occurs in otherwise healthy term infants as a result of factors that include RBC turnover, liver immaturity (eg, low levels of uridine diphosphate [UDP]-glucuronyl transferase), and increased enterohepatic circulation of bilirubin (due to delayed stooling, presence of bilirubin in meconium, and presence of glucuronidase in gut).

B. Breast-Feeding Jaundice. Distinct from breast-milk jaundice (which occurs at > 1 week of life). Breast-feeding jaundice occurs in first week of life among breast-fed infants and is believed to be due to relative lack of calories or dehydration, or both.

C. Breast-Milk Jaundice. Infant presents with indirect hyperbilirubinemia between 7 days and several months of life. Thought to be due to one or more ill-defined factors in breast milk that interfere with metabolism of bilirubin. Levels of indirect hyperbilirubinemia may be as high as 10–30 mg/dL. Temporary cessation of breast-feeding results in a drop in serum bilirubin level.

D. ABO Incompatibility. Occurs most commonly among infants born to mothers with O-type blood. Maternal antibodies (IgG) cross placenta and bind to surface of RBCs, which are subsequently destroyed in the spleen. Rh incompatibility, more severe than ABO incompatibility, is uncommon with the widespread use of Rh immunoglobulin.

E. G6PD Deficiency. An X-linked disorder that is seen in up to 10% of African-American males. G6PD helps to protect the RBC membrane from oxidant stresses. Although many cases of G6PD deficiency go undiagnosed, this diagnosis can be associated with severe hyperbilirubinemia.

F. Erythrocyte Structural Defects. Disorders such as spherocytosis and elliptocytosis are associated with RBC destruction in the spleen. Family history of splenectomy, gallbladder stones, or transfusions should raise suspicion of these disorders. Spherocytosis is due to a defect in the RBC membrane, often involving the protein spectrin.

G. Familial Disorders of Conjugation. Gilbert syndrome, associated with decreased UDP-glucuronyl transferase activity, affects up to 7% of the population and is typically diagnosed during adolescence.

Crigler-Najjar syndromes are very rare disorders, associated with structural abnormalities in UDP-glucuronyl transferase.

H. **Other Causes.** Hemolytic anemias, transfusions, and trauma associated with hematomas result in increased bilirubin load and are causes of indirect hyperbilirubinemia in any age group. Infants with galactosemia and hypothyroidism may present initially with indirect hyperbilirubinemia in the newborn period. Congenital infections (eg, cytomegalovirus, toxoplasmosis) that cause systemic illness may be associated with hemolysis and indirect hyperbilirubinemia, in addition to hepatitis and direct hyperbilirubinemia. Indirect hyperbilirubinemia may be exaggerated in the presence of the following risk factors: Asian or Native American race, prematurity, polycythemia, male sex, Down syndrome, oxytocin induction, delayed stooling, and having a sibling with a history of neonatal jaundice.

IV. **Database**
  A. **Physical Exam Key Points**
    1. **General appearance and vital signs.** May suggest infection. Patients with kernicterus may have retrocollis and opisthotonus (backward neck and back arching).
    2. **Skin.** Assess color for pallor or jaundice. Although neonatal jaundice follows a cephalocaudal progression, *do not* rely on visual diagnosis alone. Visual determination of jaundice is unreliable and imprecise and has been associated with more than several cases of kernicterus.
    3. **Abdomen.** Assess for hepatosplenomegaly, which may be seen in several infectious and metabolic processes. Splenomegaly should raise suspicion of hemolytic anemia.
  B. **Laboratory Data.** Testing should be guided by clinical suspicion. Any occurrence of jaundice in the first 24 hours of life should be followed up with a serum bilirubin level.
    1. **Transcutaneous bilirubin (icterometer) measurements.** Results vary, depending on device used. Can be helpful to assess trends and to determine if blood testing is indicated.
    2. **Total serum bilirubin.** The gold standard to determine degree of jaundice. Total and direct bilirubin levels help to distinguish indirect from direct hyperbilirubinemia. It is essential to interpret bilirubin in terms of postnatal age in hours, particularly in the first several days of life.
    3. **Direct Coombs test, blood type, and Rh type.** Recommended for any infant whose mother is Rh-negative or of unknown blood type. Consider direct Coombs testing in jaundiced newborns born to mothers with O-type blood. A negative direct Coombs test result does not rule out ABO incompatibility, which is often associated with a positive indirect Coombs test, as a cause of jaundice.

4. **CBC with smear.** Helpful in determining if anemia and evidence of hemolysis are present.

5. **Reticulocyte count.** May be helpful in determining if hemolysis is present, although results may differ from laboratory to laboratory. In the absence of significant anemia, reticulocyte count is of limited value.

6. **Liver function tests.** Should be performed in infants and children with systemic infection and sepsis to rule out hepatitis.

7. **Other workup**
   a. **Osmotic fragility test.** Used to diagnosis spherocytosis; best performed after the newborn period.
   b. **Genetic testing.** Now available for Gilbert and Crigler-Najjar syndromes.
   c. In cases of unexplained indirect hyperbilirubinemia, consider thyroid function tests (hypothyroidism) and urine for reducing substances (galactosemia).

C. **Radiographic and Other Studies.** These studies generally do not play a role in evaluating neonatal jaundice.

V. Plan

A. **General Plan.** Treatment for neonatal indirect hyperbilirubinemia is initiated to avoid neurologic sequelae and kernicterus, but in most instances jaundice is benign and self-limited. Mainstay of treatment for indirect hyperbilirubinemia is phototherapy, but exchange transfusion should be considered for severe cases, in consultation with a neonatologist. Initiate phototherapy if bilirubin rises rapidly or if level of jaundice is of concern because of patient's age in hours. American Academy of Pediatric (AAP) guidelines and nomograms are available. Avoid medications known to displace bilirubin bound to albumin (eg, ceftriaxone) to minimize risk for kernicterus when treating young infants with jaundice.

B. **Physiologic Jaundice.** Condition is self-limited, peaking at approximately 3–4 days of life for healthy term infants and resolving by 2 weeks of life.

C. **Breast-Feeding Jaundice.** Provide lactation support, if available. If infant is dehydrated, consider administering IV fluids or supplementing with formula by mouth. Breast-feeding should not be discontinued in most cases, particularly in the first weeks of life when not well established.

D. **ABO Incompatibility.** Most patients with ABO incompatibility will not have clinically significant hemolysis. For more severe cases, response to phototherapy is generally good. In very severe cases, obtain serial hematocrit and bilirubin levels. Patients with severe anemia may require packed RBC transfusions.

E. **G6PD Deficiency.** Provide family with educational materials regarding foods and medications to be avoided.

F. **Erythrocyte Structural Defects.** If spherocytosis is suspected, consult pediatric hematologist. Follow patients for pallor and jaundice. Some patients may require phototherapy in the newborn period.

G. **Familial Disorders of Conjugation.** Gilbert syndrome is benign, whereas Crigler-Najjar types 1 and 2 are associated with severe hyperbilirubinemia. Type 2 may respond to phenobarbital, but type 1 does not and is treated by phototherapy and liver transplantation.

VI. **Problem Case Diagnosis.** The 3-day-old infant was reported to be breast-feeding every 3 hours for 10 minutes on one side only. Inadequate feeding resulted in loss of 11% of birthweight and limited stooling. Final diagnosis is breast-feeding jaundice.

VII. **Teaching Pearl: Questions.** How does phototherapy work to decrease hyperbilirubinemia? What part of the brain is involved in kernicterus?

VIII. **Teaching Pearl: Answers.** Phototherapy, used to treat neonatal hyperbilirubinemia for more than 40 years, results in a number of isomers (eg, lumirubin) or photoproducts that are excreted in urine and bile. Bilirubin preferentially deposits in basal ganglia, resulting in opisthotonus, seizures, and choreoathetoid movements. The auditory system is also highly sensitive to bilirubin, and auditory neuropathy and processing disorders may be seen in patients with kernicterus.

REFERENCES

American Academy of Pediatrics Provisional Committee for Quality Improvement and Subcommittee on Hyperbilirubinemia. Practice parameter: Management of hyperbilirubinemia in the healthy term newborn. *Pediatrics* 1994;4:558–565.

Bhutani VK, Johnson L, Sivieri EM. Predictive ability of a predischarge hour-specific serum bilirubin for subsequent hyperbilirubinemia in healthy term and near-term newborns. *Pediatrics* 1999;103:6–14.

Dennery PA, Seidman DS, Stevenson DK. Neonatal hyperbilirubinemia. *N Engl J Med* 2001;344:581–590.

Gourley GR. Breast-feeding, neonatal jaundice and kernicterus. *Semin Neonatol* 2002;7:135–141.

Johnson LH, Bhutani VK, Brown AK. System-based approach to management of neonatal jaundice and prevention of kernicterus. *J Pediatr* 2002;140:396–403.

39. HYPERCALCEMIA

I. **Problem.** A 2-month-old male infant with a history of birth asphyxia is found to have a serum calcium level of 15 mg/dL (normal for this age: 9–11 mg/dL).

II. **Immediate Questions**

A. **Does patient have symptoms associated with hypercalcemia?** Symptoms usually involve the bones, kidneys, GI tract, or neuropsychiatric system; manifestations include bone pain, polyuria, polydipsia, nausea, vomiting, constipation, anorexia, fatigue, confusion, and coma.

B. Is patient dehydrated? Recognition and treatment of volume depletion in a hypercalcemic patient is the first step in management.

C. Is there a family history of hypercalcemia, hypocalcemia, or parathyroid disease? Recognition of one of the familial causes of hypercalcemia or hypocalcemia may indicate the mechanism in this patient and specify therapy.

D. What medication(s) is patient receiving? Many causes of hypercalcemia are iatrogenic.

E. Pertinent Historical Information

    1. If an infant, is there a family history of parathyroid disease or hypocalcemia? A birth history of trauma or asphyxia?

    2. Are there renal symptoms (polyuria or polydipsia)? GI complaints (eg, loss of appetite, nausea, constipation, weight loss)? CNS symptoms (weakness, fatigue, depression)?

III. Differential Diagnosis. Infantile causes of hypercalcemia are often very different from causes in childhood. The two most common causes of hypercalcemia in adults, primary hyperparathyroidism and malignancy, are relatively rare in children.

A. Neonatal Hypercalcemia

    1. Williams syndrome. Supravalvular aortic stenosis, elfin-like facies, hypercalcemia in the first year of life.

    2. Neonatal hyperparathyroidism. Several rare conditions, including a life-threatening condition associated with familial hypocalciuric hypercalcemia, a self-limited secondary hyperparathyroidism associated with maternal hypocalcemia, or, rarely, familial hyperparathyroidism syndromes.

    3. Idiopathic infantile hypercalcemia. Related to increased sensitivity to vitamin D or elevated parathyroid hormone–related peptide.

    4. Subcutaneous fat necrosis. Associated with birth asphyxia or trauma; violaceous, indurated areas on back or pressure points. Caused by increased vitamin D or prostaglandin E production.

    5. Medications. Vitamins D and A, thiazides, prostaglandin E, calcium salts.

    6. Hypophosphatemia. Major cause in premature infants.

    7. Hypophosphatasia. Rare deficiency of alkaline phosphatase.

    8. Malignancy. Rare cause in infants.

    9. Blue diaper syndrome. Tryptophan malabsorption; nephrocalcinosis, constipation, fever, failure to thrive, absence of aminoaciduria.

    10. Jansen syndrome.

B. Childhood Hypercalcemia

1. **Immobilization.** Commonly seen in adolescents weeks after severe trauma.
2. **Malignancy.** Can occur with solid tumors, lymphoma, and leukemia.
3. **Granulomatous diseases.** Sarcoidosis, tuberculosis, cat-scratch disease. Increased formation of 1,25-dihydroxyvitamin D.
4. **Medications.** Similar to those listed for infants, earlier.
5. **Hyperparathyroidism.** Often familial.
6. **Familial hypocalciuric hypercalcemia (FHH).** Heterozygous form is benign and associated with low excretion of calcium and magnesium.
7. **AIDS.**
8. **Miscellaneous endocrine disorders.** Hyperthyroidism, pheochromocytoma, Addison disease.

IV. Database

A. Physical Exam Key Points

1. **Vital signs.** Hypertension may be present.
2. **Skin.** Observe for reddish-purple, indurated areas over pressure points, with subcutaneous fat necrosis; pruritus with skin calcifications.
3. **Lymph nodes.** Sign of malignancy or granulomatous disorder.
4. **HEENT.** Elfin-like facies in infants points to Williams syndrome.
5. **Heart.** Murmur of supravalvular aortic stenosis is characteristic of Williams syndrome.
6. **Neuromuscular.** Impaired mentation, muscle weakness, and hyporeflexia.

B. Laboratory Data

1. **Total calcium and serum albumin or ionized calcium.** Each gram per deciliter of albumin changes the serum calcium level by 0.8 mg/dL. Hypercalcemia is characterized as follows:
   a. **Mild:** 10.3–11.2 mg/dL.
   b. **Moderate:** 11.2–13.5 mg/dL.
   c. **Severe:** > 13.5 mg/dL.
2. **Phosphorus.** Low serum phosphorus points to parathyroid hormone (PTH)–mediated causes, and high serum phosphorus points to vitamin D–mediated causes. Low phosphorus in a premature infant is indicative of phosphate depletion.
3. **Alkaline phosphatase.** Level is very low in hypophosphatasia but elevated in hyperparathyroidism.
4. **BUN and creatinine.** Evaluate for renal failure and dehydration as a guide for therapy.
5. **Serum PTH.** Elevated in hyperparathyroidism; suppressed by nonparathyroid diseases.
6. **Vitamin D.** Vitamin D intoxication is indicated by high 25-hydroxyvitamin D level. The level of 1,25-dihydroxyvitamin D may be elevated in granulomatous disorders or rare disorders,

especially in infants, but this value is not as useful as 25-hydroxyvitamin D level.

7. **Urine calcium, phosphorus, and creatinine.** Perform on spot sample. Low calcium points to FHH; low tubular reabsorption of phosphate is consistent with a parathyroid disorder.

8. **Other workup.** Perform studies on parents if neonatal hypercalcemia is present. Obtain maternal and paternal serum and urinary calcium levels to diagnose FHH or familial hyperparathyroidism.

C. **Radiographic and Other Studies**

1. **Bone films.** Diagnostic changes may be found in hypophosphatasia, Jansen syndrome, vitamin A intoxication, hyperparathyroidism. Diffuse osteopenia is a nonspecific sign in hyperparathyroidism. Bone scans may be positive with malignancy.

2. **ECG.** Bradycardia, shortening of QT interval, lengthening of PR interval, and AV block are characteristic of hypercalcemia.

3. **Renal ultrasound.** Look for nephrocalcinosis.

V. **Plan.** Symptomatic patients and those with severe hypercalcemia require more aggressive treatment. Recognize that most patients are volume depleted if hypercalcemia is severe or long-standing. Focus on increasing renal excretion of calcium, decreasing release from bone, or decreasing GI absorption of calcium, in that order. Diagnosis of underlying cause is often important for directing therapy. For mild hypercalcemia, the focus should be on making sure that dietary measures and medications are appropriate and ensuring that patient is mobile and hydrated.

A. **Hydration and Saline Diuresis.** Most patients with moderate to severe hypercalcemia are volume depleted because of poor intake combined with sodium and water losses from kidneys. The first step should be volume repletion, preferably with normal saline (150–250 mL/kg/day). As long as patient is volume depleted, the kidneys will avidly reabsorb sodium. Keep accurate I&Os with twice-a-day weights.

B. **Diuretics.** After patient is euvolemic, administer furosemide, 0.5–1 mg/kg per dose q6h IV, and replenish losses to prevent dehydration. Monitor Ca, Na, K, Mg, PO_4, and creatinine at least every 12 hours. Keep accurate I&Os and weights. Thiazides are contraindicated.

C. **Bisphosphonates.** Current use is off-label in children, but bisphosphonates block bone resorption and are the most powerful agents for treatment of severe hypercalcemia, especially with malignancy.

1. **Pamidronate.** Can be given IV at a dose of 0.5–1 mg/kg/day (diluted in 10 mL normal saline per milligram pamidronate) over a minimum of 4 hours; dose can be repeated. Use in infants is

described in the literature. Maximum dose in adolescents is 60–90 mg daily.

2. **Zoledronic acid.** New treatment of choice in adults and adolescents with hypercalcemia of malignancy at a dose of 4 mg given IV q15min. Avoid in patients with renal failure. Monitor for hypocalcemia.

D. **Calcitonin.** Lowers calcium level rapidly when given with pamidronate. Dose: Salmon calcitonin, 4–8 IU/kg q12h IM or SQ. Patients become refractory after a few days.

E. **Corticosteroids.** Useful in vitamin D–mediated conditions. Give methylprednisolone, 1 mg/kg/day IV, or hydrocortisone, 1 mg/kg q6h IV.

F. **Phosphorus.** Give oral phosphorus for correction of phosphorus depletion and mild hypercalcemia in phosphate-depleted premature infants; avoid in other circumstances. Contraindicated with renal failure. IV phosphorus is strictly contraindicated.

G. **Diet.** Infants with hypercalcemia can be given a low-calcium and low–vitamin D formula (CalciloXD) but need to monitor for rickets if given long term.

VI. **Problem Case Diagnosis.** The 2-month-old infant has hypercalcemia as a result of subcutaneous fat necrosis that developed after traumatic delivery. Necrosis was likely due to abnormal production of prostaglandin E or 1,25-dihydroxyvitamin D. He was treated with saline and diuretics. Corticosteroids then were used successfully as a cause-directed therapy, and infant also was placed on CalciloXD until hypercalcemia resolved.

VII. **Teaching Pearl: Question.** What causes the features seen in a hypercalcemic crisis (fever, hypertension, bradycardia, severe dehydration, stupor, bradycardia, and coma)?

VIII. **Teaching Pearl: Answer.** Excessive calcium can be associated with decreased membrane excitability, decreased membrane permeability, subsequent renal loss of water and solute, and vascular constriction.

REFERENCES

Allen SH, Goldstein DE, Miles JH, et al. Hypercalcemia in the pediatric patient: A review and case reports. *Int Pediatr* 1993;8:409.

Langman C. Hypercalcemic syndromes in infants and children. In: Favus M, ed. *Primer on the Metabolic Bone Diseases and Disorders of Mineral Metabolism,* 5th ed. American Society of Bone and Mineral Research, 2003:267–270.

Rodd C, Goodyer P. Hypercalcemia of the newborn: Etiology, evaluation and management. *Pediatr Nephrol* 1999;13:542.

Ziegler R. Hypercalcemic crisis. *J Am Soc Nephrol* 2001;12:S3.

40. HYPERGLYCEMIA

I. Problem. A 4-month-old infant with fever and a blood glucose level of 250 mg/dL is being evaluated in the pediatric clinic. Hyperglycemia is defined as a serum blood glucose level of > 100 mg/dL.

II. Immediate Questions

   A. What are the vital signs? Does patient have any mental status changes? Children with hyperglycemia due to diabetic ketoacidosis (DKA) can have mental status changes, including coma.

   B. Is patient known to have diabetes mellitus (DM)? Ask about current medications (ie, type, route, and dose) and verify most recent doses taken. Obtain information about home glucose monitoring and current illnesses.

   C. What is the serum glucose level on laboratory analysis? Serum glucose level provides the most reliable monitoring information. Glucose monitoring strips can be unreliable for many reasons, including user error, expired strips, and improper machine calibration.

   D. Is patient spilling glucose in the urine? A simple dipstick test can identify glucose in urine. Once the renal threshold has been reached, glucosuria will develop.

   E. Is patient receiving exogenous glucose and, if so, how much? Calculate the glucose infusion rate, which will indicate how many milligrams per kilogram per minute of glucose patient is receiving.

   F. Does patient have signs of sepsis or shock? Shock can result from sepsis or trauma. Patients can also develop hyperglycemia postoperatively.

   G. Are there signs of uncontrolled, new-onset DM? These signs include polyuria, polydipsia, polyphagia, weight loss, fatigue, and increased infections.

III. Differential Diagnosis

   A. Type 1 DM. Low or absent levels of endogenously produced insulin. New-onset and poorly controlled type 1 DM can both lead to hyperglycemia.

   B. Type 2 DM. Receptors on cells are resistant to insulin. Condition is exacerbated postoperatively as well as in patients who are unable to take their medications.

   C. Stress-Induced Hyperglycemia. Sepsis, trauma (especially head injury), and postoperative states can cause a stress reaction leading to decreased metabolism of glucose.

   D. TPN-Induced Hyperglycemia. Glucose is one of the major calorie sources in TPN solutions. A higher concentration of glucose is present in the solution when it is received centrally. Hyperglycemia can occur when the solution is advanced too quickly or an excessive amount is administered.

E. Medications. Pulse steroids, thiazide diuretics, theophylline, and phenytoin can induce hyperglycemia.

F. Factitious Hyperglycemia. Be sure the specimen was not drawn from or above an IV line that is infusing a solution that contains glucose. If in doubt, repeat the test.

IV. Database

A. Physical Exam Key Findings. Pay close attention to mental status, breathing pattern (Kussmaul respirations), and signs of sepsis (ie, poor perfusion, fever, lethargy) and dehydration.

B. Laboratory Data

1. **Serum glucose.** Confirm rapid strip measurement with an evaluation of serum level.

2. **Urinalysis.** Obtain urine dipstick analysis for evidence of glucose as well as infection.

3. **CBC with differential.** Evaluate for infection. If signs and symptoms of infection are present, obtain appropriate cultures (eg, blood and urine).

4. **Serum electrolytes.** Hyperglycemia can cause an osmotic diuresis and dehydration leading to electrolyte abnormalities.

5. **ABGs.** Blood pH helps to evaluate degree of acidosis (DKA).

C. Radiographic and Other Studies. If indicated by clinical presentation.

V. Plan

A. Type 1 DM. If patient is known to have type 1 DM, treat accordingly with a full evaluation for DKA, including pH, electrolytes, serum glucose, and urine. DKA exists when hyperglycemia, acidosis, and ketonemia are present. If patient is hyperglycemic without evidence of DKA, administer IV or SQ insulin and correct fluid deficits. Patients in DKA should receive isotonic bolus fluid rehydration to correct shock. Correct remaining fluid deficits slowly. Patients in DKA should also be treated with a low-dose insulin infusion that is discontinued when acidosis resolves. Correct additional electrolyte abnormalities (potassium and phosphorous), if present. Typically, hyperkalemia exists when patient is acidotic, hypokalemia and hypophosphatemia as the acidosis resolves. If patient has new-onset type 1 DM, thorough serum evaluation for cause and associated factors should be carried out. DKA can be life-threatening and must therefore be addressed promptly.

B. Type 2 DM. If patient's disease is normally controlled by diet or oral hypoglycemic agents, temporary insulin therapy may be indicated.

C. Stress-Induced Hyperglycemia. If infection is suspected, perform a thorough evaluation and initiate appropriate antibiotic therapy. If patient is postoperative without signs of infection, check to see if glucose is spilling into the urine.

D. TPN-Related Hyperglycemia. TPN may be the primary or only source of calories and nutrition; therefore, discontinuing feeding is not recommended. Consider diluting the glucose concentration (change solution to smaller dextrose concentration) or temporarily infuse insulin. Again, treatment should be initiated according to the level of hyperglycemia and whether glucose is found in the urine.

   E. Medications. Evaluate the degree of hyperglycemia and whether patient is spilling glucose into the urine. If correction is required, insulin therapy may be indicated, especially if causative medication is necessary for an underlying illness. Switching to an alternative therapeutically equivalent medicine that does not cause hyperglycemia may be appropriate.

VI. Problem Case Diagnosis. The 4-month-old infant had a high WBC count and was started on antibiotics. Blood and urine cultures obtained the next day showed a bacterial pathogen. Hyperglycemia resolved as the infection was treated.

VII. Teaching Pearl: Question. What is the difference in presentation between type 1 and type 2 DM in children?

VIII. Teaching Pearl: Answer. The incidence of type 2 DM in children and particularly adolescents is on the rise. The presentation of type 2 DM is usually more indolent than that of type 1. Acute metabolic decompensation is rare, and patients may or may not have polyuria or polydipsia. Most patients are overweight, frequently have a history of type 2 DM, and often have acanthosis nigricans on physical exam.

REFERENCES

Hay WW. Addressing hypoglycemia and hyperglycemia. Neoreviews. *Pediatr Rev* 1999;20:4e–5.

Hemachandra AH, Cowett RM. Neonatal hyperglycemia. Neoreviews. *Pediatr Rev* 1999;20:16e–24.

Nesmith JD. Type 2 diabetes mellitus in children and adolescents. *Pediatr Rev* 2001;22:147–152.

41. HYPERKALEMIA

   I. Problem. A 6-year-old boy with acute lymphocytic leukemia is undergoing chemotherapy when he begins to complain of "tingling" of the hands and feet. Serum electrolytes, which were obtained 30 minutes earlier, are urgently reported to show a potassium level of 6.9 mEq/L (normal for this age: 3.4–4.7 mEq/L).

   II. Immediate Questions
   A. What is patient's cardiac rhythm? Are ECG changes present? Hyperkalemia can produce lethal cardiac rhythm disturbances. Recognition of peaked T waves, PR prolongation, or widened QRS complex requires immediate action. Serum potassium level

may be rapidly lowered by IV administration of bicarbonate or insulin (and glucose), or both.

B. **Is potassium in any form being administered? If so, has that been stopped?** Unrecognized sources of potassium include IV fluids and blood products. Check that patient's actual fluid matches the appropriate order.

C. **What has urine output been over the past several hours?** Hyperkalemia may be a manifestation of decreased glomerular filtration rate (GFR) and may be a herald of renal failure. Continuing administration of potassium in this setting can be quite dangerous.

D. **Is laboratory result accurate?** Any hemolysis or cell lysis of a blood sample may increase potassium within the sample but may not be a true reflection of serum potassium level. Obtaining blood from a large-bore vein or an arterial sample may decrease the likelihood of hemolysis.

III. **Differential Diagnosis**

A. **Pseudohyperkalemia.** Although a cause of elevated laboratory potassium values, it is critical to rule out true hyperkalemia before concluding that the reported value is inaccurate. Because potassium is primarily an intracellular ion, any hemolysis will increase the total potassium in a blood sample. This occurs most often when blood sampling is difficult and a free-flowing sample is hard to obtain. It is significantly less likely in samples obtained from arterial puncture or central venous lines. Similarly, in patients with marked leukocytosis or thrombocytosis, enough intracellular potassium may be released in the blood sample to produce a falsely elevated level. A tourniquet applied for an extensive period of time may also produce a sample with an elevated potassium content that does not reflect the body's true serum potassium level.

B. **Redistribution.** Because only about 1–2% of the body's total potassium resides in the extracellular space, a modest shift of potassium out of the cell can produce a dramatic elevation in serum potassium. Potassium can exit the cell either by active transport or when the cell membrane becomes incompetent and cell death occurs. Redistribution of potassium to the extracellular space occurs in acidosis (metabolic or respiratory), insulin deficiency, hypertonic states, use of depolarizing neuromuscular blockade (eg, succinylcholine), β-blockers, digoxin toxicity, tumor lysis syndromes, extensive crush injuries, rhabdomyolysis, and burns. A rare autosomal-dominant disorder called *familial hyperkalemic periodic paralysis* also exists in which sudden flaccid paralysis and elevated serum potassium occurs.

C. **Aldosterone Deficiency or Unresponsiveness.** Aldosterone increases urinary excretion of potassium.

1. **Medications.** Many drugs interfere with production and action of aldosterone, including ACE inhibitors, potassium-sparing

diuretics (spironolactone), amiloride, trimethoprim, heparin, and NSAIDs.

2. Primary adrenal failure. Affects aldosterone production.

3. Hyporeninemic hypoaldosteronism and type 4 renal tubular acidosis. In these conditions, low aldosterone activity exists in the setting of a mild metabolic acidosis. Mild renal insufficiency may also be present, but GFR typically is adequate.

4. Tubular unresponsiveness to aldosterone. May occur in patients with chronic renal disease; however, plasma aldosterone levels are normal.

D. Decreased Renal Excretion. In patients with renal failure and reduced GFR, hyperkalemia can develop. It is important to consider both GFR and intake of potassium when evaluating renal failure as the source of hyperkalemia. A reduction of GFR to 20% of normal should still allow adequate excretion of a normal dietary intake of potassium. When hyperkalemia develops in a patient with renal failure, either GFR has been reduced to less than 10% of normal, or patient is receiving more potassium than is believed, or both. It is important to search for hidden sources of potassium.

IV. Database. Owing to the severe cardiac sequelae associated with hyperkalemia, it is critical to quickly confirm the diagnosis and begin therapy to lower the serum potassium level. The presence of ECG changes or physical exam findings consistent with hyperkalemia is sufficient to institute therapy while awaiting a repeat laboratory value.

A. Physical Exam Key Points. In a child with hyperkalemia, the physical exam may be completely normal.

1. Heart. Cardiac exam is likely to be completely normal despite significant ECG changes. Only when serum potassium reaches a threshold level above which the cardiac muscle cannot appropriately repolarize will the dramatic findings of a wide-complex tachycardia or ventricular fibrillation develop.

2. Other findings. The most common noncardiac findings on exam are muscle weakness and complaints of paresthesia. Child may also complain of nausea and vomiting.

B. Laboratory Data

1. Basic metabolic panel. Obtain serum and urine electrolytes, creatinine level, and serum pH.

2. CBC and serum cortisol levels. May assist in determining etiology of hyperkalemia.

3. Digoxin level (if toxicity suspected) and serum myoglobin (rhabdomyolysis or crush injuries). Obtain based on history.

4. Further workup. Pursue as necessary based on clinical presentation.

C. Radiographic and Other Studies

1. Radiographic studies. Of little help in this setting.

2. **ECG.** It is of paramount importance to obtain an ECG as quickly as possible, because cardiac manifestations may be silent on physical exam. As serum potassium level rises, the balance between intracellular and extracellular ions is disturbed, which in turn interferes with repolarization at the end of the action potential. The ECG provides excellent evidence of the degree of this disturbance, as clearly distinct changes can be seen in succession as serum potassium level rises (Table I–11).

V. **Plan.** There are multiple methods by which to lower serum potassium level. Intensity of therapy depends on child's serum level and symptoms. Typically a serum level < 6 mEq/L in an asymptomatic patient with no ECG findings requires only close monitoring, follow-up, and limitation of potassium supplied to the body. Etiology, rate of rise, and symptoms must all be taken into consideration when determining appropriate therapy. Clinician must also consider the rate at which the applied therapy will lower serum potassium.

A. **Stop Any Potassium Going to Patient.** This may seem like an obvious treatment; however, "routine" fluids containing potassium, or blood products that may have relatively high potassium content due to cell lysis, are sometimes overlooked. This action is particularly essential in patients with renal failure.

B. **Volume Expansion.** Increasing the intravascular volume with potassium-free solutions such as normal saline will dilute the relative concentration of serum potassium.

C. **Loop Diuretics.** These agents work via inhibition of a sodium-potassium-chloride co-transporter, producing increased renal excretion of potassium. In addition, increased urine output helps renal potassium excretion.

D. **Sodium Polystyrene Sulfonate (Kayexalate).** May be given orally or rectally. It serves as a potassium binder and is quite effective in reducing serum potassium; however, its effects are not immediate because absorption via the GI tract is necessary.

E. **Inhaled β-Agonist.** This therapy is easily administered if no contraindication exists. Use with caution in hyperkalemic patients who

TABLE I–11. ECG CHANGES ASSOCIATED WITH CHANGES IN SERUM POTASSIUM LEVEL

Serum K⁺ Level (mEq/L)[a]	ECG Changes
6–7	Peaked T waves
7–8	Widened PR interval, decreased P wave
> 8	Widened QRS complex, sinusoidal wave

[a] Values listed are approximate.

already demonstrate significant ECG changes. This therapy is not immediate, because administration may take several minutes.

F. **Insulin and Glucose.** Insulin causes an intracellular shift of potassium. Glucose is administered to help prevent hypoglycemia after insulin administration. Typical insulin dosing is 0.1 unit/kg with glucose, 0.5 g/kg.

G. **Sodium Bicarbonate.** Producing a metabolic alkalosis with the administration of sodium bicarbonate will cause a rapid intracellular shift of potassium. Typically 1 mEq/kg per dose of bicarbonate is given.

H. **Calcium.** Calcium therapy should be instituted in patients with ECG changes and hyperkalemia. Calcium itself will not improve hyperkalemia; however, calcium will serve to stabilize the cardiac membrane and delay development of more significant dysrhythmias. Typical calcium dosing is 10 mg/kg of calcium chloride, or 50 mg/kg of calcium gluconate.

I. **Hemodialysis.** Emergent hemodialysis is sometimes necessary to treat severe hyperkalemia. This method is typically instituted in the setting of renal failure and an ongoing expectation that dialysis will need to be continued. Peritoneal dialysis may be technically easier; however, it is not as reliable a method as hemodialysis for potassium removal.

VI. **Problem Case Diagnosis.** Serum potassium level in the 6-year-old boy became elevated as a result of massive cell death that occurred while he underwent treatment for leukemia. His earliest symptom was simple tingling of the extremities. If not treated, patient would proceed to develop a potentially lethal cardiac dysrhythmia.

VII. **Teaching Pearl: Question.** A patient has a serum potassium level of 7.1 mEq/L and peaked T waves on a cardiac monitor. The senior resident orders a calcium bolus in order to lower the serum potassium. Is this action correct?

VIII. **Teaching Pearl: Answer.** Administration of calcium to a symptomatic hyperkalemic patient is appropriate. However, calcium will act only to stabilize the cardiac myocyte membrane and delay the onset of dysrhythmia. An appropriate action would be to give calcium plus IV bicarbonate, or glucose and insulin, or both, to lower the serum potassium level.

REFERENCES

Behrman RE, Kliegman RM, Jenson HB, eds. *Nelson Textbook of Pediatrics,* 17th ed. Saunders, 2004:192–209.

Feld LG, Kaskel FJ, Schoeneman MJ. The approach to fluid and electrolyte therapy in pediatrics. *Adv Pediatr* 1988;35:497–535.

42. HYPERMAGNESEMIA

I. Problem. A 2-day-old preterm infant born to a mother with preeclampsia is found to have a serum magnesium level of 4 mg/dL (normal: 1.2–2.6 mg/dL).

II. Immediate Questions

A. Is there evidence of neuromuscular or cardiovascular effects? Hypermagnesemia can cause lethargy, decreased ventilation, and life-threatening cardiac symptoms, including heart block.

B. Was infant's mother treated with magnesium? Was maternal eclampsia, preeclampsia, or premature labor present? Parenteral magnesium sulfate is commonly used to prevent seizures in preeclampsia and to stop premature labor.

III. Differential Diagnosis

A. Renal Causes. The kidney is usually able to excrete magnesium loads; therefore, moderate to severe renal failure is associated with hypermagnesemic syndromes.

1. **Acute renal failure.** Rhabdomyolysis may be present.
2. **Chronic renal failure.** Mild hypermagnesemia is commonly seen. Look for antacid or cathartic use or magnesium-contaminated dialysate.
3. **Familial hypocalciuric hypercalcemia.** Can be associated with mild hypermagnesemia.

B. Increased Intake

1. **Magnesium compounds.** Given as laxatives, antacids, rectal enemas, or purgatives. Bowel obstruction and perforation are risk factors.
2. **Hemiacidrin.** Ureteral irrigation.

C. Neonatal Exposure

1. **Maternal treatment.** Infusions of magnesium sulfate are commonly used in treatment of premature labor, preeclampsia, and eclampsia. Symptoms in infants do not necessarily correspond to serum magnesium level, and fetal stress may contribute to lethargy.
2. **Neonatal treatment.** Experimental therapy for cerebroprotective effect.

IV. Database

A. Physical Exam Key Points

1. **Cardiovascular.** Irregular pulse and hypotension.
2. **Neuromuscular.** Decreased deep tendon reflexes.

B. Laboratory Data

1. **BUN and creatinine.** Acute or chronic renal failure is often present.
2. **Serum magnesium**
   a. **< 5 mg/dL.** Produces mild weakness and hypotension only.

        b. 5–10 mg/dL. Causes muscle weakness, hyporeflexia, and hypotension.

        c. > 10 mg/dL. Increases risk for complete heart block or paralysis.

    3. Serum calcium. Look for hypocalcemia, resulting from suppression of parathyroid hormone (PTH) secretion.

  C. Radiographic and Other Studies. Obtain ECG to look for arrhythmia, prolonged PR interval, increased QRS complex, increased QT wave, or heart block.

V. Plan. In patients with normal renal function, stopping the magnesium source is usually adequate. In those with severe hypermagnesemia, IV calcium can be used to block the effect of magnesium, and dialysis may be necessary if concomitant renal failure is present.

  A. Severe Hypermagnesemia With Cardiac or Respiratory Failure. Block effects of high serum magnesium with IV calcium.

    1. Neonates. Administer calcium gluconate, 100 mg/kg per dose (elemental calcium, 9 mg/kg per dose) IV over 20 minutes. Can repeat if necessary.

    2. Older children and adolescents. Give 100–200 mg elemental calcium IV over 5–10 minutes to acutely antagonize effect of magnesium.

  B. Hypermagnesemia With Renal Failure. Hemodialysis or peritoneal dialysis may be necessary.

VI. Problem Case Diagnosis. The 2-day-old infant had hypermagnesemia secondary to treatment of preeclampsia in the mother. Supportive care was provided; 1 week later, hypermagnesemia had completely resolved.

VII. Teaching Pearl: Question. Is hypermagnesemia or hypomagnesemia associated with suppressed PTH secretion and hypocalcemia in neonates?

VIII. Teaching Pearl: Answer. Paradoxically, both hypermagnesemia and hypomagnesemia may suppress PTH secretion and cause hypocalcemia in neonates, although by different mechanisms.

REFERENCES

Rantonen T, Kaapa P, Jalonen J, et al. Antenatal magnesium sulphate exposure is associated with prolonged parathyroid hormone suppression in preterm neonates. *Acta Paediatr* 2001:90:278.

Rude RK. Magnesium depletion and hypermagnesemia. In: Favus M, ed. *Primer on the Metabolic Bone Diseases and Disorders of Mineral Metabolism,* 5th ed. American Society of Bone and Mineral Research, 2003:292–295.

43. HYPERNATREMIA

I. Problem. A 6-week-old infant, was admitted with a history of diarrhea and fever of 2 days' duration, has a serum sodium concentration of 160 mEq/L (normal: 136–146 mEq/L).

II. Immediate Questions

A. What are the vital signs? Most children with hypernatremia are dehydrated, with typical signs and symptoms that are dependent on the degree of dehydration.

   1. Mild dehydration (3% in older children; 5% in infants). Pulse may be normal or increased, urine output is decreased, and physical exam is generally normal.

   2. Moderate dehydration (6% in older children; 10% in infants). Produces tachycardia and little or no urine output. On physical exam, eyeballs and fontanelle are sunken, with decreased tears, dry mucous membranes, loss of skin turgor, delayed capillary refill, and cool skin.

   3. Severe dehydration (9% in older children; 15% in infants). Pulse is rapid and weak, BP is decreased, there is no urine output, and on physical exam, there is accentuation of findings noted in moderate dehydration, in addition to notable skin mottling.

B. What is patient's neurologic status? Hypernatremia, even in the absence of dehydration, causes CNS symptoms that tend to parallel the degree of elevation and rate of increase in the serum sodium concentration. Patients are irritable, restless, weak, and lethargic. Some infants have a high-pitched cry. Older children complain of extreme thirst and nausea. These patients are at risk of developing brain hemorrhage (subarachnoid, subdural, and parenchymal). The etiology of the hemorrhages is related to shifting of water from the intracellular space as extracellular osmolality increases. This shift decreases brain volume, resulting in tearing of intracellular veins and bridging blood vessels as the brain moves away from the skull and meninges. Seizures and coma may ensue.

C. What is patient's sodium intake during health and now? Increased salt intake is rarely a cause of hypernatremia unless the amounts are massive. This can occur when the amount of salt ingested overwhelms the maximal osmotic clearance capacity of the kidney. Such a situation may occur, for example, if large doses of sodium bicarbonate are administered IV to correct a metabolic acidosis, or in the course of CPR. Another cause is erroneous or intentional addition of salt to infant formula. In infants, it is important to ascertain the type of milk being ingested, especially during the first 2 weeks of life. Rarely, the concentration of sodium in breast milk remains elevated, resulting in poor feeding and hypernatremic dehydration.

D. Is there a history of polyuria, polydipsia, or excessive thirst?
Diabetes insipidus or mellitus may cause hypernatremia if patient
has no access to, or poor intake of, fluids, especially water.

E. Is there a disorder of osmoregulation? Central diabetes
insipidus is caused by undetectable or low concentrations of
plasma antidiuretic hormone (ADH). Patients have sudden onset
of polyuria and a predilection for cold water. Nephrogenic diabetes insipidus has variable onset and is due to insensitivity of the
renal collecting duct to ADH. Hypodipsic essential hypernatremia
has been described in patients with cerebral lesions involving the
hypothalamus. These patients have persistent hypernatremia not
explained by apparent intravascular volume loss, ability to form
ADH, renal responsiveness to ADH, and absence or attenuation
of thirst.

**F. Does patient take any medications that could cause hyper-
natremia?** Osmotic diuretics (eg, mannitol) or osmotic cathartics
(eg, lactulose) can result in hypernatremia.

**G. What are intake and output (I&O) measurements over pre-
ceding 24–72 hours?** Elimination of water in excess of salt
through GI (diarrhea), cutaneous (excessive sweating), or renal
(obstructive uropathy) losses results in hypernatremia when
patients have limited or no access to water. These patients have
signs and symptoms of dehydration.

**H. Is patient's growth and development within normal parame-
ters?** Failure to thrive (FTT) and hypernatremia may be present in
patients with chronic renal insufficiency related to obstructive
uropathy or renal dysplasia. Hypernatremia and FTT also are
observed with ineffective breast-feeding or child neglect, or both.

**I. Is there a family history of hypernatremia and dehydration,
particularly in males, due to dehydration in early infancy?**
Congenital nephrogenic diabetes insipidus is inherited as an
X-linked recessive (most common), autosomal-recessive, or
autosomal-dominant disorder. The X-linked form manifests in
males, with females expressing variable degrees of polyuria and
polydipsia. Although the disorder is present at birth, infants are
diagnosed when they manifest hypo-osmolar urine in the face of
dehydration, hypernatremia, vomiting, and fever. Some infants
have FTT and mental retardation as a result of frequent episodes
of dehydration and hypernatremia.

J. Is there a laboratory error? Presence of hypernatremia in the
absence of pertinent history and physical findings may suggest a
laboratory error. It may be prudent to repeat the test.

K. Pertinent Historical Information
   1. If an infant, what type of formula is given, and how is it
   prepared?
   2. What are child's voiding or stooling patterns? Constipation is
   present in patients with diabetes insipidus.

3. Have similar episodes of hypernatremia occurred in the past?
4. Is there a past medical history of head trauma, brain surgery, or sickle cell anemia or trait?

III. **Differential Diagnosis.** Considers pathophysiologic processes underlying the disorder: water and sodium deficits, water losses, and sodium excess.
  A. **Water and Sodium Deficits.** Water losses are greater than sodium losses.
    1. **Renal losses (urine sodium > 20 mEq/L; urine iso-osmolality or hypo-osmolality)**
      a. Osmotic diuretics (eg, mannitol, urea, glucose).
      b. Diuretics (eg, thiazides, furosemide).
      c. Postobstructive diuresis, which occurs with relief of bilateral ureteral obstruction due to renal stones, tumors, or urethral obstruction.
      d. Polyuric phase of acute renal failure.
      e. Intrinsic renal disease.
    2. **Extrarenal losses (urine sodium < 10 mEq/L; urine hyper-osmolality)**
      a. Excessive skin losses (sweat is hypotonic).
        i. Fever (12% increase in insensible water losses for every degree increase in body temperature above 38.3°C [100.9°F]).
        ii. Exposure to high environmental temperatures.
        iii. Phototherapy.
        iv. Radiant warmers.
        v. Burns.
      b. **GI losses**
        i. Vomiting.
        ii. Diarrhea. (Stool losses due to infections are hypotonic in children. Hypernatremic dehydration is described after use of lactulose.)
        iii. Fistulae.
  B. **Water Losses.** Total body water is decreased, while total body sodium is normal.
    1. **Renal losses**
      a. **Central diabetes insipidus.** Results from inadequate production of antidiuretic hormone (ADH). If child's access to water is hampered or thirst mechanism is affected, hypernatremia occurs. May be idiopathic, hereditary (eg, Wolfram syndrome), or caused by tumors, trauma, infections (eg, meningitis), granulomas (eg, sarcoidosis), or vascular conditions (eg, cerebral aneurysm).
      b. **Nephrogenic diabetes insipidus.** Results from insensitivity of the renal collecting duct to ADH. Disease may be congenital (X-linked or autosomal dominant) or acquired due to

drugs (eg, lithium), sickle cell disease, chronic renal disease (eg, obstructive uropathy), hypokalemia, or hypercalcemia.

2. Extrarenal losses
   a. Respiratory, due to increases insensible water losses in intubated patients receiving dehumidified air or oxygen.
   b. Cutaneous, due to fever or excessive sweating.
3. Inadequate intake of water. Hypodipsic essential hypernatremia, in which patients have persistent hypernatremia not explained by extracellular volume losses, absence of thirst, partial diabetes insipidus, and normal response to ADH. Many patients have cerebral lesions in the vicinity of the hypothalamus (eg, craniopharyngioma, teratoma). The hypodipsia is attributed to a decrement in angiotensin-II–mediated thirst.

C. Sodium Excess Without Significant Change in Total Body Water (urine sodium > 20 mEq/L)
   1. Administration of hypertonic sodium
      a. Oral intake of sodium chloride tablets.
      b. IV administration of sodium bicarbonate during CPR.
      c. IV administration of hypertonic saline (3%).
      d. Ingestion of seawater, especially in infants.
      e. Improper mixing of infant formulas or enteral tube feedings.
      f. Ineffective breast-feeding.
   2. Mineralocorticoid or corticosteroid excess, in which hypernatremia is mild and clinically unimportant.
      a. Primary hyperaldosteronism.
      b. Cushing syndrome.
      c. Exogenous steroids.

IV. Database
A. Physical Exam Key Points. Children with hypernatremic dehydration tend to preserve intravascular volume better than patients with other types of dehydration because of water shifts from intravascular to extravascular space.
   1. Vital signs. Check for tachycardia (early sign of dehydration) and orthostatic changes.
   2. Skin turgor, color, perfusion. Presence of doughy skin in a dehydrated child suggests hypernatremic dehydration. Cyanosis and prolonged capillary refill suggests severe dehydration.
   3. Mucous membranes. Dry mucous membranes suggest dehydration.
   4. Neurologic findings. Irritability, lethargy, muscle twitching, and seizures may be present. Some infants have a high-pitched cry and hyperpnea. Alert patients are very thirsty; some complain of nausea.
B. Laboratory Data
   1. Serum electrolytes. Serum sodium concentration > 146 mEq/L is abnormal. Monitor serum electrolytes for hypokalemia and

hypercalcemia, which are possible etiologies of hypernatremia. Look for hypocalcemia as a sequela of hypernatremia. Follow serum sodium concentration closely.

2. **Renal studies.** Elevated BUN and creatinine may suggest intrinsic renal disease. If the BUN-to-creatinine ratio is > 20:1, dehydration is present; when the ratio is < 10:1, intrinsic renal disease is present.

3. **Serum glucose.** Mild hyperglycemia is often noted in hypernatremia. Etiology of elevated serum glucose is unknown.

4. **Urine osmolality.** Value > 700 mOsm/kg-H_2O suggests that child's renal concentrating capacity is intact, eliminating diabetes insipidus as a cause of hypernatremia.

5. **Spot urine sodium.** In the presence of hypernatremia, spot urine sodium < 10 mEq/L suggests extrarenal losses of sodium.

6. **Water deprivation test.** Performed in stable, well-hydrated patients. Serum sodium concentration and osmolality, urine specific gravity and osmolality, and weight are monitored every 2 hours. Patient is water deprived until one of the following occurs: loss of more than 3% of body weight; or serum sodium concentration > 150 mEq/L and serum osmolality > 300 mOsm/kg-H_2O. Patients with central or nephrogenic diabetes insipidus develop serum sodium concentrations ≥ 150 mEq/L in the face of urine osmolality < 150 mOsm/kg-H_2O and weight loss of 3% or more. Patients with central diabetes insipidus respond to DDAVP or vasopressin by increasing their urine osmolality and decreasing urine volume.

C. **Radiographic and Other Studies**

1. **MRI and CT scans of head.** Helpful in diagnosing tumors and other intracranial causes of central diabetes insipidus.

2. **Renal ultrasound.** Helpful in diagnosing renal causes of secondary nephrogenic diabetes insipidus.

V. **Plan**

A. **Initial Considerations.** In most patients with hypernatremia, management involves lowering the serum sodium concentration slowly (over 48–72 hours) and treating the underlying cause of hypernatremia. As hypernatremia develops, the brain increases its intracellular osmolality, which prevents loss of brain water. The process is slow and most evident when hypernatremia develops slowly. Consequently, if serum sodium concentration is corrected rapidly (with resultant decrease in serum osmolality), extracellular water will move into the intracellular space to equalize osmolality. Cerebral edema ensues, resulting in seizures, herniation, and death. It is recommended that the decrease in serum sodium concentration not exceed 0.5 mEq/L/h.

1. Restore intravascular volume. Administer isotonic saline, 20 mL/kg IV over 30–60 minutes. Several boluses may be needed to resuscitate the intravascular volume.

2. Replace deficits. Infants with hypernatremic dehydration are considered to be at least 10% dehydrated. The magnitude of free water deficit can be estimated using the serum sodium concentration. This calculation is based on the assumption that the increase in serum sodium concentration is caused solely by a decrease in total body water.

Ideal total body water × 145 mEq/L = Current total body water
× Current serum sodium

Current total body water = 0.6 × Current weight

The difference between calculated ideal body water and current total body water provides an estimate of the free water deficit. The remainder of the dehydration volume contains electrolytes, with an assumption that 60% of losses are extracellular, containing 140 mEq/L of sodium, and 40% are intracellular, containing 150 mEq/L of potassium.

3. Provide daily maintenance fluids and replace ongoing losses (eg, persistent stool losses).
4. Monitor serum electrolytes q6h.
5. Once hypernatremia and dehydration are corrected, evaluate and treat the underlying cause. If child has central diabetes insipidus, administer DDAVP. Children with congenital nephrogenic diabetes insipidus are maintained on a low-solute diet, thiazides, and indomethacin.

B. **Salt Poisoning or Overload.** The hypernatremia will correct spontaneously if renal function is normal, because the sodium excess will be excreted in urine. The following steps are instituted.

1. Eliminate the source of the sodium. Always suspect nonaccidental addition of salt to infant formulas.
2. Urinary excretion of sodium is enhanced by administering furosemide, 1 mg/kg per dose, which increases excretion of sodium and water. Water losses can be replaced by administration of D_5W. Infusion of the hypotonic solution without use of the loop diuretic will further expand the already increased intravascular volume, resulting in pulmonary edema.

C. **Patients With Concurrent Renal Failure.** Peritoneal dialysis with a hypertonic solution is recommended.

VI. **Problem Case Diagnosis.** The 6-week old infant had hypernatremic dehydration resulting from GI losses. He was treated following the guidelines for hypernatremic dehydration presented earlier (see V, A, 1–6, earlier). Patient had no complications from rehydration therapy, and sodium level normalized within 48 hours.

VII. **Teaching Pearl: Question.** The infant described in the opening problem had a BP of 90/50 (normal), heart rate of 120 (high normal), flat anterior fontanel, and diaper with evidence of urine. How can you explain these findings?

VIII. Teaching Pearl: Answer. Children with hypernatremic dehydration have better preservation of intravascular volume due to water shifts from the intracellular space. Consequently, BP and pulse may be less affected initially. These deceptive findings may lead clinicians to underestimate the degree of dehydration during treatment. Any child with a history similar to that described in the opening problem should be estimated to have a minimum fluid deficit of at least 10%.

REFERENCES

Finberg L. Hypernatremic (hypertonic) dehydration in infants. *N Engl J Med* 1973;289:196.

Meadow R. Non-accidental salt poisoning. *Arch Dis Child* 1993;68:448–452.

Rose BD, Post TW. *Clinical Physiology of Acid-Base and Electrolyte Disorders,* 5th ed. McGraw-Hill, 2001:749–761.

Strange K. Regulation of solute and water balance and cell volume in the central nervous system. *J Am Soc Nephrol* 1992;3:12–27.

44. HYPERPHOSPHATEMIA

I. Problem. A 10-year-old boy with cerebral palsy and constipation is transferred from a long-term health care facility with a serum phosphate level of 15 mg/dL (normal for this age: 3.7–5.6 mg/dL) and a serum calcium level of 6.0 mg/dL.

II. Immediate Questions

   A. Does patient have tetany or other signs of acute hypocalcemia? Many patients with acute and severe hyperphosphatemia develop hypocalcemia and tetany. The hypocalcemia must be recognized and treated while measures to bring down the phosphate level are being initiated.

   B. Does patient have acute or chronic renal failure? Renal failure is a significant risk factor for hyperphosphatemia and may dictate therapy. In acute situations, such as tumor lysis syndrome, the hyperphosphatemic patient may require dialysis.

   C. What medication(s) does patient take? Excessive amounts of Vitamin D cause increased intestinal absorption of phosphate. Phosphate-containing enemas also may increase phosphate levels.

III. Differential Diagnosis. Phosphate is similar to other compounds, such as potassium and magnesium, which are largely intracellular and levels of which are dependent on renal excretion. Hyperphosphatemia is usually the result of decrease in renal excretion, shift from intracellular to extracellular pools, and intake of amounts beyond what the kidney can regulate.

A. Decreased Renal Excretion
  1. **Renal failure**
      a. **Acute renal failure.** If associated with other mechanisms, can lead to severe, life-threatening hyperphosphatemia.
      b. **Chronic renal failure.** Phosphate retention issues are routine.
  2. **Parathyroid disorders.** Parathyroid hormone (PTH) stimulates the renal tubule to excrete phosphate. Decreased PTH effect results in hyperphosphatemia.
      a. **Hypoparathyroidism.** Can be congenital (DiGeorge syndrome) or acquired (autoimmune polyglandular candidiasis ectodermal dystrophy syndrome).
      b. **Pseudohypoparathyroidism.** Renal tubules are resistant to PTH.
  3. **Other causes**
      a. **Physiologic phosphate levels in infants.** Due to high phosphate reabsorption by proximal tubule.
      b. **Tumoral calcinosis.**

B. Transcellular Shifts From Intracellular to Extracellular Pools
  1. **Tumor lysis syndrome.** Look for hyperkalemia, hyperuricemia, and acute renal failure.
  2. **Rhabdomyolysis.**
  3. **Hemolysis.**
  4. **Malignant hyperpyrexia.** After anesthesia.
  5. **Diabetic ketoacidosis.**
  6. **Respiratory acidosis.**

C. Increased Intake of Phosphate or Vitamin D
  1. **Enteric.** Phosphate-containing laxatives and enemas.
  2. **High-phosphate formulas in newborns.** See discussion of neonatal hypocalcemia in Chapter 46, Hypocalcemia, p. 219.
  3. **Vitamin D intoxication.**

D. Miscellaneous
  1. **Intermittent hyperphosphatemia.** Rare condition.
  2. **Artifact.**

IV. Database
A. Physical Exam Key Points. See Chapter 46, Hypocalcemia, p. 220, for signs of parathyroid disorders that can also cause hyperphosphatemia.
  1. **Vital signs and general appearance**
      a. **Temperature.** Hyperthermia after anesthesia; malignant hyperpyrexia.
      b. **Respiratory rate.** Increased rate may be sign of respiratory acidosis.
      c. **Body mass.** Obesity is associated with pseudohypoparathryroidism.
  2. **Neuromuscular.** Look for tetany as a sign of hypocalcemia. Muscle tenderness may be a sign of rhabdomyolysis.

3. **Skeletal.** Look for short metacarpals, metatarsals of pseudo-hypoparathyroidism (Albright hereditary osteodystrophy). Masses around large joints are a sign of tumoral calcinosis.

B. **Laboratory Data**
   1. **Basic metabolic panel**
      a. **BUN and creatinine.** High values are signs of acute or chronic renal failure.
      b. **Potassium.** If high, consider tumor lysis, rhabdomyolysis, and hemolysis.
      c. **Glucose.** Look for diabetic ketoacidosis. Low calcium level may occur secondary to hyperphosphatemia, hypoparathyroidism, or pseudohypoparathyroidism. High serum calcium level may point to vitamin D intoxication.
   2. **Phosphorus.** Hyperphosphatemia may be missed because serum phosphorus level is not included in most chemistry panels. Serum phosphorus level is physiologically elevated in young children or infants and does not have to be treated. Normal levels are age dependent (see Section II, Phosphorus, p. 472).
   3. **ABGs.** Evaluate acid-base status; look for respiratory or metabolic acidosis.
   4. **CBC with differential.** Look for blasts in leukemia, signs of hemolysis.
   5. **Creatinine phosphokinase.** Check for rhabdomyolysis.
   6. **Vitamin D.** 25-Hydroxyvitamin D level is diagnostic of vitamin D toxicity. No need to routinely check 1,25-dihydroxyvitamin D levels.
   7. **Parathyroid hormone.** Intact PTH may be low in hypoparathyroidism, high in pseudohypoparathyroidism and renal failure.

C. **Radiographic and Other Studies.** X-ray film of hands can confirm diagnosis of Albright hereditary osteodystrophy.

V. **Plan**
   A. **Initial Management.** Treat severe hypocalcemia associated with tetany or seizures first, as described in Chapter 46, Hypocalcemia, p. 221. Correct hypocalcemia only until acute symptoms resolve, then focus on lowering phosphorus level to avoid precipitating calcium and phosphorus in soft tissues. Management may vary, depending on acuteness of patient's condition and whether renal function is normal. In conditions associated with tissue breakdown (eg, tumor lysis), address other abnormalities, such as hyperkalemia and acidosis.
   B. **Mild, Symptomatic Hyperphosphatemia (< 2 mg/dL greater than age-adjusted norm)**
      1. **Dietary restriction.** Limit phosphorus intake to 800–1000 mg/day by avoiding milk and other foods high in phosphate (obtain dietary consultation). In infants, low-phosphate formulas (Similac PM 60/40) or breast milk are useful in lowering phosphorus levels.

  2. **Phosphate binders.** Oral phosphate-binding agents are useful in blocking absorption of phosphate in food and intestinal fluids. Clinician can choose from magnesium- or aluminum-containing phosphate binders (avoid in chronic renal failure), calcium agents such as calcium carbonate or calcium acetate (avoid with hypercalcemia), and calcium-free phosphate binder (Sevelamer). These binders are best administered with meals; if patient is NPO, give at regular intervals around the clock to bind phosphorus in GI secretions.
  3. **Renal excretion.** In patients with tumor lysis syndrome and other acute release of phosphorus from cells, maintain diuresis and renal function with aggressive hydration.
  C. **Severe Hyperphosphatemia (> 2 mg/dL greater than age-adjusted norm and hypocalcemia or renal failure)**
  1. **Decrease intake and binders.** As previously described.
  2. **Dialysis.** In patients with acute or chronic renal failure, dialysis may be necessary. Phosphorus is removed rather poorly by hemodialysis, but treatment may be necessary to remove phosphorus, correct hypocalcemia, and correct other abnormalities such as hyperkalemia or acidosis. Phosphorus levels characteristically rebound 6–10 hours after dialysis until the primary process is resolved.

VI. **Problem Case Diagnosis.** The 10-year-old patient had been treated with repeated doses of a phosphate-containing enema. He developed severe dehydration with acute renal failure, hypernatremia (sodium concentration of 170 mEq/L), severe hypocalcemia, and hyperphosphatemia. Rehydration was ineffective, and acute dialysis was required to correct the abnormalities. Renal function, along with calcium and phosphorus levels, subsequently returned to normal.

VII. **Teaching Pearl: Question.** In pediatric patients with renal failure, how does clinician determine which calcium and phosphorus products to use?

VIII. **Teaching Pearl: Answer.** In patients with renal failure, avoid products in which serum calcium in milligrams per deciliter multiplied by serum phosphorus in milligrams per deciliter (calcium × phosphorus) is greater than 55. Target for other patients with chronic hyperphosphatemia is not known, but this is a reasonable goal for older children. In infants with physiologic hyperphosphatemia, this guideline does not apply.

REFERENCES

Brenner RM, ed. *Brenner & Rector's The Kidney*, 7th ed. Saunders, 2004:1058–1060.
Hruska KA, Lederer ED. Hyperphosphatemia and hypophosphatemia. In: Favus M, ed. *Primer on the Metabolic Bone Disorders of Mineral Metabolism*, 5th ed. American Society of Bone and Mineral Research, 2003:296–306.

45. HYPERTENSION

I. **Problem.** A 13-year-old girl who is significantly obese has BP of 145/90.

II. **Immediate Questions**
   A. **What is normal BP for child of this age?** Using age-specific BP percentiles (see Appendix B, p. 759), check 95th and 99th percentiles for BP appropriate to a child of this age; more urgency is required if BP exceeds 99th percentile.
   B. **Does patient have any symptoms?** Headache is rarely caused by moderate hypertension (ie, < 99th percentile). Hypertensive urgency may be indicated if headache is present and BP is > 99th percentile. Patients with symptoms (nausea, vomiting, dyspnea, mental changes, visual changes, or seizure) must be treated as a hypertensive emergency.
   C. **Past history of hypertension?** Obtain previous BP readings (including those from sports physicals, school nurses, and emergency department visits).
   D. **Past history of other illness?** Renal scarring secondary to early childhood UTI, umbilical artery catheterization, or bronchopulmonary disease can cause hypertension.
   E. **Does patient take any drugs (legal or illegal)?** Contraceptives, diet pills, cold medicine containing pseudoephedrine, antirejection drugs (particularly cyclosporine), corticosteroids, NSAIDs, erythropoietin, cocaine, amphetamine, and phencyclidine (PCP) can increase BP.
   F. **Is there a family history of hypertension or cardiovascular disease?** Ask about essential hypertension, metabolic syndrome (or syndrome X), and other familial forms of hypertension such as Alport syndrome, polycystic kidney disease, juvenile nephronephritis, glucocorticoid remediable aldosteronism, and Liddle syndrome, among others.

III. **Differential Diagnosis**
   A. **Secondary Hypertension.** The younger the child and the higher the BP, the more likely clinician will be to find a primary cause for hypertension. Starting at school age, children destined to have essential hypertension may present with mild BP elevation.
      1. **Renovascular Conditions.** This diagnosis should not be considered seriously in patients with isolated systolic hypertension. In newborns and infants, renal artery stenosis is most often due to thromboembolic events, frequently as a complication of umbilical artery catheterization. In older children, fibromuscular dysplasia is the most common cause for renal artery stenosis; neurofibromatosis and vasculitides are much less common causes.
      2. **Congenital renal malformation.** Renal dysplasia with or without cyst formation, polycystic kidney disease, and hydronephrosis can all result in hypertension.

3. **Bronchopulmonary dysplasia.** Steroid use and chronic hypoxemia-related vasoconstriction may explain the hypertension frequently seen in patients with this condition.
4. **Coarctation of aorta.** Although usually diagnosed within first years of life, an occasional adolescent patient may present with this condition.
5. **Renal parenchymal disease.** Reflux nephropathy with scar formation and different glomerulonephritides can occur in hypertensive children.
6. **Endocrine conditions**
   a. **Pheochromocytoma.** In pediatric patients, often presents as chronically elevated BP. Flushing, pallor, diarrhea, dyspnea, diaphoresis, palpitations, intermittent fever, and headaches may be present or absent.
   b. **Hyperthyroidism.** Occasionally presents with isolated systolic hypertension.
   c. **Primary hyperaldosteronism.** Not commonly seen in children; rule out in hypertensive patients with hypokalemia.
   d. **Glucocorticoid remediable aldosteronism (GRA).** Rare familial form of hypertension; aldosterone production is under adrenocorticotropic hormone control.
   e. **Cushing disease.** Rarely seen in children; consider with typical physical appearance and hypokalemic metabolic alkalosis.
7. **Drugs and other chemicals.** See discussion at II, E, earlier. Licorice and lead poisoning can also cause hypertension.
8. **Postoperative conditions.** Pain, general discomfort, immobility, and medications in postoperative period can all contribute to a *transient* elevation in BP.
9. **Gestational hypertension.** Consider in adolescent girls.
10. **Miscellaneous conditions**
    a. **Liddle syndrome.** In rare familial cases, excessive sodium reabsorption with associated hypokalemia, metabolic alkalosis, and low-renin hypertension is seen.
    b. **Apparent mineralocorticoid excess (AME).** Rare, severe, and hard-to-treat hypertension with hypokalemia. Because of an enzyme defect, local cortisol is not deactivated by mineralocorticoid receptor. Excessive amounts of cortisol byproducts are excreted in urine.
    c. **Cerebrovascular accidents.** With the exception of intraventricular hemorrhage in preterm neonates, very unusual as a cause of hypertension; neurologic signs and symptoms give clues.

B. **Essential Hypertension.** Common familial condition even in children. In childhood, BP elevation is modest and asymptomatic. BP well over the 99th percentile in a child or young adolescent is unlikely due to this condition.

C. **Office ("White Coat") Hypertension.** Needs to be excluded with mild hypertension. Some of these children later may develop fixed hypertension.

IV. Database

A. Physical Exam Key Points

1. **Vital signs.** BP must be taken with a cuff that covers 80% of patient's upper arm. Obtain measurements in both arms and, preferably, in legs. Feel for femoral pulses.
2. **Eyes.** Diagnosis of hypertensive encephalopathy largely depends on presence of papilledema. Evaluate fundus for hemorrhage, exudate, arteriolar narrowing, and arteriovenous nicking.
3. **Lungs.** Rales occur with congestive heart failure in hypertensive emergency.
4. **Heart.** Listen for murmur of aortic regurgitation or gallop rhythm due to congestive heart failure.
5. **Abdomen.** Palpate for masses and enlarged kidneys (large hydronephrosis, polycystic or multicystic kidneys, Wilms tumor).
6. **Neurologic exam.** Evaluate mental status; look for focal deficit. Disorientation and somnolence are ominous signs of hypertensive encephalopathy.

B. Laboratory Data

1. **Chemistry panel.** Serum creatinine and BUN indicate renal function; serum carbon dioxide and potassium help in diagnosing low-potassium forms of hypertension (primary hyperaldosteronism, Liddle syndrome, Cushing disease, GRA, and AME).
2. **Endocrine studies.** With extreme values, serum aldosterone and plasma renin activity are helpful in diagnosing renal artery stenosis and low-potassium forms of hypertension. Moderately abnormal values have little clinical value. Thyroid studies, urinary and serum catecholamine studies, and urinary steroid profile have a role in later stages of workup.
3. **Urinalysis.** Simple, useful study to assess for parenchymal renal disease; look for protein, RBCs, or cellular casts.
4. **CBC.** Of limited value in diagnosing secondary forms of hypertension. Anemia may indicate glomerulonephritis; schistocytes are seen in malignant hypertension.
5. **Drug screening.** Obtain in appropriate clinical setting with any adolescent hypertensive patients.

C. Radiographic and Other Studies

1. **Renal ultrasound.** Quick and easy way to assess renal anatomy. Check for hydronephrosis, renal cysts, size discrepancy, renal mass, and renal echogenicity. In older children and adolescents, Doppler extension of study assists in diagnosing renal artery stenosis.

2. **Dimercaptosuccinic acid (DMSA) renal scan.** When reflux nephropathy is suspected, this is definitive study for renal scarring.

3. **Echocardiogram.** Useful in assessing heart for possible end-organ damage and in determining how long-standing and how severe hypertension has been. Occasional unexpected finding is coarctation of aorta.

4. **Chest x-ray.** Provides an initial, quick look at heart size and diagnosis of congestive heart failure in hypertensive emergency.

5. **CT or MRI scan.** Can discover masses not seen by ultrasound (pheochromocytoma, neurofibromatosis, or Wilms tumor). In hypertensive emergencies, it is necessary to obtain an image of the head. CT angiography or magnetic resonance angiography are excellent alternatives to renal arteriography to diagnose stenosis of major renal vessels (main artery and arcuate arteries).

6. **Metaiodobenzylguanidine (MIBG) radionuclide scan.** If pheochromocytoma is strongly suspected, obtain this study in tandem with MRI scan of abdomen.

7. **ECG.** Quick and easy way to evaluate heart for left ventricular hypertrophy.

8. **Ambulatory BP monitoring.** Best way to establish the diagnosis of office hypertension. School nurses are the "poor person's ambulatory BP monitors."

V. Plan

A. **Hypertensive Emergency.** Hypertension associated with signs of end-organ damage (pulmonary edema, hypertensive encephalopathy, cerebral bleeding, or cerebral infarction) requires immediate IV treatment. Therapeutic goal for first several hours should be ~25% reduction from maximal BP. Final BP goal should be gradually achieved within 48 hours.

1. **Nitroprusside.** Very powerful drug with predictable and immediate action on BP. Starting dose is 0.3 mcg/kg/min, with maximum of 10 mcg/kg/min. BP changes occur within 1 minute during titration. Infusion set needs to be protected against light. Monitor thiocyanide and cyanide levels after 3 days (earlier, in liver or renal failure).

2. **Nicardipine.** Rapidly acting calcium channel blocker; used at 0.3–5 mcg/kg/min. Very irritating to tissue.

3. **Esmolol.** Potent β_1-adrenergic receptor antagonist. Load patient with 100–500 mcg/kg quick IV push and maintain BP control with 25–100 mcg/kg/min infusion. Can be carefully titrated up to 500 mcg/kg/min.

4. **Labetalol.** Combined α- and nonspecific β-antagonist. Can be given as boluses from 0.1–1 mg/kg; maximum 20 mg per dose. Constant infusion titrated to 0.1–1 mg/kg/min, occasionally to maximum of 3 mg/kg/min.

5. **Enalaprilat.** Effective in 5–10 mcg/kg doses q8–24h. Because neonates have a more active renin-angiotensin system, they are more sensitive to drug than older children and should be given dose in lower range. Closely monitor renal function and serum potassium level.

6. **Hydralazine.** Old but trustworthy drug given at 0.1–0.5 mg/kg as a bolus. Maximum dose per bolus is 20 mg. Can be repeated q3–4h. Monitor heart rate and hold doses if significant tachycardia. Watch for resistance to BP-lowering effect.

7. **Diazoxide.** Extremely effective; can cause precipitous drop in BP and elevate blood glucose concentration. If normal saline infusion is available at bedside to treat acute hypotension, 1–3 mg/kg quick IV push works well. Second bolus can be given within 5–15 minutes if needed, not to exceed 5 mg/kg combined dose. Effective dose can be repeated q4–24h.

B. **Hypertensive Urgency.** Symptomatic hypertension without evidence of end-organ damage. Oral treatment is acceptable, although IV medications may also be considered. Long-acting oral agents (ie, those recommended in once- or twice-daily doses) should be avoided due to delayed peak concentration.

1. **"Sublingual" nifedipine.** No excessive side effects reported in pediatric literature; frequently administered, convenient drug of choice for pediatric hypertensive urgencies if administered in appropriate dose. Conventional dose is 0.25–0.5 mg/kg per dose q3–4h, not to exceed 10 mg per dose or 3 mg/kg/day. Although labeled as sublingual, absorption takes place from stomach, so capsule needs to be opened before being swallowing.

2. **Oral hydralazine.** Doses of 0.75–1 mg/kg q4–6h may work well. Maximum one-time dose is 25 mg, with cumulative daily dose of 5 mg/kg.

3. **Minoxidil.** More powerful vasodilator than hydralazine, with more side effects. In acute situations, 0.2 mg/kg may work well. Add diuretic if treatment exceeds a few days.

4. **Propranolol.** Given in doses of 0.12–0.25 mg/kg q6–12h.

5. **Chronic hypertension.** Not within scope of this discussion, but lifestyle changes, such as low-salt diet, exercise, and weight loss, should be part of any comprehensive treatment plan for patients with chronic hypertension.

VI. **Problem Case Diagnosis.** The 13-year-old girl had modest BP elevation, which might be attributed to office hypertension, essential hypertension, or metabolic syndrome. Further investigation showed multiple high BP readings had been obtained by school nurse, and patient also had a strong family history of hypertension. Diagnosis of essential hypertension was made, and patient's BP was well controlled on salt restriction and hydrochlorothiazide, 25 mg daily.

VII. Teaching Pearl: Question. What is the only form of hypertension that will never develop into malignant hypertension?

VIII. Teaching Pearl: Answer. Coarctation of the aorta never progresses into malignant hypertension. This is the only form of hypertension in which the kidneys are sheltered from elevated systemic BP. This observation suggests the pivotal role of the kidneys in the pathomechanism of malignant hypertension.

REFERENCES

Fivush B, Neu AM, Furth S. Acute hypertensive crises in children: Emergencies and urgencies. *Curr Opin Pediatr* 1997;9:233–236.

Friedman AL. Approach to the treatment of hypertension in children. *Heart Dis* 2002;4:47–50.

National High Blood Pressure Education Working Group on Hypertension Control in Children and Adolescents. Update on the 1987 task force report on high blood pressure in children and adolescents: A working group report from the National High Blood Pressure Education Program. *Pediatrics* 1996;98:649–658.

Sinaiko AR. Hypertension in children. *N Engl J Med* 1996;335:1968–1973.

46. HYPOCALCEMIA

I. Problem. A 7-day-old infant is admitted with a history of jitteriness and poor feeding associated with total serum calcium level of 6.0 mg/dL (normal for this age: 7.6–10.9 mg/dL).

II. Immediate Questions

A. Is patient symptomatic? Hypocalcemia can be asymptomatic or associated with serious life-threatening manifestations. Severe manifestations that require immediate treatment include paresthesias, tetany, laryngospasm, and seizures. Diagnostic signs suggesting the need for immediate treatment are positive Chvostek and Trousseau signs.

B. Is low serum calcium level an artifact or reflective of low ionized calcium? Whereas total serum calcium is routinely measured, it is the ionized calcium component that is physiologically important. Ionized calcium can be measured directly or can be estimated by subtracting 0.8 mg/dL for every 1 g/dL by which serum albumin is < 4 g/dL.

C. Is serum magnesium level low? Serum calcium will not respond to correction with IV or oral calcium as long as severe hypomagnesemia remains untreated.

D. Pertinent Historical Information

1. Infants. Is there a history of parathyroid or other endocrine diseases? What is the gestational history? Pay particular attention to maternal illnesses (eg, diabetes mellitus, hyperparathyroidism), medications, birth history, and gestational age. What type of formula or supplements is infant given?

    2. Children. Is there a history of acute or chronic illnesses, medication use, or surgery? Ask about diet and sun exposure.

III. Differential Diagnosis. Causes of hypocalcemia in infants need to be distinguished from those in children. Neonatal hypocalcemia is classically divided into early (first 4 days of life) and late, which usually presents at 5–10 days of life. In children of all ages, abnormalities can be divided into those involving parathyroid hormone (PTH), vitamin D, and binding or distribution of calcium.

A. Neonatal Hypocalcemia

  1. Early neonatal hypocalcemia

    a. Preterm infants. Transiently decreased PTH secretion.

    b. Neonates with asphyxia. Possibly associated with increased calcitonin secretion.

    c. Infants of diabetic mothers. Related to maternal hypomagnesemia.

    d. Infants whose mothers had preeclampsia. Related to maternal hypomagnesemia.

  2. Late neonatal hypocalcemia

    a. Dietary phosphate loading. Results from inability of immature kidneys to excrete phosphate in infants fed cow's milk formula.

    b. Hypoparathyroidism. Transient, insufficient PTH secretion.

    c. Hypomagnesemia. Can be associated with rare defects in magnesium transport.

  3. Miscellaneous causes of hypocalcemia in infants and neonates

    a. Congenital hypoparathyroidism. Can be associated with DiGeorge anomaly or CATCH-22 syndrome (*cardiac* anomalies, *abnormal* facies, *thymic* aplasia, *cleft* palate, *hypocalcemia*, caused by deletion in chromosome *22*q11.2).

    b. "Late-late" hypocalcemia. Skeletal hypomineralization and poor mineral and vitamin D intake presenting at 2–4 months of age.

    c. Infants of hyperparathyroid mothers.

    d. Ionized hypocalcemia. Associated with exchange transfusions of citrated blood, lipid infusions, or respiratory alkalosis.

B. Childhood Hypocalcemia

  1. Parathyroid disorders

    a. Hypoparathyroidism. Associated with chromosome 22q11 abnormalities (see A, 3, a, earlier) or autoimmune syndromes such as autoimmune polyglandular syndrome.

    b. Pseudohypoparathyroidism. Disorders of activation of the cellular effects of PTH.

    c. Calcium-sensing abnormalities. Occurs when parathyroid gland is abnormally sensitive to serum calcium, causing PTH levels to be low in relation to level of calcium.

     d. Hypomagnesemia. Associated with decreased PTH secretion and PTH effect.

  2. Vitamin D disorders

    a. Vitamin D deficiency. Low levels of vitamin D due to dietary insufficiency, lack of sunshine, fat malabsorption, or liver disease.

    b. Vitamin D–dependent rickets. Block in 1,25-dihydroxyvitamin D formation (type 1) or abnormal receptor (type 2).

    c. Renal failure. Acute or chronic, with inadequate formation of 1,25-dihydroxyvitamin D.

    d. Fanconi syndrome. Proximal renal tubular dysfunction with low 1,25-dihydroxyvitamin D formation and renal phosphate wasting.

    e. Altered metabolism. Often due to drugs such as phenobarbital, phenytoin, or ketoconazole.

  3. Abnormal distribution or binding of calcium

    a. Tumor lysis syndrome. Hyperphosphatemia, hypocalcemia, and acute renal failure.

    b. Acute rhabdomyolysis. Trapping of calcium into injured muscle.

    c. Hungry bone syndrome. Shift of calcium and phosphorus into bone, often after parathyroidectomy.

    d. Drugs. Foscarnet, bisphosphonates, calcitonin, calcium chelators (citrate, phosphorus).

    e. Miscellaneous. Acute pancreatitis, toxic shock syndrome, sepsis.

IV. Database

  A. Physical Exam Key Points

    1. General appearance. Albright hereditary osteodystrophy with pseudohypoparathyroidism (short stature, obesity, round face); large-for-gestational-age infants of diabetic mothers.

    2. Skin. Mucocutaneous candidiasis with autoimmune polyglandular syndrome; alopecia with type 2 vitamin D–dependent rickets.

    3. HEENT. Facial features of DiGeorge syndrome, laryngospasm, cataracts.

    4. Skeletal findings. Evidence of bowing with rickets; short metacarpals and metatarsals with pseudohypoparathyroidism.

    5. Neuromuscular exam. Neuromuscular excitability manifested by irritability, facial grimacing, hyperactive deep tendon reflexes, muscular spasms, twitching and tetany, confusion, seizures.

    6. Heart. Cardiac abnormalities seen in DiGeorge syndrome.

    7. Specific tests for tetany of hypocalcemia

      a. Chvostek sign. Elicited by tapping on the facial nerve below the zygomatic arch and 2 cm anterior to the earlobe. Positive sign ranges from twitching of the lip at the angle of the mouth to contraction of the facial muscles.

      b. Trousseau sign. Performed by inflating a BP cuff on the upper arm to just above systolic BP for 3 minutes. With hypocalcemia, carpal spasm may occur in response to ischemia of the ulnar nerve.

B. Laboratory Data

    1. Serum electrolytes. In addition to total calcium, focus on potassium, phosphate, and magnesium levels. The latter two are not usually included in standard panels and may have to be ordered separately. Serum calcium should be interpreted in relation to serum albumin (see II, B, earlier). Hyperkalemia may be a sign of tumor lysis. Serum phosphate is elevated in renal failure, tumor lysis, rhabdomyolysis, phosphate enemas, and parathyroid disorders. It is also seen in most of the neonatal hypocalcemic disorders. Hypophosphatemia is a sign of vitamin D disorders, hungry bone syndrome, and Fanconi syndrome. Severe hypomagnesemia, < 1 mg/dL, is a cause of refractory hypocalcemia.

    2. Serum albumin. As previously described.

    3. Ionized calcium. Particularly valuable in the presence of alkalosis and chelators, which may selectively lower ionized calcium. In confusing cases, ionized calcium can help with diagnosis and management.

    4. BUN and creatinine. Signs of renal failure, acute or chronic.

    5. PTH level. Should be interpreted in relation to serum calcium level.

    6. Vitamin D levels. 25-Hydroxyvitamin D identifies deficiency or abnormalities of metabolism whereas 1,25-dihydroxyvitamin D may be helpful in patients with vitamin D–dependent states and renal disease.

C. Radiographic and Other Studies

    1. Bone films. Look for rickets, osteopenia, or renal osteodystrophy.

    2. ECG. Hypocalcemia may result in prolonged QT interval or T wave inversion.

V. Plan. Evaluate for symptomatic hypocalcemia that would necessitate immediate IV treatment with calcium and possibly magnesium. Obtain laboratory studies and initiate oral treatment after patient is stabilized.

A. Neonates

    1. Emergency treatment

        a. For symptomatic hypocalcemia or when serum calcium is < 5–6 mg/dL, give 10–20 mg elemental calcium per kilogram body weight, or 1–2 mL of calcium gluconate per kilogram body weight (10% solution). This should be given no faster than 1 mL/min under constant cardiac monitoring.

        b. Treat hypomagnesemia with 0.1–0.2 mL/kg of 50% magnesium sulfate (0.4–0.8 mEq/kg or 5–10 mg/kg) IV or IM, again under constant cardiac monitoring. May repeat magnesium dose q12–24h.

2. **Nonemergency or maintenance therapy.** Oral calcium at a dose of 50–75 mg elemental calcium per kilogram per day as calcium glubionate (23 mg/mL), calcium carbonate (100 mg/mL), or calcium gluconate (9 mg/mL). Give in 4–6 divided doses, and combine with low-phosphorus formula such as maternal breast milk or Similac PM 60/40.

3. **Vitamin D.** Daily supplement of oral vitamin D at a dose of 400–2000 IU/day.

B. **Children**

1. **Emergency treatment**

a. For acute symptomatic hypocalcemia, give 2–3 mg elemental calcium per kilogram body weight or 0.25 mL calcium gluconate per kilogram body weight (10% solution) IV at a rate of no more than 1 mL/min under constant cardiac monitoring. Can continue with a constant infusion at a rate of 50–75 mg elemental calcium per kilogram per day until hypocalcemia is corrected.

b. For hypomagnesemic hypocalcemia, give 6 mg elemental magnesium per kilogram body weight or 0.12 mL per kilogram body weight of 50% magnesium sulfate IM or IV over 1–4 hours.

2. **Chronic treatment**

a. **Calcium.** Oral calcium at a dose of 500–1000 mg elemental calcium per dose q6h. This can be given as liquid (calcium carbonate, 100 mg/mL; calcium glubionate, 25 mg/mL) or one of many tablet forms.

b. **Vitamin D.** Treat vitamin D deficiency with ergocalciferol drops at a dose of 800–8000 IU/day. Doses have been described in the literature up to 600,000 units given in a single day. For patients with renal failure, calcitriol can be given at a dose of 0.25–1 mcg/day. Patients with hypoparathyroidism, pseudohypoparathyroidism, and vitamin D–dependent rickets type 1 also require calcitriol therapy rather than ergocalciferol. This can be given orally or intravenously.

VI. **Problem Case Diagnosis.** The 1-week-old infant had late neonatal hypocalcemia, and a phosphorus level of 9.2 mg/dL. Infant was treated with IV calcium gluconate and placed on Similac PM 60/40. There was no evidence of DiGeorge syndrome or recurrence of hypocalcemia.

VII. **Teaching Pearl: Question.** In most cases of vitamin D–deficiency rickets, is the level of 1,25-dihydroxyvitamin D high, normal, or low?

VIII. **Teaching Pearl: Answer.** The 1,25-dihydroxyvitamin D levels are usually in the normal range, but this is inappropriate for the level of hypophosphatemia, hypocalcemia, and hyperparathyroidism that may be present.

REFERENCES

Carpenter TO. Neonatal hypocalcemia. In: Favus M, ed. *Primer on the Metabolic Bone Diseases and Disorders of Mineral Metabolism,* 5th ed. American Society of Bone and Mineral Research, 2003:286–288.

Koo W. Hypocalcemia and hypercalcemia in neonates. In: Umpaichitra V, Bastian W, Castells S. Hypocalcemia in children: Pathogenesis and management. *Clin Pediatr* 2001;40:305.

47. HYPOGLYCEMIA

I. **Problem.** A previously healthy 3-year-old boy is brought to the emergency department in the early morning after his parents found him difficult to arouse. The family had been traveling and the child had a prolonged fast. His blood glucose level is 28 mg/dL.

II. **Immediate Questions**
   A. **What constitutes a low serum glucose level in a patient of this age?** Hypoglycemia in children is defined as follows.
      1. **Term neonate.** Serum glucose < 50–60 mg/dL.
      2. **Infants and young children.** Serum glucose < 45–60 mg/dL.
      3. **Older children and adolescents.** Serum glucose < 60 mg/dL.
   B. **What is patient's mental status?** An unconscious patient must first be stabilized. Quickly assess ABCs (airway, breathing, and circulation) and obtain access to draw samples for laboratory analysis and provide glucose.
   C. **Is patient diabetic?** Excess insulin administration or administration of insulin in a patient who is not eating can induce hypoglycemia.
   D. **Has patient had adequate intake? Was TPN abruptly discontinued?** Often children who are sick have decreased oral intake and may not have had anything to eat or drink for several hours. Abrupt discontinuation of dextrose-containing fluids can also lead to hypoglycemia.
   E. **Is ingestion a possibility?** Many different agents can induce hypoglycemia, including salicylates, alcohol, and oral hypoglycemic agents.
   F. **Is patient a newborn, an infant of a diabetic mother, intrauterine growth retarded (IUGR), or small or large for gestational age (SGA or LGA)?** Infants of diabetic mothers are often hyperinsulinemic at birth and when glucose stores from the placenta are removed can become hypoglycemic. SGA infants (defined as < 10th percentile or < 2.5 kg at term) and LGA infants (defined as > 95th percentile or > 4.0 kg at term) are at increased risk of hypoglycemia.
   G. **What symptoms are associated with hypoglycemia?** Symptoms include anxiety, diaphoresis, jitteriness, weakness,

nausea, headache, and confusion. Infants with hypoglycemia can present with few symptoms.

III. Differential Diagnosis
A. Medications
1. **Insulin.** Check for administration error, including patient identity, dose, preparation, and route.
2. **Other medications.** Ingestion of agents such as oral hypoglycemics, salicylates, quinine, and pentamidine can lead to hypoglycemia.
3. **Ethanol.** Consider accidental ingestion of alcohol or other ethanol-containing substances such as mouthwash.

B. Inborn Errors of Metabolism
1. **Carbohydrate metabolism.** Examples include galactosemia and glycogen storage diseases.
2. **Lipid metabolism.** Examples include carnitine deficiencies; very long–, long-, medium-, and short-chain acyl-CoA dehydrogenase deficiency.
3. **Amino acid metabolism.** Examples include Maple syrup urine disease and methylmalonic acidemia.

C. Neonatal Causes
1. **Gestational diabetes.** These infants, often LGA, are hyperinsulinemic at birth and can become hypoglycemic when the placental glucose source is removed.
2. **IUGR or SGA.** These infants can have limited glycogen stores and decreased body fat and muscle protein.
3. **Perinatal stress.** Stressors such as fetal hypoxia and prematurity can lead to hypoglycemia.
4. **Genetic malformations.** Patients with Beckwith-Wiedemann syndrome may exhibit hypoglycemia.

D. Ketotic Hypoglycemia.
This is the most common form of childhood hypoglycemia and is related to prolonged fast, usually with intercurrent illness. Typical presentation is a child, aged 18 months to 5 years, who has missed dinner or breakfast and is found to be difficult to arouse. Can be associated with seizures and lead to coma.

E. Sepsis.
Hypoglycemia or hyperglycemia can occur in septic shock. Usually a sign of late infection.

F. Severe Liver Failure.
Glycogen stores are easily depleted in patients with advanced liver disease and destruction.

G. Reactive Hypoglycemia.
Can occur post-prandially in a small percentage of the population, especially in patients with dumping syndrome.

H. Endocrinopathies.
Includes adrenal insufficiency, hypothyroidism, and hypopituitarism.

I. Abrupt Discontinuation of TPN.
Rare.

      J. Factitious Hypoglycemia. Due to laboratory error (unspun blood that sits out too long) or as a result of leukocyte metabolism in a patient with markedly increased WBC count.

      K. Insulinoma or Other Neoplasms.

      L. Other Causes. Severe malnutrition, seizures, vasovagal fainting, narcolepsy, and anxiety attack.

IV. Database

A. Physical Exam Key Points

1. Assess airway, breathing, and circulation (ABCs) and vital signs.
2. Evaluate for hepatomegaly, pigmentation, short stature, and neurologic signs.

B. Laboratory Data.
Careful history and physical exam usually provide clues to diagnosis. Patients with a history of hypoglycemia may require hospital admission to induce hypoglycemia and to obtain laboratory data during an acute episode.

1. Obtain serum glucose, insulin, cortisol, and growth hormone levels, and urinalysis for ketones. If possible, also obtain C-peptide, lactate, ammonia, thyroid-stimulating hormone, and thyroxine levels.
2. Serum electrolytes, renal and liver function studies, and CBC may be helpful in evaluating some of the causes listed under differential diagnosis, earlier.

C. Radiographic and Other Studies.
May be indicated to evaluate for insulinoma, malignancy, and pituitary lesions if suggested by history, physical exam, or screening studies.

V. Plan

A. Administer Glucose.
If hypoglycemia is strongly suspected, do not wait for results of serum glucose testing.

1. **Oral.** Preferred initial therapy if patient is awake and has an intact airway. Give orange juice by mouth or via nasogastric (NG) or orogastric (OG) tube.
2. **Parenteral.** In children, give a 2 mL/kg bolus of $D_{25}W$ IV or IO. In infants, give a 2–4 mL/kg bolus of $D_{10}W$ IV or IO. After the dextrose bolus, patient should be started on maintenance $D_{10}W$ electrolyte solution to provide glucose at a rate of 6–8 mg/kg/min.
3. **Intramuscular or subcutaneous (IM or SQ).** If no IV access is available, give glucagon IM or SQ.
   a. **Neonate.** Dose is 0.3 mg/kg IM or SQ.
   b. **Child or adolescent.** Dose is 0.5–1 mg IM or SQ.
4. **Other agents.** Diazoxide, octreotide, and hydrocortisone may have a role in treatment of hypoglycemia, depending on the cause.

B. **Evaluate for Underlying Cause of Hypoglycemia.** If laboratory studies can be efficiently obtained, this should be accomplished prior to therapy.

VI. **Problem Case Diagnosis.** The 3-year-old child has ketotic hypoglycemia. (For further discussion, see Teaching Pearl: Answer, below.)

VII. **Teaching Pearl: Question:** What is the most common cause of hypoglycemia in children, and how is it treated?

VIII. **Teaching Pearl: Answer:** Ketotic hypoglycemia is the most common cause of hypoglycemia in children. Immediate treatment consists of the administration of glucose (oral glucose if patient can be aroused and airway is intact). Children with this condition are instructed to avoid fasting, especially during times of intercurrent illness, and to have frequent carbohydrate-rich meals.

REFERENCES

Behrman RE, Kliegman RM, Jenson HB, eds. *Nelson Textbook of Pediatrics,* 17th ed. Saunders, 2004:505–517.
Perkin R, Swift J, Newton D. *Pediatric Hospital Medicine: Textbook of Inpatient Management.* Lippincott Williams & Wilkins, 2003:138–139.

48. HYPOKALEMIA

I. **Problem.** A 6-month-old female infant with a ventricular septal defect is admitted with a 3-day history of poor feeding, vomiting, and diarrhea. Initial laboratory studies show serum potassium level of 2.0 mEq/L (normal for this age: 4.1–5.3 mEq/L).

II. **Immediate Questions**
A. **Is patient symptomatic?** Symptoms of hypokalemia include muscular weakness, gastric hypomotility, and cardiac disturbances (arrhythmia, premature atrial contractions [PACs], premature ventricular contractions [PVCs], flattened T waves, ST segment changes, U waves).
B. **What medication(s) does child take?** β-Agonists, penicillins, loop diuretics, steroids, laxatives, aminoglycosides, and amphotericin B may all contribute to hypokalemia. Hypokalemia can potentiate digitalis toxicity.
C. **Is there a history of hypokalemia?** A history of hypokalemia in the patient or a family member may point to associated syndromes or tumor.

III. **Differential Diagnosis.** To determine the etiology of hypokalemia, one must first decide which of five primary mechanisms exists: redistribution, renal loss, GI loss, other loss (sweating), or inadequate intake.
A. **Redistribution Hypokalemia.** Potassium is primarily an intracellular ion; hence a small shift of this ion into the cell can cause a

large change in plasma potassium concentration. Extracellular potassium can shift into the intracellular space in the setting of alkalosis, β-agonist use, catecholamine excess, insulin administration, hypothermia, and familial periodic paralysis (autosomal dominant).

B. Renal Potassium Loss. Can be differentiated based on child's acid-base status.

1. **With metabolic acidosis.** Includes such disorders as type 1 and type 2 renal tubular acidosis, and diabetic ketoacidosis.

2. **With metabolic alkalosis.** Bartter syndrome, Gitelman syndrome, diuretic therapy, and mineralocorticoid excess (hyperaldosteronism, Cushing syndrome, adrenal tumor, exogenous steroid administration).

3. **Variable.** Renal losses not associated with a specific acid-base imbalance occur with hypomagnesemia, some penicillins, aminoglycosides, amphotericin B, cisplatin, and osmotic diuresis.

C. GI Loss. The major source for extrarenal potassium loss occurs in the setting of colonic fluid loss, seen with diarrhea and laxative abuse. Severe vomiting can produce hypokalemia in patients with contraction alkalosis.

D. Other Loss. Copious sweating is the primary cause of potassium loss other than from kidney and GI tract.

E. Inadequate Intake. Produces hypokalemia over time as total body stores become depleted.

IV. Database. Data collection for hypokalemia serves two purposes. First, one must use data to determine the source of potassium depletion. Second, one must obtain data to assist in diagnosis of related disorders and to detect adverse consequences of hypokalemia. Most of the appropriate studies to perform will be based on information obtained by taking a thorough history. Review all medications child may be taking, including any home remedies administered.

A. Physical Exam Key Points

1. **Overall appearance.** Does patient appear severely dehydrated or cachectic?

2. **Heart.** Is rhythm regular and heart rate adequate?

3. **Lungs.** Is child making a good respiratory effort?

4. **GI.** Any evidence of intestinal dysmotility, ileus, or obstruction?

5. **Neurologic exam.** Is weakness, blunting of reflexes, or paresthesia present?

B. Laboratory Data

1. **Serum electrolytes.** Identify associated abnormalities that may affect treatment (hypomagnesemia) or exacerbate cardiac disturbances (hypocalcemia).

2. **ABGs.** Remember, alkalosis can cause intracellular shift of potassium. In addition, many of the renal causes of potassium

loss have an associated acid-base disturbance. Finally, an anion gap acidosis may be present in the setting of elevated lactate with severe dehydration, poor cardiac output, or sepsis. Treatment of acidosis produces a "relative alkalosis" and may exacerbate hypokalemia, so prioritize therapy.

3. **Urine.** Urine sodium, potassium, chloride, and osmolality may assist in diagnosis. Urine drug screening may be useful if amphetamine or other sympathomimetic drug overdose is suspected.

4. **Other blood testing.** Obtain based on history and index of suspicion.

   a. **Digoxin level.** May be critical in treatment of cardiac disturbances.

   b. **Adrenocorticotropic hormone, cortisol, renin, and aldosterone.** Assist in determination of underlying adrenal disorders.

C. **Radiographic and Other Studies**

   1. **Radiographic studies.** Rarely helpful in the acute setting but may help identify underlying abnormalities responsible for hypokalemia. Abdominal ultrasound or CT scan may help identify adrenal tumors, and MRI scan of the brain may identify pituitary abnormalities associated with increased cortisol release. These studies should be performed based on an index of suspicion from history and laboratory results.

   2. **ECG.** Of paramount importance, especially as serum potassium level drops below 3 mEq/L. Rapid recognition of cardiac disturbances is critical. It is also important to monitor cardiac status as therapy is instituted. (ECG changes, outlined earlier at II, A, include PACs, PVCs, flattened T waves, ST segment changes, and U waves). The classic finding of a U wave is poorly understood. It is believed to represent delayed repolarization of cardiac muscle. The U wave appears after the T wave. As hypokalemia worsens, the T wave flattens and the U wave becomes more pronounced, producing what appears to be a prolonged QT interval.

V. **Plan.** Treatment is variable, depending on severity of the potassium deficit as well as presence of symptoms and associated conditions. Serum potassium level is not a good indication of total body potassium deficit. Patients with diabetic ketoacidosis often present with a normal to high serum potassium level, yet have a severe total body deficit. In adult patients (70-kg man) an estimate of total body potassium deficit can be approximated as 150 mEq for each 1 mEq/L decrease in serum potassium from 4 mEq/L. No such physiologic studies have been performed in children to produce a reliable estimate.

A. **Mild, Asymptomatic Hypokalemia (serum K⁺ 3–3.5 mEq/L).** Depending on cause, may resolve without therapy or require oral supplementation of potassium chloride (KCl). Must consider ongoing loss when correcting serum level as well as daily requirement of 2–3 mEq/kg/day.

B. Severe or Symptomatic Hypokalemia (serum K⁺ < 3 mEq/L). Requires more rapid assessment and therapy as well as more stringent cardiac monitoring. Typically IV administration of KCl is required. Usual dose is 0.5 mEq/kg IV, to be given over 1 hour and not to exceed 40 mEq total. Infusion of as much as 1 mEq/kg/h may be used in severe, life-threatening hypokalemia. It is important to perform all infusions with appropriate cardiac monitoring and to reassess serum potassium level frequently.

C. Recalcitrant Hypokalemia. Correct serum magnesium and reconsider severity of ongoing potassium loss.

VI. Problem Case Diagnosis. Hypokalemia in the 6-month-old infant was secondary to GI loss from severe gastroenteritis. Patient responded well to IV administration of KCl.

VII. Teaching Pearl: Question. A patient has a serum potassium level of 3 mEq/L and is also anemic; a blood transfusion is ordered. How should you approach correcting the potassium level?

VIII. Teaching Pearl: Answer. Stored blood is often relatively high in potassium due to red cell hemolysis. If the patient is asymptomatic, it may be wise not to treat a mild hypokalemia when giving blood. Repeating a potassium level after transfusion may show that you have accomplished your goal.

REFERENCES

Barkin R. *Pediatric Emergency Medicine,* 2nd ed. Mosby, 1997.
Feld LG, Kaskel FJ, Schoeneman MJ. The approach to fluid and electrolyte therapy in pediatrics. *Adv Pediatr* 1988;35:497–535.

49. HYPOMAGNESEMIA

I. Problem. A 15-year-old renal transplant patient develops acute tetany. Serum calcium level is 6.5 mg/dL and serum magnesium, 0.8 mg/dL (normal: 1.2–2.6 mg/dL).

II. Immediate Questions

A. Is patient symptomatic? Important and even life-threatening neuromuscular and cardiovascular manifestations may be present.

B. Are there other important electrolyte disturbances? Hypocalcemia, hypokalemia, and metabolic alkalosis often accompany hypomagnesemia. Although these disturbances need to be recognized and treated, often it is important to correct the hypomagnesemia first (eg, hypocalcemia).

   C. Pertinent Historical Information
     1. In infants, is mother diabetic?
     2. Has patient undergone procedures that would lead to chronic GI disorder?
     3. What medication(s) does patient take?

III. Differential Diagnosis. Hypomagnesemia generally occurs as a result of GI disorders, renal losses, or dietary deficiency. It is an important contributing factor for tetany in newborns (see Chapter 47, Hypoglycemia, II, F, p. 223, for discussion of infants of diabetic mothers).

   A. GI Disorders. Often due to loss of magnesium-containing secretions.
     1. Acute or chronic diarrhea.
     2. Malabsorption syndrome.
     3. Short gut syndrome.
     4. Prolonged nasogastric suction or vomiting.
     5. Protein-calorie malnutrition or kwashiorkor.
     6. Primary intestinal hypomagnesemia (rare X-linked syndrome presenting in neonates).

   B. Renal Losses. Due to primary and secondary defects.
     1. Osmotic diuresis, recovery from acute tubular necrosis (ATN), and volume expansion. Nonspecific losses of magnesium and other electrolytes.
     2. Diuretics. Loop diuretics (in particular) and thiazides.
     3. Nephrotoxic agents. Aminoglycosides, amphotericin B, cisplatin, cyclosporine A.
     4. Hypercalcemia. Competes with magnesium reabsorption.
     5. Primary renal magnesium wasting. Bartter syndrome, Gitelman syndrome, isolated magnesium wasting. With Bartter and Gitelman syndromes, look for hypokalemia and alkalosis.
     6. Postrenal transplantation. In addition to cyclosporine A.
     7. Diabetes mellitus.

IV. Database
   A. Physical Exam Key Point
     1. Cardiovascular. Irregular heartbeat and hypertension.
     2. Neuromuscular. Check for neuromuscular excitability with Chvostek and Trousseau signs (see Chapter 46, Hypocalcemia, IV, A, 7, p. 220). Muscular tremor, weakness, and carpopedal spasm may be present. Observe for ataxia, vertigo, nystagmus, and choreiform movements. Important cause of neonatal tetany.
   B. Laboratory Data
     1. Serum electrolytes. Concurrent hypokalemia is very common, whether due to GI or renal losses (primary or secondary).

2. **Serum calcium.** Hypocalcemia is a classic sign of hypomagnesemia. May have to treat hypomagnesemia first.
3. **Fractional excretion of magnesium (FE_{Mg}).** To distinguish renal from GI causes, measure FE_{Mg} in a spot urine using the following formula:

$$FE_{Mg} = \frac{U_{Mg} \times P_{Cr}}{0.7 \times P_{Mg} \times U_{Cr}} \times 100$$

In which Cr = creatinine; FE = fractional excretion; P = plasma; U = urine.

Fractional excretion in nonrenal disorders should be < 2%; in renal disorders, it is typically > 5%. Magnesium-loading tests described in adults have not been standardized in children.

C. **Radiographic and Other Studies.** Perform ECG to look for arrhythmia (prolonged PR interval, wide QRS complex, diminished T wave).

V. **Plan.** Hypomagnesemia, especially if associated with hypocalcemia and tetany, can be a medical emergency. The magnitude of the magnesium deficit cannot be determined with accuracy, so empiric formulas are used for replacement. Acute IV doses of magnesium need to be followed by longer term enteral or parenteral therapy for full replacement.

A. **Severe Hypomagnesemia With Hypocalcemia or Tetany.** Goal for acute therapy is to increase serum magnesium above 1 mg/dL, which should stop seizures or tetany. Can give calcium as well (see Chapter 46, Hypocalcemia, p. . . .).

1. **Neonates.** Give 0.1–0.2 mL/kg per dose of 50% magnesium sulfate (0.4–0.8 mEq/kg) IV or IM slowly under constant cardiac monitoring. May repeat magnesium dose q12–24h.
2. **Older children and adolescents.** Give 0.12 mL/kg per dose of 50% magnesium sulfate (0.5 mEq/kg) over 1–4 hours by IV; can repeat q12h.
3. **Adolescents.** In case of seizures, can give 0.2 mEq/kg (up to 15 mEq or 180 mg) over 10 minutes. Alternative for severe hypomagnesemia is 50 mEq magnesium sulfate IV over 8–24 hours. Use half dose in presence of renal failure.

B. **Moderate Hypomagnesemia or Long-term Therapy.** Half of IV dose is excreted in urine, so to fully correct magnesium depletion, slow replacement over 3–5 days may be needed.

1. **Young children.** Dose is elemental calcium, 10–20 mg/kg per dose 4 times daily.
2. **Older children and adolescents.** Oral dose of 300–600 mg/day elemental magnesium can be given; divide dose to avoid diarrhea.

C. **Hypokalemia and Hypomagnesemia.** May need to treat hypomagnesemia before hypokalemia can be corrected.

VI. **Problem Case Diagnosis.** The 15-year-old patient had tetany associated with hypocalcemia and hypomagnesemia. Renal transplantation, cyclosporine A, and diuretics likely were the causes of the hypomagnesemia. IV magnesium sulfate and then PO calcium corrected the tetany. Oral magnesium supplements were needed for full correction.

VII. **Teaching Pearl: Question.** Do all diuretics cause hypomagnesemia?

VIII. **Teaching Pearl: Answer.** No; potassium-sparing diuretics decrease renal magnesium wasting and are useful in avoiding the hypokalemia and hypomagnesemia seen with loop diuretics or thiazides.

REFERENCES

Agus Z. Hypomagnesemia. *J Am Soc Nephrol* 1999;10:1616.
Rude RK. Magnesium deficiency: A cause of heterogeneous disease in humans. *J Bone Miner Res* 1998;13:749.

50. HYPONATREMIA

I. **Problem.** A 3-month-old female infant is admitted after several days of poor oral intake and significant vomiting and diarrhea. During a physical exam, she develops a tonic-clonic seizure. Laboratory values show serum sodium concentration of 114 mEq/L (normal: 136–146 mEq/L).

II. **Immediate Questions**
A. **Is patient adequately ventilated, with a safe and patent airway?** It is critical to assess the ABCs (airway, breathing, and circulation) because hyponatremia can be associated with neurologic changes and respiratory difficulty. Severe neurologic depression is likely to suppress patient's ability to protect the airway, thus increasing risk of aspiration.
B. **Does history suggest reasons other than hyponatremia that explain tonic-clonic movements?** Gastroenteritis from shigellosis can be associated with seizures. Seizures can also be seen with drug intoxication, infections (meningitis), and underlying neurologic problems.
C. **What factors contributed to patient's development of hyponatremia?** Thorough history that includes clues about the three general mechanisms (see later discussion at III, B) may expedite decision about underlying etiology and, therefore, treatment.
D. **How quickly did hyponatremia develop?** Rapid decrease in sodium is associated with cerebral edema. Acute presentation is

more likely to be associated with conditions such as gastroenteritis and acute renal failure, whereas insidious course is associated with conditions such as nephrotic syndrome, adrenal insufficiency, and cirrhosis.

E. Is there a laboratory error? Presence of hypernatremia in the absence of pertinent history and physical findings may suggest laboratory error. It may be prudent to repeat the test.

F. Pertinent Historical Information. It is important to determine patient's fluid intake and output (I&O) over past several days. Key questions should include volume and types of ingested liquids; amount, volume, and consistency of stools; and patient's ability to obtain fluid on his or her own.

1. If an infant, what type of formula is given, and how is it prepared?

2. If a hospitalized child, what are fluid orders? Confirm that appropriate IV solutions are being administered.

3. Does past history include any factors that could influence homeostatic mechanisms for water and salt balance? Medications (eg, diuretics) and disorders such as renal failure, heart failure, ascites, and intracranial masses may alter the body's normal water and salt control mechanisms.

III. Differential Diagnosis. Hyponatremia signifies an excess of intravascular free water relative to sodium. It is the most common electrolyte disturbance; seen in approximately 1.5% of all pediatric hospital admissions. The absolute serum sodium number itself indicates nothing about the degree of intravascular volume, extracellular fluid volume (ECFV), and total body sodium.

A. General Mechanisms Producing Hyponatremia. There are three general mechanisms by which hyponatremia may develop. These mechanisms may occur by themselves or in combination with one another.

1. Decreased sodium intake.

2. Increased sodium excretion.

3. Free water retention.

B. Volume Status. When attempting to identify the cause and decide treatment for a patient with hyponatremia, clinician must determine patient's volume status.

1. Increased ECFV (hypervolemic hyponatremia).

2. Decreased ECFV (hypovolemic hyponatremia).

3. Pseudohyponatremia and hyponatremia with hypertonicity.

C. Figure I–4 outlines the differential diagnosis for hyponatremia. It excludes pseudohyponatremia (increased serum lipids) and hyponatremia with hypertonicity (increased serum glucose).

IV. Database. History and physical exams are of paramount importance in determining proper course of treatment. Identifying exact causes of hyponatremia enables clinician to provide safe and appropriate

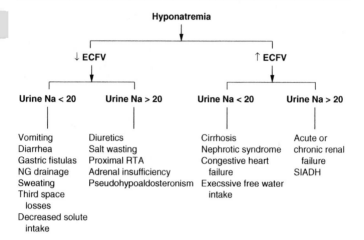

Figure I–4. Differential diagnosis of hyponatremia. (↓ = decreased; ↑ = increased; ECFV = extracellular fluid volume; Na = sodium; NG = nasogastric; RTA = renal tubular acidosis; SIADH = syndrome of inappropriate secretion of antidiuretic hormone.)

correction of serum sodium concentration. Proper treatment is of particular importance due to potential neurologic sequelae of abnormal serum sodium. Cerebral edema develops when serum sodium decreases very rapidly. In hyponatremia associated with severe intravascular volume depletion, neurologic sequelae may develop as a function of hypotension, or the development of a cerebral venous sinus thrombosis.

A. **Physical Exam Key Points**
   1. **Vital signs and general appearance.** Mental status changes, weakness, muscular cramps, and hypotension may all be associated with hyponatremia or decreased intravascular volume.
   2. **Fluid status.** Assess total body water (including both intracellular and extracellular volume). Assess volume status by checking mucous membranes, presence of tears, capillary refill, peripheral edema, ascites, jugular venous distention, tachycardia, hypotension, and murmurs.
   3. **Abdomen.** Palpate for masses or organomegaly consistent with congestive heart failure.

B. **Laboratory Data**
   1. Electrolytes, including BUN, creatinine, and glucose.
   2. Serum osmolality as compared with urine osmolality and urine sodium and creatinine.

   3. Consider serum pH, determination of anion gap, liver function tests, thyroid function tests, cortisol levels, and aldosterone levels.
   4. Plasma triglycerides are useful in identifying pseudohyponatremia. Serum glucose dilutes serum sodium because it is hyperosmolar and pulls free water into the intravascular space (hyponatremia with hypertonicity).
C. **Radiographic and Other Studies.** Radiographic studies typically are not helpful unless clinician suspects an underlying malignancy participating in the cause of hyponatremia.
   1. **Chest x-ray.** Helps to rule out heart failure, as well as identify heart size as a factor in determining volume status.
   2. **CT scan of head.** May help rule out intracranial mass, hemorrhage, or sinus thrombosis; however MRI is more sensitive for most tumor masses.
   3. **CT scan or ultrasound of abdomen.** May be helpful to determine ascites, portal hypertension, or renal or adrenal masses.

V. Plan
A. **Symptomatic Hyponatremia.** In patients such as the infant with seizures described in the opening problem, rapid but modest correction of serum sodium concentration is of paramount importance. Seizures that develop as a result of hyponatremia are difficult to treat unless serum sodium is corrected.
   1. **Initial goal.** Do not attempt to correct to a normal sodium concentration (> 135 mEq/L), but rather to raise serum sodium to a level at which seizures may be controlled (typically > 120 mEq/L). This can be performed by administration of 3% saline.
   2. **Rule for 3% saline administration.** Administration of 1 mL/kg of 3% saline will raise serum sodium by approximately 1.6 mEq/L.
   3. **Considerations.** Keep in mind that seizures may have developed due to rapid decrease in serum sodium and cerebral edema. Once seizure activity is controlled, this therapy should be held and more definitive treatment initiated. Administration of 3% saline is not appropriate for asymptomatic hyponatremia. Ideal rate of rise of serum sodium should not exceed 1 mEq/h once seizures are controlled. This management should occur in consultation with a pediatric nephrologist and intensivist.
B. **Asymptomatic Hyponatremia**
   1. **Hypovolemic hyponatremia (decreased ECFV)**
      a. Estimate total fluid deficit.
      b. Use 0.9% normal saline for maintenance fluids plus deficit.
      c. Consider ongoing losses when determining fluid rates.
   2. **Hypervolemic hyponatremia (increased ECFV)**
      a. **Low urine sodium (edematous states)**

          i. Water and sodium restriction (two-thirds maintenance).
          ii. Consider loop diuretics.
      b. High urine sodium. Water restriction (two-thirds maintenance).

VI. Problem Case Diagnosis. The 3-month-old infant had hyponatremic-induced seizures as a result of gastroenteritis. Urine sodium value was < 20 mmol/24 h (normal is 40–120 mmol/24 h). CT scan of the head was normal. Patient showed clinical improvement over the next 2 days once sodium imbalance was gradually corrected.

VI. Teaching Pearl: Question. What neurologic condition is associated with a rapid increase in serum sodium?

VII. Teaching Pearl: Answer. Central pontine myelinolysis develops in patients who experience a rapid increase in serum sodium and hence is a risk factor in treatment of hyponatremia.

REFERENCE

Verbalis JG. Hyponatremia epidemiology, pathophysiology and therapy. *Curr Opin Nephrol Hypertens* 1993;2:636.

51. HYPOPHOSPHATEMIA

  I. Problem. A 10-year-old boy with cerebral palsy and seizures who was treated with divalproex sodium is admitted with acute respiratory illness. His serum phosphate level is 1 mg/dL (normal for this age: 3.7–5.6 mg/dL).

  II. Immediate Questions
    A. Does patient have any acute symptoms related to hypophosphatemia? Patients with moderate to severe hypophosphatemia (< 1 mg/dL) may have many systemic manifestations and need to be promptly treated. Symptoms can include cardiomyopathy with heart failure; muscle weakness that can lead to rhabdomyolysis; hemolysis; and encephalopathy, seizures, and coma.
    B. Are there acute factors that have resulted in severe hypophosphatemia? Most cases of hypophosphatemia result from a shift of phosphate from extracellular to intracellular fluid. Factors causing this shift can be severe and life threatening and include refeeding syndromes and treatment of diabetic ketoacidosis (DKA).
    C. Pertinent Historical Information. Ask about diet, medications, underlying conditions, and relevant family history.

  III. Differential Diagnosis. Hypophosphatemia usually results from one of the following processes: shift of phosphate into the intracellular compartment, renal losses, or GI losses. Changes can be acute, chronic, or a combination.

A. **Transcellular Shift From Extracellular to Intracellular Compartment**
1. **Nutritional repletion or refeeding syndrome.** Can occur with enteral or parenteral nutrition in patients who are malnourished or those with anorexia nervosa or AIDS.
2. **DKA and insulin therapy.** Renal losses are also involved.
3. **Respiratory alkalosis.** Increased renal losses are also present.
4. **Sepsis.** Especially gram-negative and toxic shock syndrome.
5. **Leukemia with blast crisis.**

B. **Increased Urinary Losses**
1. **Renal tubular defects.** Fanconi syndrome (may be primary or acquired), X-linked hypophosphatemic (XLH) rickets, post–renal transplantation status.
2. **Hyperparathyroidism.** Primary (rare in children) or secondary to vitamin D deficiency or other nonrenal causes.
3. **Diuretic phase of acute tubular necrosis (ATN).**
4. **Postobstructive diuresis.**
5. **Post–renal transplantation status.**

C. **Increased GI Losses**
1. **Use of oral phosphate-binding antacids.**
2. **Decreased intake.** Starvation, anorexia nervosa, protein-calorie malnutrition. At high risk for refeeding syndrome (see III, A, 1, earlier). Premature infants require phosphate supplementation.
3. **Malabsorption syndromes.**
4. **Vitamin D deficiency.** Low levels of vitamin D due to dietary deficiency or lack of sunshine, malabsorption, or liver disease.
5. **Vitamin D–dependent rickets.** Block in 1,25-dihydroxyvitamin D formation (type 1) or abnormal receptor (type 2).

IV. **Database**

A. **Physical Exam Key Points**
1. **Vital signs and general appearance**
   a. **Temperature.** Severe hyperthermia can cause hypophosphatemia through transcellular shift. Fever may be a sign of sepsis or toxic shock.
   b. **Respiratory rate.** May be a sign of respiratory alkalosis.
   c. **Body mass.** Look for evidence of malnutrition or short stature, as well as cystinosis or congenital Fanconi syndrome.
2. **Heart.** Look for evidence of heart failure as result of severe depletion.
3. **Neuromuscular.** Assess for confusion, coma, and muscle weakness. Muscle tenderness may be a sign of rhabdomyolysis.
4. **Skeletal.** Look for bowing, rachitic rosary, and flared growth plates at wrists and knees as sign of rickets.

   5. **Skin.** Large café au lait spots may point to McCune-Albright
      syndrome.
B. **Laboratory Data**
   1. **Basic metabolic panel.** Low bicarbonate level may point to
      acidosis or changes secondary to respiratory alkalosis.
      Fanconi syndrome may be associated with low bicarbonate,
      low potassium, and possibly elevated creatinine levels. Low
      calcium level points to rickets (not XLH) or hungry bone syn-
      drome. High calcium level may point to hyperparathyroidism,
      but in children most have secondary hyperparathyroidism with
      normal or low calcium.
   2. **ABGs.** Evaluate acid-base status; look for respiratory alkalosis
      or metabolic acidosis.
   3. **CBC with differential.** Hypophosphatemia may cause hemol-
      ysis and thrombocytopeni a. Increased WBC with left shift may
      suggest sepsis.
   4. **Creatinine phosphokinase.** Check for rhabdomyolysis if
      muscle tenderness is present.
   5. **Uric acid.** Low in patients with volume overload or Fanconi
      syndrome.
   6. **Vitamin D levels.** 25-Hydroxyvitamin D is diagnostic of vitamin
      D deficiency. No need to routinely check 1,25-dihydroxyvitamin
      D levels.
   7. **Urine studies.** Spot urine for phosphorus and creatinine
      allows measurement of phosphate excretion to see if etiology
      is increased renal loss, as in Fanconi syndrome. Fanconi syn-
      drome is characterized by glucosuria, renal tubular acidosis,
      aminoaciduria, and excretion of small-molecular-weight pro-
      teins such as β_2-microglobulin.
C. **Radiographic and Other Studies.** Consider skeletal survey to
   look for changes characteristic of rickets, osteomalacia, or hyperparathyroidism. Changes may not point to exact etiology; antacid
   abuse can lead to osteomalacia.

V. **Plan.** Mild hypophosphatemia is a common finding in hospitalized
   patients, usually due to transcellular shifts of phosphate into intracellular fluid, and requires no specific therapy. Moderate
   hypophosphatemia can be treated with oral supplementation, but
   severe or symptomatic hypophosphatemia may require careful parenteral correction.
   A. **Moderate Hypophosphatemia (1–2 mg/dL in adolescents;
      2–3 mg/dL in infants and young children)**
      1. **Dietary replacement.** Milk contains 1 g inorganic phosphate
         per liter. Avoid low-phosphate formulas (Similac PM 60/40) or
         breast milk as replacement.
      2. **Enteral supplements.** Potassium phosphate can be given as
         an oral supplement at a dose of 250–750 mg q6h, depending
         on body size. Commonly available supplements are Neutra

Phos or K-Phos Neutral, which come as 250-mg tablets, capsules, or packets. Contents can be diluted with 75 mL water or taken with food. Monitor calcium to avoid hypocalcemia. Watch for diarrhea. Phosphosoda (Fleet Phosphosoda) can be given orally or as an enema at a dose of 15–30 mL three to four times daily.

B. Severe Hypophosphatemia (< 1 mg/dL in adolescents; < 2 mg/dL in children younger than 12 years)

1. **Enteral supplements.** As listed under moderate hypophosphatemia, earlier; use for asymptomatic hypophosphatemia.
2. **Parenteral phosphate.** Usually used for symptomatic hypophosphatemia. Avoid with renal failure. Potassium phosphate can be given IV at a dose of 2.5 mg (0.08 mmol)/kg body weight in $\frac{1}{2}$ normal saline (NS) over 6 hours or, for symptomatic patients, at 5 mg (0.16 mmol)/kg body weight in $\frac{1}{2}$ NS over 6 hours. Monitor calcium, phosphate, and potassium every 6 hours. Monitor BP. Stop parenteral replacement when serum phosphate is > 2 mg/dL.

C. Treatment of Primary Etiology. After emergency treatment, recognition and treatment of primary cause is important. May require vitamin D analogues (see Chapter 46, Hypocalcemia, p. 221).

VI. Problem Case Diagnosis. The 10-year-old patient has Fanconi syndrome, likely due to divalproex sodium administration. In addition to low serum phosphate level, he had low serum potassium level, metabolic acidosis, glucosuria, and a very large renal leak of phosphorus. He required large amounts of IV phosphorus and bicarbonate, but the renal tubular defect improved after stopping divalproex sodium.

VII. Teaching Pearl: Question. Why is the expression of serum phosphate as milliequivalents per liter (mEq/L) uniquely confusing as compared with other ions.

VIII. Teaching Pearl: Answer. Because the average charge of phosphate changes at physiologic pH (charge at pH 7.4 is −1.8), the valency and the value for milliequivalents per liter varies with changes in serum pH. Expression of phosphate in millimoles per liter (mmol/L) and milligrams per deciliter (mg/dL) avoids this problem.

REFERENCES

Hruska KA, Lederer ED. Hyperphosphatemia and hypophosphatemia. In Favus M, ed. *Primer on the Metabolic Bone Disorders of Mineral Metabolism,* 5th ed. American Society of Bone and Mineral Research, 2003:286–288.

Rubin MF, Narins RG. Hypophosphatemia: Pathologic and practical aspects of its therapy. *Semin Nephrol* 1990;10:536.

Subramanian R, Khardori R. Severe hypophosphatemia: Pathophysiologic implications, clinical presentations, and treatment. *Medicine* 2000;79:1.

52. HYPOTENSION

I. **Problem.** A 2-year-old boy who was admitted earlier in the day with diarrhea and dehydration now has a BP of 64/33.

II. **Immediate Questions**

   A. **What are the vital signs? Is patient adequately perfused? Are airway, breathing, and circulation (ABCs) compromised?** Hypotension represents a medical emergency and requires immediate assessment and treatment. To determine lowest acceptable systolic BP for age (represents fifth percentile for age), use the guidelines in Table I–12. If systolic BP falls below these ranges, patient is considered to be hypotensive and metabolic demands of the body for both oxygen and nutrients may not be met. As treatment is occurring, a simultaneous search for cause of hypotension should begin.

   B. **Is patient tachycardic?** Sinus tachycardia is the body's first modality to maintain adequate cardiac output in the face of hypovolemia and suggests intravascular volume depletion.

   C. **How was BP measured?** Be sure that cuff size is appropriate. Cuff that is too large may give a falsely low BP. Agitation and movement may alter result and make measurement inaccurate.

   D. **What has urine output been?** Urine output is the best noninvasive marker of end-organ perfusion and, in the presence of normal renal function, provides an accurate reflection of intravascular volume status. For pediatric patients, urine output should be at least 1 mL/kg/h.

   E. **What is patient's mental status?** The body does all it can to maintain perfusion to heart, brain, and adrenal glands in the face of hypotension or inadequate cardiac output. If mental status is not normal, assume that cerebral perfusion has been compromised. This represents an even more urgent medical emergency and may require immediate attention to airway as fluid resuscitation is occurring.

   F. **Are invasive monitors in place?** If so, measuring central venous pressure (CVP) or wedge pressure provides an objective

TABLE I–12. LOWEST ACCEPTABLE SYSTOLIC BLOOD PRESSURE FOR AGE

Age	Lowest Acceptable Systolic BP (mm Hg)
Birth–1 mo	60
1 mo–1 y	70
1–10 y	$70 + (2 \times \text{Age in years})$
10 y or older	90

assessment of intravascular volume status. Patients should receive fluid resuscitation until CVP is ≥ 10 cm H_2O or wedge pressure is ≥ 15 cm H_2O. If this is achieved and patient remains hypotensive, consider use of inotropes or vasopressors.

G. Were any medications recently given? If patient has received any sedatives or analgesics that may affect BP, this must be considered as the potential cause of hypotension. If so, antidotes may be given (eg, naloxone for opioids), but patient should still receive fluids. Consider an allergic reaction to any medication recently given.

III. Differential Diagnosis

A. Hypovolemia. Gastroenteritis is the most common cause of hypotension in children. Assess patient's intake and output (I&Os) since admission, but keep in mind that much fluid may still be present in the gut, and that third spacing of fluid may be occurring.

B. Incomplete Resuscitation. Fluid losses may continue. Despite what may appear to be adequate initial resuscitation, continue to provide fluid resuscitation if appropriate.

C. Cardiac Dysfunction. Although uncommon in pediatric patients, myocarditis may present with hypotension and sinus tachycardia. Likewise, pericarditis with pericardial effusion and cardiac tamponade may present in a similar fashion. Finally, consider other things that may impair cardiac output: tension pneumothorax, high positive end-expiratory pressure if mechanically ventilated (may impair venous return), and myocardial ischemia.

D. Sepsis. Many types of infection in children can be associated with diarrhea and subsequent hypovolemia. If child does not seem to be responding to initial efforts at resuscitation, a more serious infection must be considered. Bacterial toxins and subsequent release of circulating cytokines can decrease cardiac function and cause vasodilation, resulting in hypotension (frequently associated with lactic acidosis).

E. Neurogenic Shock. Disturbance of vasomotor tone from injury such as trauma to the spinal cord; typically results in hypotension and tachycardia.

F. Vasogenic Shock. Inappropriate loss of vasomotor tone can be seen with sepsis, anaphylaxis, adrenal insufficiency, and medications.

IV. Database

A. Physical Exam Key Points

1. **Vital signs.** High fever by itself may cause vasodilation and hypotension and should be treated with antipyretics and active cooling. If present, it should increase suspicion of a more serious infection. If patient is tachypneic without evidence of pulmonary disease, consider the presence of metabolic acidosis

and an attempt by patient to compensate with respiratory alkalosis. See also earlier discussion at II, A, regarding heart rate and BP.

2. **General appearance.** Does patient appear toxic? Is patient in distress? If so, consider serious infections and prepare to be more aggressive in therapy.

3. **Skin.** Patients in hypovolemic shock have cool, clammy skin. Look for rashes (eg, petechiae or purpura, or a diffuse erythematous rash) that may be indicative of more serious infections.

4. **Neck.** Look for jugular venous distention as evidence of right heart failure, tension pneumothorax, or pericardial tamponade.

5. **Heart.** Listen for heart sounds. If sounds are muffled, or a rub is present, consider pericardial effusion. Gallop is indicative of cardiac dysfunction. Examine ECG tracing to be sure tachycardia is sinus and that no other rhythm disturbance is present (especially supraventricular tachycardia).

6. **Lungs.** Unilateral decreased breath sounds may be indicative of pneumothorax, pleural effusion, or consolidation. Listen for crackles or rales, which are indicative of pneumonia.

7. **Abdomen.** Distention, tenseness, guarding, and hypoactive or absent bowel sounds may indicate an acute abdomen. Peritonitis with subsequent fluid sequestration may be present.

8. **Extremities.** Assess hands and feet to see if they are cool or warm. Often, if resuscitation is not yet adequate, a line of demarcation from cool to warm can be noted, and this line travels more distally until it disappears as patient is resuscitated. Assess capillary refill. If delayed, continue resuscitation. Evaluate for presence of edema that may be indicative of third spacing.

9. **Neurologic exam.** Although last in this list, this should be the first thing assessed in physical exam. Decreased mental status indicates inadequate cerebral perfusion and requires emergent attention and treatment with aggressive fluid resuscitation and consideration of airway protection.

B. **Laboratory Data**

1. **Hemoglobin and hematocrit.** Severe anemia (Hgb < 8 g/dL) has been associated with poor outcomes in patients with shock. During fluid resuscitation, hemoglobin is likely to be diluted. If hemoglobin is < 8 g/dL and patient does not respond to aggressive fluid resuscitation, consider transfusion.

2. **Electrolytes.** Hypotensive patients may present with a variety of electrolyte disturbances (too many to list here). Electrolytes should be checked initially, and then rechecked frequently during resuscitation. Frequent electrolyte assessment will allow appropriate intervention.

3. **Coagulation studies.** If sepsis is suspected, coagulation abnormalities may exist; these may require treatment with fresh frozen plasma, platelets, or cryoprecipitate.

4. **ABGs.** This evaluation is essential in determining acid-base balance. Metabolic acidosis reflects inadequate perfusion and cardiac output until proven otherwise. Compensatory respiratory alkalosis may also be seen. Evaluation of serum lactate level may be helpful; level is elevated if perfusion and cardiac output are inadequate.

C. Radiographic and Other Studies

1. **Chest x-ray.** Allows for determination of pneumothorax, pneumonia, and size of cardiac silhouette. Enlarged cardiac silhouette may indicate tamponade or failure.
2. **Measurement of CVP.** If patient is poorly responsive to fluid therapy alone, therapy with inotropes or vasopressors may be necessary. If this occurs, placement of a central venous catheter should be considered. In addition to providing central access for fluid resuscitation, the catheter enables measurement of CVP, which will help to direct further therapy. If hypotension is refractory or continuous BP monitoring is needed, consider arterial line placement.

V. Plan
A. Immediate Plan

1. Place the largest bore IV possible. If unable to obtain rapid IV access, an intraosseous (IO) needle should be inserted.
2. Immediate action consists of *rapid* infusion of at least 20 mL/kg of an isotonic solution (preferably normal saline or lactated Ringer). Aggressive and immediate fluid resuscitation is the cornerstone of management of hypotension. This requires at least 20–40 mL/kg of an isotonic solution that is pushed as rapidly as possible. If there is no response, or inadequate response, to initial fluid therapy, continue fluid boluses. Some patients may require as much as 100–120 mL/kg before stabilization occurs.
3. Administer oxygen to patient, support airway if needed, and place patient in Trendelenburg position (head 30 degrees below feet).

B. Specific Plans

1. **Hypovolemic shock.** Resuscitate with isotonic crystalloids (normal saline or lactated Ringer). Blood products may be given if hemoglobin is < 8 g/dL or coagulopathy exists. Ensure adequate fluid resuscitation before instituting therapy with inotropes or vasopressors. Place a Foley catheter to monitor urine output. If a central venous catheter is required, measure CVP and provide fluid resuscitation until CVP is at least 10 cm H_2O. If BP, perfusion, or urine output remains inadequate, consider vasopressors or inotropes.
2. **Cardiogenic shock.** A central venous catheter will be required. Consider a pulmonary artery catheter. If pericardial

tamponade is present, drainage of pericardial fluid is required. If there is evidence of myocarditis, cardiology colleagues should be consulted. Generally, medications that are both inotropes and afterload reducers are best in these situations. Consider dobutamine, milrinone, or amrinone. Dopamine may also be helpful. If patient is still poorly responsive, then norepinephrine or epinephrine may be useful.

3. **Neurogenic shock.** Initial therapy includes aggressive volume resuscitation. If hypotension persists, therapy with vasopressors or inotropes is indicated.

4. **Vasogenic shock (includes septic shock and anaphylactic shock).** Initial therapy consists of aggressive volume resuscitation; be prepared to give very large volumes of fluid. Therapy with vasopressors or inotropes may be required, but should not be started until adequate fluid resuscitation has occurred (CVP > 10 cm H_2O). If patient is poorly responsive to resuscitation with crystalloids, blood products should be considered, especially if anemia, thrombocytopenia, or coagulopathy is present. Treatment of underlying infection with appropriate antibiotics is essential. If patient is in anaphylactic shock, treat immediately with isotonic fluids and epinephrine (0.01 mL/kg of 1:1000 SQ to a maximum dose of 0.3 mL). Diphenhydramine and ranitidine may be useful adjuncts to therapy. Vasogenic shock can also be seen with an addisonian crisis, which should be treated with hydrocortisone.

VI. **Problem Case Diagnosis.** The 2-year-old patient was diagnosed with hypovolemic shock secondary to gastroenteritis. Despite initial resuscitation, he continued to have ongoing fluid losses and the need for further aggressive fluid resuscitation. He was given an additional 20 mL/kg of normal saline, which was repeated twice until the systolic BP remained adequate (> 75 mm Hg).

VII. **Teaching Pearl: Question.** Is presence of hypotension necessary to make the diagnosis of shock?

VIII. **Teaching Pearl: Answer.** No; shock is an acute syndrome characterized by inadequate circulatory perfusion of tissue to meet the metabolic demands of vital organs. It is a misconception that shock occurs only with low BP (hypotension). Through various compensatory mechanisms, hypotension may be a late finding in shock.

REFERENCES

Frankel LR, Mathers LH. Shock. In: Behrman RE, Kliegman RM, Jenson HB, eds. *Nelson Textbook of Pediatrics,* 17th ed. Saunders, 2000:296–301.

Hazinski MF, Barkin RM. In: Barkin et al, eds. *Pediatric Emergency Medicine: Concepts and Clinical Practice,* 2nd ed. Mosby, 1997:118–145.

53. HYPOTHERMIA

I. **Problem.** A 4-year-old boy is brought to the emergency department by EMS personnel after falling through the ice into a frozen pond. He was immersed in the water for less than 5 minutes, and his head was submerged for less than 1 minute. He is lethargic, with a rectal temperature of 32°C (89.6°F).

II. **Immediate Questions**

   A. **What are the vital signs? Is patient breathing?** Is there a pulse? Does patient have a cardiac arrhythmia?

   B. **What is patient's core temperature?** Hypothermia is defined as a core temperature of 35°C (95°F) or less. It occurs when the body is no longer able to sustain normal temperature. Onset of hypothermia depends on the imbalance between increased heat loss and decreased heat production. Core temperature will help determine medical therapies: passive or active rewarming, cardioversion, or drug therapy.

   C. **What is the clinical setting?** Very young children are susceptible to hypothermia as a result of environmental exposure. Alcohol ingestion also predisposes humans to environmentally induced hypothermia.

   D. **Is there a history of other medical problems?** Patients with hypoglycemia, hypopituitarism, and hypoadrenalism may present with hypothermia.

   E. **Does patient have any possible source of infection?** Septic patients may be hypothermic.

III. **Differential Diagnosis**

   A. **Contributing Factors for Hypothermia.** Children have a higher surface area to mass ratio than adults and therefore cool faster and become hypothermic at an increased rate. Environmental factors such as cold, wind, and inadequate clothing can increase heat loss. Heat production can be affected by such factors as age, trauma, medical illness, and alcohol ingestion.

   B. **Physiologic Stages of Hypothermia**

   1. **Mild hypothermia: Core temperature of 32–35°C (89.6–95°F).** Increased metabolic rate and tachypnea occur; shivering mechanism is usually preserved; BP is maintained; dysarthria, ataxia, and apathy can develop.

   2. **Moderate hypothermia: Core temperature of 28–32°C (82.4°F).** Cardiac output, respiration, and level of consciousness all decrease; shivering mechanism diminishes; atrial fibrillation and other dysrhythmias occur.

   3. **Severe hypothermia: Core temperature < 28°C (82.4°F).** Shivering is absent; loss of consciousness occurs; cerebral blood flow is decreased; acid-base balance is disrupted; there is increased susceptibility to ventricular fibrillation or asystole; significant hypotension can occur.

    C. ICU Patient. Hypothermia typically results from thermoregulatory impairment, such as drug or alcohol intoxication, massive CNS injury, burns, sepsis, or endocrinopathies.

IV. Database
A. Physical Exam Key Points
1. **Vital signs.** Core temperature, BP, and volume status should be continuously monitored. Look for shivering as a mechanism of heat production. Hypothermic patients may be vasoconstricted peripherally and have distal pulses that are difficult to palpate. Severely hypothermic patients will have paradoxical vasodilation and cutaneous erythema.
2. **Neurologic exam.** Check mental status and perform a complete neurologic exam if patient is not comatose. Assign a modified Glasgow Coma Scale score (see Appendix F, p. 765). Observe for signs of increased intracranial pressure.
3. **Secondary survey.** Observe for signs of trauma or continuing blood loss. Hemostasis and volume resuscitation may be necessary before correction of hypothermia can succeed.

B. Laboratory Data
1. **CBC.** To help rule out conditions such as sepsis, and determine hemoglobin concentration and oxygen-carrying capacity of blood.
2. **Basic metabolic panel.** Provides clues to volume status, hypoglycemia, and electrolyte disturbances. BUN is another clue in determination of volume status. Renal function can be estimated by creatinine value. Hypoglycemia and electrolyte imbalances, if present, should be corrected.
3. **Urinalysis.** Rule out rhabdomyolysis and myoglobinuria resulting from excessive shivering and cell breakdown.
4. **ABGs.** Provide acid-base, ventilation, and oxygenation status.

C. Radiographic and Other Studies
1. **Chest x-ray.** Look for pulmonary edema or aspiration.
2. **Continuous ECG monitoring.** Rule out cardiac dysrhythmia.
3. **CT scan.** Used to rule out intracranial or intra-abdominal process, especially in suspected trauma patients.
4. **Neck x-rays.** Often needed in patients with suspected head or neck trauma to evaluate the cervical spine.

V. Plan.
Management must address the underlying condition impairing thermoregulation that led to hypothermia. Hypothermic patients are at increased risk of refractory ventricular fibrillation, which may be provoked by rough handling, including chest compressions and electrical defibrillation. Aggressive volume resuscitation with isotonic fluids is a mainstay in treating hypothermia. Method chosen to rewarm patient must be tailored to the individual, and presence or absence of circulation is at least as important as patient's temperature. Most textbooks mandate active rewarming for core temperature < 28°C

(82.4°F). Patients should not be declared dead until they have been rewarmed to 32°C (89.6°F).

A. CPR. Initiate if patient is not breathing or is pulseless. Continuous ECG monitoring is necessary because pulses are very difficult to palpate in hypothermic patients. Defibrillation is typically unsuccessful until patient is warmed to 32°C (89.6°F). If initiated, CPR should be continued until patient is warmed to 32°C.

B. Passive Rewarming (Patients Who Are Shivering). Shivering mechanism is usually preserved if core temperature exceeds 30°C (86°F). As long as patient is shivering, passive rewarming techniques may be utilized. These include removing cold or wet clothing, transporting to a warm environment, and covering with dry blankets. Passive rewarming requires that patient have spontaneous heat production, which makes it useful only in mild cases of hypothermia.

C. Active Rewarming (Patients Who Are Not Shivering). Patients who are not shivering have lost their thermoregulatory drive and require active rewarming. Controversy exists over exact temperature at which to begin internal active rewarming. Decision should be made based on individual patient and institutional expertise.

  1. External active rewarming. Includes techniques such as hot packs, heating lamps, and warm water baths. These techniques are familiar, inexpensive, and readily available. External active rewarming may result in rewarming shock, decreased core temperature (afterdrop), and ventricular fibrillation. Severe hypovolemia is common in hypothermic patients due to vascular leak and a profound cold diuresis. Heat applied externally restores circulation to the coldest part of the body, which dumps cold and stagnant blood into the core. This, combined with an already depressed myocardium, dilated vascular beds, and hypovolemia, can lead to vascular collapse and a drop in core temperature. External active rewarming is unlikely to be effective in patients who do not have adequate spontaneous circulation.

  2. Internal active rewarming (core rewarming). Preferred for severe hypothermia or patients with absent or ineffective circulation. Common techniques include warm humidified oxygen, heated intravascular fluids, closed thoracic or pleural lavage with warm saline, and heated lavage of bladder, stomach, colon, or peritoneum. Open thoracotomy with mediastinal irrigation and extracorporal circulation with heating elements are also effective. Core rewarming requires invasive devices not always available at rural or community hospitals. These methods are advantageous in that they are very effective and they lessen the chance of rewarming shock, core cooling, and cardiac arrhythmias.

VI. Problem Case Diagnosis. The 4-year-old boy had mild hypothermia from environmental exposure. He maintained his ability to shiver and responded well to passive rewarming.

VII. Teaching Pearl: Question. Why are children at increased risk of developing hypothermia?

VIII. Teaching Pearl: Answer. Children have a relatively high body surface area to mass ratio, decreased subcutaneous fat, and limited thermogenic capacity, all of which contribute to an increased risk of developing hypothermia.

REFERENCES

Kiley J, Robinson MD, Seward PN. In: Furhman BP, Zimmerman JJ. *Pediatric Critical Care*, 2nd ed. Mosby, 1998:1147–1149.
Lazar HL. The treatment of hypothermia. *N Engl J Med* 1997;337:1545.

54. HYPOTONIA

I. **Problem.** An 8-month-old girl is brought to the pediatric clinic with respiratory distress. She is unable to sit without support.

II. **Immediate Questions**
   A. **Is patient experiencing impending respiratory failure?** Hypotonia, especially when associated with muscle weakness, may result in respiratory compromise. Evaluate airway patency, protection, and efficacy of respiratory effort.
   B. **Is inability to sit due to muscle weakness, hypotonia, or both?** Answer helps narrow differential diagnosis and guide immediate approach. In patients who have CNS causes of hypotonia, muscle weakness is not present; these patients have preserved deep tendon reflexes or hyperreflexia. Patients who have diseases affecting the lower motor neuron usually have both weakness and hypotonia and, if the anterior horn cell or peripheral motor neuron is involved, have diminished or absent reflexes.
   C. **Is there abnormal phasic tone, postural tone, or both?**
      1. Phasic tone is the rapid contraction of a muscle. Examining deep tendon reflexes best tests this. Determine if reflexes are present or absent. If present, determine if they are symmetric, diminished, or brisk.
      2. Postural tone is sustained or prolonged contraction against gravity. Examining child's traction response, horizontal suspension, and vertical suspension can assess postural tone. Traction response is elicited by pulling child to a sitting position from a supine position. Examiner should feel child resisting against the traction. Child should initiate lifting the head as body is raised and should attempt to keep the head erect when sitting. Significant head lag and failure to flex limbs in response to traction is indicative of hypotonia. In horizontal suspension, infant with normal tone should maintain head at midline; flex hips, knees, and elbows; and keep back straight. In vertical suspension with examiner's hands under the axilla, infant with

normal tone should allow for suspension without compressing the thorax, given normal shoulder strength. In addition, infant should hold the head erect and flex at the knees, hips, and ankles.

D. Is process acute, subacute, or chronic? This may or may not be an easy classification, because sometimes an acute event can exacerbate an underlying condition. It is one way to stratify the diagnostic possibilities. Botulism, spinal cord trauma, sepsis, intestinal obstruction, Reye syndrome, toxic encephalopathy, concussion, intracranial hemorrhage, tumors of the posterior fossa, Guillain-Barré syndrome, myasthenia gravis, and collagen vascular disease can all present with acute or subacute onset of hypotonia.

E. Does underlying process involve brain, spine, or motor unit? For normal tone to be present, patient must have intact central nervous and peripheral nervous systems.

F. What is child's developmental history? Are milestones delayed? Is the delay in motor milestones, only, or also in speech and cognitive development? Children with hypotonia from a CNS source usually present with more global developmental delay.

G. What is child's birth history? Is there a history of decreased intrauterine movement, distress, hypoxia, apnea, infection, hyperbilirubinemia, and neonatal seizures? In addition to identifying possible causes, this information helps to identify time of onset. Presence of decreased intrauterine movement, fetal distress, polyhydramnios, joint contractures, arthrogryposis, or dislocation of hips noted at birth all provide evidence of probable prenatal onset.

H. What is patient's immunization status? Was child vaccinated against polio? Is there a history of travel with possible polio exposure?

I. Are any family members nonambulatory? Is there a family history of childhood deaths? Family history helps to determine possible congenital causes (eg, glycogen storage disease, hereditary neuromyopathies, spinal muscle atrophy, Ehlers-Danlos syndrome, Tay-Sachs disease, congenital myasthenia gravis, or benign congenital hypotonia).

J. Any history of trauma? Newborn infants with spinal cord injuries can present with hypotonia. This is more common with breech vaginal deliveries but can be seen with cephalic presentations. Abnormal rectal tone, a distended bladder, lack of deep tendon reflexes with no spontaneous movement in the lower extremities, or loss of sensation below the nipple line should alert clinician to spinal cord insult.

K. Any possible exposure to *Clostridium botulinum* spores? Spores can be found in soil and honey. Exposure to soil disruption such as excavation sites or ingestion of honey would both be significant risk factors. In cases of infantile botulism, constipation usually precedes the onset of ascending hypotonia. A careful history of stooling pattern should be included.

III. Differential Diagnosis

A. Brain Disorders. Consider toxicity, metabolic encephalopathy, chromosomal disorder (eg, Prader-Willi syndrome, trisomy 21), infection, periventricular leukomalacia, cerebrovascular accident, hypoxic ischemic encephalopathy, trauma (intracranial hemorrhage), cerebral palsy, benign congenital hypotonia, mass (tumor, cyst).

B. Spinal Cord Disorders. Trauma and hypoxic ischemic insult.

C. Anterior Horn Cell Disorders. Poliomyelitis and spinal muscle atrophy.

D. Peripheral Nerve Disorders. Polyneuropathy, Guillain-Barré syndrome, trauma.

E. Neuromuscular Junction Disorders. Infantile botulism, myasthenia gravis, transitory neonatal myasthenia gravis, aminoglycoside antibiotic, hypermagnesemia.

F. Muscle Disorders. Hypothyroidism, metabolic myopathies (eg, acid maltase deficiency, phosphorylase deficiency, glycogen storage disease), muscular dystrophies, polymyositis.

G. Systemic Diseases. Malnutrition, sepsis, intestinal obstruction, cyanotic heart disease, collagen vascular disease.

IV. Database

A. Physical Exam Key Points

1. **General appearance**
   a. Does child have a recognizable congenital syndrome (eg, Down syndrome)? What is general posture? Children with hypotonia often assume a frog-leg position and have positional plagiocephaly because of their usual positioning on back with little head movement.
   b. Any signs of sepsis? Check for decreased skin perfusion, tachycardia, and prolonged capillary refill.
2. **Vital signs and respirations.** Is the airway protected? Check gag reflex. What is the respiratory effort, and is it effective? Check for grunting, flaring retractions, paradoxical respiratory movements, and overall aeration. Confirm with pulse oximetry.
3. **Neurologic findings**
   a. **Intracranial pressure.** Perform cranial nerve exam, and check for a flat fontanel and papilledema.
   b. **Evidence of trauma.** Check for stability of cervical spine, intact frenulum, bruising of skin, bony tenderness.
   c. **Deep tendon reflexes.** Are reflexes preserved, hyperreflexic, hyporeflexic, or absent? Are primitive reflexes present? Presence of primitive reflexes beyond the neonatal period reflects CNS or upper motor neuron disease.

    d. Sensation. Loss of sensation raises concern of spinal cord injury. However, inability to withdraw from a noxious stimulus may indicate severe muscle weakness. To assess this parameter more carefully, examine infant's ability to resist gravitational forces when an extremity is raised. Children with lower motor neuron disease should have preserved mental status.

    e. Tongue fasciculation. Given the generous subcutaneous tissue mass usually present on most infants, muscle fasciculation or wasting may be difficult to assess elsewhere.

  4. Musculoskeletal findings. Any arthrogryposis, contractures, or dislocations? Presence of these findings during infancy points to a prenatal onset.

B. Laboratory Data. Initial studies are guided by history and physical exam but will likely include the following:

  1. CBC with differential.

  2. Infectious workup (eg, blood culture, urinalysis, urine culture, lumbar puncture). Consider if infection is suggested by history or physical exam.

  3. Electrolytes (including glucose, calcium, potassium).

  4. BUN and creatinine.

  5. Thyroid function tests.

  6. Urine for organic acids.

  7. Creatine phosphokinase.

  8. Other tests (as appropriate)

    a. Stool studies for *Clostridium botulinum*.

    b. DNA test for spinal muscle atrophy (SMA) or myotonic dystrophy.

C. Radiographic and Other Studies

  1. CT or MRI scan of spine. Obtain acutely if there is concern of possible spinal cord injury in an infant.

  2. Electromyogram. Obtain if muscle weakness is present.

  3. MRI scan of head. Consider if laboratory studies do not support diagnosis of myopathy and there is concern of a central CNS process, including tumor, cyst, enlarged ventricles, cerebral atrophy, or congenital malformation.

  4. Chest x-ray. If respiratory symptoms are present.

V. Plan. Most children with hypotonia have a chronic or subacute presentation. It is critical to recognize an acute presentation of hypotonia. Thorough history and physical exam allow clinician to narrow the differential diagnosis based on its chronicity and anatomic classification. This in turn allows for systematic and focused evaluation of child.

A. Initial Management

  1. If child's presentation is acute or if child is experiencing an acute exacerbation of a subacute or chronic problem, it is important to anticipate respiratory compromise and be able to proceed with airway stabilization in a controlled fashion.

2. Rapid identification of child with sepsis, CNS infection, malnutrition, intestinal obstruction, cyanotic heart disease, toxicity, trauma, cerebrovascular accident, mass lesion, hypothyroidism, Guillain-Barré syndrome, or infantile botulism is important because these are all potentially treatable conditions if detected early. Infantile botulism is often treated with supportive care, although some centers use botulism antitoxin; aminoglycosides exacerbate hypotonia by competing at the neuromuscular junction.

3. Most commonly, hypotonia is related to a known CNS insult. If child has central hypotonia and no identifiable preceding insult, the hypotonia is often benign. Children with central hypotonia are also treated with supportive therapy, including physical therapy. A swallowing evaluation may be required, and feeding support such as nasogastric tube feedings may be required if children have significant sucking or swallowing difficulties.

B. **Congenital Myopathies.** Treatment of most patients with congenital myopathies is supportive. Diagnosis of spinal muscular atrophy is important to help guide future decisions regarding appropriate level of intervention, including intubation. In general, the younger the child at diagnosis, the worse will be the prognosis.

VI. **Problem Case Diagnosis.** The 8-month-old girl was diagnosed with spinal muscular atrophy, based on a DNA test demonstrating presence of *SMN* gene. Of interest, an infection with respiratory syncytial virus caused bronchiolitis, which led to the acute presentation.

VII. **Teaching Pearl: Question.** If a patient presents with hypotonia yet with vibrant facial expressions, what does this suggest?

VIII. **Teaching Pearl: Answer.** Children with neuromuscular disease often have preserved facial expressions and appear vibrant despite significant hypotonia and weakness.

REFERENCES

Fenichel GM. *Clinical Pediatric Neurology: A Signs and Symptoms Approach,* 4th ed. Saunders, 2001.

Swaiman KF Ashwal S. *Pediatric Neurology: Principles and Practice,* 3rd ed. Mosby, 1999.

55. INABILITY TO VOID (URINARY RETENTION)

I. **Problem.** A 3-year-old boy is brought to the emergency department by his parents with a complaint of no urination in the past 24 hours. He appears uncomfortable.

II. Immediate Questions

A. Is patient toilet trained? Has patient attained dryness at night and at daytime, or is patient in transition phase, still wearing pull-ups? Has the urinary stream been straight and strong or weakened and interrupted?

B. Is patient constipated? Are bowel habits regular?

C. Is there pain on urination or fever? Pain with fever suggests UTI.

D. History of trauma? Urethral rupture is an emergency.

E. What medication(s) does patient currently take? Anticholinergics (eg, imipramine) can cause urinary retention.

F. What is the prenatal history? Was a prenatal ultrasound performed and, if so, were findings normal? Abnormal urinary flow can be seen with renal dysplasia or GU obstruction.

G. Is there a past medical history of UTI? Children with GU reflux commonly present with recurrent UTIs.

H. What is the social situation? Is there a history suggestive of sexual abuse? See Chapter 15, Child Abuse: Sexual, p. 75.

I. Are there other associated signs or symptoms? Loss of weight, leg pain, and neurologic symptoms provide clues to other underlying conditions.

III. Differential Diagnosis

A. Transitional Voiding or Dysfunctional Voiding Syndromes. Intermediate stage of toilet training, fright of bathrooms.

B. Constipation. Large amounts of stool in the colon can impinge on the bladder.

C. UTI. Child with UTI can present with either urinary frequency or retention.

D. Bladder Outlet Obstruction. Posterior urethral valves in male patients.

E. Neurogenic Bladder. Occult spinal dysraphism.

F. Pelvic Malignancy. Rhabdomyosarcoma.

G. Sexual Abuse or Other Psychological Stressors.

IV. Database

A. Physical Exam Key Points

1. **General appearance.** Does child appear well or ill, comfortable or uncomfortable, playful or timid?

2. **Abdomen.** Tender, tense, smooth suprapubic mass usually indicates a distended bladder. Prominence in left lower quadrant often indicates that sigmoid colon is distended with stool.

3. **Back.** Observe for lumbosacral skin abnormalities (café au lait spots, hemangiomas, fatty appearance, skin dimple or skin tag, tuft of hair, dermal vascular malformation, or subcutaneous lipomas).

4. **Genitalia.** Phimosis (if uncircumcised), meatal stenosis, and erythema of prepuce or glans may represent acute balanoposthitis; ecchymotic areas may represent physical or sexual abuse.

5. **Rectal exam.** Perform gently with a well-lubricated small finger. Position patient on side, with legs drawn into chest. Assess anal tone and rectal vault content for the following: loose or impacted stool; indurated mass in area of prostate and bladder neck, which could represent pelvic malignancy (rhabdomyosarcoma).

6. **Neurologic exam.** Check for sensation in perineum. Examine extremities for high arched foot, discrepancy in muscle size.

B. **Laboratory Data.** Obtain basic metabolic panel, CBC with differential, urine for analysis and culture.

C. **Radiographic and Other Studies**

1. **KUB.** Useful in general assessment of bowel pattern, occult spinal dysraphism, abdominal masses, stool impaction.

2. **Renal and bladder ultrasound.** Evaluate appearance of bladder and kidneys for acute changes (bladder distention, ureteral or renal pelvis dilation) or chronic changes (bladder wall thickening and hydroureteronephrosis with parenchymal thinning and ureteral tortuosity).

3. **Voiding cystourethrogram (VCUG).** Can be performed electively if ultrasound shows hydronephrosis or bladder wall thickening to rule out bladder outlet obstruction secondary to posterior urethral valves.

4. **Urodynamic studies.** May be necessary if neurologic or functional cause is suspected.

5. **MRI scan of abdomen and lumbosacral spine.** To exclude tethered cord or bladder abnormalities.

V. **Plan.** Determine if patient needs medical intervention (eg, catheterization) or simply assistance with elimination. If patient has signs and symptoms of UTI, a neurologic disorder, or abnormalities on ultrasound, intervention is more likely to be necessary.

A. **Constipation.** Give an enema and begin bowel program (ie, mineral oil or stool softeners). See Chapter 18, Constipation, V, C, p. 91.

B. **Voiding Problems Secondary to Toilet Training Imbalance**

1. *Avoid catheterization if possible.* Give midazolam (nasally or orally, 1–5 mg/kg PO as 1 dose to a maximum of 20 mg; time of onset, 10–30 minutes) to relax patient and perform bladder massage (gently massage suprapubic area until distended bladder becomes tense, representing impending urination). Midazolam will relax external urinary sphincter, facilitating urination. Avoid ambulation, because balance may be affected.

2. If patient is still unable to void, instill 2% lidocaine solution into urethra and catheterize while still under midazolam effect, to

minimize recollection of catheterization. Remove catheter after draining bladder. Give ibuprofen, 10 mg/kg every 6 hours, to control dysuria associated with catheterization.

C. Organic Urinary Retention. Catheterize urethra to drain bladder. Try a 10 or 12 Fr Foley catheter or a 10 Fr straight catheter (smaller in younger children); a straight catheter may be more easily advanced, but it needs to be taped to the penis with clear adhesive tape (Tegaderm). Leave catheter in place and consult urology colleagues.

D. Cystoscopy and Endoscopic Valve Ablation. Consult urology colleagues if posterior urethral valves are demonstrated by VCUG.

VI. Problem Case Diagnosis. The 3-year-old boy has dysfunctional elimination syndrome with constipation and dysfunctional voiding. He responded to a bowel program of mineral oil and stool softeners.

VII. Teaching Pearl: Question. What is the bladder capacity of a 3-year-old child?

VIII. Teaching Pearl: Answer. Approximately 150 mL; a normal bladder at birth holds 30–60 mL and increases its capacity by approximately 30 mL per year until puberty. Bladder capacity can be calculated using the following formula: Volume in ounces = age in years + 2.

REFERENCES

Baskin LS, Kogan BA, Duckett JW. *Handbook of Pediatric Urology.* Lippincott-Raven, 1997.

Bauer SB. Neuropathology of the lower urinary tract. In: Belman AB, King LR, Kramer SA, eds. *Clinical Pediatric Urology,* 4th ed. Martin Dunitz, 2002:371–408.

Koff SA, Jayanthi VR. Dysfunctional elimination syndromes of childhood. In: Walsh PC, Retik AB, Vaughn ED, Wein AJ, eds. *Campbell's Urology,* 8th ed. Elsevier, 2002:2262–2280.

Wein AJ. Drug therapy for neurogenic and non-neurogenic bladder dysfunction. In: Seidmon EJ, Hanno PM, eds. *Current Urologic Therapy,* 3rd ed. Saunders, 1994:291–298.

56. INCREASED INTRACRANIAL PRESSURE

I. Problem. A 7-year-old girl with a 1-week history of headaches and vomiting presents with depressed mental status. CT scan of the head demonstrates a large mass in the posterior fossa and dilated cerebral ventricles.

II. Immediate Questions

A. Is patient maintaining a safe and patent airway? Severe neurologic depression is likely to suppress a patient's ability to protect the airway, thus increasing the risk of aspiration.

B. What are the vital signs? Patients with increased intracranial pressure (ICP) often become hypertensive. If there is significant pressure producing herniation, both hypertension and bradycardia will be present.

C. Neurologic status and results of funduscopic exam? Papilledema is a hallmark sign of raised ICP but may be absent when pressure has risen acutely.

D. Is there a history of trauma? Trauma would provide a possible source of intracranial bleeding that would require immediate evaluation and neurosurgical intervention, if present.

E. Pertinent Historical Information

1. Does patient have a frontal headache that worsens when lying down, blurred vision, and vomiting, especially in the morning without associated nausea (classic history of ICP)?
2. Is there a history of bleeding disorders or coagulation disorders, fever, problems with coordination, or underlying medical conditions?
3. What medication(s) does patient take?

III. Differential Diagnosis. Increased ICP occurs when there is an excess of cerebrospinal fluid (CSF), blood, or brain tissue within the rigid confines of the skull. Increased ICP can result from a variety of causes.

A. Anatomic Causes

1. **Hydrocephalus.** Hydrocephalus develops when there is obstruction of CSF reabsorption or flow (see Chapter 65, Macrocephaly, III, A, p. 295).
2. **Hematoma.** Traumatic brain injury or cerebral vascular accidents may produce collections of blood in any of four spaces within the skull.
   a. Extra-axial.
   b. Epidural.
   c. Subdural.
   d. Intraparenchymal.
3. **Tumor.** A mass can produce increased ICP directly or by obstructing CSF flow, producing hydrocephalus. Tumors may also cause hemorrhage.
4. **Venous drainage obstruction.** Cerebral venous sinus thrombosis, superior vena cava syndrome, or severe cor pulmonale can increase ICP.

B. Physiologic Causes

1. **Endocrine abnormalities.** Addison disease, Cushing disease, hypothyroidism, hypoparathyroidism.
2. **Infectious disease.** Meningitis, encephalitis, encephalopathies, abscess formation, Reye syndrome (aspirin associated with influenza, varicella).
3. **Autoimmune disorders.** Systemic lupus erythematosus, antiphospholipid antibody syndrome.
4. **Metabolic abnormalities?** Hypoxemia, hyperammonemia, kernicterus, lead toxicity, acute osmolar changes (diabetic ketoacidosis, hypernatremia).

    5. Medications. Steroid withdrawal, vitamin A (retinoic acid), cyclosporine, levothyroxine, lithium, sulfonamides, tetracyclines.

C. Edema. Edema of neuronal cells is the common endpoint producing increased ICP in many of the preceding conditions. There are two types of edema to consider:

    1. Cytotoxic. Sodium-potassium pump fails, as does calcium transport, causing fluid to enter cells.

    2. Vasogenic. Blood-brain barrier is defective, and fluid enters the interstitial space.

IV. Database

  A. Physical Exam Key Points

    1. Vital signs. The brain's response to increased pressure is to provide increased oxygen delivery. This initial response occurs through increased BP and tachycardia. Patient may also hyperventilate to reduce the $PaCO_2$ and vasoconstrict the cerebral blood vessels. When ICP is sufficient to produce herniation of cerebral structures, the classic Cushing triad of hypertension, bradycardia, and a pattern of irregular respiration may develop.

    2. Eyes. Pupillary exam provides a quick assessment of patient's ICP as well as an indication of which areas of the brain are affected. Papilledema occurs in response to increased ICP but may be absent if ICP rises acutely. Pupillary dilation is suggestive of herniation. Herniation of the brain can occur in a variety of ways, including downward (transtentorial), or lateral and downward (uncal, transfalx), which causes compression of the brainstem. A single dilated pupil suggests lateral herniation compressing the third cranial nerve on the affected side.

    3. Neurologic exam. Immediate assessment of patient's level of consciousness and ability to maintain adequately ventilation and protection of the airway is of primary importance. Patients should be scored according to the Glasgow Coma Scale (GCS; see Appendix F, p. 765). Patients with a GCS score < 8 should be considered at severe risk of respiratory compromise and aspiration. Overall assessment of patient's strength, tone, sensation, reflexes, and coordination is important in localizing the potential lesion as well as establishing a neurologic baseline to assess further deterioration or response to therapy.

    4. Cardiovascular system. To maximize oxygen delivery to the brain, an adequate cardiovascular response must be in place. Assess intravascular volume status, anemia, and cardiac contractility, all of which are important in allowing the body to deliver oxygen to the brain.

  B. Laboratory Data. Because the factors producing increased ICP are so diverse, laboratory data should include serum electrolytes as well as CBC. ABG measurement is useful to determine patient's $PaCO_2$. Other tests that may be useful include coagulation studies to assess for signs of disseminated intravascular coagulation (DIC), liver function studies, ammonia level, total and direct bilirubin, and blood cultures.

C. Radiographic and Other Studies. Suspicion of increased ICP should prompt an immediate CT scan of the head to determine etiology. Lumbar puncture should be deferred.

V. Plan. Rapid intervention is critical in reducing morbidity and mortality from increased ICP. Therapies differ somewhat based on etiology, although some generalizations apply. Therapy should be instituted as soon as a raised ICP is suspected. Care should be coordinated with a pediatric intensivist or pediatric neurosurgeon, or both. Immediate actions should always include proper evaluation and management of patient's airway, breathing, and circulation. Cerebral perfusion pressure (CPP) must be adequate to provide blood flow to the brain. CPP is the net driving force of blood into the brain and is a function of the mean arterial blood pressure (MAP) and the ICP or the central venous pressure (CVP), whichever is greater.

$$CPP = MAP - [ICP \text{ or } CVP, \text{ whichever is greater}]$$

Although the appropriate CPP in children has not been absolutely defined, adult patients with raised ICP from traumatic brain injury should be maintained with a CPP ≥ 60 mm Hg.

A. Position. Simple first maneuvers should include having child lay supine, with head of bed elevated to 30 degrees and child's head in a midline position. Use care when positioning the head of a trauma patient with potential cervical spine injury. When placing the cervical collar, be sure there is no compression of the jugular veins by the collar, which would decrease CPP by raising jugular venous pressure.

B. Ventilation. Maintaining adequate oxygenation and ventilation is of primary importance. Because CO_2 is a cerebral vasodilator, maintaining normal $Paco_2$ (40 mm Hg) helps decrease ICP by decreasing cerebral blood volume. Hyperventilation is indicated only in the setting of impending herniation.

C. Osmotic Therapy. Osmotic therapy consists of mannitol (typically 0.5–1 g/kg) or 3% saline (typically 3–5 mL/kg). Both agents reduce ICP in two ways.

    1. Immediate reduction in ICP is caused by the laminar effect of the osmolar load into the vascular supply. This forces blood to flow in a more laminar pattern and hence reduces the cross section of cerebral blood vessels while maintaining the same blood flow.

    2. The second effect is seen as water exits the brain cell in order to equalize the osmolar load on each side of the blood-brain barrier. This reduces cell volume and hence ICP.

D. Sedation and Seizure Control. Adequate sedation and keeping patient calm helps to reduce ICP and brain injury by reducing oxygen demand of the brain cells. However, sedation that produces hypotension may worsen CPP. In a similar fashion, control of seizure activity is beneficial both in reducing ICP and in reducing the brain's oxygen requirements. Barbiturates are often used to produce sedation, coma, and seizure control.

E. **Steroids.** Steroids have proven beneficial in reducing vasogenic edema associated with mass lesions such as tumors within the brain. However, there is no proven benefit in administering steroids to patients with traumatic brain injury.

F. **BP Management.** To maintain adequate CPP, MAP must be sufficient. Fluid administration may benefit the MAP, but at the same time may increase the CVP. Fluid administration may be given as 3% saline to expand blood volume with the benefit of osmotic therapy, or as blood if indicated secondary to anemia or blood loss. Vasoactive agents may be necessary to increase MAP enough to produce a sufficient CPP.

G. **Diuretics.** Furosemide, especially when administered with mannitol, may augment the osmolar benefits. Again, use caution to avoid hypotension. Acetazolamide, a carbonic anhydrase inhibitor, can reduce CSF production and hence delay worsening of ICP caused by hydrocephalus.

H. **Surgical Intervention.** Surgical intervention has two benefits.

  1. Introduction of appropriate intracranial monitoring devices that can monitor the ICP and the response to therapy; these include catheters placed in the ventricular space or brain parenchyma.

  2. Removal of what is in excess in the intracranial vault, including CSF, blood, or tumor mass.

VI. **Problem Case Diagnosis.** The 7-year-old child has a newly diagnosed brain tumor. The mass of this tumor was not responsible for the signs of increased ICP. However, when the mass reached sufficient size it obstructed CSF flow, producing hydrocephalus and raising ICP.

VII. **Teaching Pearl: Question.** How should a clinician approach an intubated patient with a known intracranial mass and hydrocephalus who develops progressive hypertension and bradycardia?

VIII. **Teaching Pearl: Answer.** Administer mannitol, 0.5–1 g/kg IV, and position patient midline, with the head of the bed at 30 degrees. Obtain a CT scan of the head to ensure that no new mass (eg, bleeding) has occurred to account for the sudden changes.

REFERENCES

Bhardwaj A, Ulatowski JA. Hypertonic saline solutions in brain injury. *Curr Opin Crit Care* 2004;10:126–131.

Dutton RP, McCunn M. Traumatic brain injury. *Curr Opin Crit Care* 2003;9:503–509.

Poss BW, Brockmeyer DC, Clay B, Dean MJ. Pathophysiology and management of the intracranial vault. In: Rogers MC, Nichols DG, eds. *Textbook of Pediatric Intensive Care*, 3rd ed. Williams & Wilkins, 1996:645–665.

57. INTRAVENOUS ACCESS PROBLEMS

I. **Problem.** A 6-month-old infant enters the hospital with 3-day history of vomiting and diarrhea. Rehydration is necessary, but there are no available veins for IV access.

II. **Immediate Questions**

A. **What is the nature of patient's illness, and what other locations or vascular access should be considered?** Alternative therapies or regimen may be attempted in some medical conditions or clinical situations (eg, oral or nasogastric tube rehydration can be considered in mildly dehydrated, hemodynamically stable patients). Always have a well-formulated plan for vascular access; *do not* waste time looking for small peripheral veins. Children requiring immediate IV access (eg, hypotension with shock) should undergo intraosseous cannulation or percutaneous femoral line placement in the absence of large peripheral veins (eg, saphenous or antecubital). Always consider the possibility of a bleeding diathesis or coagulopathy before inserting a central venous line.

B. **Is there a history of chronic illness, prolonged hospitalization, or known difficult IV access? What routes of access were used on other occasions?** Chronically hospitalized patients often lose usable peripheral veins after multiple IV insertions and venipunctures.

III. **Differential Diagnosis.** Peripheral IV access may be poor in the following situations:

A. **Chronic Illness** (eg, sickle cell disease).

B. **Prolonged Hospitalization.**

C. **Obesity.**

D. **Prior Chemotherapy.**

E. **Lymphedema.**

F. **Hypotension and Hypovolemia.**

G. **Chronic Steroid Use.**

H. **Skin Disorders** (eg, epidermolysis bullosis).

IV. **Database**

A. **Physical Exam Key Points**

1. **Vital signs.** Hypotension or weak peripheral pulses often cause peripheral veins to collapse. Cold ambient temperature may impede access.

2. **Extremities.** Initially look for an antecubital vein in the upper arm or a saphenous vein located anterior to the medial malleolus of the ankle if child is clinically stable.

B. **Laboratory Data.** These studies usually are not helpful in solving IV access problems. Consider obtaining hematocrit and platelet count, because even small amounts of blood loss can be significant in a child.

C. **Radiographic and Other Studies.** Follow-up chest films should be obtained after central lines are inserted to confirm their locations.

V. Plan. IV access should be approached in the following order in both emergent and elective situations.

A. **Peripheral (Arm).** Start distally and work proximally. Lower extremities can be used for infants, toddlers, or children who are nonambulatory due to underlying disease (eg, cerebral palsy). Scalp veins can be used in patients up to 18 months of age. Standard-gauge catheters for children are 24, 22, 20, and 18 gauges, depending on age of child and clinical setting. For elective IV line, application of warm towels or a heating pad on the extremity for a few minutes may dilate the vein.

B. **External Jugular.** Simple IV catheters can be placed in the external jugular vein without difficulty and with little or no risk to child. Place child in Trendelenburg (head-down) position and gently occlude vein just above the clavicle to dilate it.

C. **Intraosseous.** Attempt if child is in cardiopulmonary arrest or being treated for decompensated shock with no venous access.

D. **Central Lines**
   1. Percutaneous puncture should be attempted in the following order:
      a. Femoral.
      b. Internal jugular.
      c. Subclavian.
   2. Experience with a particular route of access, however, is also an important determinant. The femoral vein is the preferred site in emergency situations because it is relatively easy to cannulate, has fewer complications, and does not interrupt CPR. The complication rate for cannulation of the internal jugular or subclavian vein is higher when attempted by an inexperienced clinician.

E. **Cutdown.** If peripheral venous, central venous, and intraosseous cannulations are unsuccessful, venous cutdown may be attempted to gain vascular access.

VI. Problem Case Diagnosis. An intraosseous cannula was placed in this ill-appearing child who was in decompensated shock. BP stabilized and perfusion improved after administration of a 20 mL/kg normal saline bolus.

VII. Teaching Pearl: Question. In what scenarios should intraosseous cannulas be avoided?

VIII. Teaching Pearl: Answer. Avoid if patient has an overlying skin infection, a bone fracture, or at the site of previous infiltration.

REFERENCE

Hankins J, Waldman Lonsway RA, Hedrick C, Perdue MB. *Infusion Therapy in Clinical Practice.* Saunders, 2001.

58. IRRITABILITY

I. **Problem.** A 3-month-old female infant has been seen for fussiness and frequent crying spells, especially in the evening, since 2–3 weeks of age. There are no associated symptoms, and physical exam is normal. Shortly after infant is switched from a cow's milk–based formula to an elemental formula, her parents notice a significant decrease in fussiness.

II. **Immediate Questions**

A. **How old is patient?** Although meningitis, otitis media, gastroesophageal reflux disease, abuse, and other causes of irritability can occur at any age, special considerations in neonates (0–2 months of age) include colic, neonatal abstinence syndrome, metabolic disorders, and anatomic abnormalities. Colic usually begins in second or third week of life and subsides by 3–4 months of age. Persistent crying in a neonate younger than 2 weeks of age or in an older infant is unlikely to be colic.

B. **What are the vital signs?** Fever implies an infectious etiology. Tachycardia may be secondary to pain, fever, or volume depletion. Hypotension suggests volume depletion or septic shock.

C. **What is the time course of the irritability?** Acute, unexplained crying is defined as an episode lasting longer than any previous crying episode or more than 2 hours. Although infectious disease appears to be the most common cause, initially consider a broad differential diagnosis. Long-standing or chronic, persistent crying suggests colic, gastroesophageal reflux, milk-protein allergy, increased intracranial pressure, abuse, or an underlying metabolic problem.

D. **Is there a history of trauma?** Infants with subdural hematomas may present with persistent crying and not have altered mental status or seizures. Crying may also be the only clue to a long bone fracture. Clues to the diagnosis of nonaccidental injury include a history that does not adequately explain the injuries and evidence of a chaotic social situation (see Chapter 14, Child Abuse: Physical, p. 69).

E. **Any history of prenatal drug exposure?** Consider in neonates with signs and symptoms suggestive of withdrawal (eg, irritability, tachycardia, diaphoresis, and diarrhea).

F. **What medication(s) does patient take?** If child is being breast-fed, it is also important to know what medication(s) mother is taking. Antihistamines and corticosteroids can cause paradoxical CNS stimulation in young infants. Decongestants can cause irritability and insomnia. Consider accidental ingestion or environmental toxin in a toddler with irritability and change in mental status.

G. **Are there any associated symptoms to suggest GI pathology?** In a young infant, this would include poor weight gain, vomiting, crying, arching or posturing after feeding, recurrent wheezing or pneumonia, apnea, flatulence, diarrhea, constipation, or an abdominal or inguinal mass.

H. Any associated symptoms to suggest CNS pathology? In a young infant, this would include lethargy, apnea, increased or decreased muscle tone, or abnormal movements. In a toddler or older child, complaints may also include headache, behavioral or visual changes, or gait disturbance.

III. Differential Diagnosis

A. Infection. The most common cause of acute, unexplained crying behavior. Includes otitis media, viral illness (eg, gastroenteritis), herpangina, herpetic stomatitis, UTI, CNS infections (ie, meningitis, encephalitis), sepsis or bacteremia, osteomyelitis, septic arthritis, lymphadenitis, cellulitis, retropharyngeal abscess, and appendicitis or peritonitis.

B. Trauma

1. **Shaken-baby syndrome.** Produces a constellation of subdural and subarachnoid hemorrhage, traction-type metaphyseal fractures, and retinal hemorrhages. Largely restricted to children younger than 3 years of age, with majority of cases occurring during the first year of life (see Chapter 14, Child Abuse: Physical, p. 70).

2. **Subdural hematoma.** Accidental subdural hemorrhages have been reported in infants and young children after motor vehicle collisions or falls involving substantial angular deceleration. Infants with enlarged extra-axial spaces, as seen in some cases of shunted hydrocephalus, appear to be at increased risk for subdural or subarachnoid hemorrhage with lesser degrees of trauma.

3. **Fracture.** Clues to diagnosis include swelling, tenderness, and pseudoparalysis. Unexplained extracranial bony injuries or multiple fractures in different stages of healing are pathognomonic for abuse (see Chapter 14, Child Abuse: Physical, p. 70).

4. **Corneal abrasion.** Can be quite painful, with dramatic photophobia, epiphora, and resistance to opening of the eyes. Infants may present with excessive crying and not have symptoms referable to the eyes.

5. **Ocular or oral foreign body.**

6. **Hair tourniquet.** Requires close inspection of digits for diagnosis.

7. **Burn.**

8. **Bite.**

C. Drugs. Side effects of common over-the-counter medications (OTC) and prescription drugs may result in excessive crying. Includes antihistamines, OTC cough preparations, pseudoephedrine, phenobarbital, and corticosteroids. Also consider ethanol withdrawal and neonatal narcotic withdrawal.

D. Colic. Etiology is unclear. Occurs in 10–25% of otherwise healthy and well-nourished infants. Defined as paroxysmal crying beginning in the first *3 weeks of life*, lasting longer than *3 hours a day*, at least *3 days per week*, and continuing for more than *3 weeks* in infants younger than *3 months old* **("rule of 3's").** Crying is qualitatively normal, but quantitatively excessive. Generally worse in evening. Infants may be inconsolable, with facial flushing, grimacing, clenched fists, flatulence, or drawing up of legs during episodes.

E. GI disorders

   1. Constipation. Rectal exam is diagnostic and often therapeutic.

   2. Gastroesophageal reflux. May cause excessive crying, as well as frequent regurgitation or vomiting, failure to thrive, hiccups, episodes of stiffening or arching or head tilting associated with feedings (Sandifer syndrome), recurrent wheezing or pneumonia, stridor, and obstructive apnea.

   3. Milk-protein allergy. Seen in a minority of colicky infants. Other clues to the diagnosis include vomiting, diarrhea, hemepositive or grossly bloody stools, flatulence, difficulty feeding, failure to thrive, family history of allergy, eczema, or eosinophilia.

F. CNS Disorders

   1. Increased intracranial pressure (ICP)

      a. Subdural hematoma. Post-traumatic, spontaneous rupture of congenital aneurysm, or bleeding from arteriovenous malformation.

      b. Brain tumor. Clues to diagnosis include vomiting, early morning headache, behavioral changes, and gait disturbance.

      c. Meningitis or encephalitis.

      d. Pseudotumor cerebri. Consider only after imaging studies and lumbar puncture have ruled out other causes of ICP.

   2. Arnold-Chiari type 1 malformation. May present with irritability and intermittent episodes of neck arching, probably representing pain originating in the posterior fossa.

G. Metabolic Disorders

   1. Glutaric aciduria type 1. Infants may be irritable and exhibit other neurologic signs (eg, dystonia).

   2. Partial ornithine transcarbamylase deficiency. May present with excessive crying, intermittent lethargy, and emesis.

   3. Sickle cell disease. Vasoocclusive crisis, including dactylitis in older infants and toddlers, may present with crying without other constitutional symptoms.

   4. Calcium disorders. Hypercalcemia in infants with William syndrome may produce irritability, lassitude, weakness, renal stones, nausea, vomiting, or constipation. Symptoms of hypocalcemia include tetany, paresthesias, myopathy, seizures, muscle spasm, weakness, irritability, and mental status changes.

    5. Congenital hyperthyroidism. Thyrotoxicosis is associated with irritability, tachycardia, hyperthermia, hypertension, and failure to thrive.

H. Cardiac Disorders

    1. Supraventricular tachycardia. In infants, may present with irritability, poor feeding, tachypnea, and diaphoresis.

    2. Congestive heart failure. In addition to fussiness, infant may present with failure to thrive, poor feeding, tachycardia, diaphoresis, cough, or tachypnea.

I. Behavioral Disorders. Infants with certain temperaments or behavioral responses (eg, poor adaptability, withdrawal, irregular biologic functions) may cry excessively.

    1. Overstimulation. May result in persistent crying.

    2. Sleep (partial) awakenings. More common in second half of the first year.

    3. Sleep terrors. Sleep disorder common in young children.

J. Anatomic Abnormalities

    1. Incarcerated hernia.

    2. Intussusception. May present early, without vomiting or diarrhea and with only intermittent irritability.

    3. Volvulus. Usually associated with abdominal distention and vomiting.

    4. Gastric rupture. May occur after excessive, vigorous crying.

    5. Choanal atresia or other upper airway obstruction.

    6. Congenital glaucoma. Diagnostic clues include red eye, tearing, or enlarged or cloudy cornea.

K. Toxins. Include carbon monoxide, cyanide, organic solvents, lead, mercury, and arsenic.

IV. Database

A. Physical Exam Key Points

    1. General appearance. Child's mental status with regard to level of alertness and interaction with examiner and parents can be used as a measure of the seriousness of illness. Interaction between parents and infant offers insight into their coping mechanisms. Growth measurements demonstrate adequate nutrition.

    2. Vital signs. Fever suggests infection. Tachycardia may be secondary to fever, pain, volume depletion, cardiac disease, or hyperthyroidism. Bradycardia with respiratory irregularity suggests CNS dysfunction and possibly increased ICP. Hypotension can be seen in sepsis and volume depletion. Hypertension may indicate pain, increased ICP, drug effect, or hyperthyroidism.

    3. Head. Look for evidence of trauma pointing to subdural hemorrhage. Tense anterior fontanelle may signify increased ICP.

4. **Eyes.** Perform funduscopic exam for retinal hemorrhages in cases of suspected shaken-baby syndrome or abuse. Papilledema suggests increased ICP. Red eye in association with tearing or an enlarged or cloudy cornea suggests congenital glaucoma. Fluorescein staining of corneas demonstrates corneal abrasions. Eversion of the eyelids is important to rule out foreign body.

5. **Ears.** Check tympanic membranes for erythema, fullness, and decreased mobility, suggesting otitis media.

6. **Nasopharynx.** Vesicular lesions in the oropharynx indicate herpes gingivostomatitis or herpangina. Beefy red or bulging posterior pharynx associated with drooling and muffled cry suggests retropharyngeal abscess. Carefully inspect oropharynx for foreign body if infant winces when swallowing. In neonate, assess patency of nares to rule out choanal atresia.

7. **Neck.** Resistance to passive flexion of the neck suggests meningitis or subarachnoid bleeding. Positive Kernig and Brudzinski signs also indicate meningeal irritation but often are not present in neonates or young infants. Erythematous, tender neck mass indicates lymphadenitis or infected brachial cleft or thyroglossal duct cyst.

8. **Chest.** Prolonged expiratory phase with rhonchi and wheezing may be noted in infants with gastroesophageal reflux.

9. **Abdomen.** Distention, tenderness, or guarding suggests intra-abdominal pathology. Erythematous, tender, nonreducible mass in inguinal region suggests incarcerated hernia.

10. **Skin.** Examine infant with all clothes removed so subtle bruises, burns, or bites are not missed. Any bruise is abnormal in an infant, and patterns of bruising must be defined in toddlers. Hemorrhagic rash suggests meningococcal infection. Local areas of redness, warmth, induration, and tenderness indicate cellulitis or underlying soft tissue infection.

11. **Musculoskeletal system.** How infant flexes or extends an extremity may signify possible trauma. Carefully examine all extremities for tenderness or a hair tourniquet.

12. **Neurologic exam.** Abnormalities of tone suggest meningitis, seizure, or head injury. Focal findings or gait disturbance also suggest an intracranial process.

B. **Laboratory Data**

1. **Urinalysis and urine culture.** Rule out an occult UTI.

2. **CBC with differential, coagulation studies, and basic metabolic panel.** Helpful only if clinician suspects abnormalities based on history and physical exam.

3. **Blood culture.** Obtain if serious bacterial infection is suspected.

4. **Thyroid function tests.** If clinically indicated.

5. **Urine and serum toxicology screening.** Consider in neonates with suspected prenatal drug exposure or toddlers with suspected accidental ingestion.

C. Radiographic and Other Studies
1. **Lumbar puncture.** Required in any febrile neonate (0–2 months) or any older infant or child with unexplained fever and mental status alteration to evaluate for meningitis.
2. **Skeletal survey.** Required in cases of suspected nonaccidental injury or to confirm a fracture suspected during palpation of a tender extremity.
3. **CT scan of head.** Required if there is any suspicion of trauma or abuse or increased ICP, or in the presence of focal neurologic signs, seizures, retinal hemorrhages, or papilledema.
4. **Barium enema.** Consider in infant or child with bilious emesis or other signs of obstruction.
5. **pH probe.** The gold standard for diagnosing gastroesophageal reflux.
6. **ECG.** In infants with unexplained tachycardia.

V. Plan. Complete history and careful physical exam will suggest diagnosis in most cases; only those tests that confirm a diagnosis suggested by history or exam should be performed. If the cause of crying is still unclear, additional testing may be necessary. Occasionally an infant will need an extended period of observation, requiring hospitalization or close follow-up if families are known to be reliable.
A. Infection. Treat with appropriate antibiotics.
B. Trauma. If intracranial hemorrhage is present, consult neurosurgery colleagues immediately. Cases of suspected abuse should be reported immediately to child protective service agencies and police.
C. Drugs. Avoid repeated exposure.
D. Colic. Reassurance and support is usually all that is necessary. It is crucial to evaluate parents' responses to the crying, because certain responses may inadvertently increase severity of the crying. A behavior diary can be helpful in this regard. In only a minority of colicky infants is a true protein allergy or formula intolerance actually present. If infant has other symptoms suggestive of a possible allergy, a formula change may be indicated; switch to a casein-hydrolysate formula.
E. GI Disorders. Chronic constipation should be treated aggressively with stool softeners. A trial of antacid therapy may be helpful in a crying infant with suspected gastroesophageal reflux.
F. CNS Disorders. If child has evidence of increased ICP or hemorrhage, consult neurosurgery colleagues immediately.
G. Metabolic Disorders. Treat underlying defect or its secondary effects, or both.
H. Cardiac Disorders. Treat underlying cardiac problem.
I. Behavioral Disorders. Provide reassurance and suggest behavior modification techniques.
J. Anatomic Abnormalities. Consult general surgery or appropriate surgical subspecialty colleagues.

    K. Toxins. Provide supportive care. Consult poison control center or toxicologist for specific interventions.

VI. Problem Case Diagnosis. This case demonstrates the typical presentation of an infant with coli c. Patient is 3 months old, at an age when persistent crying tends to improve regardless of the mode of intervention. If elemental formula is used to treat colic, return to cow's milk–based formula later in the first year of life, unless other signs or symptoms of protein intolerance are noted.

VII. Teaching Pearl: Question. Is formula change effective in treating infantile colic?

VIII. Teaching Pearl: Answer. Although allergic reactions to cow's milk protein have been implicated as a cause of colic, it appears that only a minority of infants benefit from a formula change.

REFERENCES

Brazelton BT. Crying in infancy. *Pediatrics* 1962;29:579–588.

Forsythe BW. Colic and the effect of changing formulas: A double-blind, multiple-crossover study. *J Pediatr* 1989;115:521–525.

Moore DJ, Tao BS, Lines DR, et al. Double-blind, placebo-controlled trial of omeprazole in irritable infants with gastroesophageal reflux. *J Pediatr* 2003;143:219–223.

Poole SR. The infant with acute, unexplained, excessive crying. *Pediatrics* 1991;88:450–455.

59. JOINT SWELLING

  I. Problem. An 8-year-old girl who is brought to the emergency department has left knee swelling but minimal pain.

  II. Immediate Questions
    A. Is there a history of trauma? With any trauma, be concerned about fractures, dislocations, or damage to menisci and ligaments.
    B. How long have symptoms been present? If acute (< 1 week), think septic arthritis, trauma, Lyme arthritis, reactive arthritis, leukemia, or neuroblastoma. Chronic arthritis (> 6 weeks) points more toward juvenile rheumatoid arthritis (JRA), tuberculosis, pigmented villonodular synovitis (PVNS), discoid meniscus, synovial chondromatosis, or hemangioma.
    C. Is there a history of prior joint swelling? How recently? Perhaps the pattern is consistent with migratory acute rheumatic fever. With previous joint swelling, consider pauciarticular JRA, Lyme arthritis, PVNS, psoriasis, and inflammatory bowel disease (IBD).
    D. Are there any systemic or constitutional symptoms? Fever or systemic toxicity may point to septic arthritis, although patient may be afebrile. Weight loss and height deceleration raise concern about IBD.

E. **What is the past medical history?** Does patient have any underlying disease processes, such as sickle cell disease, coagulopathy, von Willebrand disease, hemophilia, or hypothyroidism? Inquire about rashes, preceding flulike illnesses, or gastroenteritis.

III. Differential Diagnosis

A. **Trauma.** Includes fractures, patellar dislocations, torn menisci or ligaments (eg, anterior cruciate).

B. **Infection or Infection-Associated Process.** Septic arthritis, often due to staphylococcal and streptococcal species, is the most important diagnosis to make in a timely fashion. Upper respiratory infection, with fever, rash, and polyarthritis, increases likelihood of reactive arthritis due to viral infection, (parvovirus, adenovirus, rubella, hepatitis B virus, and Epstein-Barr virus [EBV]). EBV can be monoarticular, whereas the others are more likely polyarticular. Conjunctivitis, urethritis, and polyarthritis suggest postdysenteric arthritis, although extra-articular manifestations in *Salmonella*- and *Yersinia*-related arthritis are not always seen. Swollen joint may indicate osteomyelitis of adjacent distal femur with sympathetic effusion. Lyme arthritis presents months after initial tick bite, usually involving knees, ankles, and then elbows. Often swelling out of proportion to degree of discomfort. Lyme arthritis is the most common cause of intermittent monoarthritis in school-age children in endemic areas.

C. **Hemarthrosis.** In addition to trauma, bloody effusion may be due to a bleeding disorder, such as hemophilia. PVNS and hemangioma should also be considered.

D. **Tumor.** Produces joint effusion with malignancy (eg, leukemia and neuroblastoma) in metaphyses of long bones.

E. **Inflammatory Condition.** Seen with early rheumatic disease, such as JRA, psoriatic arthropathy, or other seronegative spondyloarthropathy. Joint swelling of Henoch-Schönlein purpura can precede the rash and is usually periarticular, without warmth or erythema. Sarcoidosis may present as joint swelling in children younger than 5 years, but is usually polyarticular.

F. **Metabolic Disorder.** Hypothyroidism (especially if polyarticular).

G. **Other Causes.** Avascular necrosis associated with sickle cell disease; IBD-related arthropathy.

IV. Database

A. **Physical Exam Key Points**

1. **Vital signs.** Fever suggests septic arthritis.

2. **Cardiovascular system.** Look for pancarditis or congestive heart failure as part of acute rheumatic fever; atrioventricular block for early Lyme disease (unlikely at time of arthritis).

3. **Skin.** Look for erythema marginatum (acute rheumatic fever); conjunctivitis (with urethritis suggests postdysenteric arthritis); malar rash, oral or nasal ulcers (systemic lupus erythematosus);

scaly rash, pitted nails (psoriasis); distal extremity papules, pustules, or vesicles with reddened bases (gonococcal arthritis); hives (serum sickness or drug reaction).
   4. **Musculoskeletal system.** Tender, warm, red joint suggests septic arthritis or rheumatic fever. Septic joint is usually monoarticular and intensely red, tender, swollen and hot with restriction, rigidly guarded. Large swelling out of proportion to level of pain is indicative of Lyme arthritis. Diffuse bone pain points toward malignancy. Point tenderness over medial collateral ligament, limited extension, or instability of joint may indicate internal ligamentous or meniscal injury. It is essential to distinguish true arthritis (joint involvement) from muscle and bone problems.
B. Laboratory Data
   1. **CBC, ESR, C-reactive protein.** Useful if signs of infection are present. May also see elevated WBC count in systemic JRA. WBC count is elevated in leukemia, but atypical WBCs as well as abnormalities of other cell lines would also be expected.
   2. **Joint aspiration.** Essential if clinician suspects septic arthritis. Send fluid for cell count with differential, Gram stain, and cultures. *Caution:* Unexpectedly high WBC counts (100,000/mm^3) may be seen in Lyme arthritis. Hemarthrosis may point to anterior cruciate or other ligamentous injury.
   3. **Cultures.** If septic arthritis is suspected, obtain urine and blood cultures. If infection is suspected (eg, osteomyelitis of adjacent bone), obtain blood culture. If considering acute rheumatic fever, obtain throat culture and streptococcal antibody titers.
   4. **Other workup.** Perform Lyme ELISA and Western blot tests if in an endemic area or as suggested by history or physical exam. Rheumatoid factor and ANA are unnecessary in acute evaluation but should be obtained when there is high suspicion for JRA or systemic lupus erythematosus. If considering prolonged therapy with NSAIDs, obtain creatinine level.
C. Radiographic and Other Studies.
   1. **Plain x-rays.** Used to evaluate for tibial plateau fracture in trauma. Helpful for baseline evaluation in chronic arthritis.
   2. **Bone scan.** May be necessary if osteomyelitis of periarticular bone is suspected.

V. Plan
   A. Trauma. Traumatic injury may require orthopaedic consultation and knee immobilizer.
   B. Septic Arthritis. Obtain orthopaedic consultation for drainage, admit patient, and order IV antibiotics.
   C. Infection-Associated Arthritis. If Lyme arthritis is suspected, await ELISA and Western blot results. If positive, treat patient with amoxicillin or doxycycline (> 9 years old) for 30 days. If rheumatic fever, treat with appropriate antibiotic and salicylates and evaluate for presence of carditis.

D. Other Arthritis. If no contraindications, initial therapy is often NSAIDs and warm compresses. Consider referral to rheumatology colleague for further evaluation and management of possible connective tissue or inflammatory disease-associated arthritis.

VI. Problem Case Diagnosis. The 8-year-old patient has Lyme arthritis, characterized by large swelling of the knee with minimal pain and lack of constitutional symptoms. Although no rash is recalled, parents remember child having a flulike illness approximately 6 months earlier and transient swelling of the other knee several weeks ago.

VII. Teaching Pearl: Question. What are the most common pathogens in septic arthritis?

VIII. Teaching Pearl: Answer. Dependent on age: in neonates and infants, expect *Staphylococcus aureus,* group B streptococcus, and gram-negative bacteria; in children younger than 5 years of age, expect *S aureus* and *Haemophilus influenzae* (rare); in sexually active young adults, consider *Neisseria gonorrhoeae* and *Chlamydia trachomatis.*

REFERENCES

Ansell BM. Rheumatic disease mimics in childhood. *Curr Opin Rheumatol* 2000;12:445–447.

Cassidy JT, Petty RE. Juvenile rheumatoid arthritis. In: Cassidy JT, Petty RE, eds. *Textbook of Pediatric Rheumatology,* 4th ed. Saunders, 2001:218–321.

Levine M, Siegal LB. A swollen joint: Why all the fuss? *Am J Therapeut* 2003;10:219–224.

Till SH, Snaith ML. Assessment, investigation, and management of acute monoarthritis. *J Accid Emerg Med* 1999;16:355–361.

Towheed TE, Hochberg MC. Acute monoarthritis: A practical approach to assessment and treatment. *Am Fam Phys* 1996;54:2239–2243.

60. LEG PAIN

I. Problem. A 6-year-old boy has right hip pain and refuses to walk.

II. Immediate Questions

A. Has patient had fever? Infectious etiologies of leg pain include septic arthritis, osteomyelitis, and acute rheumatic fever (ARF). It is essential to make an early diagnosis of a septic joint to prevent destruction of cartilage.

B. Was there a recent history of lower extremity trauma? Traumatic causes of leg pain are very common and range from serious conditions (eg, fractures and joint dislocations) to strains and sprains.

C. Is there joint pain or swelling and, if so, how many joints are involved? Localizing the problem to a joint can help to narrow the differential diagnosis. Common problems caused by pathology to a single joint include slipped capital femoral epiphysis (SCFE), Legg-Calvé-Perthes disease (LCPD), and toxic synovitis. Among the causes of polyarthritis that might produce leg pain are Kawasaki disease, serum sickness, and the early stages of Lyme disease.

D. Is this an acute or a chronic problem? Long-standing lower extremity pain might be caused by a bony tumor, leukemia, juvenile rheumatoid arthritis (JRA), Osgood-Schlatter disease, LCPD, or osteochondritis dissecans.

E. Is there an associated rash? Diseases producing both a rash and limited mobility due to pain include ARF, Lyme disease, serum sickness, Kawasaki disease, systemic lupus erythematosus (SLE), disseminated gonococcal infection, and Henoch-Schönlein purpura (HSP).

III. Differential Diagnosis. The differential diagnosis is lengthy; it is helpful to attempt to stratify children into a diagnostic category.

A. Infection. Suggested by abrupt onset of symptoms and associated fever in the absence of trauma.

1. **Bacterial (septic) arthritis.** A serious cause of leg pain or refusal to walk. More common in children younger than 2 years of age. Most will have fever and severely limited range of motion of the affected joint. Septic arthritis of the hip must be recognized early to prevent joint destruction.

2. **Osteomyelitis.** Sickle cell anemia is a risk factor. Femur and tibia are the most common bones involved. Most patients have point tenderness. About 25% are afebrile.

3. **Soft-tissue infection.** Includes cellulitis, subcutaneous abscesses, or paronychia as with an ingrown toenail.

4. **Disseminated gonococcal infection.** Especially in adolescents. More than 90% have migratory arthralgia or arthritis, especially in lower extremity joints. Patients usually have fever and a rash.

5. **ARF.** Polyarthritis is the most common finding. Produces very painful arthritis of the larger joints of the lower extremities, making ambulation difficult.

6. **Lyme disease.** In early stages, children may have fever and polyarthralgia or polyarthritis. For those untreated, a monoarthritis of the knee may develop weeks to months after the initial tick bite.

7. **Postinfectious conditions.** Children may develop arthralgia 1–2 weeks after a nonspecific infectious illness. Parvovirus, Epstein-Barr virus, varicella zoster, and herpesviruses have all been implicated.

8. **Toxic or transient synovitis of the hip.** Especially in boys aged 3–8 years. Thought to be a postinflammatory synovitis. Patients are less likely to have fever and limitation of range of motion compared with those who have septic arthritis.

B. Trauma or Overuse

  1. **Fracture.** Often, there will be an obvious extremity deformity. However, so-called toddler fracture (a nondisplaced, spiral fracture of the distal tibia) frequently presents without objective findings suggestive of a fracture.

  2. **Soft tissue injuries.** These include ligamentous sprains, muscle strains, tendonitis, and contusions. A severe sprain may be associated with joint laxity.

  3. **Osgood-Schlatter disease.** Especially in boys 11–15 years of age. Causes microavulsions of proximal tibia, at the point of patellar tendon insertion. Often bilateral.

  4. **SCFE.** Especially in obese boys, in early adolescence. Capital femoral epiphysis slips posterior and inferior to the proximal femoral metaphysis. Frequently bilateral. Diagnosis is often made after trivial injury.

  5. **LCPD.** Especially in boys 4–9 years of age. Produces aseptic necrosis of the femoral head; cause is unknown.

  6. **Osteochondritis dissecans.** Especially in boys 11–15 years of age, possibly from repeat trauma or overuse. Separation of a small portion of the distal end of a long bone (eg, femur or tibia) causes knee or ankle pain.

  7. **Chondromalacia patellae.** Common in early adolescence. Produces fissures and erosions of articular cartilage of the patella. Probably caused by overuse.

  8. **Foreign body.** For example, glass or a splinter. Consider when child has localized swelling or tenderness on plantar surface of foot. Other painful conditions in this area that may cause pain include a plantar wart or a blister such as might result from poor-fitting shoes.

C. Immune-mediated Condition or Vasculitis

  1. **Serum sickness.** Mildly painful polyarthritis associated with angioedema and urticaria. Often, there is a recent history of antibiotic use.

  2. **Kawasaki disease.** In young children, fever for at least 5 days associated with four of the following five features: conjunctivitis without exudate, oropharyngeal erythema and swelling, swelling of hands and feet, a nonspecific rash, and cervical adenopathy. Associated findings include arthralgia or arthritis.

  3. **HSP.** Characteristic purpura (often palpable) predominantly located below the waist. Some children have joint swelling and discomfort.

  4. **SLE.** Especially in adolescent African-American girls. Has a variable presentation, which may include facial rash, renal disease, or arthritis.

D. Other Causes

  1. **JRA.** Also called *chronic idiopathic arthritides of childhood.* Cause unknown. One, few, or several joints may be involved, with or without systemic illness. Symptoms must be present for

at least 6 weeks to meet diagnostic criteria. Has highly variable prognosis.

2. **Complex regional pain syndrome.** Formerly called *reflex sympathetic dystrophy*. Common in adolescent girls. Cause is unknown. Produces localized swelling, sweating, color changes, and pain with light touch; especially of distal extremities.

3. **Sickle cell anemia.** Vasoocclusive crisis results in ischemia. Bony pain is often severe enough to prevent ambulation.

4. **Hemophilia.** Patients are at risk for hemarthrosis, especially after trauma.

IV. Database

A. **Physical Exam Key Points.** Certain etiologies are strongly suggested by a combination of demographic factors and physical exam findings.

1. **Lower extremity monoarthritis.** Externally rotated hip with severely limited range of motion, especially if associated with fever, suggests septic arthritis. Painful hip held in external rotation but with nearly complete active range of motion is more consistent with transient synovitis. Patients with late-stage Lyme disease often have a swollen knee with good range of motion and no fever. Chronic or recurring monoarthritis can be consistent with JRA.

2. **Polyarthritis** (Table I–13).

3. **Osgood-Schlatter disease.** Most common presentation is a boy in early adolescence with point tenderness or swelling at either (or both) tibial tubercle(s).

4. **SCFE.** Commonly presents as an afebrile obese boy in early adolescence with knee, thigh, or hip pain without arthritis; restricted range of motion, with or without preceding minor trauma.

TABLE I–13. POLYARTHRITIS AND ASSOCIATED FINDINGS

Etiology	Associated Findings
Acute rheumatic fever (ARF)	Painful arthritis, new murmur or congestive heart failure, recent group A streptococcal infection
Disseminated gonococcal infection	Fever, vesicular or pustular rash, tenosynovitis
Henoch-Schönlein purpura (HSP)	Purpuric rash below waist
Juvenile rheumatoid arthritis (JRA)	Chronic or recurrent fever and rash
Kawasaki disease	See discussion under Differential Diagnosis, earlier
Lyme disease	Polyarthralgia or polyarthritis in early stages, recent tick bite, fever, malaise
Postinfectious	Onset 1–2 weeks after gastroenteritis, often involving large, lower extremity joints
Serum sickness	Urticaria, angioedema, recent febrile illness or antibiotic use
Systemic lupus erythematosus (SLE)	Highly variable, may include skin or renal involvement

    5. LCPD. Commonly presents as a boy, aged 4–9 years, who has hip pain without arthritis but with a limp or leg-length discrepancy.

B. Laboratory Data

    1. If bony or joint infection is suspected, obtain CBC with differential, blood culture, C-reactive protein (CRP), and ESR. In equivocal cases, a normal CRP and ESR result would be reassuring, because these levels are markedly elevated in the vast majority of patients with septic arthritis or osteomyelitis. Screening tests for ARF, Lyme disease, and SLE should be ordered selectively based on the likelihood of these diagnostic possibilities.

    2. Arthrocentesis. Indicated if patient has abrupt onset of monoarthritis with significantly limited range of motion, especially in the absence of trauma. Test synovial fluid for glucose and protein, cell count and differential, Gram stain, and culture. WBC counts exceeding 50,000/mm^3 are indicative of infectious arthritis.

C. Radiographic and Other Studies

    1. Plain x-rays. Can establish or strongly suggest the diagnosis of fractures, Osgood-Schlatter disease, SCFE, LCPD, osteochondritis dissecans, chondromalacia patellae, bony tumors, and foreign body. With SCFE, the abnormality may be apparent only on the frog-leg view. With osteomyelitis, there may be no apparent abnormalities within the first 10 days of symptoms.

    2. Ultrasound. Especially helpful in detecting hip effusion and in guiding needle placement during arthrocentesis.

    3. MRI scan. Helpful in assessing soft tissue pathology, such as ligamentous sprains, and in diagnosing suspected osteomyelitis when physical exam, laboratory data, and radiographic studies are inconclusive.

    4. Bone scan. Best option for detecting osteomyelitis, especially within the first 10 days of symptoms.

V. Plan. Most children with leg pain have benign causes such as minor trauma. Signs of systemic illness, such as fever and rash, should be sought and may indicate a more serious etiology. Conditions requiring prompt diagnosis and initiation of treatment to avoid adverse outcomes include septic or gonococcal arthritis, osteomyelitis, ARF, Lyme disease, SCFE, and Kawasaki disease.

VI. Problem Case Diagnosis. The 6-year-old boy with right hip pain and refusal to walk was noted to be febrile and to have severely limited range of motion. Ultrasound revealed a hip effusion, and the synovial fluid profile was consistent with septic arthritis.

VII. Teaching Pearl: Question. What are three conditions that cause leg pain associated with polyarthritis and fever?

VIII. Teaching Pearl: Answer. Disseminated gonococcal infection, ARF, and Kawasaki disease.

REFERENCES

Pinals RS. Polyarthritis and fever. *N Engl J Med* 1994;330:769–774.
Scarfone RJ. Joint pain. In: Fleisher GR, Ludwig S, eds. *Textbook of Pediatric Emergency Medicine,* 4th ed. Lippincott Williams & Wilkins, 2000:467–471.

61. LETHARGY

I. **Problem.** A 12-year-old boy is found in a lethargic state in the school bathroom.

II. **Immediate Questions**
   A. **Is this an emergency, urgent, or routine clinical condition?** An emergency case requires the same attention to detail as a routine case; however, the pace of actions and order in which they are completed differs. Remember the ABCs (airway, breathing, circulation).
   B. **What is the clinical description of the lethargy?** Obtain a thorough description of patient's lethargy and events prior to presentation. This description should be obtained from child, parent, and a witness if possible. When did lethargy begin? Were there any associated activities such as movements of the face or body? Has child had any similar episodes previously? Were there any precipitants to this episode?
   C. **What is the cause of this alteration in patient's interaction with environment?** Lethargy can be the manifestation of a number of clinical conditions, ranging from toxic and metabolic conditions to seizures; the differential diagnosis is broad. Conditions that can present with lethargy include increased intracranial pressure, intoxication, and systemic medical, post-traumatic, vascular, behavioral, and sleep disorders.
   D. **Pertinent Historical Information.** Prenatal and neonatal course may identify risks for long-term neurologic sequelae.
      1. **Prenatal history.** Did mother receive prenatal care? Is there any history of maternal medication use or substance abuse during pregnancy? Maternal medical complications during pregnancy? Was pregnancy full term? Any complications during the delivery?
      2. **Neonatal history.** Were developmental milestones achieved at appropriate ages? Is there any significant medical or surgical history? History of trauma?
      3. **Family history.** Is there a family history of neurologic disorders?

III. **Differential Diagnosis**
   A. **Seizures**
      1. **Generalized.** Present with sudden onset of loss of consciousness, because they are a manifestation of widespread abnormal electrical discharges.

2. **Partial.** Result from localized abnormal electrical discharge and can present with altered arousal or GI symptoms, confusion, hallucinations, localized motor or sensory activity, or autonomic changes.

3. **Etiology.** Seizures have many etiologies, including cerebral malformations, hypoxia, head trauma, structural or destructive lesions (neoplasm, stroke, vascular anomalies), infections (meningitis or encephalitis), toxicity (lidocaine, theophylline, psychotropic agents, isoniazid, chemotherapeutic agents, cocaine, amphetamines, heroin, PCP, methanol, ethylene glycol, or carbon monoxide), metabolic alterations (hypoglycemia, hyponatremia, hypocalcemia, or phenylketonuria), or degenerative disorders. Systemic disorders may be associated with seizures (tuberous sclerosis, neurofibromatosis, sickle cell anemia, or acute lymphocytic leukemia).

B. **Increased Intracranial Pressure.** Lethargy may reflect the presence of increased intracranial pressure secondary to space-occupying lesions within the cranial vault (hematoma, abscess, or tumor), progressive hydrocephalus, or cerebral edema.

C. **Trauma.** A patient can remain lethargic for a variable period of time following closed head injury. There may be a transient lucid period between the traumatic event and the alteration of arousal. Trauma may be severe enough to produce intracranial hemorrhage (subarachnoid hemorrhage) or even a space-occupying hematoma (subdural or epidural), which, in turn, can lead to increased intracranial pressure and, potentially, to herniation.

1. **Concussion.** Defined as an alteration of brain function following head trauma. Classified as grade 1, 2, or 3 based on symptoms and their duration.

a. **Grade 1.** Manifested by transient confusion (not loss of consciousness) with resolution of symptoms within 15 minutes.

b. **Grade 2.** Similar to grade 1, but symptoms persist for more than 1 hour.

c. **Grade 3.** Occurs when there is any loss of consciousness.

2. **Symptoms of concussion**

a. **Early (minutes to hours).** Headache, dizziness, nausea, vomiting, and disorientation. Confusion (immediate or up to several minutes) with disturbance of vigilance, distractibility, inability to maintain a coherent stream of thought, inability to complete a sequence of goal-directed movements, and amnesia can also occur.

b. **Late (days to weeks).** Can include persistent headache (low grade), lightheadedness, poor attention and concentration, memory problems, difficulty focusing vision, fatigability, sleep disturbance, ringing in the ears, mood changes (anxiety, depression), irritability and low frustration tolerance, and intolerance to bright light and loud noises.

     c. Neurobehavioral features. Include vacant stare, delayed motor or verbal responses, inability to focus and distractibility, disorientation (time, date, place, direction), slurred or incoherent speech, incoordination, emotionality, memory deficits (eg, repeatedly asking the same question), or loss of consciousness.

D. Intoxications. Ingestion of a toxic substance (eg, alcohol or substances of abuse) may result in depression of mental status. Intoxication can also be caused by a medication (eg, anticonvulsant, antidepressant, or anxiolytic) that has been prescribed for an existing medical condition.

E. Sleep Disorders. Insufficient or inefficient sleep may result in excessive daytime sleepiness and lethargy. Sleep disorders can be an isolated diagnosis or a complication of other medical conditions (eg, obstructive sleep apnea, adverse effects of medications, behavioral disorders, or nocturnal seizures).

F. Behavioral Disorders. Inappropriate response to the environment can be the presenting feature of a behavioral disorder. A child may ignore his or her surroundings as a sign of a mood or conversion disorder. Nonepileptic seizure is a diagnosis of exclusion.

G. Migraine. Clinical presentation includes headache, nausea, and vomiting. Patients often want to go to sleep in a quiet and dark room because of associated photophobia and phonophobia.

H. Medical Disorders. Several disorders can present with an alteration in patient's level of arousal (without a seizure), including CNS infections (bacterial, viral, or rickettsial meningitis and encephalitis) or postinfectious or postimmunization encephalopathy. A child with a severe respiratory condition causing hypoxia may present with decreased arousal. Cardiac dysfunction, hypotension, and toxic effects of severe liver, kidney, endocrine, metabolic, or neurodegenerative disorders may manifest as an alteration in mental status.

I. Vascular Disorders. Hypertensive encephalopathy or vasculitic disorders (eg, systemic lupus erythematosus) can present with alteration of arousal.

IV. Database

A. Physical Exam Key Points. A complete general physical exam is important in identifying a systemic disorder, beginning with ABCs.

     1. Vital signs. Changes in heart rate and BP may reflect systemic infection, cardiac disease, intoxication, or an active seizure. Alteration of temperature may reflect an infection or effects from intoxication.

     2. General appearance. Is patient appropriately developed and nourished? Growth and development problems may reflect an underlying medical or neurologic disorder. Is patient cooperative, interactive, or in distress?

3. **Skin.** Inspect for signs of trauma, rash, and birthmarks (erythematous, hypopigmented or hyperpigmented lesions). Rash may suggest infectious or vasculitic disorder. Neurocutaneous disorders (eg, neurofibromatosis, tuberous sclerosis, Sturge-Weber syndrome, von Hippel-Lindau syndrome, and ataxia telangiectasia) may present with alteration of arousal.

4. **Head and neck.** Head circumference may reflect alteration in brain parenchyma (microcephaly or macrocephaly). Inspect for signs of head trauma. Neck stiffness (meningismus) may indicate meningitis or subarachnoid hemorrhage.

5. **Heart and lungs.** Cardiac murmur or altered cardiac dynamics may indicate cardiac dysfunction. Identify respiratory dysfunction by auscultation.

6. **Abdomen.** Hepatosplenomegaly may be seen in a variety of metabolic and neurodegenerative disorders.

7. **Neurologic exam.** Disorders of the cerebral cortex affect cognition, whereas lesions in the brainstem affect specific cranial nerves. Spinal cord lesions demonstrate motor or sensory levels, or both, on exam.

   a. **Mental status.** Assess ability to interact with the environment by speaking with and listening to patient, evaluating at an age-appropriate level.

   b. **Cranial nerves.** Pupil size and reactivity, in addition to eye movements, reflect function of upper brainstem. Symmetric movement of face, soft palate, and tongue demonstrates integrity of lower brainstem.

   c. **Motor system.** Muscle bulk, tone, and strength demonstrate function of motor pathways. Fine motor skills may suggest developmental abilities. Involuntary movements may be seen in several neurologic disorders. Assess patient's gait.

   d. **Sensory system.** Localized sensory deficits may reflect dysfunction of central or peripheral nervous system as well as functional disorders.

   e. **Deep tendon reflexes.** Demonstrate integrity of specific reflex pathways from peripheral muscle through levels of the spinal cord; rarely affected by disorders that present as staring.

   f. **Cerebellar exam.** Cerebellar dysfunction may be a sign of localized space-occupying, destructive, or degenerative disorders.

B. **Laboratory Data**

   1. **Basic metabolic panel, glucose, calcium.** Electrolyte abnormalities (hypernatremia, hyponatremia, hypocalcemia) and hypoglycemia or hyperglycemia can present with alteration of mental status. Metabolic acidosis may point to an underlying metabolic disorder or intoxication. Respiratory acidosis can be seen in intoxications with alcohol, benzodiazepines, and barbiturates.

2. **Renal and hepatic profile.** Can indicate acute or chronic end-organ dysfunction.
3. **CBC with differential.** Elevated WBC count may indicate active infection.
4. **Toxicology screening and drug levels.** Based on patient's history, order blood levels of prescription medications, ingested medications, or substances of abuse.
5. **ABGs.** Obtain if hypoxia or acid-base problems are suggested by history or physical exam.
6. **Lumbar puncture.** Perform if history and physical exam suggest an intracranial infection (meningitis or encephalitis); can also demonstrate subarachnoid hemorrhage. Do *not* perform in the presence of increased intracranial pressure or a space-occupying lesion, because of risk of herniation.

C. **Radiographic and Other Studies**
1. **Neuroimaging (CT or MRI scan).** Obtain a neuroimaging study for all patients with altered mental status. If patient has a normal exam and only a history of altered arousal, study is not needed emergently. MRI is a more sensitive exam; however, sedation is often necessary because patient must remain still for a prolonged period of time.
2. **EEG.** The gold standard for seizures; can demonstrate cerebral cortical dysfunction due to generalized encephalopathy or localized destructive or space-occupying lesion.
3. **ECG.** Obtain if a cardiac disorder is suspected.

V. **Plan**
A. **Emergency Management.** Initiate emergency treatment if patient has signs of increased intracranial pressure (bradycardia and hypertension along with mental status or papillary changes).
1. Increased intracranial pressure is a neurologic emergency. Elevate head of bed 30–45 degrees to improve jugular venous pressure.
2. Hyperventilation should *not* be used in cases of head trauma; it will rapidly result in cerebral vasoconstriction due to hypocarbia.
3. Give mannitol (an osmotic diuretic), 0.25 g/kg, 20% solution, IV. Maintain serum osmolarity < 320 mOsm.
4. If an intracranial space-occupying lesion is present, neurosurgical intervention is required.
5. Patients with severely increased intracranial pressure require an intracranial pressure monitor, intubation, and mechanical ventilation. General anesthesia may be required; often pentobarbital is used because response can be titrated and followed by continuous bedside EEG monitoring. A loading dose of 15–20 mg/kg IV is given over 1–2 hours; patient is then maintained on continuous IV infusion of 1 mg/kg/h. Infusion is weaned after 1–5 days to assess clinical effectiveness.

B. Seizures. For active convulsive seizures, place patient on his or her side, control airway, and protect from objects that may fall onto or otherwise harm patient during seizure. Antiepileptic medications are indicated if seizures are protracted or recurrent. In epileptic patients, doses may need to be adjusted or new medications prescribed.

C. Concussion. Concussions in children may occur during sports activities and competitions. On-site and follow-up management is outlined below.

1. Grade 1

a. Remove patient from sports activity and examine immediately and at 5-minute intervals at rest and exertion. Patient may return to the activity if all symptoms clear within 15 minutes.

b. If a second grade 1 concussion occurs in the same contest, have patient cease all sports activity for remainder of that day.

c. Patient may resume sports activities when asymptomatic at rest and exertion for 1 week.

2. Grade 2

a. Have patient cease sports activity for remainder of that day. Examine on site and the following day.

b. Patient may return to sports activity when asymptomatic for 1 week at rest and exertion.

c. Obtain CT or MRI scan if symptoms persist for > 1 week.

d. Following a second grade 2 concussion, patient may return to sports activity when asymptomatic for 2 weeks.

e. Advise termination of sports activity for the season in patients whose CT or MRI scan is consistent with edema or contusion.

3. Grade 3

a. Patient should be transported to the nearest emergency department if unconscious or if worrisome signs are noted. Perform thorough neurologic exam, and admit any patient with intracranial pathology on imaging or deficits on neurologic exam. Patients with persistent unconsciousness should be transported to a trauma center.

b. Obtain CT or MRI scan if symptoms persist for > 1 week.

c. Following brief (seconds) grade 3 concussion, patient may return to sports activity if asymptomatic for 1 week (at rest and exertion). Following prolonged (minutes) grade 3 concussion, patient may return to sports activity if asymptomatic for 2 weeks at rest and exertion.

d. Following a second grade 3 concussion, patient should refrain from activity for a minimum of 1 month once symptom-free.

e. Patients with any abnormal findings on CT or MRI scan (eg, edema or contusion) should terminate sports activities for remainder of the season and be discouraged from future competition.

    D. Other Conditions. Initial and subsequent therapy is based on diagnosis and severity of presenting features of the underlying conditions.

VI. Problem Case Diagnosis. The 12-year-old boy has a grade 2 concussion. According to the history, his parents had more difficulty than usual awakening him that morning, and he was sleepy on the school bus and during first period in school. No involuntary movements or prior spells had been noted. Patient had been hit in the head while playing basketball the night before. He complained of headache and nausea but did not have a medical evaluation following the incident. His prenatal, birth, developmental, family, and past history was otherwise unremarkable. Physical exam was significant for frontal ecchymosis, stiff neck, and occipital scalp hematoma. Neurologic exam was significant for lethargy, in addition to memory, thinking, and concentration problems. Drug toxicology screening and head CT scan were normal.

VII. Teaching Pearl: Question. Is a neuroimaging study the most useful way to monitor a patient's progress after a concussion?

VIII. Teaching Pearl: Answer. Microscopic changes in the brain may not be evident on neuroimaging studies; therefore, history and neuropsychological exam are the most useful tools to follow a patient's progress after concussion.

REFERENCES

Adelson PD, Kochanek PM. Head injury in Children. *J Child Neurol* 1998;13:2–15.
Fenichel GM. Altered states of consciousness. In: *Clinical Pediatric Neurology: A Signs and Symptoms Approach,* 4th ed. Saunders, 2001:47–76.
Kelly JP, Nichols JS, Filley CM, et al. Concussion in sports: Guidelines for the prevention of catastrophic outcome. *JAMA* 1991;266:2867–2869.

62. LEUKOCYTOSIS

I. Problem. A 7-year-old girl is brought to the emergency department with lymphadenopathy and fever of 2 days' duration. CBC shows a WBC count of 35,000/mm^3.

II. Immediate Questions

    A. What is patient's clinical status? Elevated WBC count can be a sign of serious infection. Look for fever and signs of shock, including hypotension or tachycardia.

    B. Is there a history of underlying systemic illness? Prolonged illness, which might include fevers, night sweats, weight loss, and bone or joint pain, suggests a more chronic process (eg, malignancy or collagen vascular disease), whereas acute onset of symptoms in a previously healthy child suggests an infectious process. Some systemic illnesses, such as immunodeficiency syndromes, malignancy, or sickle cell disease, place patients at higher risk for certain types of infection. Splenectomized patients are at increased risk for serious infection from encapsulated organisms such as *Streptococcus pneumoniae.*

C. What medication(s) does patient take? Certain medications, such as growth factors used to stimulate WBC production in patients treated for malignancy, can cause a marked increase in WBC count. Glucocorticoids can cause leukocytosis due to demargination of leukocytes.

D. Are there any prior blood counts for comparison? In certain situations, such as sickle cell disease or splenectomized patients, the baseline WBC count is 10,000–25,000/mm^3.

E. Has patient traveled or had any infectious exposures? Some infections are endemic to certain areas. A history of tick exposure could lead to a diagnosis of Lyme disease or Rocky Mountain spotted fever.

III. Differential Diagnosis. Leukocytosis must be diagnosed based on the normal WBC count for age. Average WBC count in a neonate is 18,000–23,000/mm^3; that for an older child or adolescent is 7400/mm^3 (range: 4500–11,000/mm^3). Leukocytosis carries a broad differential, including a multitude of infectious etiologies and systemic illnesses such as malignancy or collagen vascular disease.

A. Acute Leukocytosis

1. **Acute bacterial infection.** Bacterial infections may be localized, as in abscess, cellulitis, or pneumonia. They may affect almost any area of the body, including bones or joints, urinary tract, and CNS, or may be systemic, as in bacteremia or sepsis. Risk of occult bacteremia in highly febrile children is higher if WBC count is > 15,000/mm^3 or < 5000/mm^3, and increases as WBC count and temperature increase.

2. **Viral infection.** Viral infections are common in children but usually do not result in as severe a leukocytosis as do bacterial infections. Viral infections such as pertussis can result in a marked lymphocytosis.

3. **Other infections.** May include mycobacteria, fungi, rickettsiae, or spirochetes.

4. **Acute hematologic disorder.** Patients with leukemia or lymphoma can present with elevated WBC count. Some patients with acute leukemia have hyperleukocytosis, defined as WBC count > 100,000/mm^3. This represents an oncologic emergency, because serious complications may arise from sludging of WBCs in the microvasculature.

5. **Medications.** Including corticosteroids and granulocyte colony-stimulating factor.

6. **Vasculitis.** Possibilities include juvenile rheumatoid arthritis and Kawasaki disease.

7. **Ischemia.** Acute ischemic events with tissue necrosis, such as a thromboembolic event or intussusception, can cause leukocytosis.

8. **Emotional or physical stress.** Exercise and acute physical or emotional stress can cause a rapid rise in WBC count by demargination, which is a shift of cells from the marginal (vascular wall) to the circulating pool.

B. **Subacute or Chronic Leukocytosis**

1. **Persistent or partially treated infection.** Diagnoses include osteomyelitis, subacute bacterial endocarditis, or intra-abdominal abscess.

2. **Mycobacterial or fungal infection.** These infections tend to be more insidious and might result in sustained leukocytosis, possibly with low-grade fever.

3. **Rheumatologic or inflammatory disorders.**

4. **Malignant disorders.** These include leukemias (acute lymphoblastic leukemia, acute myelogenous leukemia, chronic myelogenous leukemia), myeloproliferative disorders, or solid tumors infiltrating the marrow.

5. **Leukemoid reaction.** Infants with Down syndrome can develop a transient leukemoid reaction with extremely high WBC count, consisting mostly of neutrophils and immature myeloid elements, which resolves spontaneously. Blood smear can resemble that seen in chronic myelogenous leukemia.

6. **Asplenia.**

7. **Medications.** Same as for acute leukocytosis (see A, 5, earlier).

IV. **Database**

A. **Physical Exam Key Points**

1. **General appearance.** This is critically important in gauging illness severity. Is a young child running around the room playing or lying quietly, allowing strangers to examine him or her without protest?

2. **Vital signs.** Fever (or hypothermia) can accompany infection, neoplasia, or rheumatologic disorder. Tachycardia may suggest more severe illness, and with hypotension and fever suggests septic shock.

3. **Lymph nodes.** Enlarged lymph nodes can accompany infection, inflammation, or infiltrative disorders. Tender, mobile nodes are more likely to be reactive; firm, fixed, or matted nodes, malignant. Nodes up to 1 cm are usually not pathologic in children. Fluctuance suggests abscess. Location is important. Look for a source of infection in an area draining into the nodal region. Enlarged supraclavicular nodes suggest malignancy and should prompt immediate investigation.

4. **Lungs.** Look for signs of pulmonary infection (eg, rales, rhonchi, egophony, or decreased breath sounds). Pleural rub

may accompany an infectious, malignant, or rheumatologic disorder.

   5. Skin and mucosa. Petechiae, bruising, or mucosal bleeding suggests concurrent thrombocytopenia or coagulopathy, which might accompany a malignant hematologic disorder or disseminated intravascular coagulation from severe infection. Also look for rashes, which may help identify an infection or rheumatologic diagnosis.
   6. Heart. New murmur in a patient with a high WBC count and fever can indicate bacterial endocarditis or rheumatic fever.
   7. Abdomen. Tenderness, guarding, or rebound with leukocytosis suggests an acute abdominal process (eg, appendicitis) and would necessitate emergency surgical consultation. Hepatosplenomegaly may suggest an infiltrative disorder.
   8. GU system. Pelvic pain or vaginal discharge in a sexually active girl can indicate pelvic inflammatory disease.
   9. Neurologic exam. Irritability or lethargy, seizures, or cranial nerve palsies can indicate CNS infection such as meningitis or encephalitis or CNS infiltration with leukemic cells.
B. Laboratory Data
   1. Hemoglobin and platelets. Leukocytosis accompanied by anemia or thrombocytopenia suggests leukemia, although infection and certain medications can sometimes cause cytopenias with leukocytosis.
   2. Blood smear and differential. Always examine the blood smear to look for malignant cells in a patient with leukocytosis. Atypical lymphocytosis often accompanies viral infection, particularly Epstein-Barr virus. Neutrophilia with bandemia suggests bacterial infection. Eosinophilia accompanies connective tissue disease, hypersensitivity, parasitic infection, or malignancy. Pertussis causes extreme lymphocytosis.
   3. Urinalysis with microscopic analysis. WBCs, nitrates, or leukocyte esterase in urine indicate UTI.
   4. LDH and uric acid. Elevated uric acid or LDH can accompany leukemia or lymphoma.
   5. Cultures. Cultures of blood, urine, cerebrospinal fluid, throat, or stool are critical in diagnosing infection. Whenever possible, cultures should be obtained prior to antibiotic administration.
   6. ESR and C-reactive protein. These studies are nonspecific and can be elevated in many situations causing leukocytosis. May be useful as a baseline to follow progression of patient's condition.
   7. Thyroid function. Hyperthyroidism can sometimes cause leukocytosis.
   8. Rheumatologic studies. ANA, rheumatoid factor, complement levels, and other, more specific, tests can point toward a rheumatologic diagnosis.
C. Radiographic and Other Studies

1. **Chest x-ray.** Can diagnose pulmonary infection, mediastinal adenopathy, or pleural effusion.
2. **CT scan or ultrasound.** Can be useful in diagnosing infection within abdomen and pelvis, as well as malignant infiltration of lymph nodes, liver, or spleen.
3. **Bone marrow aspirate and biopsy.** Should be performed in patients suspected of having a marrow infiltrative disorder; occasionally can be useful in diagnosing certain infectious processes (eg, toxoplasmosis).
4. **Lumbar puncture.** Consider in patients with headache or meningismus. Cerebrospinal fluid (CSF) should be sent for cell count, protein, and glucose, as well as culture. If malignancy is a concern, also obtain cytology. If brain abscess, increased intracranial pressure, or mass-occupying lesion is suspected, order head CT scan before obtaining CSF.

V. Plan. The etiology of leukocytosis should guide therapy. Patients with infectious etiologies should be managed with antibiotics, if appropriate, or followed expectantly. Patients in whom appendicitis or abscess are suspected should undergo immediate surgical consultation. Patients with possible malignancy or rheumatologic disorders should be referred to appropriate consultants. Acutely ill patients are admitted to the hospital. When the etiology is not readily identified, despite initiation of an appropriate evaluation, follow-up is critical.

VI. Problem Case Diagnosis. The 7-year-old girl suffered from acute streptococcal pharyngitis. Throat exam showed exudate and palatal petechiae. She had anterior cervical lymphadenopathy, and all nodes were tender and less than 1 cm. Rapid strep test was positive.

VII. Teaching Pearl: Question. CBC is obtained for an apparently healthy, full-term newborn at 12 hours of age. The infant's total WBC count is 23,000/mm^3. What action is indicated at this time?

VIII. Teaching Pearl: Answer. No specific action is indicated. The mean WBC count for an infant of this age is 22,800/mm^3 (range: 13,000–38,000/mm^3).

REFERENCES

Dinauer MC. The phagocyte system and disorders of granulopoiesis and granulocyte function. In: Nathan DG, Orkin SH, Ginsberg D, Look AT, eds. *Nathan and Oski's Hematology of Infancy and Childhood,* 6th ed. Saunders, 2003:923–1010.

Ezekowitz RA, Stockman JA. Hematologic manifestations of systemic diseases. In: Nathan DG, Orkin SH, Ginsberg D, Look AT, eds. *Nathan and Oski's Hematology of Infancy and Childhood,* 6th ed. Saunders, 2003:1759–1809.

Lichtman MA. Classification and clinical manifestations of neutrophil disorders. In: Beutler E, Lichtman MA, et al, eds. *Williams Hematology,* 6th ed. McGraw-Hill, 2001:817–822.

63. LEUKOPENIA AND NEUTROPENIA

I. **Problem.** A full-term 1-day-old infant boy has an absolute neutrophil count (ANC) of 100/mm³. His mother has lupus but is currently well. Pregnancy history and labor and delivery were otherwise unremarkable. The infant appears well and is afebrile. Physical exam findings are normal.

II. **Immediate Questions**
   A. **What is an ANC?** ANC is a value obtained by multiplying WBC count by the total number of polymorphonuclear neutrophils (PMNs) and bands: ANC = WBC × (PMNs + bands). Thus, if WBC count is 6000/mm³, with 20% PMNs and 5% bands, ANC = 6000 × (0.20 + 0.05) = 1500/mm³. Neutropenia is defined as a decrease in the number of circulating neutrophils.
   1. **Mild (1000–1500/mm³).**
   2. **Moderate (500–1000/mm³).**
   3. **Severe (< 500/mm³).** Only severe neutropenia is associated with a significant risk of infection.
   B. **Does child appear ill or febrile?** Neutropenic patients can present quite suddenly with serious infections, despite a negative history. Some of these patients need to be diagnosed and treated immediately with antibiotics. Immunocompromised children with infections can be seriously ill, even without fever.
   C. **Are there signs or symptoms of pneumonia?** Pneumonia is a common infection in patients with neutropenia.
   D. **Is there need for immediate treatment?** In some cases, hospitalization and treatment with IV antibiotics are needed immediately.
   E. **If hospitalization is not needed, does patient need antibiotics?** Many patients with known neutropenia and a well-defined clinical history can be safely treated as outpatients.

III. **Differential Diagnosis**
   A. **Causes of Neutropenia in Children**
   1. **Viral.** Most common cause of transient neutropenia in childhood; typically lasts 3 days to 1 week. Causes include hepatitis A and B, parvovirus, respiratory syncytial, Epstein-Barr, cytomegalovirus, HIV, influenza A and B, and varicella viruses.
   2. **Benign ethnic neutropenia.** Racial variation is seen in normal WBC counts. For children aged 2 weeks to 1 year, the lower limit of normal is 1000/mm³ for white infants and 500/mm³ for black infants. Similarly, for white and black children older than 1 year of age, the lower limits of normal are 1500/mm³ and 1000/mm³, respectively.
   3. **Drug-induced.** Abrupt drop in ANC to < 500/mm³ usually occurs 1–2 weeks after exposure to drug. Spontaneous recovery is the

rule, but in some patients neutropenia can last for months. Drugs commonly associated with drug-induced neutropenia include:

   a. Indomethacin, ibuprofen.
   b. Penicillins, sulfonamides.
   c. Phenytoin, carbamazepine.
   d. Hydralazine.
   e. Phenothiazines.
   f. Cimetidine, ranitidine.
   g. Chemotherapeutic agents.

4. **Cancer.** Results in infiltration and replacement of normal marrow with malignant cells.

   a. Leukemias. Acute lymphoblastic leukemia and acute myelogenous leukemia (neutropenia alone is rarely a presenting sign).

   b. Solid tumors metastatic to bone marrow. Rhabdomyosarcoma, retinoblastoma, or neuroblastoma; it would be very unusual to see neutropenia alone as sole presenting sign of these tumors.

5. **Severe congenital neutropenia.** Patients are younger than 1 year of age with neutropenia and severe infections. May be autosomal dominant or autosomal recessive (Kostmann syndrome). ANC is usually < 200/mm^3; often 0. Platelets and hemoglobin are usually normal.

6. **Cyclic neutropenia.** Rare, relatively benign disorder with oscillations of ANC. Often patients have remarkably regular 21-day cycles. ANC nadir is usually < 100/mm^3; often 0. Reticulocytes and platelets may cycle, too. Patients may have fever, malaise, and mucositis. Diagnosis is made by checking CBC 2–3 times per week for 2–3 months.

7. **Shwachman-Diamond syndrome.** Very rare exocrine pancreatic insufficiency with neutropenia. Patients present in early childhood with short stature and failure to thrive. Neutropenia may be chronic or cyclic. Patients may also have anemia or thrombocytopenia.

8. **Reticular dysgenesis.** Very rare congenital absence of neutrophils. Patients present in infancy with severe immunodeficiency, absence of lymph nodes and tonsils, and thymic shadow. Most patients die by 6 months of age.

9. **Chronic idiopathic neutropenia.** Diagnosis of exclusion; may be difficult to differentiate from autoimmune neutropenia. Most patients have mild disease.

10. **Fanconi anemia.** Autosomal-recessive inheritance; 80% of patients have phenotypic anomalies (including skeletal anomalies of thumb). Initial blood problem is usually thrombocytopenia, not neutropenia.

11. **Myelokathexis.** Very rare, moderately severe neutropenia with increased myeloid elements in marrow but decreased circulating

neutrophils. Primarily affects females. Patients have frequent airway infections and pneumonia.

12. **Familial benign neutropenia.** Rare, often autosomal-dominant, mild neutropenia. Patients have no significant increased risk of infections.

13. **Chédiak-Higashi syndrome.** Rare, moderate neutropenia associated with partial albinism and neuropathy.

14. **Acquired aplastic anemia.** Neutropenia alone, as the only manifestation of aplastic anemia, would be unusual.

15. **Autoimmune neutropenias.** The most common causes of chronic neutropenia in childhood. Approximately one in five patients has a positive ANA finding. Serious infections are rare. Patients usually have an ANC < 500/mm^3. Almost all patients recover fully within months to 2 years. May be triggered by infections, drugs, other autoimmune disorders, or cancer.

16. **Splenic sequestration.** Patients rarely have neutropenia as the sole manifestation.

17. **Metabolic diseases.** Very rare causes of neutropenia are Barth syndrome and glycogen storage disease type IB.

B. **Neonatal Neutropenias**

1. **Sick or septic newborns, including premature infants.** Newborns have fewer mature neutrophils and neutrophil precursors per kilogram. Sick newborns are slow to upregulate the number of circulating neutrophils during infection.

2. **Alloimmune neutropenia of newborn.** Neonatal neutropenia caused by maternal antibodies against paternal WBC antigens. Analogous to neonatal anemia caused by Rh incompatibility; 40% of mothers have had miscarriages. Maternal antibodies are most commonly generated to paternal WBC antigens NA1 and NA2. Associated with fevers and serious infections (eg, pneumonia or omphalitis).

3. **Neonatal autoimmune neutropenia.** Occurs in infants of mothers with autoimmune neutropenia as a result of passive transfer of ANA from mother to child. Profound neutropenia can last 2–4 weeks.

4. **Autoimmune neutropenia of infancy.** Similar to idiopathic thrombocytopenic purpura or autoimmune hemolytic anemia. Acquired disorder, unrelated to maternal or paternal antigen incompatibility. Typically seen at 3–30 months of age. Clinically mild disorder; probably many cases are undiagnosed. Median duration of illness is 2 years, and 95% of patients recover by age 4.

5. **Infants of preeclamptic mothers.** Half of these infants have neutropenia (up to 80% if intrauterine growth retardation is present).

IV. **Database**

A. **Physical Exam Key Points.** Pay particular attention to vital signs, mucositis, infections, lung exam, and growth parameters. Observe for physical anomalies, with special attention to thumb, wrist, and forearm.

B. Laboratory Data. Obtain CBC, differential with ANC, smear, and ANA test (if autoimmune neutropenia is suspected).

C. Radiographic and Other Studies. Obtain chest x-ray to screen for other associated abnormalities (eg, pneumonia).

V. Plan

A. Initial Management

1. Most important intervention is to quickly determine whether patient is at risk for severe infection or sepsis while assessing ABCs (airway, breathing, circulation). Careful history and physical exam with several sets of vital signs establishes this initial risk evaluation. Hematology consultation with bone marrow aspirate and biopsy is often required to narrow the differential diagnosis.

2. Once determination is made about urgent need for hospitalization, antibiotics, and granulocyte colony-stimulating factor (G-CSF), a more careful workup can begin. History and physical exam can be very informative. A detailed history can uncover prior infections, drug use, hospitalizations, sick siblings, or relatives who died young from infection. Careful physical exam can detect important clues (eg, skeletal malformations of thumb and forearm in Fanconi anemia). Sequential CBCs are critical. Often rechecking the CBC once or twice a week for several weeks points the way to the correct diagnosis. Start with the common diagnoses in the differential and go from there to the more unusual.

B. Specific Management

1. **Severe congenital neutropenia.** Administer G-CSF, > 5 mcg/kg/day, rarely up to > 100 mcg/kg/day.

2. **Cyclic neutropenia.** Administer G-CSF, > 3 mcg/kg/day.

3. **Shwachman-Diamond syndrome.** Administer enzyme replacements and G-CSF.

4. **Reticular dysgenesis.** Bone marrow transplantation; G-CSF is not useful.

5. **Chronic idiopathic neutropenia.** Administer G-CSF for infants with severe disease and infections.

6. **Autoimmune neutropenias.** Administer G-CSF.

7. **Sick or septic newborns, including premature infants.** There is no role for G-CSF or granulocyte-macrophage colony-stimulating factor (GM-CSF) in treatment of sick or septic newborns; growth factors increase ANC, but not survival.

8. **Alloimmune neutropenia of newborn.** Administer antibiotics and G-CSF, 5 mcg/kg/day, even if neonate appears well.

9. **Infants of preeclamptic mothers.** G-CSF increases ANC but not survival in sick infants with neutropenia.

VI. Problem Case Diagnosis. The 1-day-old infant has neonatal autoimmune neutropenia. His mother, who has an autoimmune disease (lupus), has had chronic benign neutropenia for years without significant infections. Her ANC is typically 400-600/mm³.

VII. Teaching Pearl: Question. A newborn infant has omphalitis and neutropenia. What tests should be ordered to confirm the likely diagnosis?

VIII. Teaching Pearl: Answer. The infant should be tested for presence of ANAs. Parents' blood should be sent for WBC antigen determination (ie, NA1 and NA2). It is likely that this infant has alloimmune neutropenia of the newborn. The presence of antigens on paternal, but not maternal, WBCs clinches the diagnosis.

REFERENCES

Dale DC, Cottle TE, Fier CS, et al. Severe chronic neutropenia: Treatment and follow-up of patients in the Severe Chronic Neutropenia International Registry. *Am J Hematol* 2003;72:82–93.

Dinaver MC. The phagocytic system and disorders of granulopoiesis and granulocyte function. In: Nathan DG, Orkin SH, Ginsberg D, Look AT, eds. *Nathan and Oski's Hematology of Infancy and Childhood,* 6th ed. Saunders, 2003:932–1010.

Lehrnbecher T. Haematopoeitic growth factors in children with neutropenia. *Br J Hematol* 2002;116:28–56.

Maheshwari A, Christensen RD, Calhoun DA. Immune-mediated neutropenia in the neonate. *Acta Paediatr Suppl* 2002;438:98–103.

64. LIMP

I. Problem. A 4-year-old girl is brought to the emergency department with a limp of 2 days' duration.

II. Immediate Questions

A. Was onset sudden or insidious? When is limp most noticeable? Sudden appearance of limping suggests traumatic or infectious cause. Insidious limps are of greater concern, and often associated with gradual weakness from neuromuscular or metabolic disease. Always ask about delay or regression in developmental milestones; this is an ominous sign of serious disease. Neoplastic processes such as leukemia and neuroblastoma may also present with bone pain and periarticular pain, leading to limp. Morning "stiffness" causing a limp is more likely in rheumatic diseases such as juvenile rheumatoid arthritis (JRA), whereas evening symptoms are more suggestive of muscle fatigue, possibly from an orthopedic or a neurologic cause.

B. Is there a history of trauma? Trauma is one of the most common causes of limp in childhood. It may be misleading, however, because children from toddlerhood through adolescence are constantly exposed to trauma. If history and location fit, the differential diagnosis will be narrowed. Always consider nonaccidental trauma, particularly when history or physical exam, or both, are suspicious.

C. History of illness? May suggest immune complex–mediated disease, such as postinfectious arthritis (eg, Henoch-Schönlein purpura [HSP], acute rheumatic fever, Epstein-Barr virus, or parvovirus), transient synovitis of the hip, or arthritis or arthralgia associated with serum sickness (associated with more systemic features after medications such as cephalosporins or minocycline).

D. Are there associated constitutional symptoms? Constitutional symptoms (eg, fever and weight loss) are consistent with systemic diseases, including malignancy and infection. Patients with emergency diagnoses such as septic arthritis or osteomyelitis may present with new onset of fevers. Malignancy may be associated with lingering fevers or fevers without an obvious source. Specific rashes are associated with many rheumatologic conditions, such as dermatomyositis, systemic-onset JRA, and systemic lupus erythematosus (SLE).

E. Is limp secondary to pain? Where does pain originate? Starting distally, consider foot, ankle, tibia or fibula, knee, quadriceps or hamstrings, hip, groin, abdomen, and spine. Do not omit referred pain from abdomen, pelvis, testicles, spine, retroperitoneum, and hip.

III. Differential Diagnosis

A. Infectious Disease. *One of the most important categories to rule out.* Differential includes septic arthritis (true medical emergency), osteomyelitis (bacterial or tuberculous), diskitis, myositis (viral or pyogenic), cellulitis, and postinfectious arthralgia or arthritis.

B. Orthopaedic Condition. More urgent diagnoses include fracture, slipped capital femoral epiphysis (SCFE), developmental dysplasia of the hip (DDH), and avascular necrosis, such as Legg-Calvé-Perthes disease (LCPD). Other orthopedic syndromes, such as Osgood-Schlatter disease, osteochondritis dissecans, and chondromalacia patellae, may contribute to a limp. Check for leg length inequality.

C. Inflammatory Condition. Transient synovitis of the hip, a diagnosis of exclusion, is commonly seen after viral infection or trauma. Less common diagnoses associated with arthritis or muscle weakness include JRA, acute rheumatic fever, SLE, juvenile dermatomyositis, HSP, Sjögren syndrome, and inflammatory bowel disease.

D. Neoplastic Disorder. Benign conditions include osteochondroma and osteoid osteoma (typically associated with nighttime pain and relief with acetylsalicylic acid). Local malignant conditions include osteogenic sarcoma and Ewing sarcoma, both with typical radiologic appearance. Patients with leukemia and neuroblastoma may present with constitutional symptoms such as fatigue, weight loss, and fever, with pain out of proportion to physical findings. Also consider metastases, Langerhans cell histiocytosis, and spinal cord tumors.

E. Neuromuscular Disorder. Rarely, weakness manifests for the first time as limp. Conditions to consider are muscular dystrophy, Guillain-Barré syndrome, and tick paralysis. Previously undiagnosed mild cerebral palsy may cause limp secondary to contracture or hypertonicity, which is not recognized until child ambulates.

F. Other Causes. Consider referred pain from abdomen, retroperitoneum, testicles, and spine. Sickle cell disease may lead to avascular necrosis of the femoral or humoral heads, and hemophilia may lead to hemarthrosis. Ligamentous laxity or hypermobile joints contribute to evening aches and pains that may lead to limp. Consider nonaccidental trauma and poorly fitting shoes.

IV. Database

A. Physical Exam Key Points

1. **General appearance, including vital signs.** Fever may occur with infectious, inflammatory, and neoplastic processes.
2. **Skin.** Observe for Still's rash in patients with JRA; Gottron papules in those with dermatomyositis; or cellulitis.
3. **Musculoskeletal system.** Check long bones for point tenderness (fracture, osteomyelitis). Check joints for warmth, tenderness, effusion, or restriction of full range of motion. Hip pathology manifests on exam with the hip joint flexed, abducted, and externally rotated to decrease mean articular pressure. Observe for muscle atrophy and leg length discrepancy.
4. **Neurologic exam.** Check for symmetric strength, reflexes, and tone. Watch gait for clue to pain or weakness. Running may intensify an abnormal gait.
5. **Referred pain.** Evaluate for areas of referred pain in abdomen, genital area, and spine.

B. Laboratory Data.
Obtain CBC, ESR, and C-reactive protein (CRP). Abnormal findings help identify infectious or inflammatory etiology. Serial results help clinician track progress of treatment. Obtain culture of blood, joint fluid, or bone if septic joint or osteomyelitis is suspected. CRP is more sensitive than ESR for early osteomyelitis and therefore more likely to be abnormal earlier in disease process.

C. Radiographic and Other Studies

1. **X-rays.** Obtain two views in perpendicular planes. Particularly helpful when child is younger than 2 years of age, because screening X-rays of bilateral lower extremities reveal fractures in 20% of cases. In children, growth plates are weaker than ligamentous attachments; thus, occult fractures through the growth plate are more common. X-rays show sclerotic changes of some bone tumors and osteomyelitis. Periosteal reaction or lytic changes can be seen in infections (> 10 days).

   2. **Ultrasound.** Quick and easy method of evaluating for joint effu-
      sion, particularly in the hip joint.
   3. **Bone scan.** More sensitive than other tests for early
      osteomyelitis and useful if multiple areas are suspected or
      when site of problem is unclear.
   4. **CT and MRI scans.** Usually not needed acutely. Obtain CT
      scan for definition of bones, MRI scan for definition of soft
      tissues and effusions. Useful if presentation is atypical or diag-
      nosis is difficult.

V. Plan. Start with careful history of limp and constitutional symptoms.
   A. If patient has high fever or other features of infection, locate the
       source: bone, joint, muscle, skin. Consider CBC with differential,
       ESR, CRP; abnormalities may also suggest malignancy. Culture
       potential sources of infection and start empiric antibiotics if
       warranted.
   B. Determine if there was trauma. Could this be abuse? Point ten-
       derness on growth plate may suggest fracture. Consider obtaining
       x-rays of the area. Bone pain suggests fracture, local bone tumor,
       or leukemia. X-rays showing fractures, sclerotic rings, or leukemic
       lines will support the diagnosis.
   C. Carefully evaluate hip joint. Remember that referred pain to the
       knee may originate in the hip. Permanent damage may result
       from increased pressure within the joint capsule. Consider
       DDH in younger kids, LCPD in school-age boys, SCFE in over-
       weight adolescents, and septic arthritis in everyone (medical
       emergency).

VI. Problem Case Diagnosis. This 4-year-old girl had fever of 5 days'
    duration and point tenderness over the left distal tibia. A plain x-ray
    was normal, but increased uptake was seen on bone scan in the
    left tibial metaphysis. Diagnosis of osteomyelitis was made. Bone
    biopsy was performed, and culture was positive for *Staphylococcus
    aureus.*

VII. Teaching Pearl: Question. Why does knee pain occur in patients
    with hip pathology?

VIII. Teaching Pearl: Answer. The anterior branch of the obturator nerve
    passes close to the hip joint and, if irritated, may send a painful sen-
    sation to the medial side of the knee.

REFERENCES

Leet A, Skaggs D. Evaluation of the acutely limping child. *Am Fam Physician*
    2000;61:1011–1018.
Renshaw T. The child who has a limp. *Pediatr Rev* 1995;16:458–465.
Rose C, Doughty RA. Limp. In: Fleisher G, Ludwig, S, eds. *Pediatric Emergency
    Medicine.* Williams & Wilkins, 1993:304–309.

65. MACROCEPHALY

I. **Problem.** During a routine health maintenance visit, macrocephaly is noted in a 6-month-old male infant.

II. **Immediate Questions**
   A. **Is this an emergency, urgent, or routine clinical condition?** Determine if this is an emergency. Remember the ABCs (airway, breathing, and circulation).
   B. **Is there a family history of macrocephaly?** Macrocephaly can be familial, unassociated with an underlying abnormality, or associated with an array of other problems, as in neurocutaneous disorders.
   C. **Does patient have an associated developmental delay?** Many conditions (eg, hydrocephalus, neurocutaneous disorders, metabolic disorders) can present with macrocephaly and developmental delay.
   D. **Pertinent Historical Information.** Information about child's prenatal and neonatal course may identify risks for neurologic disorders or sequelae.
      1. Did mother receive prenatal care?
      2. Was prenatal ultrasonography performed?
      3. Was there any history of maternal medication use or substance abuse during pregnancy?
      4. Were there any maternal medical complications during pregnancy?
      5. Was pregnancy completed to term?
      6. Were there any complications during delivery?
      7. Were developmental milestones achieved at appropriate ages?
      8. Is there any significant medical or surgical history?
      9. Any history of head trauma?
      10. Any family history of neurologic disorders?
      11. Is patient appropriately developed and nourished? Growth and development problems may reflect an underlying medical or neurologic disorder.
      12. Is patient cooperative, interactive, or in distress?

III. **Differential Diagnosis**
   A. **Hydrocephalus.** Occurs as a result of impaired production, flow, or absorption of cerebrospinal fluid (CSF) within the cranial vault.
      1. **Noncommunicating (obstructive) hydrocephalus.** Caused by physical blockade of CSF flow from the ventricular system within the brain to the subarachnoid space surrounding the brain. This results in increased pressure within the intracranial space. Intracranial mass lesions (tumors, abscesses, vascular anomalies, and hamartomas) are often the cause of noncommunicating hydrocephalus. The most common cause in early

infancy is aqueductal stenosis, which can be inherited or caused by infectious conditions and posthemorrhagic complications of prematurity. Other cerebral developmental disorders that can cause noncommunicating hydrocephalus include Dandy-Walker malformation, Chiari malformation, Klippel-Feil syndrome, and Warburg syndrome.

2. **Communicating (nonobstructive) hydrocephalus.** May occur following intracranial infection or hemorrhage, in addition to benign enlargement of subarachnoid space. Typically resolves by 2 years of age. A rare cause of hydrocephalus is overproduction of CSF by choroid plexus papilloma.

B. **Neurocutaneous Disorders.** These disorders include cardinal features within CNS and skin. Several of these disorders may present with macrocephaly, including neurofibromatosis (the most common of these conditions) and tuberous sclerosis. Other neurocutaneous disorders include hypomelanosis of Ito, linear nevus sebaceous syndrome, and incontinentia pigmenti.

C. **Metabolic Disorders.** Several metabolic disorders result in the storage of substances within the brain. These disorders include Alexander disease, Canavan disease, gangliosidoses, and mucopolysaccharidoses. Head circumference of a patient with one of these disorders typically is normal at birth but increases as the storage material builds up, causing child to regress neurologically.

D. **Disorders of Skull Thickening.** Disorders of bone that may result in thickening of the skull include rickets, osteogenesis imperfecta and hyperphosphatemia, to name a few. These disorders present as macrocephaly, without enlargement of CNS (brain).

E. **Familial Macrocephaly.**

IV. **Database**

A. **Physical Exam Key Points.** Complete general physical exam is important in identifying a systemic disorder. Assess ABCs to avoid missing an emergency condition.

1. **Vital signs.** Heart rate and BP changes may reflect systemic infection, cardiac disease, or intoxication, or even suggest increased intracranial pressure. Alteration of temperature may reflect infection or effects of intoxication.

2. **Skin.** Inspect for signs of trauma, rash, and birthmarks (erythematous, hypopigmented, or hyperpigmented lesions). Rash may suggest infectious or vasculitic disorder. Look for signs of a neurocutaneous disorder such as neurofibromatosis (café au lait spots and family history), tuberous sclerosis (hypopigmented macules on trunk or limbs, café au lait spots, and seizures, in addition to cysts or tumors of kidney, cardiac rhabdomyomas, and retinal tumors), hypomelanosis of Ito (large hypopigmented lesion), or linear nevus sebaceous syndrome (unilateral linear nevus on face or scalp with ipsilateral hemihypertrophy).

3. **Head and neck.** Head circumference may reflect alterations in brain parenchyma (microcephaly and macrocephaly), hydrocephalus, or even skull thickening. Inspect for signs of head trauma. Neck stiffness (meningismus) may indicate meningitis or subarachnoid hemorrhage.

4. **Heart and lungs.** Listen for cardiac murmur or altered cardiac dynamics. Respiratory dysfunction or abnormal breathing patterns may be a sign of neurologic disease.

5. **Abdomen.** Hepatosplenomegaly may be seen in a variety of metabolic and neurodegenerative disorders.

6. **Neurologic exam.** Detailed neurologic exam allows clinician to localize the condition to specific regions of central and peripheral nervous systems. Disorders of the cerebral cortex affect cognition, whereas lesions in the brainstem affect specific cranial nerves. Spinal cord lesions demonstrate motor or sensory levels on examination, or both.

   a. **Mental status.** Ability to interact with the environment is assessed by observing, speaking with, and listening to patient. This must be carried out at an age-appropriate level.

   b. **Cranial nerves.** Pupil size and reactivity in addition to eye movements reflect function of portions of the upper brainstem. Symmetric movement of face, soft palate, and tongue demonstrates integrity of the lower brainstem.

   c. **Motor system.** Muscle bulk, tone, and strength demonstrate function of the motor pathways. Fine motor skills may suggest developmental abilities. Assess patient's spontaneous, voluntary, and involuntary movement. Involuntary movements may be seen in a variety of neurologic disorders.

   d. **Sensory system.** Localized sensory deficits may reflect dysfunction of central or peripheral nervous system, or they may be seen in functional disorders.

   e. **Deep tendon reflexes.** These reflex arcs demonstrate integrity of specific reflex pathways from the peripheral muscle through the levels of the spinal cord.

   f. **Cerebellar exam.** Cerebellar dysfunction may be a sign of localized space-occupying, destructive, or degenerative disorders.

B. **Laboratory Data**

1. **Basic metabolic panel, glucose, calcium.** Electrolyte abnormalities can be seen in patients with acute cerebral disorders and with increased intracranial pressure.

2. **Renal and hepatic profile.** These tests can indicate acute or chronic end-organ dysfunction.

3. **CBC with differential.** Elevated WBC count may indicate active infection.

4. **ABGs.** Obtain if hypoxia or acid-base problems are suggested by history or physical exam.

C. **Radiographic and Other Studies**
1. **Neuroimaging (CT or MRI scan).** A neuroimaging study should be performed on all patients with macrocephaly. If patient is stable on exam and only has a physical finding of macrocephaly, the study may not need to be obtained emergently. MRI scan is a more sensitive exam; however, this test requires that patient remain still for a prolonged period of time and therefore often requires sedation.
2. **EEG.** If seizure or clinical feature of encephalitis is present.
3. **ECG.** If cardiac disorder is suspected.
4. **Lumbar puncture.** Helpful if history or physical exam suggests intracranial infection (meningitis or encephalitis) or subarachnoid hemorrhage. Do *not* perform in the presence of increased intracranial pressure because of the risk of herniation.

V. **Plan**
A. **Emergency Management.** If patient demonstrates signs of increased intracranial pressure on presentation, perform a complete assessment expeditiously, along with urgent neuroimaging.
B. **Neurosurgery Consultation.** If acute signs of increased intracranial pressure are noted, arrange neurosurgical consultation. Emergent placement of ventriculostomy or ventriculoperitoneal shunt may be indicated.
C. **Evaluate for Underlying Etiologies.** If suggested by history, physical exam, or laboratory evaluation.
D. **Follow-up.** Patients with macrocephaly and hydrocephalus need frequent follow-up. Patients are seen regularly for signs of increased intracranial pressure (before shunting is required or for shunt failure) in addition to developmental and cognitive follow-up.

VI. **Problem Case Diagnosis.** The 6-month-old infant was found on examination to have macrocephaly and mild gross motor delay. His prenatal history was significant for ventriculomegaly, noted during the third trimester. Family and past medical histories were unremarkable, as was physical exam (no neurocutaneous stigmata or organomegaly). Neurologic exam was significant only for macrocephaly and mild gross motor delay. Head circumference was above the 98th percentile for a 6-month-old male infant, which is 50th percentile for a 2-year-old child. Nonemergent MRI scan of the brain demonstrated hydrocephalus, cystic dilation of the fourth ventricle, and cerebellar hypoplasia: the Dandy-Walker malformation. No other intracranial abnormalities were noted. This case is not a medical emergency because the macrocephaly is not associated with any symptoms at this time; however, patient will require frequent follow-up.

VII. **Teaching Pearl: Question.** Does the presentation of Dandy-Walker malformation vary depending on age of diagnosis?

VIII. **Teaching Pearl: Answer.** The disorder presents with the triad of hydrocephalus, cystic dilation of the fourth ventricle, and cerebellar hypoplasia (complete or partial agenesis of the cerebellar vermis). Hydrocephalus can develop in utero or during early childhood (typically, first year of life). In older children, the disorder can present with signs of increased intracranial pressure (lethargy, headache, and vomiting) or cerebellar dysfunction (ataxia). Other CNS anomalies may be present, including agenesis of the corpus callosum, heterotopias, congenital tumors, and aqueductal stenosis.

REFERENCES

Bernard JP, Moscoso G, Renier D, Ville Y. Cystic malformation of the posterior fossa. *Prenat Diagn* 2001;21:1064–1069.

Niesen CE. Malformations of the posterior fossa: Current perspectives. *Sem Pediatr Neurol* 2002;9:320–334.

Pascual-Casatroviejo I, Velez A, Pascual-Pascual S, et al. Dandy-Walker malformation: Analysis of 38 cases. *Child Nerv Sys* 1991;7:88–97.

66. METABOLIC DISEASES

I. **Problem.** A full-term neonate, who previously appeared well, presents with rapidly increasing lethargy after 3–4 days of poor feeding.

II. **Immediate Questions**
   A. **Is there a family history of neonatal losses?** Such a history is highly suspicious for metabolic disease caused by enzyme deficiencies. These diseases typically are transmitted in an autosomal-recessive or occasionally X-linked fashion, making the recurrence risk for these families significant.
   B. **Is there associated vomiting?** Can be nonspecific, or excessive with hyperammonemia.
   C. **Does patient have an unusual odor?** Organic acids are volatile and thus can be associated with an unusual odor of sweat, urine, or earwax. Maple syrup urine disease (MSUD) is often suspected from sweet-smelling earwax. A foul "sweaty feet" or "cat urine" odor can occur in several of the organic acidemias.
   D. **If available, what were the newborn screening results?** Newborn screening studies in many states include many of the organic acidemias, fatty acid oxidation defects, and urea cycle defects. Check screening results of child or other family member, if available. Because of limitations of screening tests, a negative study cannot be relied on to rule out disease (specifically, several urea cycle defects and energy production defects). Due to residual enzyme function, a sample obtained before the onset of symptoms may be normal, even in an affected patient. Abnormal results must be verified with acute samples (see later discussion under V, Plan).

III. **Differential Diagnosis**
   A. **Sepsis.** Always consider in acutely ill or febrile neonates. Conversely, metabolic diseases are probably as common as true

sepsis and should be considered in all acutely sick neonates. In all suspicious cases, obtain appropriate cultures (eg, blood, cerebrospinal fluid, and urine) and consider appropriate antibiotics. Because infection can exacerbate metabolic disease, it should be considered even when a metabolic disorder is likely.

B. Organic Acidemia. Most often caused by enzyme or cofactor deficiencies in the catabolism of branched chain amino acids (valine, leucine, and isoleucine). Organic acid and a positive gap acidosis develop from metabolites built up behind the enzymatic block. Other effects of metabolite excess include inhibition of enzymes of the urea cycle with secondary hyperammonemia. Many of these metabolites have direct CNS toxicity. Marrow suppression and altered glucose metabolism (hyperglycemia or hypoglycemia) also can occur as secondary effects.

C. Primary Urea Cycle Defects. Typically result in hyperammonemia without acidosis. Hallmark of these disorders is respiratory alkalosis in an ill-appearing child; hyperammonemia affects the respiratory centers, causing deep and rapid breathing (hyperpnea) with resultant drop in carbon dioxide.

D. Disorders Involving Energy Production

    1. Glycogen storage disorders. Patients classically present with enlarged liver and subsequent preprandial hypoglycemia and may manifest acute hypoglycemia with intercurrent illness or fast. Lactic acidosis from the chronic energy depletion state provides a source of energy for the brain, and often the hypoglycemia goes unnoticed until an illness occurs. Long-term sequelae can include liver adenomas, progressive renal insufficiency, and gout.

    2. Fatty acid oxidation (FAO) defects. Involve enzymatic defects in fatty acid β-oxidation. In fasting states, when glycogen stores are depleted, fats must be mobilized for energy production. If β-oxidation is impaired, hypoglycemia develops with relative hypoketosis or aketosis. Metabolites are organic acids, with resultant positive gap acidosis, and may have a direct toxic effect on the CNS. Myopathy, cardiomyopathy, retinopathy, and other systemic manifestations can occur over time in some patients with FAO defects.

    3. Primary lactic acidosis. Typically thought of as disorders of gluconeogenesis, Krebs cycle, or the electron transport chain. Patients often present acutely with positive gap acidosis due to lactate or pyruvate, or both. Hypoglycemia is variable.

E. Structural cardiac defects. Suggested by history and physical exam.

F. Trauma. Altered mental status or vomiting can occur with head or abdominal trauma.

G. Toxic Exposure (eg, organophosphates).

H. Dehydration. From intercurrent GI illness or formula intolerance.

IV. Database
A. Physical Exam Key Points
1. **Vital signs.** Tachypnea is a common reaction to stress in the neonate. When acidosis or hyperammonemia, or both, are present, hyperpnea (deep and rapid breathing) is often seen. Fever suggests infection, which can occur as a primary or secondary phenomenon in metabolic disease.
2. **HEENT.** A full fontanelle can accompany meningitis and hyperammonemia (secondary to cerebral edema). Altered pupillary reactions with subsequent herniation can occur if untreated. If cataracts are present, consider galactosemia. Dry mucous membranes can indicate dehydration from poor feeding of any etiology.
3. **Abdomen.** Transient hepatomegaly can accompany many of the metabolic disorders. It is typical in disorders of energy production (eg, FAO defects and disorders of gluconeogenesis), resolving when metabolic stability is attained. Progressive hepatomegaly can be seen in the glycogen storage disorders.
4. **Neurologic exam.** Mental status changes are a common finding in neonates in distress. Metabolic considerations include hypoglycemia, hyperammonemia, and severe acidosis. Hyperreflexia and clonus can result from hyperammonemia-induced cerebral edema.

B. Laboratory Data
1. **Glucose**
   a. **Hypoglycemia.** Ketotic hypoglycemia is seen in endocrine disorders, some organic acidemias, primary lactic acidoses, and some glycogen storage diseases. Hypoketotic or aketotic hypoglycemia is seen in hyperinsulinism. Hypoglycemia is seen in metabolic disorders, including type I ("classic") glycogen storage disease (Von Gierke), and is the hallmark of FAO defects. When considering hypoglycemia due to energy production disorders, the length of the fast may be helpful: glycogen is a fuel that is necessary shortly after meals (~3–4 hours); fatty acid metabolism is the next obligatory fuel (~4–8 hours); and gluconeogenesis is utilized thereafter. Prolonged fast or intercurrent vomiting and diarrheal illness is typical of hypoglycemia with FAO defects; whereas a short fast (3–4 hours) may result in hypoglycemia in patients with glycogen storage disease. Fasting tolerance increases with age.
   b. **Secondary hyperglycemia.** Can also accompany organic acidemias. Ketosis may be seen in these disorders as well, making the presentation difficult to distinguish from neonatal diabetic ketoacidosis.
2. **Urine ketones.** Neonates make and use ketones highly efficiently, so they are a rare finding before 2–3 months of age.

Ketosis in a neonate suggests an organic acidemia. Outside of the neonatal period, inappropriate ketones in the face of a normal or elevated blood glucose level suggests organic acidemia. Conversely, absence of ketones in a hypoglycemic child suggests glycogen storage disease and FAO defects. See earlier discussion.

3. **Electrolytes.** Low bicarbonate suggests acidosis. ABGs should be obtained to confirm this, because hyperpnea caused by hyperammonemia can result in hypocarbia and compensatory renal wasting of bicarbonate.

4. **ABGs.** Metabolic acidosis is typically seen in acutely ill neonates, often due to lactic acidosis with respiratory or circulatory compromise. Organic acidemias or lactic acidosis from metabolic disease should be considered. Respiratory alkalosis is unusual in an acutely ill child and is typical of the primary urea cycle defects (see III, C, 3, earlier).

5. **Anion gap.** Calculated as follows: $Na - (Cl + HCO_3)$; normal anion gap is 12–15. In confirmed acidosis, an elevated anion gap is seen the presence of an unmeasured ion, such as an organic acid, lactate, excessive ketones, or toxic ingestion.

6. **Blood ammonia.** Typically significantly elevated in primary urea cycle defects. May be secondarily elevated in organic acidemias. Mild to modest elevations can be seen in FAO defects or primary lactic acidosis.

7. **CBC.** Elevated WBC count can suggest infection. Bone marrow suppression can occur in some organic acidemias and severe infections.

8. **Liver function tests.** May be elevated in many metabolic disorders (see IV, A, 3, earlier).

9. **BUN.** In urea cycle disturbances (primary or secondary), patients are unable to make urea; therefore, BUN is low even in the presence of dehydration.

10. **Lactic acid.** Can be elevated in tissue hypoxia from sepsis, seizure, and trauma. Often excessive in mitochondrial disease, primary lactic acidoses, and glycogen storage diseases.

11. **Pyruvate.** Lactate and pyruvate are in equilibrium, depending on the redox potential of the cell. In lactic acidosis, pyruvate elevations and lactate-to-pyruvate ratios may help to localize the enzymatic defect. These levels should be obtained simultaneously.

12. **Uric acid.** May be elevated in energy-deficient states such as the primary lactic acidoses, FAO defects, and glycogen storage diseases. Often excessive in glycogen storage diseases due to both overproduction and underexcretion.

C. **Radiographic and Other Studies**

1. **MRI and CT scans.** May show evidence of cerebral edema when hyperammonemia is present.

2. **Abdominal ultrasound.** Microvesicular fatty infiltration is consistent with FAO defect. Hepatomegaly due to glycogen storage

is nonspecific on ultrasound; biopsy is usually required to identify glycogen.

V. Plan. Exact diagnosis may be made after the initial presentation using specimens obtained acutely. Such studies, including urine organic acids, plasma amino acids, and acylcarnitine profile, require specialized laboratories. For practical purposes, samples of acute urine and plasma (with cellular portion spun off and discarded) can be frozen and remain stable for days to months. If other samples cannot be obtained, a newborn screening filter paper dotted with blood and air-dried can be most helpful. Because some children with metabolic diseases appear biochemically normal when well, obtaining samples acutely is critical in establishing a diagnosis.

A. Hemodialysis. For extreme acidosis or hyperammonemia with mental status changes, hemodialysis is the fastest method of ammonia removal. If medical center does not have this capability, emergent transfer is recommended. When cerebral edema is present, mannitol, hyperventilation, and ventilatory support may be used if herniation is suspected or impending. Correcting ammonia level and removing organic academia will resolve the cerebral edema in most situations.

B. Stop Offending Agent. In primary urea cycle defects and the common organic acidemias, stopping protein intake is essential.

C. Intravenous Dextrose. Essential in acute treatment of hypoglycemia of any etiology. Ensuring a constant source of glucose until an appropriate diet can be established for FAO defects and glycogen storage disorders can prevent further hypoglycemic episodes. Providing an energy source to stop catabolism can prevent worsening of the clinical status in disorders involving protein metabolism (urea cycle disorders and organic acidemias). For neonates, 8–10 mg/kg/min, and for children, 6–8 mg/kg/min of IV dextrose is recommended. In organic acidemias, FAO defects, and primary urea cycle defects, a forced diuresis may help to rid the body of toxic metabolites, which are excreted in the kidneys. If a central line has not yet been established or in children with known metabolic disease presenting with acute exacerbations but without significant mental status changes, D_{10} at 2 times maintenance with appropriate electrolytes may suffice. This treatment is appropriate in all of the common metabolic disorders, with the exception of the primary lactic acidemias and mitochondrial disease, because excess glucose may increase lactate production. Use dextrose cautiously with appropriate fluid hydration in these situations.

D. Ammonia Scavengers. Sodium phenylbutyrate and sodium phenylacetate provide a route for ammonia removal in primary urea cycle disorders. These are orphan drugs and should be used only with the help of a metabolic specialist.

E. Insulin. With large amounts of glucose used to stop catabolism, patients may develop hyperglycemia and associated fluid losses.

Hyperglycemia may be a presenting feature of some organic acidemias. To ensure that glucose given is being used to stop or prevent catabolism and promote anabolism, an insulin drip may be used. Insulin and growth hormone have both been used to promote anabolism in patients who are not responding to the usual measures.

F. Vitamin or Cofactor Therapy. Until a diagnosis is established, treatment with cofactors for the most likely enzymes can be beneficial. Biotin, vitamin B_{12}, is the cofactor most likely involved in the organic acidemias; thiamine and biotin in the primary lactic acidemias. MSUD, which is often apparent due to the typical odor, may respond to thiamine.

G. L-Carnitine. Rarely available or used acutely. Provides a method of organic acid removal via esterification and renal clearance. Supplementation prevents a secondary carnitine deficiency. Caution should be used in treating certain FAO defects.

H. Transfusion. For marrow suppression or excessive blood loss. Concern always exists of increasing the protein load in patients with disorders of protein metabolism. Usually well-tolerated, but monitor closely.

I. Albumin and Fluid Resuscitation. Concern always exists of increasing the protein load in patients with disorders of protein metabolism. Although patients should be closely monitored, when necessary, this treatment is usually well-tolerated.

J. Unexplained Death. In the case of potential metabolic disease, certain specimens may be most helpful in establishing a post-mortem diagnosis. Most of these disorders are autosomal recessive and thus pose a significant recurrence risk to families. Acute samples of plasma and urine may be sent for metabolic studies if kept frozen. A filter paper sample can provide metabolic information and is also a very stable source of DNA for future studies such as mutation analysis. If possible, premorten or immediate postmortem biopsy specimens from liver and muscle, flash frozen and stored at $-40°C$, may be used for enzyme analysis, DNA, and so forth. A fibroblast line established from a skin biopsy sample obtained using sterile technique premorten or immediately post-mortem may be used similarly, although at the current time, not all enzymes can be studied in fibroblasts. Samples can be placed in sterile saline and refrigerated until proper medium for culture can be obtained.

VI. Problem Case Diagnosis. Physical exam of this term neonate was unremarkable. Laboratory workup was significant for hypoglycemia, acidosis, ketosis, and hyperammonemia. Results of bacterial cultures were negative. Diagnosis is methylmalonic acidemia.

VII. Teaching Pearl: Question. What is the most likely cause of illness in an 11-month-old, previously healthy infant with a 3-day history of symptoms of upper respiratory infection, diarrhea of 24 hours' duration, and poor oral intake? Liver is palpable on exam. Electrolytes are as follows: Na 140, K 5.0, Cl 106, T_{CO_2} 12. Glucose level is 23 mg/dL. VBGs show pH of 7.29 and CO_2 of 28. AST is 112 and ALT, 86. Urinalysis shows 1+ ketonuria.

VIII. Teaching Pearl: Answer. FAO defect; medium-chain acyl CoA dehydrogenase (MCAD) is the most common of these defects and the most likely to present in a previously healthy child without other system involvement.

REFERENCES

Fernandes J, Saudubray J-M, van den Berghe G, eds. *Inborn Metabolic Diseases: Diagnosis and Treatment,* 3rd ed. Springer, 2000.

Rimoin DL, Connor JM, Pyeritz Re, Korf BR, eds. *Emery and Rimoin's Principles and Practice of Medical Genetics,* 4th ed. Churchill Livingstone, 2002.

Scriver CR, Beaudet AL, Sly WS, Valle D, eds. *The Metabolic & Molecular Basis of Inherited Disease,* 8th ed. McGraw-Hill, 2001.

67. NASOGASTRIC TUBE MANAGEMENT

I. Problem. A 3-year-old boy has bloody output from his nasogastric (NG) tube 2 days after undergoing small bowel resection for intussusception.

II. Immediate Questions

A. What are the vital signs? Hypotension and tachycardia, in the presence of bleeding, are indicative of volume loss that requires prompt correction.

B. What is the character of the NG bleeding? Lightly blood-tinged fluid or "coffee-ground" emesis is less worrisome than fresh red blood.

C. How much bloody drainage has there been? Large amounts of bloody drainage are of concern. Blood volume in children aged 1–3 years is approximately 75 mL/kg.

D. Has patient had recent or remote GI surgery? If surgery was recent, there may be bleeding from a new anastomotic site, or there may be a marginal ulcer at an old anastomotic site.

E. Is patient passing flatus or stool? What is the character of the stools? Often, decreased NG output correlates with return of bowel function. Abdominal obstruction or ileus may result in decreased passage of gas or bowel movements. Fresh red blood from the rectum along with bloody NG drainage is very serious. Melena suggests upper tract or small bowel bleeding. Stools that are normal in appearance and occult blood–positive are suggestive of slower GI bleeding. Stools that are negative for occult blood suggest very early or insignificant bleeding.

F. How long has NG tube been in place? A tube that has been recently placed may have a small amount of bloody drainage secondary to the insertion. A tube that has been in place for

> 48 hours may cause oozing from gastric or esophageal mucosal irritation.

G. Is patient receiving antacids, H₂ blockers, or proton pump inhibitors (PPIs)? What is the pH of the drainage? Presence of acidic gastric secretions may predispose to formation of gastritis and "stress" ulcers. Gastric pH > 4 may enhance mucosal protection.

H. Is there associated abdominal distention? If patient develops ileus or obstruction, the amount of aspirate may increase.

 I. Is output bilious? Bilious NG output indicates bile reflux into the stomach, or NG tube that has been placed distal to the pylorus.

J. Is tube functioning? Tubes often become obstructed with mucous or medications. While the tube is on suction, listen for a whistle, which indicates patency.

K. Is patient taking, or being given, extra fluid by mouth? Often, excessive amounts of ice chips are given to patients with NG tubes. This can lead to high NG outputs. Careful questioning of family and caregivers can identify this possibility.

L. Are there any respiratory symptoms? If NG tube is misplaced in the esophagus or oropharynx, patient may have a cough or complain of throat pain.

III. Differential Diagnosis
A. Bloody NG Drainage
1. **Insertion trauma.** Usually nasopharyngeal.
2. **Mucosal irritation.** Often results from a tube that has been in place for > 48 hours; there is usually an associated acidic pH.
3. **Swallowed pharyngeal blood.** Posterior nosebleeds may not be clinically obvious.
4. **Suture line disruption or hemorrhage.** More likely in a patient who has had recent surgery.
5. **Gastric or duodenal ulceration.** More common in severely ill patients (eg, premature infants, burns, sepsis, head injury, steroid use, pancreatitis).
6. **Gastric erosion or gastritis, esophagitis or Mallory-Weiss tear, esophageal varices.** Mallory-Weiss tears are more frequent in patients who have had forceful vomiting or retching. Esophageal varices can result in severe GI bleeding.
7. **Aortoenteric fistula.** Severe GI bleeding; may be secondary to foreign body ingestion or occur after aortic surgery.
8. **Coagulopathy.**

B. Change in Output of NG Drainage
1. **Increased output**
   a. **Tip of tube distal to pylorus.** NG tube aspirates all biliary and pancreatic solutions, as well as gastric output.
   b. **Gastric outlet or small bowel obstruction.** NG tube can irritate the pylorus and create edema or a pyloric channel ulcer.

       c. **Surreptitious fluid ingestion.**
   2. **Decreased output**
       a. **Return of normal bowel motility and function.**
       b. **Obstructed or kinked tube.**
       c. **Medications.** Agents that improve motility and gastric emptying, such as metoclopramide.
       d. **Tip of tube in esophagus.** Above the GE junction or coiled in the esophagus.

IV. Database
A. Physical Exam Key Points
   1. **Vital signs.** Tachycardia, hypotension, hypoxemia, and fever are suggestive of substantial bleeding or sepsis, or both.
   2. **Mouth.** Check that tube is not kinked in the mouth or throat. Look for evidence of oral, nasal, or pharyngeal bleeding.
   3. **Abdomen.** Look for distention, tenderness, and peritoneal signs. Listen for bowel sounds. Absence of bowel sounds indicates obstruction. Distention occurs with ileus or obstruction.
   4. **Rectal exam.** Is stool present? Absence of stool may reflect an anatomic obstruction. Check stool for occult blood. Assess color and character of stool (normal versus melena versus fresh blood).
   5. **Tube.** Check patency and function by flushing with air or water. Check gastric fluid pH if tube is patent; pH < 4 promotes bleeding.

B. Laboratory Data
   1. **CBC with platelets.** Check for anemia as well as evidence of inflammation or infection.
   2. **PT and PTT.** Evaluates clotting ability.
   3. **Type and crossmatch.** For significant bleeding.
   4. **Amylase and lipase.** Screen for pancreatitis.
   5. **Blood cultures.** For fever, tachycardia.
   6. **Serum electrolytes.** Carefully monitor patient's hydration, as well as potassium and bicarbonate levels, during continuous suction.
   7. **NG aspirate.** A pH > 6 indicates use of antacids or H_2 blockers or that tip of the tube is distal to the pylorus.

C. Radiographic and Other Studies
   1. **Chest x-ray and abdominal obstruction series.** Look for free intraperitoneal air or obstruction. Mediastinal air suggests esophageal perforation. Upright chest x-ray may show a large stomach bubble, indicating poor gastric emptying. Check position of the tube. Upright and flat abdominal x-rays may show distended bowel, indicating ileus or obstruction.
   2. **Contrast swallow study.** To identify gastric outlet obstruction or partial small bowel obstruction, order a Gastrografin or dilute barium swallow study. Contrast should not be used in patients with ileus or complete obstruction.

V. Plan. First, determine stability of patient and whether bleeding, if present, is serious enough to require aggressive therapy. Determine if NG tube is functioning properly and is in correct position. **Note:** *Do not* reposition an NG tube without a full understanding of why the tube was placed and, if applicable, details of surgery performed.

A. Bloody NG Drainage

1. For serious upper GI bleeding, obtain IV access and start fluids. Hypotensive patients may require fluid and blood replacement. Transfer to ICU for careful monitoring.

2. Irrigate NG tube with room-temperature water. Avoid ice water lavage, which may contribute to tissue ischemia. Lavage probably will not stop bleeding but it can help clinician to assess status of bleeding. Lavage also clears the stomach of clots, making endoscopy more effective.

3. **Medical therapy.** Attempt to maintain gastric pH > 4. This may be accomplished by antacids, 0.5 mL/kg per dose (to maximum of 30 mL) every 2 hours. Vomiting patients may not tolerate antacids. Sucralfate, as a protective barrier, may be helpful. IV H_2 blockers or PPIs may also be helpful. IV somatostatin analogues have been useful in patients with severe upper GI bleeding.

4. Consider upper endoscopy when bleeding persists.

5. Presence of peritoneal signs or new, free intra-abdominal air requires emergency laparotomy.

B. Change in Output of NG Drainage

1. **Position.** Tube should be in the stomach without a kink.

2. **Function.** Sump tubes should whistle continuously on low suction. Most tubes need to be flushed with water (5–30 mL, depending on size of child) every 3–4 hours to maintain patency. Flush tube with 5–30 mL (depending on size of child) of air while auscultating over gastric area to determine its functioning and position.

3. **Increased output**

   a. **Poor gastric emptying (no obstruction).** Try metoclopramide, 0.1 mg/kg per dose to a maximum of 5 mg IV every 6 hours. Erythromycin can also be used.

   b. **Distal obstruction.** Continue NG suction; consider further evaluation or surgery, or both, to relieve obstruction.

   c. **Ileus.** Patience and a period of observation are necessary, especially if this occurs in the immediate postoperative period. Correct electrolyte abnormalities, including hypokalemia, with IV therapy. Continue NG suction. Look for an intra-abdominal abscess if ileus persists, especially if patient has fever.

4. **Decreased output**

   a. Correlate this return with physical exam and passage of flatus and stool. The latter usually indicates return of bowel function.

      b. Remove NG tube, if appropriate.

      c. Irrigate tube to clear it, or advance tube into the stomach if it is not positioned correctly.

VI. Problem Case Diagnosis. The 3-year-old boy who had bloody NG tube drainage after surgery for intussusception underwent gastric lavage, which revealed fresh blood and "coffee ground" residue. Hemoglobin remained stable. Stool was not grossly bloody and was negative for occult blood. ENT exam revealed a posterior nosebleed, arising from the nostril containing the NG tube.

VII. Teaching Pearl: Question. What type of intestinal obstruction usually cannot be relieved with NG suction?

VIII. Teaching Pearl: Answer. Patients with colonic obstruction and a competent ileocecal valve, or patients with a closed (or "blind") bowel loop obstruction are poorly decompressed by NG suction. If a patient on NG suction develops increased abdominal pain and distention along with worsening of bowel dilation on abdominal obstruction series, surgical intervention may be necessary.

REFERENCES

Glick MI. Intestinal obstruction. In: Snape WJ, ed. *Consultations in Gastroenterology.* Saunders, 1996:490–495.

Heitlinger LA, McClung HJ, Gastrointestinal hemorrhage. In: Wyllie R, Hyams JS, eds. *Pediatric Gastrointestinal Disease: Pathophysiology, Diagnosis, Management.* Saunders, 1999:64–72.

68. NECK SWELLING AND MASSES

  I. Problem. A 3-year-old girl has right-sided neck swelling.

 II. Immediate Questions

    A. Does patient have any pain? Pain suggests inflammation and may be seen with infectious causes of neck swelling, including isolated bacterial lymphadenitis and reactive adenopathy and lymphadenitis associated with other head and neck infections (eg, pharyngitis, gingivostomatitis, and peritonsillar, dental, and retropharyngeal abscesses). It is essential to ask about pain in young children because it may affect their overall activity and demeanor and interfere with oral intake.

    B. How long has swelling been present? Acute onset is seen with bacterial cervical lymphadenitis (most common cause of lymph node enlargement in children). Gradual onset is seen with atypical mycobacterial infection, tuberculosis, Epstein-Barr virus (EBV), cytomegalovirus (CMV), cat-scratch disease, reactive adenopathy, and malignancies. Intermittent swelling might be seen with congenital cystic lesions, such as thyroglossal duct and branchial cleft cysts. A solitary, swollen lymph node persisting more than 6–8 weeks raises suspicion of malignancy.

C. Has patient had a fever? Fever may be seen with viral and bacterial infections as well as malignancies and other inflammatory processes.

D. Has any redness been noted? Redness is seen with trauma and infections.

E. Is patient having difficulty swallowing? Difficulty swallowing secondary to pain and swelling may be seen with pharyngitis, and peritonsillar and retropharyngeal abscesses. Affected patients may have drooling from inability to swallow secretions, and decreased oral intake and dehydration.

F. What are associated symptoms? Sore throat, drooling, decreased oral intake, and neck stiffness may be seen with retropharyngeal abscess, peritonsillar abscess, and pharyngitis. Constitutional symptoms suggest an infectious, malignant, or other systemic etiology.

III. Differential Diagnosis

A. Cervical Lymphadenopathy. Any viral or bacterial infection in the head and neck may be associated with reactive cervical adenopathy that is often bilateral.

B. Acute Cervical Lymphadenitis With or Without Abscess. Typically unilateral; seen in any age group but more commonly in children aged 1–4 years. Group A β-hemolytic streptococcus and *Staphylococcus aureus* account for 80% of cases. Probably occurs as a result of bacteria from oropharynx and upper respiratory tract seeding the draining lymph nodes. Viral cervical adenitis is usually self-limited and bilateral. Unilateral, solitary cervical node enlargement may be present in 50–70% of patients with Kawasaki disease.

C. Chronic or Subacute Cervical Lymphadenitis

1. **Nontuberculous mycobacteria (*Mycobacterium avium-intracellulare scrofulaceum* [MAIS] complex).** Typically chronic, with symptoms lasting weeks or months, although it may also present acutely. Infection with MAIS complex occurs in young school-aged children and produces a mildly tender, erythematous, rubbery mass.

2. **Other causes of chronic lymphadenitis.** These include *Mycobacterium tuberculosis* and cat-scratch disease. Cat-scratch disease typically produces tenderness, erythema, warmth, and induration; history of contact with a cat or kitten is present in over 90% of cases.

3. **Parinaud oculoglandular syndrome.** Concurrent granulomatous conjunctivitis and ipsilateral preauricular or submandibular lymphadenopathy that is most often due to *Bartonella henselae* but also may be seen with tuberculosis, EBV infection, and syphilis.

D. Retropharyngeal Cellulitis or Abscess. Presents as a neck mass in up to 58% of patients and generally occurs in children younger than 5 years of age as an extension of nasopharyngeal and middle ear infections. Retropharyngeal abscesses are less common in older children and adolescents but may occur following penetrating trauma to the area. Bacterial agents involved in this infection include *Streptococcus pyogenes* (group A streptococcus), *S aureus, Haemophilus influenzae,* and anaerobes. Complications include airway compromise, sepsis, aspiration of abscess contents, and thrombophlebitis.

E. Congenital Cysts

    1. Branchial cleft cyst. Typically of second branchial cleft origin.

    2. Pyriform cysts. Very rare and always found in the left neck; may be mistaken for branchial cleft cysts.

    3. Thyroglossal duct cyst. Most common congenital neck mass; seen with a persistent thyroglossal duct, which is normally obliterated during fetal development. Typically, these midline lesions are diagnosed in children 2–10 years old.

F. Dermoid Cyst. May be found in the midline of the neck and mistaken for a thyroglossal duct cyst; contains sebaceous material, hair follicles, and connective tissues.

G. Cystic Hygroma. Benign, multiloculated, cystic, lymphatic malformation seen in 1 in 12,000 births. Majority of cases are diagnosed by age 3 years and usually the malformation grows as the child grows. Complications include infection, airway compromise, and extension into the mediastinum and chest. Other benign tumors include lipoma and hemangioma.

H. Torticollis

    1. Neonatal. Also known as fibromatosis coli or fibroma of the sternocleidomastoid muscle. May present as a fibrous mass in a 2- to 8 week-old infant with a head tilt; occurs as a result of collagen and fibrous tissue deposition around atrophied muscle fibers of the sternocleidomastoid muscle.

    2. Older children. Typically present with complaints of neck stiffness rather than neck mass.

I. Lymphoma (Hodgkin and non-Hodgkin), Rhabdomyosarcoma, and Other Malignant Tumors. Tend to be painless, solid, and fixed. Systemic symptoms may be present, but their absence should not rule out malignancy. In children 6 years of age or younger, the most commonly encountered tumors in the head and neck region include neuroblastoma, Hodgkin and non-Hodgkin lymphoma, and rhabdomyosarcoma. In older children, lymphoma, thyroid carcinoma, and rhabdomyosarcoma should be considered. Noninflammatory (tumoral) adenopathy may be seen in children with leukemia or lymphoma.

J. Uncommon Diagnoses

    1. Ludwig angina. Used to describe infection beginning at the floor of the mouth and rapidly spreading to involve bilateral sublingual and submandibular spaces without abscess formation or lymphatic involvement. Fever, drooling, neck stiffness, and swelling are typical.

2. **Lemierre syndrome.** Typically seen in adolescents and adults; refers to thrombophlebitis of the internal jugular vein, which is thought to occur as a result of oropharyngeal infection. Patients typically present with neck pain and swelling, fever, and rigors; infection is due to *Fusobacterium necrophorum,* bacteroides, and streptococcal and lactobacillus species.

3. **Kimura disease.** Rare, inflammatory disorder, typically seen in Asian males and characterized by painless unilateral cervical adenopathy or subcutaneous head and neck masses, eosinophilia, and elevated immunoglobulin E (IgE) levels.

IV. Database

A. Physical Exam Key Points.
Perform a complete physical exam to assess for generalized lymphadenopathy or hepatosplenomegaly, which would raise suspicion of systemic infection or malignancy.

1. **General appearance.** Determine if signs of respiratory distress (tachypnea, stridor, or wheezing) are present. Children with bacterial infections may appear quite ill and have fever and irritability. Some children with a retropharyngeal infection may present with torticollis or limited neck movement. Drooling is usually a sign of peritonsillar or retropharyngeal abscess but may be seen in other children with severe oropharyngeal pain.

2. **Quality of voice.** A "hot-potato" voice is seen with peritonsillar abscess, and a muffled voice may be seen with retropharyngeal cellulitis or abscess.

3. **Oropharynx.** Assess carefully and thoroughly to determine presence of ulcerations, gingivitis, pharyngeal irritation, tonsillar hypertrophy and exudate, and posterior pharyngeal bulging.

4. **External neck.** Check for a palpable mass. Familiarity with anatomic location of the anterior and posterior cervical and occipital nodes is crucial. Swelling along the lymph node chain may represent reactive adenopathy, lymphadenitis, lymph node abscess, or lymphoma. Branchial cleft cysts may present as fluctuant masses in the anterior neck along the sternocleidomastoid muscle; if infected, there may be erythema, warmth, and tenderness. Thyroglossal duct cysts are midline lesions that may be infected on presentation. Cystic hygromas are soft, nontender, and cystic, and are commonly found in the posterior triangle of the neck.

5. **Reexamination.** Essential to determine response to therapy, particularly in cases of suspected bacterial cervical lymphadenitis.

B. Laboratory Data

1. **CBC with differential.** May show an elevated WBC count in infectious processes, including cervical adenitis, retropharyngeal

abscess, and peritonsillar abscess. This test should also be performed if malignancy is suspected.

2. **Blood chemistries, including renal and hepatic function tests and urinalysis.** Perform if malignancy is suspected.

3. **Blood culture.** Can help guide antibiotic therapy if positive.

4. **Gram stain, aerobic and anaerobic cultures of abscess contents.** Obtained through needle aspiration or incision and drainage; may reveal causative agent in the diagnosis of acute cervical lymphadenitis or abscess and retropharyngeal abscess. Avoid if *M tuberculosis* is suspected (leads to chronic drainage).

5. **Purified protein derivative skin testing.** Recommended for children with subacute or chronic cervical lymphadenitis to rule out *M tuberculosis,* especially if risk factors are present or there is poor response to initial treatment.

6. **Other laboratory tests.** Depending on history and clinical suspicion, consider other tests, including *B henselae* and *B quintana* titers for cat-scratch disease, and Monospot and antibody titers for EBV. Warthin-Starry silver stain may be used to identify bacilli in cat-scratch disease, but this test is not specific for *B henselae.*

7. **Histopathologic evaluation of tissue.** Perform following excisional biopsies to determine if malignancy is present.

C. **Radiographic and Other Studies**

1. **Lateral neck X-ray.** Obtain during inspiration with patient's neck hyperextended. Widening of prevertebral soft tissues suggests retropharyngeal infection, although flexion and expiration may give false-positive results. An air-fluid level may be seen in some patients with retropharyngeal abscess.

2. **Ultrasonography.** Can be useful for soft, fluctuant masses (to differentiate lymphangiomas, hemangiomas, and lipomas) and suspected thyroglossal duct cyst (to identify presence or absence of normal thyroid tissue). Color-flow Doppler imaging is helpful to assess blood flow through certain lesions (eg, increased blood flow may be seen in tumoral lymphadenopathy). In fibromatosis coli, ultrasound will demonstrate an oval echogenic mass within the body of the sternocleidomastoid muscle.

3. **CT scan of neck with contrast or MRI scan.** May show inflammation in retropharyngeal cellulitis or a ring-enhancing abscess in patients with a cervical lymph node or retropharyngeal abscess, and helpful in distinguishing cellulitis from abscess. CT or MRI scans typically are used when malignancy is suspected.

IV. **Plan**

A. **General Management**

1. **Airway management.** Essential if the degree of neck swelling results in airway obstruction. Patients with severe airway

obstruction should be intubated and transferred to a pediatric ICU.

2. **Hydration.** Should be provided by IV fluids in patients unable to take oral fluids and in those who present with dehydration.

3. **Pain relief.** Pain should be treated with analgesics, such as acetaminophen and ibuprofen. If pain is severe, consider use of codeine or parenteral analgesics.

4. **Antibiotic therapy.** Used to treat cervical adenitis, retropharyngeal cellulitis and abscess, and peritonsillar abscess. Antibiotic selection should be based on the causative agents and generally includes use of one or more of the following: nafcillin, ampicillin, ampicillin-sulbactam, clindamycin, cefuroxime, and ceftriaxone. Improvement should be seen within 48 hours.

5. **Needle aspiration.** May be helpful in the treatment of fluctuant lesions, but avoid if mycobacterial infection is suspected. Needle aspiration may also be used in cat-scratch disease if lesions are particularly painful.

6. **Incision and drainage of cervical and retropharyngeal abscesses.** Generally performed by a trained pediatric otolaryngologist. Need for surgical drainage should be determined by the degree of respiratory compromise, patient's response to antibiotic therapy, and reaccumulation of fluid following needle aspiration (eg, with cervical abscesses). Gauze packing typically is used to allow for healing by secondary intention.

B. **Specific Management**

1. **Cervical lymphadenopathy.** Typically self-limited; provide reassurance.

2. **Acute cervical lymphadenitis.** Administer antibiotic therapy to prevent worsening of infection, including cellulitis and abscess formation. Antibiotic treatment should cover *Staphylococcus* and *Streptococcus.* Use a first-generation cephalosporin (eg, cephalexin) for 7–10 days. For ill-appearing or young children, consider IV antibiotics and inpatient hospitalization.

3. **Subacute or chronic lymphadenitis**
   a. **Atypical mycobacterium.** Treatment is complete excision of the affected lymph node if spontaneous resolution does not occur.
   b. **Infection due to *M tuberculosis.*** Administer antituberculous mediations for 9–12 months; clinical response should be seen by 3 months.
   c. **Cat-scratch disease.** Usually self-limited, with resolution after 2–4 weeks. Bactrim, rifampin, and ciprofloxacin are effective, but optimal therapy is not known and treatment is only uniformly recommended for immunocompromised hosts.

4. **Retropharyngeal abscess.** Requires hospitalization and IV antibiotics. If there are signs of airway compromise, or if there is lack of clinical response to IV antibiotics, intraoral or surgical

drainage may be necessary; this should be performed only by a trained otolaryngologist.

5. **Branchial cleft cyst.** Surgical excision should be performed shortly after diagnosis and when infection (if any) has resolved. Recurrent infection is common. Infected cysts require antibiotic treatment and warm compresses.

6. **Thyroglossal duct cyst.** Treatment is complete surgical excision of uninfected lesions. If infected, treatment includes warm compresses, antibiotic treatment, and, at times, incision and drainage.

7. **Dermoid cyst.** Treatment is surgical excision.

8. **Cystic hygroma.** Rarely regress spontaneously, and surgical excision is recommended. Some cystic hygromas are so complex that surgical excision is not an option; sclerosing agents, such as bleomycin and OK-432, may be helpful in these cases.

9. **Neonatal torticollis.** Treatment includes range-of-motion exercises and other physical therapy. If facial asymmetry occurs, surgical intervention may be necessary.

10. **Lymphoma (Hodgkin and non-Hodgkin), rhabdomyosarcoma, and other malignant tumors.** Consultation with a pediatric oncologist is necessary for management and treatment of these diagnoses.

11. **Uncommon diagnoses.** Ludwig angina and Lemierre syndrome occur as a result of bacterial infection and must be treated with IV antibiotics appropriate to pathogens mentioned earlier. In Lemierre syndrome, anticoagulation therapy with heparin is recommended, particularly if extensive thrombosis occurs. Kimura disease is often diagnosed based on surgical biopsy. Although excision may be curative, lesions may recur.

V. **Problem Case Diagnosis.** The 3-year-old girl had bacterial cervical adenitis, causing pain, swelling, tenderness and erythema. Because of the extent of infection, she was admitted. IV antibiotics were provided, and patient showed clinical improvement after 48 hours.

VI. **Teaching Pearl: Question.** An anterior neck mass moves up and down during swallowing and with protrusion of the tongue. What lesion does this suggest, and why?

VII. **Teaching Pearl: Answer.** A thyroglossal duct cyst; during fetal development, the thyroid diverticulum descends along the anterior neck from the base of the tongue, forming the thyroid gland in the anterior neck. In normal development, the thyroglossal duct is obliterated; however, in some individuals the duct persists and results in the formation of a cyst or sinus.

REFERENCES

Brown RL, Azizkhan RG. Pediatric head and neck lesions. *Pediatr Clin North Am* 1998;889–905.

Elden LM, Grundfast KM, Vezina G. Accuracy and usefulness of radiographic assessment of cervical neck infections in children. *J Otolaryngol* 2001;30:82–89.

Lee SS, Schwartz RH, Bahadori RS. Retropharyngeal abscess: Epiglottitis of the new millennium. *J Pediatr* 2001;138:435–437.

Long SS, ed. *Principles and Practice of Pediatric Infectious Diseases,* 2nd ed. Churchill Livingstone, 2003:161–162, 170, 494.

Swischuk LE, John SD. Neck masses in infants and children. *Radiol Clin North Am* 1997;35:1329–1340.

69. NUTRITION IN THE PEDIATRIC PATIENT

I. **Problem.** A 1-year-old male infant with severe failure to thrive is brought to the clinic by his parents. The infant, who was born full term after an uncomplicated pregnancy, initially did well on breast milk. At 3 months of age, he was switched to cow's milk–based formula. Infant cereal was started at 4 months of age, with fruits and vegetables. There has been no excessive vomiting. Stools are slightly loose, not oily or grossly bloody, yet intermittently contain mucus. There is no history of chronic fevers. The infant has a dry rash on the malar surfaces. His weight curve began to drift at 6 months of age; length remained steady until 2 months ago.

II. **Immediate Questions**

A. **Does patient have problems with feeding, swallowing, or choking?** These problems may suggest gastroesophageal reflux, swallowing dysfunction, congenital abnormalities, or inappropriate feeding practices.

B. **How much does patient ingest orally in a 24-hour period?** Using the term *daytime* may cause parents or other caretakers to underestimate child's total caloric intake.

C. **If an infant, how does parent mix formula?** Distinguish formula preparation (ready-to-feed, concentrate, or powder). Check recipe for caloric density.

D. **Does water used for mixing formula come from a well?** Well water may be a source of an infectious agent (eg, *Giardia*).

E. **Is there a family history of food allergies, cystic fibrosis, or metabolic disease?** These conditions may be associated with malabsorption and poor weight gain.

F. **Are there associated symptoms?** For example, cyanosis may suggest cardiac disease; diarrhea suggests infection, malabsorption, or food allergy.

III. **Differential Diagnosis**

A. **Inadequate Intake.** May result from a swallowing problem, formula mixing error, lack of access to formula or other foods due to limited finances, inappropriate substitution of other liquids (eg, juice) for formula, or neglect.

B. **Excessive Losses Due to Diarrhea.** Consider infectious agents (bacterial, *Giardia*), HIV, cystic fibrosis, or inflammation due to food allergies.

C. **Increased Needs Due to Hypermetabolism or Increased Work of Breathing.** Consider cystic fibrosis, hyperthyroidism, and cardiac disease.

D. **Metabolic or Genetic Abnormalities.** Consider inborn errors of metabolism and chromosomal abnormalities.

IV. Database

A. **Physical Exam Key Points**

1. **Growth charts.** With chronic inadequate calories and nutrients, patient's weight drifts first, then height falls off the curve, and finally head circumference. It is important to evaluate weight-for-height, a measure of body leanness, or the body mass index (BMI = weight in kg × height in meters squared). It is critical to obtain accurate and consistent measurements with nude weights of all infants and toddlers, and weight in underpants or gown in older children.

2. **Head circumference.** Measure in children until 24–36 months.

3. **Abdomen.** May be distended and full of gas in malnourished children, particularly if they are malabsorbing nutrients.

4. **Musculoskeletal system.** Check for muscle wasting in extremities and buttocks.

5. **Anthropometrics.** Tests such as skinfold thickness evaluate body energy stores; midarm muscle circumference evaluates lean body stores when compared with norms.

6. **Other findings.** Other signs of malnutrition and nutrient deficiency include sparse, dry, pluckable hair; dry scaly skin; red and swollen gums or tongue; cheilosis; diaper rash; and pale or spoon-shaped nail beds. Advanced vitamin deficiencies may lead to neurologic symptoms such as ataxia and dementia.

B. **Laboratory Data.** Should be guided by history and physical exam findings.

1. **CBC with differential.** To assess for anemia, evaluate lymphocyte (HIV) and eosinophil (allergy) counts.

2. **Albumin and visceral proteins.** Albumin is somewhat useful for assessing chronic protein depletion. Its half-life is 18–20 days; affected by stress, infection, nephrosis, colitis or overhydration. Serum levels of visceral proteins (prealbumin, transferrin, and retinol-binding protein) with shorter half-lives are more sensitive indicators than albumin.

3. **Other workup.** Complete metabolic panel with liver and kidney function tests plus electrolytes, thyroid function studies, celiac panel, immunoglobulins, and sweat test (cystic fibrosis) may be indicated.

C. **Radiographic and Other Studies**

1. **Radiographic tests.** Based on clinical findings.

2. **Calculations of energy needs.** Estimate kilocalorie needs using formulas designed for children. The World Health

TABLE I–14. WORLD HEALTH ORGANIZATION PEDIATRIC FORMULA TO PREDICT RESTING ENERGY EXPENDITURE (REE)

Age	Male	Female
0–3 y	$(60.9 \times$ wt in kg$) - 54$	$(61 \times$ wt in kg$) - 51$
3–10 y	$(22.7 \times$ wt in kg$) + 495$	$(22.5 \times$ wt in kg$) + 499$
10–18 y	$(17.5 \times$ wt in kg$) + 651$	$(12.2 \times$ wt in kg$) + 746$

wt = weight.

Organization pediatric formula to predict resting energy expenditure (REE) is provided in Table I–14. The REE value is multiplied by factors to predict estimated kilocalorie needs, as shown in Table I–15.

V. Plan

A. Initial Management. Evaluate height, weight, weight-for-height, vital signs, and signs of dehydration. If patient is dehydrated or severely malnourished, hospital admission may be advisable. Goals of nutrition support must be delineated. Calculate child's energy needs. Can patient be enterally fed? If so, with what solids or formula products, and by which route?

B. Enteral Nutrition. Can be delivered by mouth; nasogastric, nasoduodenal, or nasojejunal tube; or gastric or jejunal tube.

1. Infant formulas (Table I–16). Typically provide 20 kcal/oz, mimicking breast milk. Most infants tolerate either cow's milk–based or soy-based formulas. There are hypoallergenic products in which the proteins have been broken down into peptides (Nutramigen, Pregestimil, Alimentum). Children with severe allergies may require products with free amino acids (Neocate, Elecare). Many specialized products for metabolic

TABLE I–15. ESTIMATION OF KILOCALORIE NEEDS USING RESTING ENERGY EXPENDITURE (REE) VALUE

Estimated Kcal Needs	Patient Considerations
REE × 1.0–1.1	Well-nourished child, or child who is sedated on ventilator; ECMO; minimal stress
REE × 1.3	Well-nourished child with decreased activity or minor surgery
REE × 1.5	Ambulatory child with mild-to-moderate stress; inactive child with sepsis, cancer, trauma, or extensive surgery; minimally active child with malnutrition and catch-up growth needs
REE × 1.7	Active child with catch-up growth requirement; active child with severe stress

ECMO = extracorporeal membrane oxygenation.

TABLE I–16. GENERAL CONTENTS OF COMMONLY USED FORMULAS

Formula	Lactose	Protein	Medium-Chain Triglycerides
■ **COW'S MILK—BASED**			
Enfamil	Yes	Whey	No
Similac	Yes	Casein	No
■ **SOY-BASED**			
Isomil	No	Soy	No
ProSobee	No	Soy	No
■ **HYPOALLERGENIC**			
Nutramigen	No	Amino acid hydrolysate (AAH)	No
Alimentum	No	AAH	Yes
Pregestimil	No	AAH	Yes

diseases are also available. Children with fat malabsorption (cystic fibrosis or cholestatic liver disease) should be given formulas with a high percentage of fat as medium-chain triglycerides (Pregestimil, Alimentum).

2. **Formulas for children older than 1 year.** Primarily provide 30 kcal/oz; designed as a meal replacement and available as low-osmolality, low-lactose products. Hypoallergenic formulas contain either peptides or free amino acids. Many formulas have modified fat, protein, or carbohydrate content targeting special disease states. Properties such as the osmolality of the product will affect its tolerance and rate of delivery. Hypoallergenic products are often unpalatable and may require tube feeding. Generally the more specialized the product, the higher is the cost.

C. **Parenteral Nutrition Support.** May be necessary if oral or enteral feeding is not feasible or tolerated.

1. **Peripheral intravenous nutrition.** Limited by osmolality of solution. In general, do not give > 10% dextrose solution with 2% amino acids. Higher concentrations cause frequent infiltration of IV fluid. Lipid solutions are well tolerated in peripheral IV lines and may significantly increase delivered kilocalories.

2. **Central line parenteral nutrition.** Should be written by a trained health care provider for safety and optimization of nutrient content. Complications include infection, hyperglycemia, and long-term issues such as hepatic steatosis and cirrhosis.

VI. **Problem Case Diagnosis.** The 1-year-old patient had celiac disease, diagnosed by serum antibody panel and duodenal biopsies. Growth failure after introduction to solid foods is a classic sign of either celiac disease or food allergy. Patient's growth improved with removal of the offending protein (gluten).

VII. Teaching Pearl: Question. Why can electrolyte imbalances occur when refeeding a severely malnourished child?

VIII. Teaching Pearl: Answer. Watch for refeeding syndrome when repleting a malnourished child. Severely malnourished children should be fed approximately 50% of estimated kilocalorie needs, and advanced slowly over several days with daily monitoring of serum electrolytes, especially potassium, phosphorus, calcium, and magnesium, to avoid cardiac instability.

REFERENCES

Duggan C. Nutritional assessment and requirements. In: Walker WA, Durie PR, Hamilton JR, eds. *Pediatric Gastrointestinal Disease: Pathophysiology, Diagnosis and Management.* Decker, 2000:1691–1703.

Gunn VL, Nechyba C, eds. *The Harriet Lane Handbook.* Mosby, 2002.

Olsen IE, Mascarenhas MR, Stallings VA. Clinical assessment of nutritional status. In: Walker WA, Watkins JB, Duggan C, eds. *Nutrition in Pediatrics.* Decker, 2003:6–16.

Shulman RJ, Phillips S. Parenteral nutrition in infants and children. *J Pediatr Gastroenterol Nutr* 2003;36:587–607.

70. PAIN MANAGEMENT

I. Problem. A 10-year-old boy with a history of sickle cell disease presents to the emergency department with acute pain in both lower extremities and in his right arm. The pain started suddenly 3 hours ago.

II. Immediate Questions

  A. How does patient characterize the pain? Is it acute? If recurrent, how frequent are the acute painful episodes? How many times has patient sought medical attention for pain in the past year? How often has patient required hospitalization for painful episodes? Have painful episodes been managed with oral or parental therapies? What has been the typical frequency and duration of painful episodes?

  B. Is this episode similar to previous episodes? If a patient describes the pain as being different, it should raise suspicion of a different etiology of the pain. Most patients with chronic pain, such as that caused by sickle cell crisis or disease, are able to recognize their typical painful episode.

  C. What medication, if any, has been tried? Is patient taking pain medication(s) at home (prescription or over-the-counter)? What dose and for how long? Is pain medication effective? What medications have worked in the past? This information gives clinician a starting point for ascertaining how well the pain is typically controlled and which analgesics to start with in current treatment. Chronic or recurrent opioid therapy leads to opioid tolerance, requiring usually higher doses to attain pain relief.

D. Pain Assessment

1. **Can patient identify characteristics of the pain (stabbing, shooting, throbbing, aching, burning)?** Determine the intensity of each site of pain using an appropriate validated pain scale; self-report is preferred. Behavioral-observational pain scales are used for preverbal or neurologically impaired children.

2. **When did this painful crisis begin? Can patient identify any aggravating or alleviating factors? Has pain limited patient's ability to function (sleep, eat, go to school)?** Breakthrough painful episodes in children with sickle cell disease are treated as acute pain. Because of the recurring and life-long nature of this pain, however, principles of chronic pain management are also necessary, such as behavioral-cognitive, psychological, and physical modalities.

E. Are there any precipitating factors? Fever, dehydration, hypoxemia, stress, and fatigue are common precipitating factors of pain in patients with sickle cell disease.

III. Differential Diagnosis.
There is a broad differential diagnosis of pain in children. For example, sources of pain in patients with sickle cell disease include vasoocclusion caused by the sickling process, osteomyelitis, avascular necrosis, trauma, tumor, and somatization disorder. This chapter is not intended to provide a review of the medical management of sickle cell disease, but rather a focused discussion of acute pain management. See Table I–17 for definitions of terms relating to pain and dependency.

IV. Database
A. Physical Exam Key Points

TABLE I–17. TERMINOLOGY RELATING TO PAIN AND DEPENDENCY

Term	Definitions
Somatic pain	Nociceptive pain from skin, bones, joints, ligaments, and muscle
Visceral pain	Pain from nerve endings in viscera responding mostly to stretch; often referred to other areas of body
Neuropathic pain	Pain from nerve injury, compression, or disease; in central or peripheral nervous system
Tolerance	Decreased analgesic effect, or need to increase opioid dosage to maintain same analgesic effect
	Tolerance develops at different rates and is dependent on drug, dosage, frequency, and duration
Physiologic dependence	Need to continue medication administration to prevent signs or symptoms of physical withdrawal
Psychological dependence or addiction	Compulsive drug use characterized by continued drug craving and need to use opioids for effects other than pain relief

1. **Vital signs.** Tachycardia and tachypnea may occur with pain, or they may indicate other diseases such as infection.
2. **Hydration status.** Dehydration precipitates pain in sickle cell disease.
3. **Chest.** Listen for crackles and observe for cyanosis or other signs of infection. Consider the chest as a source of pain, particularly in patients with sickle cell disease (acute chest syndrome, pneumonia).
4. **Abdomen.** Evaluate as a source of pain. Examine for tenderness, guarding, or rigidity.
5. **Neurologic exam.** Observe mental status, and assess ease with which patient can be distracted from the pain.
6. **Extremities.** Look for localized tenderness, decreased range of motion, deformities, areas of erythema, warmth, and swelling.

B. **Laboratory Data.** Consider infection; obtain CBC with differential, C-reactive protein, ESR, blood culture, and urinalysis, if febrile.

C. **Radiographic and Other Studies.** Studies are based on the location, quality, and intensity of pain. In a patient with sickle cell disease, consider obtaining a chest X-ray if acute chest syndrome is suspected or plain X-rays of extremities if warranted. Focal abdominal pain often warrants an ultrasound.

V. **Plan**

A. **Opioid Use for Moderate to Severe Pain.** Consider opioids (IV versus oral), if severe pain. Tailor analgesic regimen to meet patient's needs (Table I–18).

1. For moderate to severe pain, start treatment with IV morphine. Patient may require repeated doses every 15–30 minutes, titrated to achieve pain relief. Patients on home oral opioids may be opioid tolerant and require higher doses of morphine (1.5–2 times or more standard starting dose); titrate dose by assessing between each dose.

2. If patient is unable to tolerate morphine due to adverse effects, hydromorphone is an alternative. When switching from one

TABLE I–18. OPIOID DOSING FOR PAIN IN INFANTS, CHILDREN, AND ADOLESCENTS

Opioid Drug	Parenteral Dosing Range	Oral Dosing Range
Morphine	0.05–0.1 mg/kg q3–4h	0.15–0.3 mg/kg q3–4h
Hydromorphone	0.01 mg/kg q3–4h	0.05 mg/kg q3–4h
Fentanyl	0.5–1.5 mcg/kg q30min	NA
Oxycodone	NA	0.1–0.2 mg/kg q3–4h
Codeine	NA	0.5–1 mg/kg q3–4h

NA = not applicable.

opioid to another, decrease dose of new opioid because tolerance to the new opioid may be less.

3. Avoid meperidine in patients with sickle cell disease, renal failure, or renal disease. Accumulation of normeperidine metabolite may precipitate seizures.

4. If patient experiences adequate pain relief with 1–2 doses of IV
opioids, consider giving acetaminophen-codeine or acetamin-
ophen-oxycodone every 4 hours. Oxycodone alone may be
used if there is concern over total acetaminophen dose.

5. Oral route is preferred whenever possible, unless patient is
unable to take oral medication or pain is severe enough to
require rapid management.

6. If multiple doses of IV opioids are needed to achieve pain relief,
initiate IV morphine or hydromorphone around-the-clock or
start patient-controlled analgesia (PCA), if patient is cognitive-
ly, developmentally, and physically able to manage.

B. PCA. Consider intermittent PCA versus intermittent PCA plus
basal infusion (Table I–19).

1. PCA allows patients to self-titrate to an acceptable level of
comfort, giving them some control in their care. Children with
sickle cell disease who are known to be opioid tolerant will
need a larger PCA intermittent dose to obtain analgesia.

2. A low-dose basal infusion given with PCA helps maintain analgesia during sleep, minimizing patient waking due to severe
pain. Opioid-tolerant patients handle basal infusions well, but
use caution in opioid-naïve patients because the basal infusion
bypasses the inherent safety mechanism that occurs when an
awake patient titrates his or her analgesia. See Table I–19 for
PCA dosing guidelines.

C. Conversion to Oral Opioids (Table I–20). Remember when converting oral to parenteral opioid administration, or vice versa, that
lower parental narcotic doses are required compared with oral
doses. It is important that patients receive adequate oral opioid
doses to maintain analgesia after discharge. Codeine is a relatively weak opioid, and between 4% and 12% of patients lack the
enzyme that converts codeine to morphine, which is the source of

TABLE I–19. PCA DOSING FOR OPIOID-NAÏVE PATIENTS WITH PAIN (INFANTS, CHILDREN, AND ADOLESCENTS)

Opioid	PCA Dose	Lockout Time	Basal Rate[a]	1-Hour Maximum
Morphine	0.02 mg/kg	6–12 min	0–0.02 mg/kg/h	0.1 mg/kg
Hydromorphone	0.003–0.004 mg/kg	6–12 min	0.003–0.004 mg/kg/h	0.02 mg/kg
Fentanyl	0.5 mcg/kg	6–12 min	0–0.5 mcg/kg/h	2.5 mcg/kg

PCA = patient-controlled analgesia.
[a] As continuous infusion.

TABLE I-20. COMPARISON OF NARCOTIC ANALGESICS USED FOR PAIN IN INFANTS, CHILDREN, AND ADOLESCENTS

Analgesic	IV Equianalgesic Comparison (mg)	PO Equianalgesic Comparison (mg)	Parenteral Oral Ratio
Morphine	10	30	1:3
Hydromorphone	1.5	7.5	1:5
Fentanyl	0.1–0.2	NA	NA
Codeine	NA	200	NA
Oxycodone	NA	30	NA

NA = not applicable.

the analgesic effect. Oxycodone or hydrocodone may be better alternatives. Around-the-clock dosing of oral opioids is preferred over prn.

D. Management of Opioid Side Effects. Respiratory depression is a serious and important side effect of opioid administration. Ensure appropriate clinical monitoring and assessment. Have naloxone available. Be prepared to manage opioid-induced side effects promptly with antiemetics, antipruritics, and laxatives or stool softeners.

E. Adjuvant Analgesics

  1. NSAIDs. An important mainstay and first step adjunct in management of pain, NSAIDs are used in many painful disorders (eg, juvenile rheumatoid arthritis, but not as extensively in sickle cell disease). Monitor for side effects.

  2. Tricyclic antidepressants. Used for analgesia and sleep in chronic pain situations; not for acute pain management.

  3. Anticonvulsants. Carbamazepine and gabapentin; used for neuropathic pain.

  4. Anxiolytics. Benzodiazepines; use for anxiety and not as a substitute for opioids.

  5. Other medications. Stimulants, SSRIs, steroids, topical patches, and α_2-blockers are valuable adjuvants in many situations, but not in acute pain.

  6. Epidural analgesia. Specialized technique, and only indicated when pain is severe and refractory to oral and parenteral analgesics.

F. Nonpharmacologic Modalities. These methods can be very important in long-term management of recurring pain in conditions such as sickle cell disease. Include behavioral (eg, biofeedback, deep breathing), psychological (eg, distraction, hypnosis education), and physical (hydration, physical therapy) modalities.

VI. Problem Case Diagnosis. This patient was experiencing an acute breakthrough pain episode from sickle cell disease. Because oral opioids had been used at home, hydration and pain management were given intravenously to control symptoms.

VII. Teaching Pearl: Question. Are patients with sickle cell disease more likely to become addicted to opioids because of their frequent need for opioid analgesia?

VIII. Teaching Pearl: Answer. No; patients on opioids may become tolerant to opioids and require gradual weaning to avoid opioid withdrawal (no more than 20% dose reduction per day). Opioid addiction is a psychological dependence on opioids that is unrelated to pain.

REFERENCES

Benjamin LJ, Dampier CD, Jacox AK, et al. *Guideline for the Management of Acute and Chronic Pain in Sickle Cell Disease.* American Pain Society, 1999.

Dampier C, Shapiro BS. Management of pain in sickle cell disease. In: Schecter NL, Berde CB, Yaster M, eds. *Pain in Infants, Children, and Adolescents.* Lippincott Williams & Wilkins, 2003:489–516.

Finley GA, McGrath PJ, eds. *Acute and Procedure Pain in Infants and Children.* IASP Press, 2001. *Progress in Pain Research and Management;* vol 20.

Latta KS, Ginsberg B, Barkin R. Meperidine: A critical review. *Am J Therapeut* 2002;9:53–68.

Schechter NL, Berde CB, Yaster M, eds. *Pain in Infants, Children, and Adolescents.* Lippincott Williams & Wilkins, 2003.

71. PHARYNGITIS

I. Problem. An 8-year-old boy presents with fever and sore throat. Over the past several days he has had progressive difficulty swallowing and difficulty opening his mouth.

II. Immediate Questions

   A. What are the vital signs? Fever and tachycardia are common to many conditions included in the differential diagnosis, but associated hypotension may signify sepsis or group A β-hemolytic streptococcal (GABHS) toxic shock syndrome. Significant tachypnea and respiratory distress can be associated with upper airway obstruction from enlarged tonsils, deep neck abscesses, epiglottitis, and bacterial tracheitis.

   B. How old is patient? Different pediatric diseases are more common in children of different ages. Group A streptococcal pharyngitis is more prevalent between ages 5 and 15 years; retropharyngeal abscesses are rare after the age of 5 years because the retropharyngeal nodes involute.

   C. What is respiratory status and patient position? Patients with upper airway obstruction often sit in the tripod and sniffing position to alleviate compression of the trachea.

   D. Was there a preceding illness? Deep neck abscesses often follow nonspecific mild upper respiratory illnesses. Bacterial tracheitis usually follows croup.

E. Has patient been immunized? *Haemophilus influenzae* type b (Hib) immunization, and patient age in this case, makes epiglottitis unlikely.

III. Differential Diagnosis

A. Pharyngitis

1. **GABHS.** Patient presents with fever, sore throat, and tender cervical adenopathy. Headache, nausea, vomiting, and abdominal pain are common. Marked erythema of throat is present, with hyperemic, exudative tonsils and palatal petechiae. Nasal congestion and rhinorrhea is usually absent. More common in late winter and early spring.

2. **Epstein-Barr virus (EBV).** Can cause severe exudative pharyngitis with fever, palatal petechiae, posterior cervical lymphadenopathy, periorbital edema, and splenomegaly. Coinfection with GABHS is common.

3. **Adenovirus.** Commonly causes exudative pharyngitis or pharyngoconjunctival fever. Ipsilateral preauricular adenopathy is a helpful clue to diagnosis.

4. **Coxsackievirus.** Typically occurs in summer and early fall. Causes herpangina with multiple small vesicles on tonsils and soft palate. Coxsackievirus A16 causes so-called hand-foot-mouth disease, characterized by small ulcers on tongue and buccal mucosa, and vesicles on hands, feet, and occasionally buttocks.

5. **Herpes simplex virus (HSV).** Can cause pharyngitis with fever and lymphadenopathy or severe gingivostomatitis in young children.

6. **Other causes.** The most common viral cause of pharyngitis is rhinovirus (approximately 20%). Coronavirus, influenza, parainfluenza, and cytomegalovirus are other viral causes. Patients with HIV acute retroviral syndrome often present with sore throat, fever, lymphadenopathy, lethargy, and nonexudative tonsillitis. Other bacterial causes include mycoplasma, *Neisseria gonorrhea,* and *Chlamydia pneumoniae.*

B. Retropharyngeal Abscess.
Insidious onset of fever, dysphagia, and neck stiffness follows mild upper respiratory infection. Signs of upper airway obstruction may be present if abscess is compressing trachea. Most common in children younger than 2 years (50%); rare in children older than 5 years (because retropharyngeal nodes involute).

C. Lateral Neck or Parapharyngeal Abscess.
Occurs in later childhood; patient presents with fever, throat pain, and trismus if anterior compartment is involved. Posterior compartment contains cranial nerves IX through XII, carotid artery, and cervical sympathetic trunk. Infection in this area, although uncommon, can affect all of these structures.

D. **Peritonsillar Abscess.** The most common deep neck infection in children. Occurs in older children and younger adolescents. Initial presentation is fever and sore throat followed by gradual onset of dysphagia, dysphonia ("hot-potato" voice), drooling, and unilateral focus to the pain. Trismus (due to an inflamed pterygoid muscle) is often present and may be a helpful clue. Uvula deviates to contralateral side.

E. **Epiglottitis.** Has become rare since development of Hib vaccine. Patient presents with fairly rapid onset of fever, sore throat, odynophagia, and drooling, which progresses to respiratory distress from upper airway obstruction. Most common in children between ages 2 and 6 years.

F. **Bacterial Tracheitis.** Rapid onset of high fever, worsening stridor, and respiratory distress following viral laryngotracheitis. Usually caused by *Staphylococcus aureus*. Most common in children between ages 4 and 6 years.

IV. Database
A. Physical Exam Key Points
1. **Vital signs.** Fever and tachycardia are common to all conditions in differential diagnosis, but presence of hypotension may signify sepsis or toxic shock syndrome. Significant respiratory distress can be associated with upper airway obstruction from enlarged tonsils, deep neck abscesses, epiglottitis, and bacterial tracheitis.

2. **HEENT.** Enlarged, erythematous, exudative or nonexudative tonsils and an erythematous pharynx are fairly nonspecific findings when attempting to identify causative organism of pharyngitis. Drooling may be noted with any infection that causes dysphagia. Palatal petechiae are often associated with GABHS and EBV. Coxsackievirus often causes small ulcers on soft palate and buccal mucosa. HSV causes vesicles and ulcers on lips and gingival mucosa. Asymmetric tonsillar enlargement and a deviated uvula are present with peritonsillar abscesses. Posterior pharyngeal fullness and fluctuance may be noted with retropharyngeal abscess. Trismus may be noted with lateral neck or peritonsillar abscesses.

3. **Neck.** Tender anterior cervical lymphadenopathy is often present with GABHS pharyngitis. Posterior cervical nodes are often present with EBV. A preauricular node ipsilateral to the side of conjunctivitis is a clue to adenovirus. Asymmetric neck fullness may be felt with lateral pharyngeal infections. Torticollis is often present with retropharyngeal abscesses or peritonsillar abscess.

4. **Skin.** Sandpaper or scarlatiniform rash may be noted with GABHS scarlet fever. Nonspecific morbilliform rash can occur after amoxicillin is given to a patient with EBV. Erythroderma may signify toxin-mediated disease.

      5. Abdomen. Splenomegaly is associated with EBV.
- **B. Laboratory Data**
    1. **Rapid streptococcal antigen and throat culture.** Perform on patients with a stable airway who have fever and pharyngitis. It is important to diagnose GABHS pharyngitis due to numerous suppurative (deep neck abscesses) and nonsuppurative (see VIII, Teaching Pearl: Answer, later) complications. Obtain throat culture if rapid antigen test is negative, because reported sensitivities of some rapid streptococcal tests are as low as 60%.
    2. **CBC.** Elevated WBC count with predominance of neutrophils suggests bacterial infection. Atypical lymphocytosis suggests EBV or CMV.
    3. **ESR and C-reactive protein.** Marked elevation suggests bacterial process.
    4. **Blood culture.** Obtain if invasive or toxin-mediated disease is suspected.
    5. **Other workup.** Obtain culture and Gram stain of an abscess if surgical therapy is warranted.
- **C. Radiographic and Other Studies**
    1. **Neck x-ray.** Widening of prevertebral soft tissue space may be seen with retropharyngeal abscess. Width of prevertebral soft tissue space at fourth vertebrae should be less than half the width of vertebral body. Be sure patient's neck is in full extension for lateral neck film to avoid an increase in false-positive readings for retropharyngeal abscesses. Neck films can also identify the so-called thumbprint sign of an edematous epiglottis in epiglottitis and "shaggy-looking" trachea in bacterial tracheitis.
    2. **CT scan of neck.** Diagnostic test of choice for retropharyngeal and lateral neck abscesses.

V. Plan. Tempo of diagnostic evaluation and treatment should be dictated by severity of patient's illness. If clinician suspects epiglottitis or if patient is in severe respiratory distress, *do not* compromise airway by examining oropharynx or *do not* send patient for radiographs before securing airway. Patients with significant respiratory distress regardless of cause may need endotracheal intubation.
- **A. Pharyngitis**
    1. Treatment for GABHS pharyngitis is 10 days of penicillin or amoxicillin. Supportive care is the mainstay of therapy for viral pharyngitis.
    2. Patients with HSV or coxsackievirus infections may need IV hydration due to oropharyngeal pain.
    3. Patients with EBV and acute airway obstruction may benefit from steroids. Those with EBV infections and splenomegaly should avoid contact sports.
- **B. Retropharyngeal Abscess**

   1. Treatment consists of antibiotic coverage against the most common pathogens and, usually, surgical drainage. Most abscesses are polymicrobial and contain a combination of GABHS, anaerobic bacteria, and *S aureus*. Less common pathogens include Hib, *Klebsiella pneumoniae,* and *Streptococcus pneumoniae.*

   2. Combination therapy with clindamycin and a third-generation cephalosporin or single therapy using ampicillin-sulbactam is an excellent choice for initial coverage. Further therapy should be guided by sensitivities of organism(s) obtained on culture.

C. Lateral Neck or Pharyngeal Abscess. Treatment consists of antibiotic coverage against the most common pathogens (see preceding discussion). Surgical therapy is dictated by size of the abscess and space involved.

D. Peritonsillar Abscess. Almost always caused by GABHS or oral anaerobes, or both. Penicillin is the drug of choice; clindamycin is an alternative. Surgical intervention with needle aspiration, incision, and drainage, or tonsillectomy may be necessary.

E. Epiglottitis. Endotracheal intubation is frequently necessary, and IV antibiotic therapy should target Hib. Use third-generation cephalosporin or ampicillin-sulbactam because of increasing ampicillin resistance of *H influenzae. S aureus, S pneumoniae,* and GABHS are occasionally isolated.

F. Bacterial Tracheitis. Endotracheal intubation is frequently necessary, and antibiotic therapy should target *S aureus*, GABHS, *Moraxella catarrhalis,* and *S pneumoniae.*

VI. Problem Case Diagnosis. On physical examination, the 8-year-old boy had asymmetric peritonsillar tissue with displacement of the uvula to the right. CT exam confirmed the diagnosis of peritonsillar abscess.

VII. Teaching Pearl: Question. What are three nonsuppurative complications of GABHS pharyngitis?

VIII. Teaching Pearl: Answer. Acute rheumatic fever, poststreptococcal glomerulonephritis, and toxin-mediated disease (GABHS toxic shock syndrome).

REFERENCES

Bisno AL. Primary care: Acute pharyngitis. *N Engl J Med* 2001;344:205–211.

Bisno AL, Gerber MA, Gwaltney JM, et al. Diagnosis and management of group A streptococcal pharyngitis: A practice guideline. *Clin Infect Dis* 1997;25:574–583.

Middleton DB. Community acquired respiratory infections in children: Pharyngitis. *Prim Care* 1996;23:719–739.

Nicklaus PJ, Kelley PE. Pediatric otolaryngology: Management of deep neck infection. *Pediatr Clin North Am* 1996;43:1277–1296.

72. PHLEBITIS

I. **Problem.** A 3-year-old girl is hospitalized with pyelonephritis. On day 4 after admission, she develops pain and erythema at the site of the IV catheter.

II. **Immediate Questions**

  A. **What are vital signs?** Fever and tachycardia, with or without hypotension, can indicate infectious cause. Persistent tachycardia without fever may indicate ongoing dehydration and signify continued need for IV hydration.

  B. **What medications are being infused?** Vancomycin, amphotericin, acyclovir, cephalosporins, oxacillin, meropenem, potassium chloride, phenytoin, and various chemotherapeutic agents are among the many medications that may irritate the vein wall and contribute to phlebitis.

  C. **How long has the peripheral IV catheter been in place?** In adults, rates of bacterial colonization and phlebitis increase if peripheral IV catheters are left in place for more than 72–96 hours. Similar studies in children, however, have concluded that rates of bacterial colonization and phlebitis *do not* significantly increase after 72 hours. The Centers for Disease Control and Prevention (CDC) recommend leaving the peripheral catheter in place in children until IV therapy is completed or a complication, such as phlebitis, occurs.

  D. **Are there comorbid conditions?** Neutropenia, immunosuppression, and malnutrition can delay onset of symptoms and increase risk for phlebitis. Patients with peripheral neuropathies may be unaware of the pain associated with phlebitis.

  E. **Does patient still need the IV catheter?** Peripheral catheters should be removed when no longer essential.

III. **Differential Diagnosis**

  A. **Phlebitis (Noninfectious).** Phlebitis occurs in 1–70% of patients receiving IV infusion therapy. Symptoms, which occur as a result of inflammation of a cannulated vein, include localized pain, erythema, edema, and thrombus formation (superficial thrombophlebitis). To minimize phlebitis, evaluate catheter site daily by palpation through the dressing and by inspection if dressing is transparent.

   1. **Mechanical.** Any substance placed in the lumen of a vein or that causes damage to the interior wall of the vein has the potential to activate the inflammatory cascade, causing erythema and edema. When using peripheral IV catheters, type of catheter, dwell time, size, location, and method of securement all are important factors. The safest catheter is one that has the smallest circumference for its intended purpose, is less rigid (eg, newer polyurethane catheters), in an appropriate location (not over a bony prominence), and adequately secured.

2. **Chemical.** Many medications increase risk of phlebitis by causing damage to the vein wall. Both pH and osmolarity of the infused substance play a role. Acidic solutions (eg, vancomycin) and basic solutions (eg, phenytoin) cause higher rates of infusion-related phlebitis. Solutions with osmolarities > 450 mOsm/kg have a greater incidence of phlebitis and may need to be infused via central route (eg, TPN with a higher concentration of dextrose and lipids).

3. **Postinfusion.** Phlebitis can occur up to 4 days after removal of a peripheral IV catheter, reflecting the continuum of inflammatory response initiated when catheter was in place. Patients may present to the emergency department wondering if a piece of catheter has been left in the arm. This is rare; more likely a small thrombus due to phlebitis is the culprit.

B. **Suppurative Thrombophlebitis.** Suppurative thrombophlebitis indicates infection within the lumen of the vein that can lead to bacteremia, sepsis, and death. Bacterial colonization of peripheral venous catheters occasionally leads to severe localized infection and systemic disease, especially in immunocompromised patients and those with burns. It should be suspected in these patients when the following findings are present: fever, extreme tenderness, marked local erythema, and suppurative catheter site.

C. **Extravasated Medication.** Extravasation is defined as leakage of IV infusate into surrounding tissue. Many medications that increase risk for phlebitis due to their pH or osmolar properties can also cause severe damage if infused into surrounding tissue.

IV. **Database**

A. **Physical Exam Key Points**

1. **Vital signs.** Initial vital signs are helpful; however, they must be interpreted with consideration of underlying illness. Phlebitis is a local phenomenon and usually not associated with fever. Suppurative thrombophlebitis often causes fever and tachycardia.

2. **Skin.** Assess peripheral IV site for erythema, warmth, tenderness, edema, and a palpable cord. If any of these symptoms is present, remove catheter and assess for signs of a suppurative infection. Assess surrounding skin for signs of extravasated medication: marked tenderness, edema, and possibly skin breakdown surrounding catheter site.

B. **Laboratory Data.** None needed unless suppurative thrombophlebitis is suspected. In that case, obtain CBC, blood culture, and culture of catheter tip.

C. **Radiographic and Other Studies.** None needed.

V. **Plan.** Removal of catheter is first step. Assess need for continued IV therapy. If indicated, place another catheter in a different site, preferably a smaller catheter in a larger vein to minimize chance of recurrence.

A. **Phlebitis (Mechanical or Infusion).** Elevate and place warm, moist compresses on site after removal of catheter. Topical, oral, or IV antibiotics are not necessary.

B. **Suppurative Thrombophlebitis.** After immediate removal of catheter, start broad-spectrum antibiotics to cover gram-negative rods and gram-positive cocci. Obtain surgical consultation, because surgical excision of affected vein is often necessary.

C. **Extravasated Medication.** If patient experiences pain during an infusion, stop infusion immediately. Attempt to aspirate several milliliters of blood or infusate from catheter site. Remove peripheral IV catheter if placement in subcutaneous tissue is suspected. Elevate and place cold compresses on affected area. Occasionally, warm compresses or antidotes, or both, are indicated for chemotherapeutic agents. In severe cases, skin breakdown will occur and surgical debridement may be necessary.

VI. **Problem Case Diagnosis.** The insertion site of the catheter in this 3-year-old girl was erythematous and tender to palpation. Otherwise, she was afebrile and had no other findings. Diagnosis is phlebitis. The catheter was removed and warm soaks were applied to the site.

VII. **Teaching Pearl: Question.** Is it safe to place a peripheral IV catheter in the foot?

VIII. **Teaching Pearl: Answer.** Although there has been a higher risk of phlebitis and infection in peripheral IV catheters placed in lower extremities of adults, this is not the case in children. The CDC states that hand, dorsum of foot, and scalp can all be used safely in pediatric patients.

REFERENCES

Macklin D. Phlebitis. *Am J Nurs* 2003;103:55–60.

O'Grady NP, Alexander M, Dellinger EP, et al. Guidelines for the prevention of intravascular catheter-related infections. *MMWR Morb Mortal Wkly Rep* August 2002;51(RR-10).

Shimandle RB, Johnson D, Baker M, et al. Safety of peripheral intravenous catheters in children. *Infect Control Hosp Epidemiol* 1999;20:736–740.

Stein JM, Pruitt BA. Suppurative thrombophlebitis. A lethal iatrogenic disease. *N Engl J Med* 1970;282:1452–1455.

73. PNEUMOTHORAX

I. **Problem.** A previously healthy 16-year-old boy develops acute, sharp, right-sided chest pain and dyspnea while sitting in a car in the school parking lot.

II. **Immediate Questions**

A. **What are the vital signs?** Tachycardia, tachypnea, and hypertension may reflect compensatory mechanisms. Negative intrapleural pressure and blood vessel torsion from mediastinal shifts leads to reduced venous return to the right atrium and hypotension.

B. Is patient cyanotic? Cyanosis indicates severe hypoxemia and acute respiratory distress.

C. Can patient communicate? Inability to communicate indicates airway obstruction and impending acute respiratory failure.

D. What was patient doing immediately prior to onset of chest pain? Pneumothorax can occur at rest as well as with activities, including chest wall trauma (eg, ball injury, wrestling, automobile accident, air bag deployment), blunt abdominal trauma, wheezing, coughing, laughing, crying, and injection of drugs into the internal jugular or subclavian veins.

E Does patient have a history of chest pain? The chest pain of pneumothorax may be recurrent and repetitive in quality and location.

F. Any history of wheezing, asthma, or chronic lung disease? Partial airway obstruction causing wheezing can result in air trapping and alveolar rupture.

G. Has patient had a recent pulmonary infection? Inflammation secondary to pulmonary infection can cause pneumothorax.

H. Does patient smoke cigarettes? Airway inflammation associated with cigarette smoking is accompanied by an increased incidence of pneumothorax.

I. If female, does patient have her menses? A pneumothorax associated with the beginning of the menstrual flow is known as catamenial pneumothorax.

III. Differential Diagnosis. Acute chest pain can be a result of pleuritic or nonpleuritic processes and occurs with diseases of the chest wall, lungs, heart, GI tract, and mediastinum.

A. Pleuritic Chest Pain

    1. Causes. Stimulation of nerves and parietal pleura resulting from diseases of chest wall, diaphragm, parietal pleura, lungs, and mediastinum.

        a. Chest wall. Rib and sternal fractures; blunt trauma; contusion; muscle tear, spasm, or irritation from severe coughing; stimulation of intercostal nerves or nerves in parietal pleura; diaphragmatic irritation; subdiaphragmatic abscess; bone infarction associated with acute chest syndrome of sickle cell disease; and leukemic infiltration of ribs and sternum.

        b. Lungs. Pneumothorax; pleural effusion associated with lobar pneumonia, tuberculosis, or small pulmonary embolism; pulmonary infarction; pulmonary laceration; tracheal rupture; and Wegener granulomatosis.

        c. Mediastinum. Mediastinitis (acute, chronic).

    2. Location and quality of pain. Typically pleuritic pain is lateral or posterior and superficial in location; is localized; and radiates to the ipsilateral shoulder. It is sharp or stabbing in quality;

severe; accentuated by coughing, sneezing, laughing, and inhaling deeply; and diminished by splinting affected side of the chest and breath holding. Pleuritic pain may be associated with friction rub. Pneumothorax causes pleuritic chest pain.

B. Nonpleuritic Pain. Caused by diseases of chest wall, lungs, heart, and GI tract and by anxiety. It is central and usually deep in location; is nonlocalized; and may radiate to the contralateral shoulder, arms, back, and neck. It is dull in quality and constant.

C. Types of Pneumothorax

1. **Primary spontaneous.** Occurs without underlying pulmonary disease; often results from rupture of apical cystic lesions in upper lobes of lung.

2. **Secondary spontaneous.** Occurs as a complication of underlying pulmonary disease (eg, asthma, cystic fibrosis, chronic lung disease, tuberculosis, *Pneumocystis carinii* pneumonitis, meconium aspiration, and neonatal respiratory distress syndrome).

3. **Tension.** Occurs when intrapleural pressure is higher than atmospheric pressure, such as with partial airway obstruction creating air trapping during expiration (and sometimes during inspiration). Causes reduced venous return and cardiac output, severe hypoxemia, and acute cardiorespiratory decompensation.

4. **Catamenial.** Occurs at onset of the menstrual flow; often preceded by anxiety or stress.

5. **Neonatal.** Likely associated with alterations in lung and chest wall mechanics during initiation of air breathing.

IV. Database

A. Physical Exam Key Points

1. **General appearance.** Note whether habitus is tall and thin. Primary spontaneous pneumothorax occurs more frequently during rapid growth associated with adolescence and in boys.

2. **Vital signs.** Assess for presence of dyspnea while patient is talking.

3. **Skin.** Examine for cyanosis. Trauma may result in bruises, lacerations, or hematomas on chest wall.

4. **HEENT.** Examine for crepitations indicative of subcutaneous emphysema, which can accompany pneumothorax, and tracheal deviation, which occurs on contralateral side of the pneumothorax.

5. **Chest.** Examine for asymmetry (chest bulge or prominence on side of the pneumothorax), alterations in configuration and contour (scoliosis, kyphosis, fused ribs), retractions, and rib and sternal tenderness.

   a. Pneumothorax is associated initially with pleuritic pain, which diminishes and even subsides following separation of the two layers of pleura.

   b. Rib or sternal fracture is suggested by bone crepitations and localized tenderness on palpation.

      c. Osteomyelitis is associated with tenderness to palpation, fever, and leukocytosis, whereas periostitis is accompanied by extreme tenderness and sharp pain accentuated by movement. Costochondritis is characterized by dull pain of acute or insidious onset, tenderness at junction of cartilage and rib (usually second rib), variable swelling in cartilage, erythema of overlying skin, and absence of radiographic changes. Pain is accentuated by inspiration and movement of ipsilateral upper extremity.

      d. Intercostal myositis is accompanied by severe aching pain accentuated by movement, tenderness to palpation, and induration and nodules in the affected muscle.

      e. Herpes zoster viral intercostal neuralgia presents with acute pain, unilateral cutaneous vesicular lesions along the nerve pathway, and burning and erythema of involved skin.

      f. Pleurodynia, usually caused by coxsackievirus B, is characterized by acute, severe, sharp, thoracic and abdominal pain that lasts a few days; systemic symptoms (fever, headache); and absence of leukocytosis.

      g. Mediastinitis is accompanied by neck and chest pain, dyspnea, tachypnea, fever, chills, and dysphagia.

      h. Hamman sign, or "mediastinal crunch," is a loud, crunching sound in the precordial area that results from movement of air in interstitial spaces during inspiration and indicates the presence of a pneumomediastinum.

  6. Lungs. With pneumothorax, there is ipsilateral hyperresonance to percussion; amphoric breathing (whistling); absence of tactile fremitus, pectoriloquy (whispered breath sounds), egophony, and bronchophony; and diminished or absent breath sounds. A pleural friction rub caused by movement of visceral against parietal pleura may be heard.

  7. Extremities. Examine peripheral pulses (radial, dorsalis pedis, femoral), capillary refill time, and for presence of digital clubbing.

  8. Neurologic exam. Identify level of consciousness, alertness, and ability to communicate.

B. Laboratory Data. Obtain oxygen saturation by pulse oximetry and ABGs.

  1. Hypoxemia indicates mismatch of ventilation (V) with perfusion (Q) and shunting of blood. Hypoventilation may accompany severe pain and contribute to hypoxemia. Atelectasis of lung contiguous to pneumothorax occurs.

  2. PaO_2 is reduced with V/Q imbalance because ventilation is diminished and overall perfusion is maintained. PaO_2 may be normal until shunting and more widespread V/Q imbalance result.

C. Radiographic and Other Studies. Obtain upright views of chest, if possible with both anteroposterior and lateral views.

Volume of pneumothorax is relatively greater during expiration than inspiration.

1. Chest x-ray. May show:

    a. Air in pleural space, mediastinum (pneumomediastinum), subcutaneous tissues (subcutaneous emphysema), pericardium (pneumopericardium), and peritoneum (pneumoperitoneum). Air appears as a relative lucency with absent lung markings.

    b. Contralateral mediastinal shift.

    c. Ipsilateral depression of diaphragm.

    d. Increased distance between ribs on ipsilateral side.

    e. Cystic lesions in lung parenchyma, a possible site of rupture, particularly in apices of upper lobes.

    f. Atelectasis near pneumothorax.

    g. Fractured or dislocated ribs or sternum.

V. Plan

A. Oxygen. Administer supplemental oxygen by nasal cannula, face mask, or rebreather mask to maintain oxygen saturation > 92%.

B. Pain Control. Administer appropriate pain medication for age and weight to control pain without sedation and secondary hypoventilation.

C. Resolution of Pneumothorax

    1. If pneumothorax is < 15%, administer humidified 100% oxygen through rebreather mask for up to 15–30 minutes to try to reduce the pneumothorax by washing out nitrogen in alveoli and pleural capillaries and enhance diffusion of intrapleural gases into capillaries.

    2. If pneumothorax is > 20%, place needle with three-way stopcock and 50-mL syringe in the second anterior intercostal space in the midclavicular line to remove air in the pleural space. If lung reexpansion does not occur, insert a chest tube at the second anterior intercostal space in the midclavicular line or below nipple in the midaxillary line directed toward apical portion of pneumothorax and connected to underwater seal or closed water suction.

    3. If pneumothorax does not resolve by 7–10 days despite presence of chest tube and suction, video-assisted thoroscopic surgery (VATS) with pleurodesis by mechanical abrasion of parietal pleura, and possibly parietal pleurectomy, is performed.

D. Recurrence of Pneumothorax. Recurrence is likely, particularly if blebs or bullae are present. If a second pneumothorax occurs in the presence of parenchymal blebs and bullae, cystic lesions are removed surgically by VATS, and pleurodesis is performed. Patient should be instructed to seek medical care immediately if chest pain recurs.

E. Prevention
1. Contact sports are discouraged for 5–6 months following a pneumothorax.
2. Pulmonary function testing should not be performed for at least 6 months to prevent alveolar rupture if lesions have not completely healed.

VI. Problem Case Diagnosis. The 16-year-old patient has right-sided pneumothorax, confirmed by chest x-ray. The chest pain was preceded by a laughing episode and worsened with deep breaths. No history of trauma was noted.

VII. Teaching Pearl: Question. Does a pneumothorax more often occur at rest or with activity?

VIII. Teaching Pearl: Answer. Pneumothorax occurs more often at rest.

REFERENCES

Light RW. Management of spontaneous pneumothorax. *Am Rev Respir Dis* 1993;148:245–248.

Sahn SA, Heffner JE. Spontaneous pneumothorax. *N Engl J Med* 2000;342: 868–874.

Schramel FMNH, Postmus PE, Vanderschueren RGJRA. Current aspects of spontaneous pneumothorax. *Eur Respir J* 1997;10:1372–1379.

74. POISONING AND OVERDOSES

I. Problem. A 2-year-old boy is brought to the emergency department for evaluation after being found near an empty unlabeled bottle of medicine.

II. Immediate Questions

A. What should clinician do first? Assess and treat patient's airway, breathing, and circulation (ABCs). When indicated, place child on cardiac monitor and establish IV access; this may be carried out while obtaining history and performing physical exam. Obtain initial, brief history, including product name, active ingredients, amount ingested, and time of ingestion (see later discussion). A detailed history should be obtained once patient is stabilized. In many cases, history is inaccurate, and ingested substance may not be known. A focused exam also assesses pupillary size, pupillary response to light, and neuropsychiatric status.

B. How severe is patient's condition? Evaluation of severity of poisoning is based on knowledge of ingested substance, maximum possible intake, and clinical condition. Once this information is gathered, poisoning case can be categorized as immediately life threatening, potentially toxic, or nontoxic. If an unknown substance has been ingested, integration of data from history, vital signs, and physical exam into various toxic syndromes (toxidromes) can suggest exposure to a toxin or a certain class of toxins. Consultation with poison-control center can be informative and should be initiated **(telephone hotline: 800-222-1222).**

III. **Differential Diagnosis.** Presentation depends on ingested substance(s), amount ingested, time lapsed, and any underlying medical conditions, among other factors. Distinct toxicologic syndromes are associated with groups of toxins; however, many other toxic exposures have nonspecific presentations. Keep in mind that there are more nontoxic than toxic exposures. Substances that are commonly associated with altered mental status are discussed in Chapter 6 (see p. 29).

   A. **Common Toxicologic Syndromes (Toxidromes)**
      1. **Anticholinergic syndrome**
         a. **Findings.** Elevated temperature; delirium; mumbling speech; tachycardia; dry, flushed skin; dry mucous membranes; urinary retention; decreased to absent bowel sounds; mydriasis; and blurred vision. Seizures and coma may also occur.
         b. Mnemonic for many of the features of this toxidrome: **"Hot** as a hare, **blind** as a bat, **dry** as a bone, **red** as a beet, **mad** as a hatter, **bloated** as a bladder."
         c. **Agents.** Drugs and toxins that block acetylcholine at muscarinic receptors; especially, atropine and atropine-like agents. These include several commonly used over-the-counter cold medications containing antihistamines, antiparkinson medications (benztropine, trihexyphenidyl, topical mydriatics), antispasmodics (Donnatal, dicyclomine), muscle relaxants (cyclobenzaprine, orphenadrine), and belladonna alkaloids (scopolamine, hyoscyamine). Cyclic antidepressants also cause anticholinergic symptoms. Plants that contain belladonna alkaloids include jimson weed (*Datura stramonium*), deadly nightshade (*Atropa belladonna*), and henbane (*Hyoscyamus niger*).
      2. **Sympathomimetic syndrome**
         a. **Findings.** Hypertension, diaphoresis, tachycardia, tachypnea, hyperthermia, and mydriasis. Restlessness, agitation, excessive speech, tremors, and insomnia also occur. Severe cases are associated with dysrhythmias and seizures.
         b. **Distinguishing features.** May be difficult to distinguish from anticholinergic syndrome. Sweating and normal to hyperactive bowel sounds are associated with sympathomimetic overdose, whereas anticholinergic toxidrome manifests with dry skin and diminished bowel sounds.
         c. **Agents.** Sympathetic agonists such as cocaine and amphetamine. Sympathomimetic effects may also be caused by over-the-counter decongestants such as phenylpropanolamine (no

longer available legally), ephedrine, and pseudoephedrine. Theophylline and caffeine may cause many of these findings by enhancing catecholamine release. Overdoses with β_2-adrenergic receptor agonists, methylphenidate, and *Ephedra* species such as ma huang cause sympathomimetic symptoms.

3. **Opioid syndrome**
   a. **Findings.** Classic triad of opioid intoxication is mental status depression, respiratory depression, and pinpoint pupils. Bradycardia, hypotension (rare), hypothermia, hyporeflexia, and needle marks may be present.
   b. **Agents.** Morphine, heroin, designer fentanyls, oxycodone, hydromorphone, and propoxyphene are commonly associated with this toxidrome. Meperidine, pentazocine, and dextromethorphan may cause CNS and respiratory depression but are often associated with dilated pupils. Central α_2-receptor agonists (eg, clonidine, guanabenz, guanfacine, and imidazoline derivatives) act on the locus ceruleus of the CNS and cause many of the same symptoms in the overdose setting.

4. **Anticholinesterase syndrome**
   a. **Organophosphates.** Commonly available as insecticides, and readily absorbed through skin, mucous membranes, and respiratory and GI tracts. Organophosphates inactivate cholinesterase enzymes, resulting in accumulation of acetylcholine at receptor sites and overstimulation of muscarinic, nicotinic, and central acetylcholine receptors.
   b. **Other causes of cholinesterase inhibition.** Carbamates and therapeutic cholinesterase inhibitors (eg, physostigmine, pyridostigmine, neostigmine, edrophonium). Clinical findings suggestive of acute anticholinesterase intoxication include muscarinic effects as well as muscle weakness, fasciculations, altered mental status, seizures, and coma.
   c. As a mnemonic to recall many of the muscarinic effects, remember **DUMBELS: D**efecation, **U**rination, **M**iosis, **B**ronchorrhea, **B**ronchospasm, **B**radycardia, **E**mesis, **L**acrimation, and **S**alivation.

5. **Sedative-hypnotic syndrome**
   a. **Findings.** Overdoses are associated with hypotension, bradypnea, hypothermia, mental status depression, slurred speech, ataxia, and hyporeflexia. Patients with ethanol intoxication may also present with many of these symptoms. Bullous lesions have been reported in some patients with sedative-hypnotic overdoses. Paradoxical excitement is seen with some sedative-hypnotics, especially in very young and elderly patients.

   b. **Agents.** Sedative-hypnotic group includes barbiturates, benzodiazepines, buspirone, paraldehyde, chloral hydrate, meprobamate, methaqualone, ethchlorvynol, glutethimide, and zolpidem. Ingestion of neuroleptics, cyclic antidepressants, and skeletal muscle relaxants may also cause significant sedation.

B. **Common Pediatric Ingestions.** Only a handful of chemical and medicinal products (ie, those substances commonly available in the household) is implicated in the vast majority of poisonings in children.

   1. **Medicinal**

      a. **Analgesics**

         i. **Acetaminophen.** Nausea and vomiting are common and may progress to hepatotoxicity and hepatic failure. Acute renal failure and hyperamylasemia are less common. Coma, metabolic acidosis, myocardial injury, and acute respiratory distress syndrome may occur with severe overdose (Figure I–5). **Onset:** Hepatotoxicity occurs within 24–36 hours of ingestion. **Toxic dose:** > 150 mg/kg (child) or > 7.5 g (young adult); malnourished patients may be at risk at lower doses.

         ii. **Ibuprofen.** Most overdoses are asymptomatic. Mild effects (common) include abdominal pain, nausea and vomiting, lethargy, drowsiness, headache, tinnitus, and ataxia. Moderate to severe effects (rare) include apnea, metabolic acidosis, coma, seizures, acute renal failure, hypotension and hypothermia. **Onset:** Within 4 hours. **Toxic dose:** With ingestion of < 200 mg/kg, significant toxicity is unlikely; ingestion of > 400 mg/kg places patient at risk for serious effects. **Young adults:** Overdoses up to 48 g have been well tolerated by healthy adults.

         iii. **Aspirin.** Aspirin ingestion and overdose is less commonly encountered today than a decade ago. Symptoms of acute severe poisoning include hyperventilation, fever, restlessness, ketosis, respiratory alkalosis, and metabolic acidosis. Depression of CNS may lead to coma; cardiovascular collapse and respiratory failure may also occur. In children, drowsiness and metabolic acidosis commonly occur; hypoglycemia may be severe. **Toxic dose:** > 120 mg/kg.

      b. **Decongestants.** See III, A, 2, earlier, for discussion of sympathomimetic syndrome.

      c. **Antihistamines.** See III, A, 1, earlier, for discussion of anticholinergic syndrome.

      d. **Iron.** Iron overdose has a wide range of severity. With severe toxicity, stupor, shock, acidosis, GI bleeding, coagulopathy,

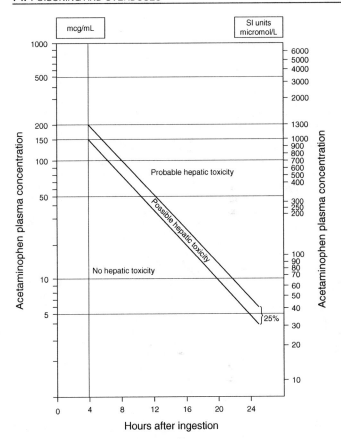

Figure I–5. Semilogarithmic plot of plasma acetaminophen levels versus time. This nomogram is valid for use after acute single ingestions of acetaminophen. Need for treatment cannot be extrapolated based on a level before 4 hours. (Reproduced from Gunn VL, Neckyba C. *The Harriet Lane Handbook*, 16th ed. Mosby, 2002; from Jones AL. Mechanism of action and value of *N*-acetylcysteine in the treatment of early and late acetaminophen poisoning: A critical review. *J Toxicol Clin Toxicol* 1998;36:277–285.)

hepatotoxicity, and coma occur. Mild to moderate toxicity produces nausea, vomiting and diarrhea; lethargy; leukocytosis; and hyperglycemia. Ingestions of iron with multivitamins appear to have slightly different toxicity than iron alone;

symptoms are often less dramatic, and there are fewer corrosive effects. **Toxic dose:** In children, toxicity is likely following ≥ 60 mg/kg elemental iron; < 20 mg/kg is generally
not toxic. **Estimated lethal dose:** 0.3 g/kg body weight for
ferrous iron. Five clinical phases can be observed.

- i. **Phase 1, 0–2 hours.** Nausea, vomiting, diarrhea;
  abdominal pain; if severe, lethargy, shock, GI bleeding,
  and acidosis.
- ii. **Phase 2.** Apparent recovery.
- iii. **Phase 3, 2–12 hours later.** Acidosis and hypotension.
- iv. **Phase 4, 2–4 days.** hepatotoxicity.
- v. **Phase 5, days to weeks.** GI strictures.

- e. **Multivitamins.** Toxicity is estimated by evaluating amounts
  of vitamin A and D individually.
  - i. **Vitamin A toxicity.** Acute poisoning is rare in children
    and is reported with ingestion of 300,000 IU. Symptoms
    are caused by increased intracranial pressure and may
    include bulging fontanelles, vomiting, headache, blurred
    vision, and irritability. Exfoliation of skin has also been
    reported.
  - ii. **Vitamin D toxicity.** Symptoms of acute poisoning include
    anorexia, nausea, vomiting, and weight loss. Many of the
    other effects of chronic vitamin D toxicity are due to
    induced hypercalcemia. Polyneuropathy may be seen.

2. **Nonmedicinal**
   - a. **Personal care products.** Some substances may be irritating or corrosive, depending on concentration, molarity, and
     other factors. In general, serious esophageal injury is associated with ingestion of products with pH ≥ 11.5. Alkaline
     corrosive ingestion may produce burns to oropharynx,
     upper airway, esophagus, and occasionally stomach.
     Spontaneous vomiting may occur. It is important to recognize that absence of visible oral burns does not reliably
     exclude presence of esophageal burns. Stridor, vomiting,
     drooling, and abdominal pain are associated with serious
     esophageal injury in most cases.
   - b. **Cleaning agents.** Serious injuries are associated with
     caustic substances with high pH. See preceding discussion.
   - c. **Plants.** Most plants have mild skin irritant effects or mild GI
     symptoms (eg, nausea, vomiting, diarrhea, or abdominal
     pain).
   - d. **Pesticides.** Two main groups of chemical are usually
     encountered: organophosphates (see earlier discussion of
     anticholinesterase syndrome, at III, A, 4) and carbamates.
     Carbamate syndrome may be indistinguishable from that
     seen after organophosphate poisoning. Generally, clinical
     effects are not as severe as those seen with organophosphate poisoning; carbamates do not penetrate CNS as

effectively as do organophosphates; thus, they produce more limited CNS toxicity.

   e. Hydrocarbons. Low-viscosity, highly volatile hydrocarbons (eg, kerosene, gasoline, liquid furniture polish) are associated with aspiration hazards. Parenchymal pulmonary injury, transient CNS depression or stimulation, and secondary effects of hypoxia, infection, pneumatocele formation, and chronic lung dysfunction can occur. Cardiac complications are rare.

C. Small, But Serious Pediatric Ingestions. Quantity of ingested substance in most cases is proportional to severity of induced toxicity. When possible, calculation of milligram-per-kilogram dose of ingestion is helpful to prognosticate outcome. In toddlers, however, a small dose can be lethal. For examples, see Table I–21.

D. Nontoxic Ingestions. Approximately 70% of all pediatric poisoning are nontoxic. Examples include oral antibiotics, antacids, chalk, crayons, hydrogen peroxide, and zinc oxide.

IV. Database. Onset of symptoms can be immediate or delayed for several hours or a few days due to latency of effect of toxin or slow release of active form. Signs and symptoms are variable and related to pharmacologic properties of toxin. Significant ingestions commonly affect vital signs, neuropsychiatric status, GI tract, and pupillary size and reactivity to light. Other less common manifestations are specific odors, skin discoloration, and disturbances of exocrine glands.

A. History Key Points. History is often inaccurate and should be interpreted cautiously. In case of suicidal attempt in a teenager or unresponsiveness where poisoning is considered, an investigative-type approach to history may be warranted.

   1. Ingestion history. Initial, brief history should include product name, active ingredients, amount ingested, and time of ingestion.

TABLE I–21. PEDIATRIC POISONS AND LETHAL DOSES

Drug	Lethal Dose per Kg	Unit-Dose	Lethal Amount
Antimalarials	20 mg	500 mg	1 tab
β-Blockers	~10 mg	25–100 mg/tab	1–2 tabs
Calcium channel blockers	15–20 mg	240 mg/tab	1 tab
Camphor	100 mg	1 g/tsp	1 tsp
Chlorpromazine	25 mg	200 mg/tab	1–2 tabs
Clonidine	< ~1 mg	0.3–7.5 mg/tab	1 tab or patch
Imipramine	15 mg	150 mg/tab	1 tab
Methyl salicylate	200 mg	7 g/tsp	< 1 tsp

tab = tablet.

    a. Obtain all prescription bottles and other containers when possible. Perform a pill count. Be sure bottles contain medications listed. Identify any unknown tablets.

    b. Contact prescribing physician(s) or pharmacy as listed on bottles to determine previous overdoses or other medications patient may have available. Identify underlying medical and psychiatric disorders and medication allergies. Review past medical records.

    c. Talk to patient's family and friends in the emergency department. If necessary, call patient's home to ask questions of others. Persons providing important elements of history should be identified in chart.

    d. Search patient's belongings for drugs or drug paraphernalia. A single pill hidden in a pocket, for example, may provide *the most* important clue to diagnosis.

    e. Have family members (or police) search patient's home, including medicine cabinet, clothes drawers, closets, and garage; this may also provide clues that enable diagnosis to be made. This step has added benefit of involving family in patient's care.

    f. Estimate maximum possible intake. In case of prescription and over-the-counter medications, calculate milligram-per-kilogram dose of ingestion.

  2. Review of systems. Focus on symptoms of vomiting, visual disturbances, palpitations, sweating, abdominal pain, breathing difficulty, and skin discoloration or rash.

  3. Past medical history. Asthma, cardiac disease, or seizure disorder is particularly important.

B. Physical Exam Key Points. The following clinical observations provide clues for toxidromes and are crucial during management decision-making process.

  1. Vital signs. Increase or decrease in temperature, heart rate, BP, or respiratory rate. Attention to pattern of breathing: slow shallow or rapid and deep. Provide 100% oxygen in case of respiratory distress.

  2. Neuropsychiatric status. Lethargy and coma require administration of IV dextrose (0.5–1.0 g/kg or 2–4 L/kg of $D_{25}W$) and naloxone (2 mg IV q2–5min until clinical response; to maximum of 10.0 mg). This is a therapeutic as well as a diagnostic measure. Treat agitation and seizure with benzodiazepines (IV diazepam, 0.1 mg/kg).

  3. Airway. Assess presence of gag and cough reflex; if absent, endotracheal intubation is indicated.

  4. Eyes. Assess pupillary size and reactivity to light.

  5. Abdomen. Absence of bowel sounds may signal presence of ileus.

  6. Musculoskeletal exam. Assess muscle tone; observe for tremors, weakness, nystagmus, or seizure.

C. Laboratory Data. Consider the following studies, depending on ingested substance and clinical circumstances. (*Do not* obtain workup for nontoxic ingestions.)

1. **Blood chemistry.** Obtain serum glucose level (including bedside test), ABGs, carboxyhemoglobin, methemoglobin, electrolytes, BUN, creatinine, liver function tests, serum osmolality, CBC, metabolic screening, and anion gap.

2. **Toxicology screening.** Obtain specific blood level of ingested or potentially ingested substance when pertinent. If time of ingestion is known, then proper timing of sampling is important.

3. **Drug screening.** Of limited use in immediate management. Useful to support clinical impression of ingestion of certain drug or class of drugs.

4. **Other workup.** Includes urine $FeCl_3$ (for salicylates).

D. Radiographic and Other Studies. Abdominal x-ray can identify iron, lead-based paint chips, or ileus from opioids.

V. Plan. Figure I–6 outlines an algorithmic approach to the poisoned child.

A. Supportive Care

1. Maintain airway and ventilation.
2. Correct acid-base and electrolyte abnormalities.
3. Correct fluid deficits and properly manage fluid therapy.

B. Prevention of Further Absorption (Decontamination)

1. **Skin.** Remove contaminated clothes; wash with warm water and soap.

2. **Eye.** Provide continuous irrigation with normal saline for 20 minutes. Remove contact lenses before flushing. Fluorescein staining may be indicated after irrigation.

3. **GI decontamination**

a. **Emesis.** Outcome studies showed no advantage. Contraindicated in infants younger than 6 months of age and in patients with potentially altered mental status, poor gag reflex, and caustic or hydrocarbon ingestions. Ingested substance and time of ingestion are two important factors to consider when deciding to induce emesis. Emesis is less likely to be helpful 1 hour after ingestion unless toxin delays gastric emptying. In rare cases when syrup of Ipecac is indicated, dose is 10 mL in patients aged 6–12 months, 15 mL in those 1–12 years, and 30 mL in those older than 12 years of age. This is followed by 1–3 ounces of water. Response is usually seen in 20 minutes.

b. **Gastric lavage.** Ineffective in most clinical scenarios. Contraindicated in caustic and hydrocarbon ingestions. If mental status is altered, trachea should be intubated with cuffed tube before lavage. Use large-bore orogastric tube, 28–40 Fr gauge. Lavage with 50–200 mL aliquots of normal

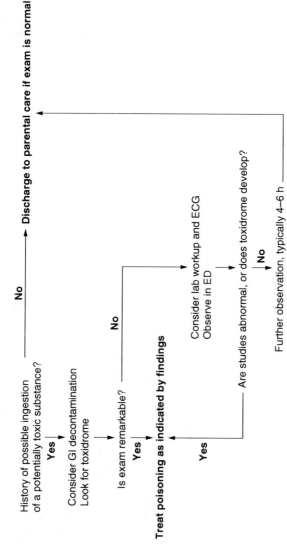

Figure I-6. Algorithmic approach to the poisoned child. (ECG = electrocardiogram; ED = emergency department; GI = gastrointestinal.)

saline until return is clear. Before removal, tube may be used to administer charcoal (see next entry).

c. **Activated charcoal.** Universal antidote. Most effective gastric decontamination method for most chemicals. Contraindicated in intestinal obstruction. Not effective against iron, lithium, alcohol, and magnesium. Dose is 1 g/kg mixed with water to form slurry; give orally or via nasogastric (NG) tube. Charcoal may be repeated to enhance adsorption and gut dialysis (extraction of toxins from mesenteric circulation by lowering intraluminal concentration). Second and subsequent doses are given as 0.5–1.0 g/kg every 2–4 hours.

d. **Cathartics.** No clear evidence of effectiveness. Decreases transit time. Contraindicated in intestinal obstruction and renal failure (for magnesium-containing cathartics). Use 70% sorbitol solution (0.5–1.0 g/kg) with first dose of charcoal, only. Do not repeat cathartics.

e. **Whole bowel irrigation.** Idea is to rinse bowel. Use GoLYTELY (polyethylene glycol electrolyte solution is not absorbed from GI tract and does not produce electrolyte imbalance). Give solution orally or via NG tube at a rate of 0.5–2 L/h until effluent is clear, usually in 6–8 hours. Excellent method for gastric decontamination in patients who have ingested concretion-forming drugs (iron, barbiturates, salicylates) or sustained-release products.

C. Enhancement of Elimination

1. **Diuresis.** Unproven efficacy. Requires normal renal and cardiopulmonary status. Avoid fluid overload.

2. **Alkalinization.** Best results are obtained in patients with salicylate and phenobarbital ingestions. Use IV sodium bicarbonate, 1–2 mEq/kg over 1 hour; can be repeated every 3–4 hours. Goal is urinary pH of 7.5–8.0. Adequate ventilation and serum potassium supplementation and monitoring are important.

3. **Dialysis.** Hemodialysis is more effective than peritoneal dialysis. Many factors affect feasibility of these methods, including molecular weight, solubility, and tissue- and plasma protein–binding abilities.

4. **Hemoperfusion and hemofiltration.** These methods are applied for selective cases of serious ingestions.

D. Specific Treatment (Antidotes). Many agents have antidotes that can prevent toxic injury or mortality. Table I–22 lists substances that are commonly ingested in overdose, and antidotes available. Antidotes should be used when cause of overdose is known and possible toxicity is determined to be severe enough that benefits of therapy outweigh risks of antidote. If clinician is unsure of how to manage an overdose or ingestion of a specific toxin, local poison-control hotline can be extremely helpful.

TABLE I-22. ANTIDOTES OF POISONINGS[a]

Poison (toxic dose)	Antidote	Dose	Comment
Acetaminophen (140 mg/kg)	N-Acetylcysteine	140 mg/kg PO or NG, then 70 mg/kg q4h × 17 doses	Use nomogram (Figure I–5) when levels available. Can be used up to 48 h after ingestion; most effective within 8 h. Treat nausea and vomiting with IV metoclopramide, 0.1 mg/kg. Could use with charcoal; bioavailability not affected
Anticholinergics	Anticholinergics	0.02 mg/kg slow IV push over 1 min and q5–10min until response. Maximum: 2–4 mg	**Caution:** Therapy is hazardous; may induce dysrhythmia, seizures, or bronchospasm; use only with significant anticholinergic symptoms. Treat physostigmine overdosage with atropine, 0.025–0.05 mg/kg. Do not use for tricyclic antidepressants
β-Blockers (variable)	Glucagon	0.15 mg/kg IV bolus, then 0.1 mg/kg/h as continuous infusion	Improves refractory hypotension (inotropic and chronotropic effects). Nausea, vomiting, and hyperglycemia are expected
Benzodiazepines (variable)	Flumazenil	0.2–0.3 mg/kg IV q1min. Maximum: 1–3 mg	Reverses respiratory depression. Can cause nausea and vomiting, headache, and withdrawal seizures
Carbon monoxide (CO)	Oxygen	100% O₂ via nonrebreather mask	Consider hyperbaric oxygen for severe symptoms, or with CO level > 25%
Clonidine (0.1 mg)	Naloxone	2.0 mg IV; up to 5–10 mg may be used	Improves hypotension and mental status. Response is variable. Aggressive supportive care should be applied
Cyanide	1. Amyl nitrite 2. Sodium nitrite 3. Sodium thiosulfate	1 ampule to inhale until IV established 0.33 mL/kg IV slow push 1.6 mL/kg IV slow push	Adjust initial dose according to patient Hgb level. Follow package insert tables. Adjust initial dose according to patient Hgb level. Follow package insert tables
Digoxin (4 mg)	Digibind	40 mL (1 vial) IV for every 0.6 mg of digoxin load	Digoxin load = 80% of ingested amount or SDC (ng/mL) × 5.6 (L/kg) × body weight (kg)
Iron (60 mg/kg)	Deferoxamine	Test dose: 30 mg/kg IM or IV, to maximum of 1 g. Then: 15 mg/kg/h IV slow infusion with NS. Maximum: 6 g/day	Serum iron > 300 mcg/dL or test dose resulting in vin rosé urine is indication for treatment. Hypotension may occur with fast infusion rate
Isoniazid (15 mg/kg)	Pyridoxine	25–75 mg/kg IV	Other measures to control seizures might be indicated
Lead	Succimer	10 mg/kg PO q8h × 5 days, then 10 mg/kg q12h × 14 days	For asymptomatic patients with lead level > 25 mcg/dL

348

		50–75 mg/kg/24 h by continuous IV infusion or deep IM q4–8h	For patients with lead level > 25 mcg/dL and positive EDTA mobilization test
	Calcium EDTA		
	BAL	3–5 mg/kg IM q4h	For patients with lead level > 70 mcg/dL Give 4 h prior to EDTA Avoid in G6PD-deficient patients
Methanol and ethylene glycol	Ethanol	750 mg/kg IV loading dose as 5% solution, then 100 mg/kg/h	Adjust to maintain blood level at 100 mg/dL. Consider hemodialysis
Nitrites, other methemoglobinemic agents	Methylene blue	1–2 mg (0.1–0.2 mL/kg of 1% solution) IV over 5 min	Treat if patient has dyspnea, severe symptoms, or methemoglobin level > 20–30%; repeat in 30 min Exchange transfusion if patient has persistent symptoms or is G6PD deficient Causes nausea and vomiting, headache, dizziness, and suprapubic pain
Opiates	Naloxone	2.0 mg IV, IO, or ET (dilute with 2 mL NS when given ET) Repeat q2min to maximum of 10 mg	May require frequent repetitions of total effective dose or continuous infusion
Organophosphates	Atropine	0.05 mg/kg IV, IO, or ET (dilute with 2 mL NS when given ET) Maximum: 2 mg	For muscarinic effects
	Pralidoxime (2-PAM)	25–50 mg/kg IV, slow push Maximum: 1 g	For nicotinic effects May repeat dosage q8–12h or more often if necessary
Phenothiazines	Diphenhydramine	0.5–1.0 mg/kg IV or IM Maximum: 50 mg	For extrapyramidal effects and dystonic reaction If effective, follow with 5 mg/kg PO q6h for 24–72 h
	Or Benztropine	0.02 mg/kg Maximum: 1 mg	
Salicylates (150 mg/kg)	Urine alkalinization	Start with 1–2 mEq/kg NaHCO₃ IV bolus over 1 h Then 1½ × maintenance of D5 with 30 mEq KCl and 120 mEq NaHCO₃/L If acidosis is severe (pH < 7.15), use additional NaHCO₃ Strive for urine pH of 7.5–8.0	Avoid fluid overload Pulmonary or cerebral edema may occur with severe salicylate toxicity See nomogram (Figure I-8)

BAL = British antilewisite; EDTA = ethylenediamine tetra-acetic acid; G6PD = glucose-6-phosphate-dehydrogenase; Hgb = hemoglobin; NS = normal saline; SDC = serum digoxin concentration.
ª Call poison-control center for consultation before use (telephone hotline: 800-222-1222).

    E. Psychosocial Evaluation. Obtain in all cases of illicit drug use and suicidal attempts.

    F. Prevention. Provide anticipatory guidance during routine well-baby visits as well as counseling following any incidence of poisoning or potential poisoning.

VI. Problem Case Diagnosis. Examination of this 2-year-old patient revealed mental status depression, respiratory depression, and pinpoint pupils consistent with opioid syndrome. Patient was given naloxone and showed clinical improvement. History revealed that patient's father had had recent spinal surgery and was taking oral oxycodone. Patient was observed for 6 hours and showed no further signs of opioid intoxication or requirement for naloxone. Toxicology screening was positive for opioids. Family was given anticipatory guidance to prevent further ingestions and accidents.

VII. Teaching Pearl: Question. How long should a patient with the toxidrome of opioid overdose be observed following administration of naloxone?

VIII. Teaching Pearl: Answer. Length of observation and treatment following opioid ingestion is dependent on clinical symptoms and duration of action of opioid ingeste d. The opioid reversal agent naloxone has a short duration of action (~20 minutes), which may necessitate giving multiple doses. In the problem case scenario described earlier, patient ingested oxycodone (duration of action: 4–6 hours). Patient was observed for several hours following treatment with naloxone, and no further treatment was required. Ingestion of narcotics with a long duration of action (eg, methadone or some sustained-release tablets) often requires multiple doses of naloxone or naloxone infusion. An alternative to naloxone infusion for overdose with long-acting narcotics is nalmefene. Nalmefene has an effective duration of action (opioid antagonism) significantly longer than that of naloxone. Dose is 0.5–1 mg/70 kg IV. It also could be administered intramuscularly, subcutaneously, or orally. Nalmefene is not approved for use in children.

REFERENCES

AACT and EAPCCT joint position statement on gastrointestinal decontamination. *J Clin Toxicol* 1997;35:695–762.

Shannon M. Ingestion of toxic substances by children. *N Eng J Med* 2000;342:186–191.

Tenenbein M. Recent advances in pediatric toxicology. *Pediatr Clin North Am* 1999;46:1179–1188.

75. POLYURIA

  I. Problem. A 4-year-old boy has frequent urination.

  II. Immediate Questions

    A. Does patient have urinary frequency and urgency? Consider voiding dysfunction (most common diagnosis) and UTI.

    B. Nocturnal enuresis or nocturia? Lack of nocturnal involvement usually excludes organic etiology.

    C. Does patient drink excessively? Is there nocturnal polydipsia (patient awakened by thirst)? Drinking large amounts of fluid during the day often is a habit but may have an organic etiology.

    D. Is there a history of GU problems? Conditions that may result in kidney damage and secondary polyuria include renal maldevelopment, posterior urethral valves, and pyelonephritis.

III. Differential Diagnosis

  A. Urinary Frequency and Urgency
1. Voiding dysfunction.
2. Transitional voiding.

  B. Excessive Drinking (Polydipsia)
1. **Organic.** High serum osmolarity; common presentation is a thirsty child. Renal conditions that prevent normal urinary concentrating ability and high solute loss (as in diabetes mellitus) may present with polyuria and polydipsia.
2. **Behavioral (psychogenic or compulsive).** Normal serum osmolarity; this presentation is unlikely in young children.

  C. Diabetes Insipidus. Large volume of diluted urine.
1. **Renal or nephrogenic.** Kidney is insensitive to vasopressin.
   - a. Renal dysplasia (congenital maldevelopment).
   - b. Obstructive nephropathy.
   - c. Interstitial nephritis (pyelonephritis).
   - d. Renal insufficiency.
   - e. Renal tubular acidosis.
   - f. Sickle cell nephropathy.
2. **Neurogenic (central).** Loss of antidiuretic hormone (ADH) secretion secondary to tumor, trauma, or, rarely, iatrogenic causes.

  D. Diabetes Mellitus. Polyphagia and glucosuria are evident.

IV. Database

  A. Physical Exam Key Points
1. Assess general appearance.
2. Observe for signs of dehydration.
3. Measure body weight and BP.
4. Exclude abdominal mass.

  B. Laboratory Data
1. **Metabolic panel.** Obtain serum electrolytes, glucose, creatinine, and BUN.
2. **Urinary evaluation.** Urinalysis with specific gravity, urine culture, and serum osmolarity (urine specific gravity > 1.020 excludes a concentrating defect).
3. **CBC.** To exclude sickle cell disease, as clinically indicated.

C. **Radiographic and Other Studies.** Consider based on findings from history, physical exam, laboratory studies, and clinical course. Imaging of urinary tract will identify patients with renal maldevelopment or obstructive uropathy.

1. **Ultrasound of abdomen.**
2. **Voiding cystourethrogram (VCUG).**
3. **CT scan of head.** Obtain if central lesion suspected.
4. **Urinary concentrating ability (water deprivation test).** In young children, this test should be completed in-hospital to allow for monitoring of body weight and electrolytes (exclude hypernatremia). Impose water restriction while assessing urine osmolality, body weight, and vital signs. Terminate test if tachycardia or hypotension develops. In these children, if administration of nasal desmopressin acetate (DDAVP)causes an increase in urine osmolality, a search for central or neurogenic cause of ADH insufficiency is indicated.

V. Plan. Keep a voiding diary (volume and timing of each urination during typical day). Initial evaluation with urinalysis and urinary volumes will differentiate patients with normal urinary volume yet abnormal urinary patterns secondary to voiding dysfunction from those with polyuria secondary to poor concentrating ability or osmotic polyuria (glucosuria).

A. **Voiding Disorder.** In children with normal urinary volumes, urine specific gravity and osmolarity, and urinary tract imaging, management consists of timed voiding to empty bladder, anticholinergic medication (oxybutynin, tolterodine), and behavioral modification.

B. **Renal Maldevelopment.** Refer to pediatric nephrologist.

C. **Obstructive Nephropathy.** Refer to pediatric urologist.

D. **Neurogenic Diabetes Insipidus.** Refer to pediatric neurologist.

VI. Problem Case Diagnosis. The 4-year-old boy had renal insufficiency secondary to obstructive uropathy (posterior urethral valves). There was no history of excessive fluid intake. Abdominal ultrasound scan showed hydronephrosis, and VCUG showed posterior urethral valves. Patient underwent transurethral ablation of valve leaflets.

VII. Teaching Pearl: Question. What is the difference between nephrogenic and neurogenic diabetes insipidus?

VIII. Teaching Pearl: Answer. Nephrogenic diabetes insipidus results from impaired tubular response to vasopressin and can be hereditary (X-linked or autosomal) or acquired (sickle cell disease, obstructive nephropathy, interstitial nephritis, renal insufficiency). Neurogenic diabetes insipidus result from vasopressin insufficiency, caused by a CNS lesion such as tumor, infection, or trauma. This form of diabetes insipidus responds to exogenous vasopressin (DDAVP).

REFERENCES

Breault DT, Majzoub JA. Diabetes insipidus. In: Behrman RE, Kliegman RM, Jenson HB, eds. *Nelson Textbook of Pediatrics,* 17th ed. Saunders, 2004:1853–1855.

Chevalier R, Howards SS. Renal function in the fetus, neonate, and child. In: Walsh PC, Retik AS, Vaughn ED, and Wein AJ, eds. *Campbell's Urology,* 8th ed. Saunders, 2002:1765–1780.

76. PROTEINURIA

I. Problem. A 14-year-old boy is found to have 3 + proteinuria during routine physical exam.

II. Immediate Questions

A. Does patient have any previously documented urinalysis? This is an important question, because most cases of incidentally discovered proteinuria resolve within a few weeks.

B. Any history of facial swelling, increased abdominal girth, or leg edema? Any of these symptoms would raise the possibility of nephrotic-range proteinuria, which, in turn, is a sign of significant renal disease.

C. Any history of constitutional symptoms or signs (intermittent fever, rash, abdominal pain, mouth sores, lymphadenomegaly, joint symptoms, weight gain or loss)? These symptoms and signs could be features of significant underlying disease causing proteinuria (eg, systemic lupus erythematosus, hemolytic uremic syndrome, Henoch-Schönlein purpura, among others).

D. Has patient ever had gross hematuria (red, brown, or pink urine)? History of brownish urine, along with proteinuria, should be considered as a sign of glomerular renal disease until proven otherwise. Fresh blood (red or pink, with or without clots) is most likely of lower urinary tract origin and is probably unrelated to presence of protein. Only a large amount of blood in urine will cause noticeable proteinuria; never microscopic hematuria.

E. Does patient have a history of recent strep throat or skin infection? Acute postinfectious glomerulonephritis (APIGN) can go unnoticed and may cause persistent proteinuria for up to 4–6 months.

F. Is there a family history of kidney disease? The few familial renal conditions that may need to be considered are Alport disease, juvenile nephronophthisis, polycystic kidney disease, and, in newborns and infants only, congenital nephrotic syndrome.

III. Differential Diagnosis

A. Normal Protein Excretion. Normal daily urinary protein excretion is < 4 mg/m^2/h. This may result in 1+ proteinuria (~30 mg/100 mL) in concentrated urine (specific gravity > 1.020 g/mL).

B. Transient Proteinuria. Most cases of incidentally discovered proteinuria resolve within a few weeks. Transient proteinuria can be the result of common febrile illnesses, exercise, and clinically undiagnosed mild, resolving APIGN.

C. **Orthostatic (Postural) Proteinuria.** Daytime (upright) protein excretion is elevated, but nighttime (supine) urine has little or no protein in it (< 50 mg/8 h). Daily protein excretion rarely exceeds 1 g. Typical patient with this condition is a thin adolescent boy experiencing a growth spurt; younger children and girls may also have this overall benign condition.

D. **Fixed (Persistent) Proteinuria**

1. **Nephrotic-range proteinuria.** A value of 3 + to 4 + proteinuria on urine dipstick, random urine protein-to-creatinine ratio > 2 (when concentrations are measured in grams per deciliter), and daily protein excretion > 2 g (some consider > 3 g) is consistent with nephrotic-range proteinuria. In younger children, proteinuria > 40 mg/m^2/h is considered nephrotic range. Nephrotic-range proteinuria usually is accompanied by peripheral edema, hypoalbuminemia, and hypercholesterolemia—a clinical condition termed *nephrotic syndrome.*

   a. **Minimal change disease (MCD).** Most common cause of nephrotic-range proteinuria in children: > 90% in preschool children, ~50% in adolescents. Urine sediment may contain hyaline casts and some RBCs, but cellular casts are absent.

   b. **Focal segmental glomerulosclerosis (FSGS).** This form of nephrotic syndrome is seen with increasing frequency in children; in some studies, as many as 30% of all newly diagnosed cases of nephrotic syndrome were due to FSGS. Incidence of FSGS in African Americans is nearly 50% higher than in Caucasians. Frequently, resistance to steroid treatment is the first warning sign that nephrotic syndrome is due to FSGS rather than to MCD. Other warning signs are hypertension and renal insufficiency.

   c. **Membranous nephropathy.** This form of nephrotic syndrome is uncommon in young children but is seen with increasing frequency in older children, adolescents, and young adults.

   d. **Glomerulonephritides.** Nearly all variants of glomerulonephritis (see discussion of nonnephrotic-range proteinuria that follows) can present with nephrotic-range proteinuria. In such cases, hypertension, decreased renal function, and active urinary sediment (RBCs, WBCs, and cellular casts) can be seen, in addition to typical findings of nephrotic syndrome. Of note, prognosis of any patient with glomerulonephritis involving a high degree of proteinuria is more guarded than that of a patient with the same nephritis but nonnephrotic-range proteinuria.

2. **Nonnephrotic-range proteinuria**

   a. **Glomerular proteinuria.** Although the conditions listed here can all present with nephrotic-range proteinuria in their more severe forms, typically proteinuria is only moderate.

       i. **APIGN.** Elevated urinary protein can be seen for up to 6 months following acute episode; hypertension can be present.

      ii. **IgA nephritis.** Proteinuria can be intermittent.

     iii. **Membranoproliferative glomerulonephritis (MPGN).**

     iv. **Henoch-Schönlein purpura (HSP).** In most cases proteinuria eventually disappears, although it may reappear with recurrences.

      v. **Hemolytic uremic syndrome (HUS).** Complete resolution of proteinuria occurs in most cases.

     vi. **Lupus nephritis.** Degree of proteinuria tends to follow disease activity and may completely resolve during full remission.

    vii. **Diabetic nephropathy.** Microalbuminuria is first sign of this condition. Because diabetic nephropathy usually takes many years to develop, this form of proteinuria is mostly seen in adolescents.

  b. Tubular proteinuria. Normal renal tubules have the capacity to reabsorb nearly all small-molecular-weight proteins that pass through an intact glomerular basement membrane. In this form of proteinuria, tubules are unable to reabsorb these proteins, causing excessive excretion of mostly small proteins (eg, β_2-microglobulin). Because urine dipstick strips are optimized to detect albumin in urine, this form of proteinuria will be underestimated by a simple urine dipstick test, or not detected at all.

IV. Database

  A. Physical Exam Key Points

    1. Vital signs. BP measurement is essential to detect nephritis.

    2. Skin. Observe for facial swelling; and for pitting edema of legs and sacral area if patient is nonambulatory. Look for vasculitic rash and sores on the buccal mucosa. If lupus is suspected, check lymph nodes.

    3. Lungs. If patient has generalized edema, carefully listen for crackles and rhonchi as signs of pulmonary edema.

    4. Abdomen. Evaluate for possible ascites; look for fluid waves and percuss for fluid shift.

    5. Joints. Thorough exam of joints is necessary if lupus or HSP is suspected.

  B. Laboratory Data. In young children with typical nephrotic syndrome, extensive workup beyond routine laboratory studies (CBC, creatinine, and serum albumin) is not needed.

    1. Urinalysis. RBCs can be present in 20–30% of patients with MCD. Hyaline casts alone have little significance, but granular and cellular casts (typically both red and white cell casts) indicate glomerulonephritis.

2. **CBC.** Anemia alone may indicate glomerulonephritis. Anemia with schistocytes and thrombocytopenia is expected in HUS. Leukopenia, usually with anemia and sometimes with thrombocytopenia, is frequent finding in lupus. HSP does not have characteristic findings on CBC.
3. **Serum chemistry.** Occasionally, elevated BUN and creatinine can be seen in MCD (if patient has severe edema and renal hypoperfusion). These findings, however, usually point to FSGS or glomerulonephritis. Hypoalbuminemia (< 3 g/dL) and high cholesterol indicate nephrotic syndrome.
4. **Serum serology.** Low C3 is expected in lupus, APIGN, and MPGN. Moderately elevated ANA (1:80–1:160) is frequently seen without vasculitis, but higher titers should raise the suspicion of lupus.
5. **ESR.** In the presence of hypoalbuminemia, ESR is moderately elevated, but values > 100 must be considered highly suspicious for systemic vasculitis.

C. **Radiographic and Other Studies**
1. **Renal ultrasound.** Findings are rarely specific. In nephrotic syndrome, kidneys are typically enlarged with decreased corticomedullary differentiation, because of interstitial fluid accumulation. Increased echogenicity is seen in any form of glomerulonephritis, even without nephrotic syndrome. Hydronephrosis may be detected in some forms of secondary FSGS that result from reflux nephropathy.
2. **Chest x-ray.** May be warranted in severe generalized edema or when respiratory symptoms are noted.

V. **Plan**
A. **Prednisone.** In a young child with nephrotic syndrome, initiate a therapeutic trial with prednisone. If there is a response, diagnosis of MCD is very likely. Prednisone is the cornerstone of treatment for many other conditions resulting in proteinuria.
B. **Diuretics.** In uncomplicated nephrotic syndrome, diuretics should not be used routinely (due to risk of further intravascular volume depletion and thromboembolic phenomenon, as well as hypotension); loop diuretics may be justifiable in severe cases of edema. Increase dose gradually to avoid acute hypovolemia.
C. **Antihypertensive Medications.** Acute and chronic control of BP is important in most conditions associated with proteinuria. Acute nephritis (eg, APIGN) can lead to hypertensive encephalopathy, whereas sustained hypertension accelerates progression of any underlying renal disease. Because of their antiproteinuric effect, ACE inhibitors and angiotensin II receptor blockers are drugs of choice for chronic treatment.
D. **Other Medications.** References for this chapter contain information about treatments for steroid-resistant nephrotic syndrome and several forms of glomerulonephritides.

VI. Problems Case Diagnosis. The 14-year-old patient had no other significant clinical findings: past medical and family histories were negative, urine sediment was absent, and results of serum chemistry and CBC analyses were normal. The urinary protein-to-creatinine ratio was 0.8 in the daytime and 0.05 in the first morning urine. Diagnosis is orthostatic proteinuria.

VII. Teaching Pearl: Question. Does a urine dipstick test that is negative for protein rule out diabetic nephropathy?

VIII. Teaching Pearl: Answer. No; the first sign of diabetic nephropathy is microalbuminuria, which results in excretion of urinary albumin in an amount that is below the sensitivity of the dipstick.

REFERENCES

Constantinescu AR, Shah HB, Foote EF, Weiss L. Predicting first-year relapses in children with nephrotic syndrome. *Pediatrics* 2000;105:492–495.

Fakhouri F, Bocquet N, Taupin P, et al. Steroid-sensitive nephrotic syndrome form childhood to adulthood. *Am J Kidney Dis* 2003;41:550–557.

Hogg RJ, Portman RJ, Milliner D, et al. Evaluation and management of proteinuria and nephrotic syndrome in children: Recommendations from a pediatric nephrology panel established at the National Kidney Foundation conference on proteinuria, albuminuria, risk, assessment, detection, and elimination (PARADE). *Pediatrics* 2000;105:1242–1249.

Hogg RJ, Portman RJ, Milliner D, et al. Recognizing and treating the nephrotic syndrome: Avoid unnecessary delays. *Cont Pediatr* 2000;17:84–93.

77. RECTAL PROLAPSE

I. Problem. A 2-year-old boy is brought to the emergency department by his mother, who reports that his "insides came out" after a bowel movement today. She describes the mass as soft and red. It is no longer present when the pediatrician evaluates him later that day in the office. There is no prior history of this problem.

II. Immediate Questions

A. Is pain associated with the mass? Most children are not in pain at the time of rectal prolapse. There may be some discomfort associated with bowel movements. In some cases, abdominal pain may have preceded rectal prolapse; often this occurs in cases of diarrhea-related rectal prolapse.

B. Are there any associated symptoms? Vomiting and irritability may be reported if intussusception is present. Painless rectal bleeding may occur with prolapse. A history of hard, infrequent stooling may be elicited. Anal pruritus can be a clue to pinworm.

C. Is bleeding associated with the mass? Traces of blood occur with rectal prolapse. More significant bleeding is seen with polyps.

D. Pertinent Medical History

1. **Is patient younger than 4 years of age?** Most cases occur in children aged 4 or younger, with peak incidence in first year of life.

2. **Is there a prior history of similar episodes? Chronic constipation and straining with stools? Does patient have cystic fibrosis or symptoms compatible with this diagnosis?** Straining at stools or with urination can predispose to rectal prolapse. Children with chronic constipation or cystic fibrosis are at risk for recurrence of rectal prolapse.

3. **Any history of surgery for imperforate anus? Prior history of polyps? Does patient have spina bifida?** Patients with pelvic floor weakness (eg, those with myelomeningocele) often have paralysis of the levator ani muscle in addition to increased intra-abdominal pressure.

4. **Is patient malnourished?** It is thought that malnourished children are at higher risk for rectal prolapse because of the decrease in ischiorectal fat that reduces perirectal support.

III. Differential Diagnosis
A. Causes of Rectal Prolapse
   1. Trauma.
   2. Cystic fibrosis.
   3. Increased abdominal pressure caused by straining (eg, constipation, protracted coughing, excessive vomiting, chronic straining during urination).
   4. Acute or chronic diarrheal disease (eg, giardiasis, shigellosis).
   5. Parasitic disease with infestations (eg, pinworm, whipworm).
   6. Neoplasms.
   7. Malnutrition.
   8. Pelvic floor weakness secondary to neurologic disorders.
   9. Sexual abuse.
   10. Other causes include Ehlers-Danlos syndrome and congenital hypothyroidism.
B. Prolapsing Rectal Polyp. Rare condition; patient presents with a darker, smaller mass than that seen in rectal prolapse.
C. Ileocecal Intussusception Protruding Through Anus. Much less common than rectal prolapse.
D. Rectal Polyp. Common cause of painless rectal bleeding in young children. Patient is unlikely to have a history of rectal prolapse.

IV. Database
A. Physical Exam Key Points
   1. **General appearance and vital signs.** Most children appear well and have normal vital signs at time of presentation.
   2. **Abdomen.** Exam is usually normal; some tenderness may be present.
   3. **Anal area**
      a. **Attempt to visualize prolapse.** If prolapsed rectum is not visualized, examine child in squatting position. If prolapse is not seen, digital exam may reveal dilated anal orifice with poor tone. If prolapse is seen, ascertain whether a finger

can be passed into the space between the anal wall and the mucosa of the protruding mass. If so, this may be an intussusception or a rectal polyp. Rectal prolapse will not allow passage of a finger between the protruding mass and the anal wall. If mass is plum colored, it is likely to be a rectal polyp.

b. **Determine whether prolapse is complete or incomplete.** In complete rectal prolapse, the full thickness of the rectum prolapses through anus. In this situation, concentric mucosal rings may be seen. Incomplete prolapse is limited to two layers of mucosa and reveals radial folds. If more than 5 cm of rectum is emerging, it is most likely a complete prolapse.

B. Laboratory Data

1. **CBC.** Consider in presence of significant blood loss.
2. **Electrolytes.** Obtain in presence of malnutrition.

C. Radiographic and Other Studies

1. **Sweat test.** To rule out cystic fibrosis.
2. **Stool culture for bacterial and parasitic infections.** If diarrhea is present.
3. **Tape test.** If pinworm infestation is suspected.
4. **Proctosigmoidoscopy.** Consider in patients who have recurrent rectal prolapse of no known etiology.
5. **Other studies.** Obtain based on history and physical exam findings.

V. Plan

A. Reduction of Rectal Prolapse

1. If rectal prolapse is noted on exam, attempt reduction by grasping protruding bowel with a lubricated glove and gently pushing it back in.
2. If it is difficult to reduce prolapse due to bowel edema, provide firm gentle pressure for several minutes to reduce swelling and enable reduction.
3. Perform a rectal exam after reduction to ascertain that prolapse is completely reduced.
4. Teach parents how to reduce prolapsed rectum.
5. If prolapse recurs rapidly, reduce again and tape buttocks together for several hours.
6. Inability to reduce rectal prolapse may lead to venous stasis. Edema and ulceration also may occur.

B. Surgical Consultation. Consider in the following situations.

1. Recurrent prolapse.
2. Mucosal ulceration.
3. Failure to obtain reduction despite sedation.
4. Full-thickness prolapse in patients with meningomyelocele or those who have had pull-through procedures for imperforate anus and Hirschsprung disease.

   C. **Evaluation for Predisposing Conditions.** Treat underlying
      causes (ie, constipation, diarrhea, cystic fibrosis).
   D. **Follow-up.** Contact with child's primary care physician is crucial
      to ensure prevention of recurrence.

VI. **Problem Case Diagnosis.** The 2-year-old patient, who has a chron-
    ic history of constipation, is diagnosed with simple rectal prolapse. It
    is noted to occur while squatting. After reduction of the prolapse,
    therapy for the underlying constipation is begun.

VII. **Teaching Pearl: Question.** How can a polyp be differentiated from
     rectal prolapse on examination?

VIII. **Teaching Pearl: Answer.** A polyp usually is plum colored and does
      not fill the entire anal circumference.

REFERENCES

Garner LM. Rectal prolapse. *eMedicine Journal* 2002;3(12). Available at:
   http://author.emedicine.com/ped/topic1897.htm
Schwartz MW, ed. *The 5 Minute Pediatric Consult.* Lippincott Williams & Wilkins,
   2000:686–687.
Siafakas C, Vottler TP, Andersen JM. Rectal prolapse in pediatrics. *Clin Pediatr*
   1999;38:63–72.
Zitelli BJ, Davis HW. *Atlas of Pediatric Physical Diagnosis,* 4th ed. Mosby, 2002:
   607–608.

78. RENAL FAILURE, ACUTE

I. **Problem.** A 2-year-old boy has had diarrhea for about 5 days. The
   diarrhea has improved, but he has not had a wet diaper in the past
   24 hours.

II. **Immediate Questions.** A medical history is essential in evaluating
    and treating patients with oliguria or acute renal failure (ARF).
    A. **Is patient in distress?** Does child appear ill or hemodynamically
       unstable? Oliguria may be an early manifestation of shock; evalu-
       ate airway, breathing, and circulation (ABCs).
    B. **Are any other serious or life-threatening conditions present?**
       ARF can be associated with hypotension, shock, hyperkalemia,
       acidosis, uremia, heart failure, and pulmonary edema.
    C. **What are patient's latest serum chemistry values? Is patient
       in renal failure? Are other electrolyte abnormalities present?**
       ARF if a clinical syndrome in which a sudden deterioration in renal
       function results in inability of the kidneys to maintain fluid and
       electrolyte homeostasis. The ratio of BUN to creatinine and
       degree of creatinine elevation are helpful in identifying the pres-
       ence and type of renal dysfunction. BUN-to-creatinine ratio > 20
       often indicates a prerenal cause (see later discussion). The higher

the creatinine value, the more likely it is that the patient has advanced renal damage.

D. What is the urine output?

1. Although urine output does not always correlate with the degree of renal failure, it may help to guide early and late treatment.

   a. **Anuria.** Output < 0.25 mL/kg/h.

   b. **Oliguria.** Output < 1 mL/kg/h.

   c. **Nonoliguric renal failure.** Output > 1 mL/kg/h.

   d. **High-output renal failure.** Output > 2 mL/kg/h.

2. The preceding loose guidelines may help to point to an etiology.

   a. Patients with nephritis and vascular events usually have little output.

   b. Those with acute tubular necrosis (ATN), interstitial nephritis, or obstruction have variable output.

   c. Those in prerenal states may have increased urine output with fluids.

E. Does patient have an underlying disease that could result in renal failure? Heart failure, liver failure, nephrotic syndrome, and recent surgery, trauma, or burns can result in decreased renal perfusion and a prerenal state. An autoimmune condition, recent infection, or leukemia can affect kidney function.

F. Does patient have signs or a condition leading to hypovolemia? Hypovolemia is the most common cause of ARF and oliguria in children. Prompt treatment is critical, because a prolonged prerenal state will eventually lead to ATN. Diarrhea, vomiting, blood loss, prolonged fever, decreased intake, low BP, skin and mucous membrane changes, and positional dizziness are all associated with hypovolemia.

G. Is there a history of urologic problems or manipulation that could be related to bladder outlet obstruction? Has a Foley catheter recently been inserted or a voiding cystourethrogram (VCUG) performed? Was an antenatal ultrasound abnormal, or does patient have a history of urologic problems?

H. Any history of hematuria, proteinuria, or other kidney problem? Does patient have underlying kidney disease that could shift into rapidly progressive nephritis?

I. Are symptoms of abdominal or flank pain present? Has patient had kidney stones, UTIs, or a history of a vascular event?

J. Has patient been exposed to nephrotoxic agents or medications? These include antibiotics (aminoglycosides, amphotericin, vancomycin); radiocontrast agents; chemotherapeutic agents (cisplatin, cyclophosphamide); immunosuppressive agents (cyclosporine, tacrolimus); NSAIDs; and crystal-forming agents (acyclovir, sulfonamides, methotrexate).

III. Differential Diagnosis. Acute renal failure is best categorized for both diagnosis and treatment into prerenal, intrinsic renal, and postrenal causes.

A. Prerenal Causes
   1. True volume depletion
      a. GI loss (dehydration).
      b. Blood loss (trauma).
   2. Decreased effective vascular volume
      a. Sepsis (vessel dilation and vascular leak).
      b. Trauma, surgery, burns (third space, sequestration).
      c. Hepatorenal syndrome.
      d. Nephrotic syndrome.
   3. Diminished cardiac output
      a. Myocardiopathy.
      b. Cardiac arrest.
      c. Postcardiac surgery.
B. Intrinsic Renal Causes
   1. Intrarenal vascular disease
      a. Hemolytic uremic syndrome (HUS).
      b. Vasculitis
         i. Polyarteritis nodosa.
         ii. Hypersensitivity vasculitis.
         iii. Scleroderma.
         iv. Henoch-Schönlein purpura (HSP).
      c. Renal venous thrombosis or artery thrombosis.
   2. Glomerulonephritis
      a. Postinfectious (post-streptococcal).
      b. Membranoproliferative.
      c. Rapidly progressive
         i. Idiopathic.
         ii. Systemic lupus erythematosus (SLE).
         iii. Goodpasture syndrome.
   3. Acute interstitial nephritis
      a. Drug related.
      b. Infectious
         i. Direct invasion (pyelonephritis: bacterial, viral, mycobacterial).
         ii. Indirect effects (postinfectious or post-streptococcal).
      c. Infiltrative
         i. Lymphoma, leukemia.
         ii. Sarcoidosis.
   4. Tubular
      a. ATN
         i. Anoxia, ischemia.
         ii. Nephrotoxic insult.
      b. Intratubular obstructive process
         i. Uric acid.
         ii. Myoglobin, hemoglobin.
      c. Oxalate.
C. Postrenal Causes

1. **Congenital**
   a. **Posterior urethral values.** Bladder outlet obstruction.
   b. **Upper tract obstruction.** Must be bilateral to cause renal failure.
      i. Ureterovesical junction.
      ii. Ureteropelvic junction.
2. **Acquired**
   a. **Intrinsic**
      i. Kidney stones.
      ii. Clots.
   b. **Extrinsic.** Tumors (neuroblastoma, sarcoma).

IV. **Database**
   A. **Physical Exam Key Points.** Physical exam may help determine cause and some of the complications of ARF. Evaluate and monitor previous and ongoing fluid inputs and all output (urine, stool, gastric), by keeping accurate daily intake and output measurements (I&Os) along with daily measurement of weight.
   1. **Vital signs**
      a. **Temperature.** Fever points to infection.
      b. **Heart rate.** Elevated with dehydration, volume depletion, or volume shifts.
      c. **BP**
         i. **Hypertension.** Usually seen in acute nephritis or with fluid overload.
         ii. **Hypotension.** Common in patients with sepsis syndrome leading to shock. Renal hypoperfusion (which initially results in a prerenal state), if ongoing, will progress to ATN. Most common cause of intrinsic renal failure in children is a prolonged prerenal state of hypoperfusion.
   2. **Skin.** Signs of dehydration or hypovolemia include dry mucous membranes, lack of tears, and poor capillary refill. Rashes suggest HSP, purpura related to decreased platelets (HUS), allergic drug reactions, or SLE.
   3. **Chest and cardiovascular.** Rales suggest heart failure or volume overload. Presence of third heart sound (S3) suggests heart failure. Murmurs suggest congenital heart disease with failure or emboli. New-onset murmur suggests endocarditis with associated nephritis.
   4. **Abdomen.** Ascites suggests nephrotic syndrome, liver failure, or heart failure. Distended bladder or mass suggests obstruction.
   5. **GU system.** Congenital abnormalities of genital system may be associated with urinary tract obstruction.
   6. **Extremities.** Edema suggests nephrotic syndrome or heart failure. Color and temperature may suggest perfusion states. Observe for lower extremity rash of HSP, and joint abnormalities of lupus or other immune-type diseases.

TABLE I–23. DIFFERENTIAL DIAGNOSIS OF ACUTE RENAL FAILURE: URINARY INDICES

Index	Prerenal Cause	Intrinsic Renal Cause
Specific gravity	> 1.020	≤ 1.010
Units of sodium	< 20 mmol/L	> 40 mmol/L
Fractional excretion of sodium (newborn) (%FE_{Na})[a]	< 1% (2%)	> 1% (2%)

[a] %FE_{Na} = $(U_{Na} + S_{Na})/(U_{Cr} + S_{Cr}) \times 100$. (Cr = creatinine; Na = sodium; S = serum; U = urine.)

    B. Laboratory Data. Refer to Table I–23 for urinary indices used to separate prerenal from intrinsic renal disease.

        1. Urinalysis. Not always helpful; can be normal with ARF.

            a. Specific gravity. If high; suggests volume depletion, contrast exposure, or nephritis.

            b. Hematuria and proteinuria. Large volume of blood and protein suggest nephritis.

            c. Microscopic findings

                i. RBCs. Finding of RBCs that are too numerous to count (TNTC; ie, > 50) suggests renal vein thrombosis or stone.

                ii. WBCs. Presence of many WBCs suggests infections.

                iii. Eosinophils. Presence suggests interstitial nephritis.

                iv. Casts. Granular casts suggest ATN; red cell, acute nephritis; white cell, pyelonephritis.

        2. Serum chemistries. Critical for identifying electrolyte abnormalities associated with renal failure, including hyponatremia and hypernatremia, hyperkalemia, low bicarbonate (metabolic acidosis), hyperphosphatemia, and hypocalcemia. If BUN and creatinine are elevated, a BUN-to-creatinine ratio > 20–30:1 could indicate a prerenal state, obstruction, GI bleeding, or catabolic state. A ratio < 10–15:1 more likely indicates an intrarenal cause. However, ratios are less accurate in children because of lower baseline creatinine levels.

        3. Urine electrolytes and creatinine. These are key findings in distinguishing prerenal states from other types of renal failure (see Table I–23). Urine sodium < 20 mmol/L suggests a prerenal state, as does fractional excretion of sodium (%FE_{Na}) < 1% (or < 2% for a newborn). %FE_{Na} is the more accurate test, and excretion < 1% (2% in newborn) is a strong indication to use aggressive fluid replacement. %FE_{Na} > 1% (2% in newborn) suggests intrinsic renal damage and more careful use of fluid replacement.

    C. Radiographic and Other Studies

        1. Renal ultrasound. Probably the single most useful study. If cause of renal failure is postrenal or obstructive, significant hydronephrosis is usually present. Hydronephrosis may be absent or less significant if patient is dehydrated. Renal ultrasound also produces good estimates of renal size and anatomy. Doppler flow ultrasound can be used to evaluate blood flow of renal artery and vein. Ultrasound studies can be helpful in identifying kidney stones, evaluating size and thickness of the bladder, and finding a site of obstruction and are safe under all conditions because no contrast is used.

2. **KUB.** This simple, fast test may locate a stone or identify a GI–related issue.

3. **CT scan, intravenous pyelogram, angiography.** Avoid if possible because these studies require use of contrast. CT scan is most useful in evaluating patients after traumatic injury, identifying kidney stones, and looking at renal artery and vein. MRI or magnetic resonance angiography may be used to evaluate renal vascular system; dye used in these studies is less toxic than that used in CT, but images may not be as clear.

4. **VCUG, retrograde pyelogram.** Useful to determine point of obstruction.

5. **Chest x-ray.** To evaluate heart size, pulmonary edema, and lung findings. Can serve as a quick test of overall fluid status when deciding whether to continue aggressive fluid replacement.

6. **Central venous pressure line.** May be needed for more accurate assessment of intravascular volume status

7. **ECG.** Useful to evaluate effect of hyperkalemia.

8. **Echocardiogram.** To evaluate left ventricular function and pericardial effusion that may affect cardiac outflow.

9. **Renal biopsy.** Useful in renal failure of unknown etiology and long duration, or if clinician suspects rapidly progressive nephritis or vasculitis.

V. Plan. Remember that during initial evaluation and management phases of ARF, medications, fluids, and radiographic procedures that use contrast may need to be modified, depending on degree of renal failure and urine output.

A. Early Diagnostic and Therapeutic Maneuvers. It is still debated whether prerenal renal failure that may be progressing to ATN can be reversed or prevented by any of these early and aggressive therapeutic maneuvers, but it may be possible to shift from an oliguric to a nonoliguric state.

1. **Urinary catheter.** If already placed, make sure catheter is patent by flushing with 20–50 mL of sterile saline. If not in place and patient is anuric or oliguric, placement of a Foley catheter will allow urine culture and urine chemistries to be obtained. It also will allow for accurate output measurements in response to therapeutic maneuvers. Once either good urine output is established and renal function is improving or patient remains anuric, remove catheter as soon as possible to prevent infections.

2. **Fluid challenge.** Consider even if child does not appear dehydrated, unless rales, increased heart size, pulmonary edema

on chest x-ray, or severe hypertension is present. Use 20 mL/kg of normal saline (up to 1 L), and repeat if patient is clinically dehydrated, %FE_{Na} is < 1%, urine sodium is < 20 mmol/L, or patient is hypotensive. This is the single most effective maneuver to prevent progression of prerenal renal failure state to permanent state of intrinsic renal failure or ATN.

3. **Loop diuretics.** Can improve both renal blood flow and tubular flow rate and may help to initiate diuresis. Consider dose of 1–4 mg/kg up to a maximum of 80 mg (given over 30 minutes to decrease any ototoxic effect). Use after at least one fluid challenge. May repeat once in 2–4 hours if no response. If effective, diuretic may be continued in lower doses to maintain urine output.

4. **Dopamine.** Dopamine may improve renal blood flow at low doses (2–5 mcg/kg/min). May need higher doses or other inotropic agents to support BP.

5. **Mannitol.** Increases tubular flow and is most useful in rhabdomyolysis, hemolysis, uric acid nephropathy, and dysfunction resulting from contrast and other nephrotoxic agents. Most effective if given before toxic event. Use with care in oliguric states, because if drug is not excreted, it will increase hyperosmolarity and volume overload of renal failure.

6. **Treat or remove initiating event or toxin if possible.**
   a. Improve cardiac output if needed with inotropic agents.
   b. Treat infections (eg, pyelonephritis or sepsis); may need to adjust antibiotic dose for renal failure.
   c. Remove all nephrotoxic agents that may be associated with interstitial nephritis.
   d. Consider starting immunosuppressive therapy for acute nephritis; this usually requires a kidney biopsy.
   e. Take great care with all medications that are excreted via kidney, and with x-rays that require contrast, because they may worsen primary renal injury.

B. **Management of Specific Causes of Renal Failure**
   1. **Prerenal.** Be sure patient is volume replete (central venous pressure > 10, and adequate systemic BP) before reducing IV fluids to insensible loss and ongoing output.
   2. **Postrenal.** Attempt to bypass site of obstruction.
      a. For obstruction at bladder outlet, bypass by placing Foley catheter; for higher obstruction, with nephrostomy or stent. These should always be managed with urologic consultation.
      b. Relief of obstruction may resolve cause of renal failure but produce significant postobstruction diuresis that will require careful fluid and electrolyte replacement.
   3. **Intrinsic renal.** Treat specific cause if known.
      a. Administer antibiotics for pyelonephritis and sepsis.
      b. Use immunosuppressive agents for rapidly progressive nephritis.

      c. Attempt to lower uric acid levels with allopurinol, cell pheresis, or hemodialysis.

C. Management of Primary Complications of ARF

  1. Fluid overload. Diuretics may or may not work. Use loop diuretics such as furosemide, 1–2 mg/kg, and stop if no response after first few doses. Institute fluid restriction after initial fluid challenge and replacement. Replace insensible loss (free water such as D_5 or D_{10} at about 35% of maintenance) plus output. Urine output usually is replaced with half-normal saline solution plus bicarbonate. **Do not use potassium unless serum electrolytes demonstrate need.**

  2. Hypertension. Elevated BP usually is related to volume overload, except in patients with nephritis.

    a. Nitroprusside. Give 0.5–5 mcg/kg/min IV; most potent vasodilator.

    b. Hydralazine. Give 0.1–0.5 mg/kg per dose IV, or 0.25–1 mg/kg per dose PO; weak vasodilator.

    c. Labetalol. Give 0.5–2 mg/kg per dose IV over 1 hour; α- and β-antagonist that works well with vasodilators listed above.

    d. Furosemide. Give 1–2 mg per dose IV if patient has urine output; second-line drug for hypertension that may be helpful after use of vasodilators or in patients with clear-cut volume overload states.

  3. Hyperkalemia. Serum potassium > 6 mEq/L; ECG changes make the diagnosis. (See also Chapter 41, p. 196)

    a. Calcium gluconate (10%). Give 0.2–0.5 mL/kg IV; provides direct membrane stabilization.

    b. Sodium bicarbonate. Give 1 mEq/kg; facilitates movement of potassium into cells.

    c. Albuterol nebulization. Give 1.25–5 mg per treatment, based on age; β-agonist that facilitates quick but transient movement of potassium into cells.

    d. Glucose plus insulin. Administer glucose, 0.5 g/kg, plus insulin, 0.2–0.3 unit/g of glucose, IV; facilitates movement of potassium into cells.

    e. Kayexalate. Give PO or per rectum, mixed 4:1 with sorbitol; exchanges sodium for potassium in gut. Use of 1 g/kg should lower serum potassium by about 1 mEq/L but will increase serum sodium.

  4. Hyponatremia or hypernatremia. (See also Chapters 43 and 50, pp. 203 and 232.)

    a. Hyponatremia (serum sodium < 130 mEq/L) occurs secondary to excess free water. Managed by decreasing intake.

    b. Hypernatremia (serum sodium > 150 mEq/L) usually occurs secondary to administration of IV fluids with sodium or medications. Managed by restricting sodium intake. Very little sodium is usually needed in patients with ARF.

5. **Hypocalcemia.** Serum calcium < 8.6 mg/dL; treat if symptoms are present. Manage carefully, because phosphorous level is usually high, and raising serum calcium may raise calcium-phosphorous product (calcium × phosphorus in milligrams per deciliter) to > 70, which can lead to systemic calcifications. (See also Chapter 46, p. 221.)

6. **Hyperphosphatemia.** (For age-adjusted normal values, see Section II, Phosphorus, p. 211.) Attempt to control with diet and phosphate binders, such as calcium carbonate, 2–10 g/day orally. Give with food 3 or 4 times daily. (See also Chapter 44, p. 211.)

7. **Metabolic acidosis.** Serum bicarbonate < 15 mEq/L; treat with sodium bicarbonate, 1–4 mEq/kg/day, up to maximum of 100 mEq/day.

8. **Uremia and diet.** Related to catabolic states and intake. Keep protein intake to 10% of total calorie intake or 0.5–1 g/kg/day, and try to maximize calorie intake PO or IV.

D. **Management of Secondary Complications of ARF**

1. **Infections.** Often related to catheters and results in sepsis. Treat aggressively with antibiotics but *do not* use prophylactic antibiotics. Remove catheters as early as possible.

2. **GI bleeding.** Related to stress and platelet dysfunction in uremia.
   a. **Proton-pump inhibitors.** No dose adjustment is necessary; give omeprazole, 1 mg/kg.
   b. **H$_2$ antagonist.** Need to reduce dose by 50%.

3. **Anemia.** Usually well tolerated and often related to blood drawing. Epogen is of limited use.

E. **Indications for Dialysis**

1. Fluid overload that is refractory to medical therapy and is associated with heart failure or severe hypertension.

2. Hyperkalemia or metabolic acidosis that is refractory to medical management.

3. Severe hyponatremia or hypernatremia that cannot be corrected medically.

4. Symptomatic uremia (drowsiness, nausea and vomiting, irritability) usually seen as BUN exceeds 100 and approaches 150 mg/dL or is rapidly rising at > 30 mg/dL/day.

5. Supportive dialysis for fluid removal to allow adequate nutritional support.

VI. **Problem Case Diagnosis.** The previously healthy 2-year-old boy had visited a petting zoo 1 week before becoming ill. On admission, he was irritable with hepatosplenomegaly and petechiae. CBC was remarkable for hemoglobin of 8.2 g/dL and platelet count of 50,000/mm^3. Urinalysis was positive for blood and protein. *E coli* O157:H7 was isolated from the heme-positive stool. The child was diagnosed with HUS (acute renal failure, hemolytic anemia, and thrombocytopenia).

VII. Teaching Pearl: Question. What additional organ system may be involved in HUS?

VIII. Teaching Pearl: Answer. CNS is involved in 20–30% of patients with HUS, causing stupor, seizures, cerebral infarct, or coma. Pancreatic insufficiency, myocarditis, and cardiomyopathy can also occur.

REFERENCES

Andreoli SP. Acute renal failure. *Curr Opin Pediatr* 2002;14:183–188.

Chan JC, Williams DM, Roth KS. Kidney failure in infants and children. *Pediatr Rev* 2002;23;47–59.

Gouyon JB, Guignard JP. Management of acute renal failure in newborns. *Pediatr Nephrol* 2000:14;1037–1044

Williams DM, Sreedhar SS, et al. Acute kidney failure: A pediatric experience over 20 years. *Arch Pediatr Adolesc Med* 2002;156:893–900.

79. RESPIRATORY DISTRESS

I. Problem. A 6-month-old girl is admitted with nasal congestion, tachypnea, and wheezing. She requires supplemental oxygen.

II. Immediate Questions

A. Does patient have impending respiratory failure or a life-threatening condition that requires immediate attention (eg, tension pneumothorax)? Respiratory failure leads to respiratory arrest if early recognition and intervention are lacking. Prognosis is poor in children who undergo respiratory arrest.

B. Is patient apneic, hypoxic, or hypoventilating? Differential diagnosis and management are shaped by this distinction.

C. What clinical features are associated with respiratory distress in this patient? Fever suggests an infectious etiology. Symptoms of upper respiratory infection are consistent with viral cause. Anaphylaxis is a consideration if distress is temporally associated with a particular food or medicine.

D. Has patient or a family member had a similar episode? This type of pattern can be seen with asthma.

III. Differential Diagnosis

A. Conditions That Can Lead to Respiratory Distress

1. Hypoxia. There are four types: hypoxic hypoxia (decreased PaO_2), anemic hypoxia, ischemic hypoxia, and histotoxic hypoxia (tissues cannot use oxygen, secondary to effects of toxins). Although carbon dioxide plays the dominant role in ventilation control, hypoxia from any cause increases ventilatory drive through stimulation of peripheral chemoreceptors found in carotid and aortic bodies. Changes in ventilation occur when arterial PaO_2 decreases to < 50 mm Hg. Causes of hypoxia include, but are not limited to, pneumonia, acute respiratory distress syndrome (ARDS), hemothorax, pleural effusion, and pneumothorax.

2. **Acidosis.** Attempts to compensate for metabolic acidosis may result in tachypnea. Classic example is a patient with diabetic ketoacidosis who develops tachypnea when the body attempts to correct metabolic acidosis by increasing ventilation (respiratory compensation).

3. **Pain.** Inadequately treated pain, from any site, may cause patient to splint chest area during ventilation, resulting in ineffective rapid, shallow breathing.

4. **Fever and hypermetabolic states.** All serious infectious diseases can have associated tachypnea.

5. **Upper airway obstruction.** Upper airway obstruction can result in tachypnea, which may be accompanied by paradoxical motion of the chest and abdomen. Causes of upper airway obstruction include, but are not limited to, laryngotracheitis (croup), tracheitis, airway foreign body, vocal cord disease, and postextubation tracheal edema.

6. **Reactive airway disease.** Risk factors such as an atopic family history often are present.

7. **Systemic inflammatory response syndrome or sepsis.** Especially when complicated by ARDS.

8. **Neurogenic problems.** Neurologic abnormalities and head injury may result in abnormal central respiratory drive.

9. **Neuromuscular disease or weakness.** Neuromuscular diseases, including myopathies, spinal cord disease (eg, spinal muscle atrophy), peripheral motor nerve disease (eg, Guillain-Barré syndrome, phrenic nerve disorders), diseases of neuromuscular junction (eg, botulism), and skeletal muscle disease (eg, muscular dystrophy) may cause hypoxia secondary to weakness and hypoventilation.

10. **Pulmonary edema or congestive heart failure.**

11. **Intra-abdominal pathology that restricts lung expansion.** Examples include massive ascites or intra-abdominal space-occupying lesion.

12. **Other causes.** Salicylate overdose, methanol, pulmonary embolism, caffeine, cocaine, pleural effusion, pneumothorax, pulmonary hypertension, anxiety, pain, carbon monoxide poisoning.

B. **Respiratory Distress and Failure**

1. **Respiratory distress.** A compensated state in which normal gas exchange is maintained at the expense of increased work of breathing. Typically this manifests as tachypnea and increased work of breathing. When adequate oxygenation, ventilation, or both cannot be maintained, respiratory failure ensues. Ventilation is a complex physiologic process, primarily controlled by carbon dioxide. Other influences come from peripheral chemoreceptors that sense changes in blood pH, carbon dioxide, and Po_2. Pulmonary stretch receptors, irritant receptors, and J receptors can all influence ventilation in certain circumstances.

a. **Dyspnea.** Subjective sensation of difficult, labored, and uncomfortable breathing. Children may not be able to report or describe dyspnea. There are pulmonary and nonpulmonary causes; in children, most causes are pulmonary.

b. **Tachypnea.** An objective measurement of increased respiratory rate for age. Healthy newborns typically breathe 24–40 times per minute. Normal respiratory rate decreases with age to adult normal value of 14–20 breaths per minute.

2. **Respiratory failure.** Inability of respiratory system to supply body with adequate oxygen and to remove carbon dioxide. Can be divided into two categories: failure to oxygenate (hypoxemic) and failure to ventilate (hypoventilatory). Both can be seen in pediatric patients and may occur together. Ventilatory support is indicated when adequate gas exchange cannot be independently achieved or maintained.

a. **Hypoxemia and hypoxemic respiratory failure**

i. **Findings.** Hypoxemia describes a decreased oxygen tension in the blood (PaO_2). Oxygenation can be determined by measurement of pulse oximetry (SpO_2) or partial pressure of oxygen in arterial blood (PaO_2). By evaluating PaO_2 in context of fraction of inspired oxygen (FiO_2) employed, objective criteria for hypoxemic respiratory failure can be established. Ratio of PaO_2 to FiO_2 (P/F ratio) is used to characterize hypoxemia. P/F ratio < 200 is consistent with ARDS, whereas a ratio between 200 and 300 is consistent with acute lung injury. Patients with P/F ratio < 300 or SpO_2 < 90–93% (in absence of cyanotic heart disease) require additional support, especially if they demonstrate signs of inadequate oxygen delivery (eg, tachycardia, metabolic acidosis, or end-organ dysfunction). Although these patients may be managed initially with high oxygen delivery systems, their disease may progress to a point at which ventilatory support is required. Because of their physiologic instability and potential need for advanced therapies, these patients should be closely monitored in a pediatric intensive care unit. Worsening of respiratory status necessitates prompt intubation and ventilatory support. Prototype disease for hypoxemic respiratory failure is ARDS, in which high shunt fraction leads to refractory hypoxemia.

ii. **Pulmonary causes. Absolute (true) shunt:** Blood passes from right to left heart without being exposed to alveolar oxygen; no response is shown to increased FiO_2; examples include capillary shunting (eg, ARDS, pneumonia, atelectasis) and anatomic shunting (eg, congenital heart defect, arteriovenous malformations). **Relative shunt (venous admixture):** Ventilation-perfusion (V/Q) mismatch (perfusion in excess of ventilation); for example, asthma. **Hypoventilation:** Carbon dioxide replaces oxygen in lungs. **Diffusion defects:** Alveolar-capillary membrane can be widened significantly without resultant hypoxemia. If it thickens (eg, fibrosis), diffusion may be reduced to the extent of resulting hypoxemia. This is unusual. In most interstitial lung diseases (eg, interstitial pneumonitis), hypoxemia is due to V/Q mismatch rather than diffusion defects.

  iii. **Nonpulmonary causes.** Decrease in cardiac index. Decrease in oxygen-carrying capacity (hemoglobin/RBCs). Increase in oxygen consumption (VO_2).

b. Hypoventilatory respiratory failure

  i. **Findings.** $Paco_2 > 50$ mm Hg indicates ventilatory failure; however, many patients have chronic ventilatory failure with renal compensation (retaining HCO_3^-). Clinical exam and absolute pH is a better guide than $Paco_2$ to determine need for ventilatory assistance. Significant acidemia suggests acute respiratory acidosis or acute decompensation of chronic respiratory acidosis. Respiratory acidosis with rapidly falling pH or absolute pH < 7.24 is an indication for ventilatory support.

  ii. **Causes.** Prototype of pure ventilatory failure is patient with a drug overdose in whom there is sudden loss of central respiratory drive with uncontrolled hypercarbia. Patients with central hypoventilation, Werdnig-Hoffmann disease (anterior horn cell disease), Guillain-Barré syndrome (peripheral motor nerve disease), botulism (disease of neuromuscular junction), obstructive pulmonary disease, and sepsis may have hypercarbic ventilatory failure. Neuromuscular failure is a category of ventilatory failure that deserves special mention. A progressive rise in respiratory rate, increased work of breathing, and abdominal paradox (inward movement of abdominal wall during inspiration rather than normal outward motion), decreased vital capacity, or decreased negative inspiratory force (> –25 cm H_2O) implies impending respiratory failure.

c. Mixed respiratory failure. Many patients have failure of both ventilation and oxygenation. An example is patient with neuromuscular disease and pneumonia. Indications for ventilatory support remain the same. Threshold for initiating ventilatory support is even lower for patients with ventilation and oxygenation failure, because oxygen management may further compound hypercarbia.

IV. Database
  A. Physical Exam Key Points

1. **General appearance and vital signs.** Assess general appearance, respiratory rate, oxygen saturation, heart rate, and BP.
2. **Cardiopulmonary system.** Assess pattern of breathing. Look for chest deformities and retractions. Evaluate for signs of impending respiratory failure or tension pneumothorax. Signs and symptoms of impending respiratory failure include use of accessory muscles, diaphoresis, inability to speak, cyanosis, and pallor. Evaluate for hypoxia: Look for cyanosis or pallor by examining lips, nail beds, and skin. Evaluate for adequate ventilation by evaluating breath sounds, chest movement, and expansion. Assess equality and adequacy of breath sounds; listen for rales and wheezes. Auscultate heart sounds and listen for muffled heart sounds, new gallops, or murmurs.
3. **Other findings.** Assess neurologic status and muscle strength. Look for petechiae and rashes. Evaluate extremities for adequate perfusion.

B. **Laboratory Data**
  1. **ABGs.** Assess oxygenation and provide information about Pco_2 and pH status.
  2. **Hemoglobin.** Obtain to rule out anemic hypoxia.
  3. **Pulse oximetry and end-tidal CO_2.** May be helpful.
  4. **Other workup.** Consider obtaining cultures, respiratory syncytial virus (RSV) rapid antigen test, or other studies based on presenting features.

C. **Radiographic and Other Studies**
  1. **Chest x-ray.** Look for infiltrates, pleural effusion, pneumothorax, or pulmonary edema.
  2. **Other radiographic studies.** CT scan may be helpful to evaluate subtle conditions. Although uncommon in children, if pulmonary embolus is suspected, consider CT, V/Q scan, or pulmonary arteriogram in consultation with radiologist.

V. **Plan**
A. **Immediate Management**
  1. Evaluate airway, breathing, and circulation (ABCs).
  2. Evaluate and treat life-threatening conditions (eg, impending respiratory failure, tension pneumothorax). Regardless of cause, consider intubation and mechanical ventilation if patient shows signs of impending respiratory failure.
  3. Evaluate for hypoxemia and provide supplemental oxygen as necessary.
  4. Evaluate for adequate ventilation. Patient may be tachypneic with good air movement in an attempt to compensate for metabolic acidosis. Alternatively, tachypnea may result from inability to achieve adequate tidal volume, a condition that is more ominous.

   5. Alleviate airway obstruction. Perform jaw-thrust or chin-lift maneuver immediately, then consider use of oropharyngeal airway, nasopharyngeal airway, and continuous or bilevel positive airway pressure. Administer racemic epinephrine or steroids for airway edema.
   B. Management of Specific Conditions
   1. Treat underlying conditions (eg, pleural effusion, pneumothorax, sepsis, pneumonia, anaphylaxis, residual neuromuscular blockade, narcotic overdose).
   2. Treat reactive or inflammatory airway disease. Consider inhaled B_2-receptor agonist, steroids, magnesium, heliox, anticholinergics.
   3. Treat fluid overload. Initiate diuresis appropriately as clinical condition warrants.
   4. Correct acidosis and conditions leading to acidotic state.
   5. Treat pain or anxiety when other serious conditions have been ruled out.
VI. Problem Case Diagnosis. The 6-month-old patient had a positive result on RSV antigen testing and was diagnosed with bronchiolitis. (For further discussion, see VII and VIII, below.)

VII. Teaching Pearl: Question. What is the treatment for RSV bronchiolitis?

VIII. Teaching Pearl: Answer. Treatment is largely supportive care (supplemental oxygen and hydration). Other therapies to consider that remain controversial include inhaled bronchodilators and racemic epinephrine for select and severe cases in children with underlying disorders. In general, steroids are not considered effective. Passive immunization and interruption of transmission are important. Further studies are needed to confirm efficacy of these therapies.

REFERENCES

Darville T, Yamauchi T. Respiratory syncytial virus. *Pediatr Rev* 1998;19:55–68.
Haist SA, Robbins JB. *Internal Medicine on Call,* 3rd ed. Lange, 2002.
Marino PL. *The ICU Book,* 2nd ed. Lippincott Williams & Wilkins, 1998.

80. SCROTAL SWELLING

   I. Problem. A 3-year-old boy is brought to the emergency department because of scrotal swelling.

   II. Immediate Questions
   A. Is swelling painful? Painful swelling is associated with torsion, infections, and incarcerations, whereas nonpainful swelling may suggest testicular tumor.
   B. Is there a history of trauma? Keep in mind that traumatic injuries in younger children are more likely to go unwitnessed.

    C. Is swelling acute or chronic? Epididymal torsion is usually associated with gradual discomfort; testicular carcinoma can present either gradually or acutely.

III. Differential Diagnosis
A. Painful Swelling
1. **Torsion of epididymal or testicular appendage.** Produces gradual discomfort, with periods that are relatively pain free. Progression of inflammation by involvement of epididymis results in steady scrotal pain. Patients often relate having experienced testicular pain a few days earlier, followed by pain-free period; scrotal inflammation and pain may worsen with increased physical activity.
2. **Torsion of cord (testis torsion).** Most commonly occurs in early puberty (prenatal or neonatal period is second most common time of presentation). Characterized by intense, escalating pain. Patient is unable to find a comfortable position. Nausea and vomiting are common.
3. **Incarcerated hernia.** More common in infants. May be associated with vomiting as incarceration progresses. These are indirect inguinal hernias due to a persistence of patent processus vaginalis. Usually noted during periods of increased abdominal pressure, during straining or crying.
4. **Epididymitis.** Rare in childhood; initially produces mild, diffuse tenderness that progresses to involve entire hemiscrotum.

B. Nonpainful Swelling
1. **Hydrocele.** May be communicating (persistent processus vaginalis) or noncommunicating (rare in children; occurs mostly in adolescents and adults). Occasionally brought on during a viral illness.
2. **Testis tumor.** Nonpainful enlargement that may be slow or rapid in growth. Leads to noticeable discrepancy in scrotal appearance.

IV. Database
A. Physical Exam Key Points
1. **Torsion of testis or epididymal appendage.** Localized scrotal erythema, pinpoint tenderness in apex of testis (testis otherwise normal), and indurated and tender appendix. Early on, "blue dot sign," or torsed ischemic appendix, may be visible below noninflamed scrotal skin. Reactive hydrocele and progressive epididymal involvement and inflammation (secondary epididymitis) may preclude determination of this condition on physical exam, and may resemble torsion of testis cord on examination. Scrotal wall edema prevents transillumination as condition progresses.
2. **Torsion of cord.** Indurated, high-riding testis with possible transverse lie; diffuse tenderness. Does not transilluminate.

3. **Incarcerated hernia.** Enlarged, tender inguinal bulge that extends into scrotum.
4. **Epididymitis.** Tenderness is maximal at base of epididymis. Progressive involvement obliterates epididymal-testicular landmarks. Must exclude UTI.
5. **Hydrocele.** May be evident as nontender, bluish, fluid-filled sac surrounding testis. Hydrocele can be decompressed by gently pressing on its walls. Transilluminates readily.
6. **Testis tumor.** Indurated, firm, nontender mass; 20% of patients have an associated hydrocele. If tumor is hormonally active, physical findings suggestive of precocious puberty may be present.

B. **Laboratory Data**
   1. **Urinalysis, Gram stain, urine culture.** Positive in epididymitis secondary to UTI.
   2. **CBC, C-reactive protein.** Elevated in epididymitis.
   3. **α-Fetoprotein.** Obtained in patients with suspected tumor; elevated in yolk sac tumors.
   4. **Human chorionic gonadotropin (β-HCG).** Elevated in patients with tumors containing syncytiotrophoblast populations.

C. **Radiographic and Other Studies**
   1. **Scrotal ultrasound.** Instrumental in differentiating tense hydroceles from testicular tumors. Doppler flow analysis is also essential to distinguish testicular torsion (diminished or absent flow) from torsion of appendix or epididymitis (increased flow). Combination of parenchymal visualization and testicular blood flow makes ultrasound the ideal radiologic study for evaluation of scrotal swelling.
   2. **Nuclear testicular scans (technetium).** Useful in cases of possible testicular torsion, although seldom used if Doppler flow sonography is available.
   3. **CT scan.** Of minimal use in evaluating scrotal swelling, but necessary in evaluating retroperitoneum and chest of patients with testicular tumors.

V. Plan. Most important determination is to exclude spermatic cord torsion, which is a surgical emergency; delay in diagnosis and management may lead to loss of testis. Most testes can be salvaged if detorsed within 6 hours of onset. Management of torsed appendages is primarily supportive. Hernias must be repaired surgically if they cannot be reduced. Epididymitis is treated with antibiotics in addition to supportive therapy if there is evidence to support bacterial infection.

VI. Problem Case Diagnosis. The 3-year-old patient had communicating hydrocele associated with viral illness. The viral illness caused an increased volume of peritoneal fluid and cough, which lead to increased intra-abdominal pressure, with fluid directed into the hydrocele.

VII. Teaching Pearl: Question. To what does the term *bell-clapper deformity* refer?

VIII. Teaching Pearl: Answer. The bell-clapper deformity refers to an anatomic anomaly in which the spermatic cord twists inside the tunica vaginalis due to its high insertion on the cord. This is the usual etiology of adolescent testicular torsion. Deformity is bilateral; therefore, bilateral testicular fixation is recommended at the time of surgical detorsion.

REFERENCES

Davenport M. ABC of general surgery in children: Acute problems of the scrotum. *BMJ* 1996;312:435–347.

Figueroa TE, Casale P. Hydroceles and varicoceles. In: Mattei P, ed. *Surgical Directives: Pediatric Surgery.* Lippincott Williams & Wilkins, 2003:719–722.

Packer MG, Zaontz MR. Torsion-testicular. In: Gomella L, ed. *The 5-Minute Urology Consult.* Lippincott Williams & Wilkins 2000:538–539.

81. SEDATION AND ANALGESIA

I. **Problem.** A 4-year-old boy is crying and struggling during an attempted lumbar puncture.

II. **Immediate Questions**
   A. **Is patient a candidate for procedural sedation?** Sedation is considered for procedures that are painful and when child must lie immobile. Patients who undergo procedural sedation must undergo presedation assessment focusing on potential complications. Screening should include review of patient's medical history, allergies, medications, prior sedation history, and last food intake. Physical exam should assess for potential airway obstruction and respiratory compromise.
   B. **Does patient have risk factors for adverse events during sedation?** Risk factors include positive history for snoring or sleep apnea, reactive airways disease, or other chronic pulmonary disease; congenital or acquired heart disease; hypertension; gastroesophageal reflux or vomiting; and neurologic disease, such as muscle weakness or poorly controlled seizures.
   C. **Any underlying medical conditions?** Hepatic or renal disease may affect metabolism of sedative agents. Patients with active upper or lower tract respiratory infections, vomiting, dehydration, and recent head or multisystem trauma are at increased risk for sedation complications.
   D. **Has patient had any previous experience or problems with sedation or analgesics?** True allergies to agents of sedation and analgesia are rare; avoid using agent or class of agents that patient has not tolerated well in the past. Some patients react paradoxically to midazolam with increased agitation rather than relaxation. Patients receiving procedural sedation multiple times

over several days may develop tolerance to medications, requiring increased dosing or change of agent for effective results.

E. What medications does patient currently take? Certain medications, most commonly antiepileptic and behavioral modification medications, may affect sedation. In general, it is best to have patient continue on his or her usual medication regimen, and to titrate sedatives accordingly.

F. When did patient last eat? Although fasting for procedural sedation is still considered desirable, a nonfasting state is not an absolute contraindication to procedure. Mounting evidence suggests that risk of vomiting is not related to time of last enteral intake.

G. Is setting appropriate for procedural sedation? Safe procedural sedation requires personnel who are skilled in airway management and resuscitation. Staffing should allow for a dedicated patient observer who is not responsible for performing procedure.

III. Indications. Choice of sedative agent or combination of agents is dependent on several key questions. Is procedure painful? How long will procedure take? Does patient need to be completely immobile, or is some movement acceptable? Figure I–7 lists indications for specific sedation agents.

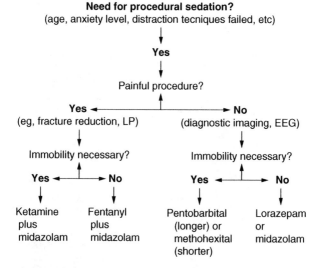

Figure I–7. Selection of procedural sedation agents. (EEG = electroencephalogram; LP = lumbar puncture.)

IV. Database
  A. Physical Exam Key Points
    1. **Airway, breathing, circulation (ABCs).** Focus on the ABCs. Is airway patent? Check for potential obstruction (eg, copious secretions, loose teeth, large tongue, small jaw, tonsillar hypertrophy). Children with certain genetic syndromes, such as trisomy 21 and Pierre-Robin sequence, pose intrinsic increased risk based on their anatomy.
    2. **Cardiopulmonary findings.** Check for wheezing, rales, tachypnea, and work of breathing. Check cardiac rate and rhythm, perfusion, and BP.
    3. **Mental status.** Document prior to sedation to ensure a return to baseline prior to discharge or discontinuation of postsedation monitoring.
  B. Monitoring. Adequate monitoring is essential, including a minimum of continuous pulse oximetry and noninvasive BP measurement. Capnography and cardiorespiratory monitoring are indicated for moderate to deep levels of sedation. Resuscitation equipment such as airway adjuncts, supplemental oxygen, bag-mask ventilator, and suction should be immediately available, and reversal agents, resuscitative medications, and defibrillator should be nearby. Be aware that once a painful procedure is finished, a patient who is suddenly lacking potent noxious stimuli may relax into hypoxia and hypoventilation. Monitor patient appropriately until he or she reaches baseline level of alertness, vital signs, and ability to retain fluids.

V. Plan. Figure I–7 depicts a useful algorithmic approach to choosing a drug regimen, and Table I–24 summarizes dosing, administration route, and timing. Common pitfalls include failure to predict and prepare for complications, failure to recognize a problem as it occurs, pharmacologic errors, and failure to monitor patient adequately postsedation. Underdosing may lead to poorly sedated, agitated patients, which in turn may lead to polypharmacy (repeated use of an agent or use of more than two agents). Avoid polypharmacy whenever possible, because complication rate increases dramatically with use of multiple agents.
  A. Sedative-Hypnotics. Sedative hypnotic-agents include chloral hydrate, benzodiazepines, and barbiturates. All provide anxiolysis and sedation but have no effect on pain.
    1. **Chloral hydrate.** Somewhat unpredictable in onset (10–30 minutes) and duration (30 to > 120 minutes); generally reserved for painless imaging procedures in infants and young toddlers; often will not produce sleep in older children. Has very bitter taste, can be administered orally or rectally, and is not reversible.
    2. **Benzodiazepines (includes midazolam, diazepam, and lorazepam).** Midazolam is the agent of choice due to its

TABLE I-24. PROCEDURAL SEDATION DRUG DOSAGE RECOMMENDATIONS

Drug	Clinical Effect	Indications	Dose[a]	Onset (min)	Duration (min)	Reversible	Comments
Sedative-Hypnotics Chloral hydrate	Sedation, sleep, motion control	Imaging or painless diagnostic studies (CT, EEG, ABR)	50–100 mg/kg PO or PR (max 100 mg/kg or 2 g)	10–30	30–120	No	Works best in young infants (<10 kg); unpredictable onset and duration; terrible taste
Midazolam	Sedation, anxiolysis	Shorter procedures, anxiolysis, mild sedation when used alone	IV 0.05–0.1 mg/kg IN 0.2–0.4 mg/kg IM 0.1–0.2 mg/kg PO/PR 0.5 mg/kg (Halve dose for >8 y, may repeat q5–10min to max of 0.5 mg/kg IV)	IV 1–2 IN 2–5 IM 5–15 PO 15–20 PR 10–15	IV 45–60 IN 15–30 IM 60–120 PO/PR 60–90	Yes (flumazenil)	Use lower doses in combination with narcotics; may produce paradoxic irritability (see text)
Pentobarbital	Sedation, sleep, motion control	Longer painless procedures (MRI, bone scan)	IV 2–6 mg/kg, titrated at 1–2 mg/kg q2–3min IM 2–6 mg/kg PO/PR 3–6 mg/kg (max 200 mg)	IV 3–5 IM 10–15 PO/PR 15–60	IV 30–90 IM 60–120 PO/PR 60–240	No	Younger children are often restless before sleep is induced; avoid in patients with porphyria

Drug	Indication	Procedure	Dose	Onset (min)	Duration (min)	Reversible	Comments
Methohexital	Sedation, sleep, motion control	Shorter painless procedures (CT)	IV 1 mg/kg, PR 20 mg/kg	IV 1–2, PR 10–15	IV 15–30, PR 30–60	No	Avoid in patients with temporal lobe epilepsy and porphyria
Analgesics							
Fentanyl	Analgesia	Shorter, moderately painful procedures	IV 1–2 mcg/kg; may increase by 1 mcg/kg q3–5min to desired effect	IV 1–2	IV 30–60	Yes (naloxone)	Chest wall rigidity may occur with rapid IV push
Ketamine[b]	Analgesia, dissociation, amnesia, motion control	Shorter, moderately to severely painful procedures	IV 1–1.5 mg/kg, IM 4–5 mg/kg (use concentrated 100 mg/mL formulation) PO 10 mg/kg	IV 1–2, IM 3–5, PO 10–30	IV 15–30, IM 30–90	No	Contraindicated in patients with increased ICP, IOP, psychosis, thyroid disease
Nitrous oxide (NO)	Mild analgesia, sedation, amnesia	Mildly painful procedures	No reported max Inhaled 30–50% NO mixed with oxygen	1–3	<5 min	No	Contraindicated in patients with trapped gas pockets
Reversal Agents							
Naloxone	Narcotic reversal		IV/IM 0.1 mg/kg (max 2 mg/dose) May repeat q2min	IV 2–3, PR 10–15	IV 20–40, IM 60–90	—	Sedative may outlast reversal agent
Flumazenil	Benzodiazepine reversal		IV 0.02 mg/kg per dose May repeat q1min to max of 1 mg	IV 1–2	IV 30–60	—	Sedative may outlast reversal agent

ABR = auditory brainstem response; CT = computed tomography; EEG = electroencephalogram; ICP = intracranial pressure; IOP = intraocular pressure; MRI = magnetic resonance imaging.

a Doses are generalizations only; dosing must be individualized in all cases. Dosing may be altered by age or degree of illness. Neonatal dosing may differ. All PO/PR/IM dosing is difficult to titrate—use caution and monitor for oversedation. Judicious use of local anesthetic may lessen dose requirements for systemic analgesia.

b Administer with atropine, 0.01 mg/kg (min 0.1 mg, max 0.5 mg), to blunt hypersalivation response. Some believe that administration with midazolam may ameliorate emergence phenomenon. All three drugs may be mixed together for IM administration.

pharmacokinetics and exceptional amnestic properties. Short-acting agent (varies by route of administration and dosage), with rapid onset (1–2 minutes IV, 2–20 minutes transmucosally or enterally). Given alone, it is unlikely to induce sleep, although it will create a relaxed state in most children. Serves as an excellent adjunct to local anesthetic or concomitant narcotic or dissociative agents for painful procedures. Midazolam, as with all benzodiazepines, produces dose-dependent respiratory depression that is significantly exaggerated by use with narcotics. Up to 10% of children experience a paradoxic hyperexcited, irritable state that can be blunted with increased dosing or flumazenil. Adolescents are more susceptible and should not be dosed on a per-kilogram basis (see Table I–24). Midazolam is reversible with flumazenil.

3. **Barbiturates.** Barbiturates depress reticular activating system and serve as very good sleep-inducing agents. Commonly used agents include pentobarbital, methohexital, and thiopental. Pentobarbital has a slower onset and longer duration compared with methohexital. Thiopental is an ultra–short-acting agent with potential for significant hypotension and is generally reserved for situations requiring profound sedation, such as rapid sequence intubation. Barbiturates are not reversible.

B. **Analgesics.** Procedural analgesics include narcotics, ketamine, and nitrous oxide. Narcotics include fentanyl, morphine, and meperidine. Fentanyl has become the favorite due to its potency, lack of histamine release and hypotension, and pharmacokinetics.

1. **Fentanyl.** Agent is 100 times as potent as morphine, and careful attention should be paid to its microgram dosing. Takes effect within 1–2 minutes of IV administration and lasts for 30–60 minutes. Potential adverse effects include so-called stiff chest syndrome (rigidity of chest wall seen with rapid administration of large doses), requiring naloxone or neuromuscular blockade to reverse. Respiratory depression is very common, especially when administered with a benzodiazepine. Vomiting and facial pruritus are also common. Fentanyl is reversible with naloxone.

2. **Ketamine.** Dissociative anesthetic that induces a unique catatonic state with profound sedation, amnesia, and analgesia. Has a rapid onset (1–2 minutes IV) and short duration (15–30 minutes). Respiratory drive and protective airway reflexes are maintained. Side effects include hypersalivation, tachycardia, hypertension, and increased intracranial pressure, in addition to possibility (5–10%) of an "emergence reaction" with agitation on awakening. Vomiting on emergence has also been reported. Side effects may be blunted by concomitant administration of a benzodiazepine and an antisialagogue, such as atropine or glycopyrrolate. It is helpful to tell patient to expect a dreamlike state with changes in visual perception (double vision is common), and to tell parent to expect to see nystagmus and flushing. Ketamine is not reversible.

3. **Nitrous oxide.** The only inhaled sedative-analgesic commonly available outside of anesthesia department. Produces state of euphoria and mild sedation and analgesia within 2–3 breaths and wears off almost instantly as well. Administered using demand-valve mask via blender capable of administering up to 50% nitrous oxide and 50% oxygen. Due to environmental contamination and concerns about toxicity in health-care workers with chronic exposure, a scavenger system must be in place to retrieve stray gas. Side effects include nausea and potential for diffusion of nitrous oxide into enclosed cavities; thus, use is contraindicated in patients with pneumothorax or obstructed bowel.

4. **Reversal agents.** Although these agents should be available whenever reversible agents are employed for procedural sedation, they are not routinely recommended at the conclusion of procedures. Duration of action of sedative-analgesic regimen may outlast that of reversal agent, raising risk of temporary reversal with later resedation. When a reversal agent is used in the setting of oversedation, patient should be monitored for duration of action of original agent, or at least 2 hours after administration of reversal agent. Reversal agents include naloxone, a narcotic antagonist that competes for opiate receptors, and flumazenil, which antagonizes effect of benzodiazepines. (See Table I–24 for dosing information.)

VI. Problem Case Diagnosis. The 4-year-old patient was screened and found to have no risk factors for sedation. He was monitored adequately; received midazolam, 2 mg IV (0.1 mg/kg), and fentanyl, 20 mcg (1 mcg/kg); and slept lightly through the procedure, which resulted in diagnosis of aseptic meningitis.

VII. Teaching Pearl: Question. What is the sedative agent of choice when a pediatric patient needs to be sedated for a long diagnostic imaging study (eg, MRI scan of spine)?

VIII. Teaching Pearl: Answer. Such procedures are painless, require complete immobilization, and take about 1 hour; therefore, IV pentobarbital at a dose of 3–6 mg/kg (maximum, 200 mg) is the agent of choice.

REFERENCES

American Academy of Pediatrics, Committee on Drugs. Guidelines for the monitoring and management of pediatric patients during and after sedation for diagnostic and therapeutic procedures: Addendum. *Pediatrics* 2002;110:836–838.

Krauss B. Management of acute pain and anxiety in children undergoing procedures in the emergency department. *Pediatr Emerg Care* 2001;17:115–123.

Krauss B, Green S. Sedation and analgesia for procedures in children. *N Engl J Med* 2000;342:938–945.

Proudfoot J. Pediatric procedural sedation and analgesia (PSA): Keeping it simple and safe. *Pediatr Emerg Med Rep* 2002;7:13–24.

82. SEIZURES, FEBRILE

I. **Problem.** A 2-year-old boy who attends day care is brought to the emergency department with a fever and a history of seizure-like activity.

II. **Immediate Questions**

   A. **Did patient have a seizure?** The first step is to decide if patient actually had a seizure. It is important to obtain a history from someone who witnessed the event. This may be difficult if seizure occurs when parents or other caretakers are not present. Ask for a description with special attention to extremity movements, eye deviations, lip smacking, and cyanosis; this information usually allows clinician to determine if child actually experienced a seizure.

   B. **What type of febrile seizure occurred?** Febrile seizures are classified as either simple (typical) or complex. A simple febrile seizure lasts less than 15 minutes, is generalized in onset, and occurs only once in a 24-hour time period. In contrast, a complex febrile seizure lasts longer than 15 minutes, is focal, or there is more than one seizure in 24 hours.

   C. **Does patient have a history of seizures?** A child with a prior history of nonfebrile seizures does not undergo the same workup or treatment as an otherwise healthy child. Similarly, children with known CNS abnormalities, developmental delay, and metabolic disorders are not included in the definition of febrile seizures.

   D. **Are there any signs of CNS infection?** It is of extreme importance to differentiate seizure with fever and febrile seizures. Meningitis and encephalitis are two potentially life-threatening infections that commonly present with seizure and fever.

   E. **Is there a history of trauma?** Head trauma is a common occurrence in young children. It is important to elicit any such history in a child presenting with seizure and fever, because these children will require a different evaluation.

   F. **Any toxic ingestion?** Children younger than 6 years of age account for more than half of poisonings in any given year. Questions regarding possible drug exposure at home or where child is cared for are essential.

III. **Differential Diagnosis.** Febrile seizures occur in infancy or early childhood, usually between 3 months and 5 years of age. The seizure activity is associated with fever but lacks evidence of intracranial infection or defined cause. Seizures with fever in children who have suffered a previous nonfebrile seizure are excluded. However, it is important to remember that fever is very common in this age group and that presence of fever may be unrelated to cause of the seizure.

   A. **Infection.** CNS infections are one of the most common causes of seizure with fever. Bacterial or viral meningitis or encephalitis must be considered. In addition, *Shigella* gastroenteritis and roseola as well as other infectious etiologies may present with seizure as a symptom.

B. Trauma. Recent head injury, with or without loss of consciousness, can lead to seizures. Nonaccidental trauma should also be considered in this age group as a cause of seizures with incidental fever.

C. Toxins. Many drug exposures may lead to seizure activity. Certain toxic ingestions commonly present with seizure and fever, including cocaine, tricyclic antidepressants, and amphetamines. In addition, children with a history of seizure disorder may have anticonvulsant levels that are too high or too low, leading to seizures with incidental fevers.

IV. Database
A. Physical Exam Key Points.
Physical exam in children with febrile seizures should be directed at finding a source for the fever as well as evaluating for other possible sources of seizure.

1. **Vital signs.** Note temperature peak, because some studies show that risk of febrile seizure recurrence is greater with lower temperatures. Hypotension is common in septic children.

2. **HEENT.** Inspect head for signs of trauma. Assess fontanelle in children in whom it is still open. Bulging fontanelle could indicate intracranial infection, such as meningitis or encephalitis, or increased intracranial pressure from other causes. Depressed fontanelle may indicate dehydration, with subsequent electrolyte abnormalities leading to fever and seizure. Lack of cooperation in infants and young children may make it difficult to evaluate papilledema. Inspect ears and throat for sources of fever.

3. **Skin.** Inspect for rashes (eg, viral exanthems and petechiae) and other skin findings indicative of underlying neurologic disorders that could account for seizure (ie, ash-leaf spots, café au lait lesions, or port-wine stains).

4. **Neurologic exam.** Careful attention to this aspect of exam is important. Prolonged altered level of consciousness or change in child's general appearance requires more aggressive evaluation. Similarly, any focal neurologic deficit demands further workup beyond the scope of simple febrile seizure evaluation.

B. Laboratory Data
1. **Blood studies.** According to a policy statement from the American Academy of Pediatrics (AAP), routine blood studies are not indicated in the workup of a first simple febrile seizure and should only be performed as part of the evaluation for a source of the fever.

2. **Lumbar puncture (LP).** In a policy statement from the AAP, recommendations regarding LP with a first simple febrile seizure are as follows:

   a. LP should be strongly considered in infants younger than 12 months of age.

    b. LP should be considered in children between 12 and 18 months of age.

    c. In children older than 18 months, LP is not routinely warranted and is only recommended in presence of meningeal signs.

    d. LP is usually indicated in children who present with complex febrile seizure after mass-occupying lesion and increased intracranial pressure have been ruled out.

C. Radiographic and Other Studies. Routine neuroimaging studies (eg, CT or MRI scan) are not recommended in evaluation of simple febrile seizure. Similarly, there is no evidence to support obtaining routine EEG. EEG does not help predict recurrence or later development of epilepsy in children with febrile seizures.

V. Plan. Febrile seizures are self-limited and, typically, very short events. Because of this, most seizures will have terminated before coming to medical attention and patients will not require stabilization. Patients with persistent seizures require airway management and more aggressive treatment of seizure activity with medications, as discussed in Chapter 84 (see p. 391). Long-term care of children with febrile seizures is directed primarily at parental reassurance, as discussed below.

A. Antipyretics. Antipyretics such as acetaminophen and ibuprofen do not prevent recurrences of febrile seizures when given with future episodes of fever.

B. Anticonvulsants. The ability of several anticonvulsants to prevent recurrent febrile seizures has been studied. However, given the benign nature of febrile seizures, side effects of most of these medications generally outweigh benefits. Oral diazepam given at the onset of future febrile illnesses may be indicated when parental anxiety about seizures is severe.

C. Parental Reassurance. This is perhaps the most important aspect of care for children with febrile seizures. Parents need to be informed that simple febrile seizures do not cause brain damage and that risk of child having nonfebrile seizures in future is only slightly greater than that of the general population. It is also important to prepare parents for the fact that approximately one third of children with febrile seizures will experience a future febrile seizure (50% recurrence risk if first episode occurs before the age of 12 months).

D. Hospitalization. Admission to the hospital is only necessary if clinician has a suspicion of underlying disease, there is a recurrent or prolonged seizure episode, or parents seem unable to cope with the seizure.

VI. Problem Case Diagnosis. On evaluation in the emergency department, the 2-year-old boy was alert and playful. Physical exam was normal, except for rectal temperature of 102°F (38.8°C). The seizure was described as generalized, lasting 5 minutes. Developmentally the child is normal, with no previous history of seizures. Diagnosis is febrile seizure.

VII. Teaching Pearl: Question. What are the risk factors for recurrence of febrile seizures?

VIII. Teaching Pearl: Answer. Risk factors for febrile seizures include young age of first febrile seizure (before 6–12 months), family history of febrile seizures, short duration of fever before initial seizure, and relatively lower fever at time of initial seizure. Children with febrile seizures are not at increased risk for mental retardation or epilepsy.

REFERENCES

American Academy of Pediatrics. Provisional Committee on Quality Improvement, Subcommittee on Febrile Seizures. Practice parameter: The neurodiagnostic evaluation of the child with a first simple febrile seizure. *Pediatrics* 1996;97:769–775.

Depiero AD, Teach SJ. Febrile seizures. *Pediatr Emerg Care* 2001;17:384–387.

Hirtz DG. Febrile seizures. *Pediatr Rev* 1997;18:5–8.

Rosman NP, Colton T, Labazzo J, et al. A controlled trial of diazepam administered during febrile illnesses to prevent recurrence of febrile seizures. *N Engl J Med* 1993;329:79–84.

Warden CR, Zibulewsky J, Mace S, et al. Evaluation and management of febrile seizures in the out-of-hospital and emergency department settings. *Ann Emerg Med* 2003;41:215–222.

83. SEIZURES, NONFEBRILE

I. Problem. A 7-year-old boy is noted to have periods of inattention during the second week of school.

II. Immediate Questions

A. Is this an emergency, urgent, or routine clinical condition? Clinician must determine if care needs to be administered emergently. An emergency case requires the same attention to detail as a routine case; however, the pace and order in which actions are completed differs. Remember the ABCs (airway, breathing, circulation).

B. What are the associated symptoms? Depending on the location of the electrical discharge, a variety of clinical phenomena can be manifested, including GI symptoms (nausea), fear, unusual sensations (eg, hallucinations), localized motor or sensory activity, or autonomic changes (heart rate and BP alterations). Associated symptoms can also give clues to underlying etiology. Diarrhea, for example, can be a clue to shigellosis.

C. Does patient have a history of similar episodes? If patient has had similar events in the past, it is much less likely that this is an urgent medical or surgical condition.

D. Did patient lose consciousness? There are two basic types of seizures: generalized and partial. Generalized seizures present with sudden onset of loss of consciousness, because they are a manifestation of widespread abnormal electrical discharges involving both hemispheres. Partial seizures are due to a localized abnormal electrical discharge and no loss of consciousness occurs. Partial seizures can secondarily generalize.

E. What is the clinical description of patient's seizure or episode of inattention? How long did event last? What time did it occur (daytime, during sleep)? Were there any associated activities, such as movements of face or body? What was child doing before and after episode (eg, interrupted speech)? Were there any precipitants to episode? One type of generalized seizure—absence seizures—classically presents with staring spells. These seizures typically last < 30 seconds and have no associated alteration of arousal before or immediately after the event. Staring is also a common manifestation of a complex partial seizure. Complex partial seizures typically last 1–3 minutes and may be followed by an alteration of arousal (postictal state).

F. Pertinent Birth, Medical, or Family history. Many situations, including prematurity, developmental delay, underlying neurocutaneous disorders, cocaine use, intracranial bleeding, and family history of epilepsy, place children at risk for nonfebrile seizures.

1. Birth history. Did mother receive prenatal care? Was there any history of maternal medication use or substance abuse during pregnancy? Were there any maternal medical complications during pregnancy? Was pregnancy completed to term? Were there any complications during delivery?

2. Medical history. Were developmental milestones achieved at appropriate ages? Is there any significant medical or surgical history? Does patient take any medications? Is there a history of head trauma?

3. Family history. Is there any family history of neurologic disorders?

III. Differential Diagnosis

A. Idiopathic Seizures. No etiology identified; common.

B. Congenital Anomalies, Structural or Destructive Lesions, and Medical Conditions. Includes cerebral malformations, tuberous sclerosis, neurofibromatosis, sickle cell anemia, acute lymphocytic leukemia, neoplasm, stroke, vascular anomalies, and degenerative disorders. Severe respiratory condition with hypoxia may present with staring and decreased arousal.

C. Birth Problems or Trauma. Hypoxia or head trauma.

D. Infections. Includes meningitis, encephalitis, and neonatal infections, including TORCH.

E. Metabolic Problems. Includes hypoglycemia, hyponatremia or hypernatremia, hypocalcemia, and inborn errors of metabolism.

F. Medications. Anticonvulsants, antidepressants and anxiolytics, lidocaine, theophylline, psychotropic agents, isoniazid, chemotherapeutic agents, cocaine, amphetamines, heroin, PCP, and carbon monoxide.

G. Disorders of Sensation. Child may present with staring spells in school if he or she is unable to see or hear normally. With deficits in special sensory stimulation, child may not know when to respond to environmental stimuli.

H. Disorders of Cognition. If child is unable to understand information presented by his or her surroundings, it is common for child to appear to ignore information. Multilingual children may initially have difficulty understanding the expressive language of their environment if it is different from the language spoken at home.

I. Intoxications. Ingestion of a toxic substance, such as alcohol (methanol, ethylene glycol) or a variety of medications may result in depression of mental status, staring, seizures, or all of these findings.

J. Sleep Disorders. Insufficient or inefficient sleep may result in excessive daytime sleepiness and subsequent alteration of arousal; this may be an isolated diagnosis or a complication of other medical conditions such as obstructive sleep apnea.

K. Behavior Disorders. Child may ignore his or her surroundings as a sign of a mood or conversion disorder. Children with attention-deficit/hyperactivity disorder often present with inattention and apparent staring or daydreaming.

L. Migraine. Children with confusional migraine can present with staring.

IV. Database

A. Physical Exam Key Points. Complete general physical exam is important for identification of systemic disorders. Evaluate ABCs to avoid missing an emergency condition.

1. **Vital signs.** Changes in heart rate and BP may reflect systemic infection, cardiac disease, intoxication, or active seizure. Alteration of temperature may reflect infection or effects of intoxication.

2. **General appearance.** Growth and development problems may reflect underlying medical or neurologic disorder.

3. **Skin.** Inspect for signs of trauma, rash, and birth marks (erythematous, hypopigmented, or hyperpigmented lesions). Rash may suggest infectious or vasculitic disorder. Neurocutaneous disorders (eg, neurofibromatosis, tuberous sclerosis, Sturge-Weber syndrome, von Hippel-Lindau syndrome, and ataxia telangiectasia) may present with alteration of arousal.

4. **Head and neck.** Head circumference may reflect alteration in brain parenchyma (microcephaly or macrocephaly). Inspect for signs of head trauma. Neck stiffness (meningismus) may indicate meningitis or subarachnoid hemorrhage.

5. **Heart and lungs.** Cardiac murmur or altered cardiac dynamics may indicate cardiac dysfunction. Respiratory dysfunction may be identified by auscultation.

6. **Abdomen.** Hepatosplenomegaly may be present in a variety of metabolic and neurodegenerative disorders.

7. **Neurologic exam.** Detailed exam allows clinician to localize condition to specific regions of central and peripheral nervous systems. Cerebral cortex disorders affect cognition; brainstem lesions affect specific cranial nerves. Spinal cord lesions demonstrate motor or sensory deficits, or both.

   a. **Mental status.** Ability to interact with environment is assessed by speaking with and listening to patient. This must be carried out at an age-appropriate level.

   b. **Cranial nerves.** Pupillary size and reactivity, in addition to eye movements, reflect function of portions of upper brainstem. Symmetric movement of face, soft palate, and tongue demonstrates integrity of lower brainstem.

   c. **Motor system.** Muscle bulk, tone, and strength demonstrate function of motor pathways. Fine motor skills may suggest developmental abilities. Involuntary movements may be seen in various neurologic disorders.

   d. **Sensory system.** Localized sensory deficits may reflect dysfunction of central or peripheral nervous system, or they may be seen in functional disorders.

   e. **Deep tendon reflexes.** Reflex arcs demonstrate integrity of specific reflex pathways from peripheral muscle through levels of spinal cord and are rarely affected.

   f. **Cerebellar exam.** Cerebellar dysfunction may be a sign of localized space-occupying, destructive, or degenerative disorders.

B. **Laboratory Data**

   1. **Basic metabolic panel, glucose, calcium.** Electrolyte abnormalities (hypernatremia, hyponatremia, hypocalcemia) and hypoglycemia or hyperglycemia can present with alteration of mental status. Metabolic acidosis is seen with underlying metabolic disorders or intoxication. Respiratory acidosis may be seen in other intoxications (alcohol, benzodiazepines, and barbiturates).

   2. **Renal and hepatic profile.** Can indicate acute or chronic end-organ dysfunction.

   3. **CBC with differential.** Elevated WBC count may indicate active infection.

   4. **Toxicology screening or drug levels.** Obtain blood levels of prescription medications, ingested medications, or substances of abuse, as indicated, based on patient's history.

   5. **ABGs.** Obtain if hypoxia or acid-base problems are suggested by history.

   6. **Lumbar puncture.** Perform if intracranial infection (meningitis or encephalitis) or subarachnoid hemorrhage is suspected. *Do not* complete procedure if increased intracranial pressure or mass-occupying lesion is noted, because of risk of herniation.

C. Radiographic and Other Studies

1. **Neuroimaging (CT or MRI scan).** Perform on all patients with altered mental status. Not needed emergently if patient's exam findings are normal and history indicates only altered arousal. MRI is a more sensitive exam and visualizes posterior fossa better than CT scan; however, MRI requires that patient remain still for a prolonged period of time and therefore often requires sedation.
2. **EEG.** The gold standard for seizures, because it is the only study that demonstrates cerebral electrical activity (physiologic cause of seizures). In addition, EEG can demonstrate cerebral cortical dysfunction due to a generalized encephalopathy or localized destructive or space-occupying lesion.
3. **ECG.** Obtain if cardiac disorder is suspected.

V. Plan

A. Emergency Management

1. Assess ABCs. If an active convulsive seizure occurs during assessment, place patient on side, control airway, and protect from objects that may fall onto or otherwise harm patient during seizure. *Do not* place any object into patient's mouth during seizure. Status epilepticus is defined as a seizure, or recurrent seizures, lasting more than 30 minutes, during which patient does not regain consciousness. Any type of seizure can progress to status epilepticus. Patients with an established seizure disorder may have been prescribed a rectal benzodiazepine medication that can be given to terminate a seizure.
2. Establish IV access (for medication administration) and obtain appropriate blood tests (see IV, B, earlier).
3. Give patient 50% dextrose solution IV for possible hypoglycemia.
4. Treat active convulsive seizure with lorazepam, 0.05–0.1 mg/kg IV, over 5 minutes (maximum of 4 mg per dose). Watch for respiratory depression. If IV access is not available, diazepam may be given rectally at a dose of 0.2–0.5 mg/kg, depending on patient's age.
5. If seizure persists, load with fosphenytoin, 20 phenytoin equivalents (PE)/kg IV or IM, over 10 minutes. Fosphenytoin (5–10 PE/kg) can be repeated if seizure persists. If seizure persists after repeated doses of fosphenytoin, load with phenobarbital, 20 mg/kg, over 20 minutes. Watch for respiratory depression. Patients who are already receiving valproic acid can be loaded with valproate sodium IV infusion, 15–25 mg/kg.
6. Patients with seizures that persist despite these interventions may require intubation, mechanical ventilation, and general anesthesia. Agent most often utilized in this setting is pentobarbital, because response can be titrated, followed by continuous

bedside EEG monitoring. Load patient with 15–20 mg/kg IV, over 1–2 hours, and then maintain on continuous IV infusion of 1 mg/kg/h. Infusion is weaned after 1–5 days to assess clinical effectiveness.

B. Seizure Control. Anticonvulsant medications are mainstay of management for seizures. Decision to initiate anticonvulsant medication is based on history and EEG findings. Most patients will not start an anticonvulsant medication until they have had at least two clinical events.

  1. Partial seizures. First-line anticonvulsant is carbamazepine; other effective agents include sodium valproate, levetiracetam, and phenytoin.

  2. Generalized seizures. First-line anticonvulsant is sodium valproate; other effective agents include levetiracetam and lamotrigine.

  3. Absence seizures. First-line agent is ethosuximide; other agents include sodium valproate and lamotrigine.

  4. Adverse effects. All anticonvulsant medications have potential adverse effects, and patient and family should be familiarized with these. Routine blood testing can identify some adverse effects, but blood tests are not predictive of impending adverse effects.

C. Follow-up. Patients who take anticonvulsant medications are followed regularly. Typically anticonvulsants are continued for at least 2 seizure-free years.

VI. Problem Case Diagnosis. The 7-year-old boy had spells of inattention that lasted between 5 and 10 seconds, with no other associated activity. Physical exam and prenatal, developmental, and past medical histories were unremarkable. Patient's older sister had similar spells at same age. EEG demonstrated frequent generalized, bilaterally synchronous, 3-Hertz spike-and-slow-wave complexes, lasting 2–10 seconds. Patient was diagnosed with childhood absence epilepsy and was effectively treated with ethosuximide.

VII. Teaching Pearl: Question. What is the typical age of onset for absence seizures, and is it beneficial to initiate treatment early?

VIII. Teaching Pearl: Answer. This disorder typically presents between ages 5 and 9 years (average, 5.7 years). Treatment is not a medical emergency, but early intervention can prevent academic and social difficulties.

REFERENCES

Arzimanoglou A. Treatment options in pediatric epilepsy. *Epileptic Disord* 2002;3:217–225.

Jack CR. Magnetic resonance imaging in epilepsy. *Mayo Clin Proc* 1996;71:695–711.

Murphy JV, Dehkharghani F. Diagnosis of childhood seizure disorders. *Epilepsia* 1994;35(suppl):S7–S17.

Pearl PL, Holmes GL. Absence seizures. In: Pellock JM, Dodson WE, Bourgeois BFD, eds. *Pediatric Epilepsy: Diagnosis and Therapy*, 2nd ed. Denios, 2002: 219–232.
Wirrel EC, Camfield CS, Camfield PR, et al. Long-term prognosis of childhood absence epilepsy: Remission or progression to juvenile myoclonic epilepsy. *Neurology* 1996;47:912–918.

84. STRIDOR

I. **Problem.** A 15-year-old boy states that he coughed and choked after chewing on a throat lozenge. He has biphasic stridor.

II. **Immediate Questions**

A. **Is patient in significant respiratory distress? Is there significant respiratory difficulty or increased work of breathing?** Respiratory collapse may be imminent and urgent control of airway needed if patient is significantly uncomfortable or becoming fatigued. Look for sternal retractions, nasal flaring, and appearance of exhaustion or terror.

B. **How long has patient had stridor?** Under what circumstances did stridor begin? Did it begin acutely? Was event witnessed (eg, choking)? What evaluation and treatment took place, during this episode and previously, and what were the results? Recent or previous airway manipulation (eg, intubation) or trauma may cause subglottic stenosis or other laryngeal lesions. If acute in onset, stridor may progress from partial to complete airway obstruction (eg, aspirated foreign body, infection, trauma).

C. **Is patient hoarse?** Listen to voice or cry. Lesions that cause significant dysphonia (severe hoarseness) can cause sudden, complete airway obstruction (eg, laryngeal papillomas, exudative infections, aspirated foreign bodies).

D. **How severe is stridor?** Episodes of cyanosis or apparent life-threatening event (ALTE) suggest a severe problem.

E. **Is there additional relevant history?** If aspiration, coughing, or choking has occurred with feeding, evaluate for local or generalized neurologic problems (eg, paralyzed vocal fold, general hypotonia) or anatomic abnormalities (eg, tracheoesophageal fistula). When difficulty breathing interferes with feeding, the problem is severe. Acute respiratory infections can cause airway problems (eg, croup) or exacerbate underlying problems (eg, subglottic stenosis). Significant cardiac, neurologic, or pulmonary abnormalities may indirectly cause airway problems or interfere with child's ability to compensate.

III. **Differential Diagnosis.** Stridor is a sign, not a discrete diagnosis, suggesting partial airway obstruction, generally in the larynx, trachea, or bronchi.

A. **Laryngomalacia.** Collapse of supraglottic structures during inspiration. Can be congenital (infants), generally improving over time, or acquired (children with neurologic problems).

B. **Subglottic Narrowing.** Most commonly from subglottic stenosis, usually acquired, especially after prolonged or traumatic intubation; but can be congenital. Other causes include subglottic hemangiomas and subglottic cysts.

C. **Aspirated Foreign Body.** Sometimes history or radiographic findings provide evidence of an aspirated foreign body. However, coughing may subside or, in a young or developmentally delayed child, episode may not be witnessed. Radiographs may be nondiagnostic. Endoscopy should be considered if there is a suggestive history, despite lack of physical findings, or a suggestive radiograph, despite lack of history.

D. **Ingested (Esophageal) Foreign Body.** Can cause extrinsic compression of airway.

E. **Croup.** Viral illness causing subglottic narrowing from subglottic edema. Onset occurs over a few days, and child has low-grade fever.

F. **Epiglottitis.** Inflammation and edema of structures immediately superior to vocal folds. Infectious epiglottitis has rapid onset, and child appears toxic, with high fever. Can be caused by mechanical, chemical, or thermal trauma.

G. **Vocal Fold Paralysis.** Dynamic cause of airway obstruction. If unilateral, child has mild stridor and weak cry; if bilateral, more severe stridor. Can be caused by central lesion (eg, Chiari malformation) or peripheral lesion (eg, trauma to recurrent laryngeal nerve during cardiac surgery). Can be congenital or acquired.

H. **Exudative Tracheitis.** Staphylococcal or other bacterial infection of trachea and larynx; may follow viral infection. Can cause sudden, complete airway obstruction.

I. **Recurrent Respiratory Papilloma.** Viral lesion with predilection for vocal folds; often presents with hoarseness preceding stridor. Can cause sudden, complete airway obstruction.

J. **Vascular Ring or Sling.** Congenital malformation of major vessels (eg, double aortic arch), causing extrinsic compression of trachea.

IV. **Database**

A. **Physical Exam Key Points**

1. **Characteristics of stridor.** May help localize site of airway narrowing. Stridor that is primarily inspiratory is generally caused by extrathoracic lesions; stridor that is primarily expiratory, by intrathoracic lesions. Biphasic stridor may be caused by tracheal lesions, or severe airway narrowing in any location. Stridor may be primarily high or low pitched.

2. **Wet sounds.** Anatomic or neurologic inability to clear secretions.

3. **Hoarseness.** Lesion includes, but is not necessarily limited to, true vocal folds.

4. **Pectus deformity.** Airway obstruction is long-standing or severe.

      5. Unilateral decreased breath sounds. Suggestive of decreased airflow to that side.

  B. Laboratory Data. Normal pulse-oximetry reading does not rule out significant airway lesion.

  C. Radiographic and Other Studies

    1. Lateral neck x-ray. May show subglottic narrowing from subglottic stenosis, croup, or other lesions.

    2. Chest x-ray (lateral and AP or PA). May demonstrate the following.

      a. Radiodense foreign body. More often, x-ray does not demonstrate foreign body but may show its sequelae. If there is partial airway obstruction, x-ray may demonstrate air trapping; if complete obstruction, postobstructive atelectasis.

      b. Abnormal tracheal anatomy. From vascular ring or other extrinsic tracheal compression.

      c. "Steeple sign." Narrowing of subglottic airway from croup.

    3. Inspiratory and expiratory x-rays or decubitus x-rays. May demonstrate air trapping that may not be evident on erect x-rays.

    4. Airway fluoroscopy. Useful if radiographic findings are subtle or patient is uncooperative.

V. Plan

  A. Acute Airway Management. May include various combinations of airway endoscopy as well as medical and mechanical control of airway. In some cases, observation is sufficient. Other options include ventilation using a bag-mask system, laryngeal mask airway, intubation with endotracheal tube or ventilating bronchoscope, or, rarely, tracheotomy.

  B. Endoscopic Evaluation of Airway. May include fiberoptic or rigid (direct) laryngoscopy or bronchoscopy, or both. Rigid endoscopy, using telescopes and ventilating bronchoscopes, allows control and manipulation of airway and provides ventilation capabilities.

  C. Adjunctive Medical Interventions. May include administration of steroids, nebulized racemic epinephrine, nebulized steroids, oxygen or helium-oxygen combinations, or antibiotics.

VI. Problem Case Diagnosis. Lateral neck x-ray demonstrated a radiolucent foreign body in midtrachea of the 15-year-old boy. The foreign body was removed endoscopically under general anesthesia. Although patient described aspirating an edible item, he actually had aspirated a chewed-up pen cap.

VII. Teaching Pearl: Question. Can a patient with stridor be in significant respiratory distress while displaying a normal pulse-oximetry value?

VIII. Teaching Pearl: Answer. Yes; patients may be able to maintain normal oxygenation until the moment of respiratory collapse. Look for other signs of respiratory failure.

REFERENCES

Bluestone CD, Stool SE, Alper CM, et al. *Pediatric Otolaryngology*, 4th ed. Saunders, 2003.

Snow JB Jr, Ballenger JJ. *Ballenger's Otorhinolaryngology Head and Neck Surgery*, 16th ed. BC Decker, 2003.

85. SYNCOPE

I. **Problem.** A 14-year-old girl has had two episodes of fainting in the past 2 months.

II. **Immediate Questions**

A. **Did patient actually have syncope?**

1. **Syncope** is a temporary loss of consciousness and postural tone resulting from abrupt, transient, and diffuse cerebral malfunction. Patients may say that they fainted or "passed out" when in fact they never lost consciousness. **Good rule of thumb:** If patients heard what was going on around them during the episode, they were not unconscious.

2. **Near-syncope** or dizzy spells usually are more benign than true syncope.

B. **What was patient doing when syncope occurred?** Syncope during exertion is a red flag for cardiac cause. Syncope immediately after exertion is of less immediate concern and origin may be neurally mediated. Patients with neurally mediated syncope typically are sitting or standing when syncope occurs. Commonly, they have changed positions quickly, from recumbent to upright, just prior to episode. Other common preceding activities including standing in line or sitting while having hair groomed. Syncope that occurs in supine position is more likely to be neurologic in origin or related to an arrhythmia. Patients with long QT syndrome often lose consciousness following a sudden loud noise or sudden strong emotion. Ask about activities such as coughing, micturition, or sudden turning of the head immediately prior to syncope.

C. **Were there preceding symptoms?** Absence of premonitory symptoms or presence of prodrome of palpitations or crushing chest pain raises red flags for possible cardiac origin. Neurally mediated syncope typically is preceded by symptoms such as nausea, sweating, lightheadedness, and vision changes. Dizziness or vertigo prior to syncope often is associated with psychogenic causes.

D. **How long was patient unconscious? Was CPR performed? When consciousness was regained, was patient oriented?** Loss of consciousness for more than 1 minute or need for resuscitation, or both, suggest cardiac etiology. Confusion or headache on awakening is typical of postictal state. Patients with other types of syncope generally awaken rapidly to full consciousness.

E. **Did observers note any tonic-clonic movements? Incontinence? Pallor?** Tonic-clonic movements or incontinence point to neurologic etiology. In all cases of syncope, transient change in cerebral circulation occurs, and seizure activity can develop secondarily. Pallor is seen in patients with neurally mediated and cardiac syncope.

F. **Did any observer obtain vital signs?** Bradycardia and hypotension occur with neurally mediated syncope but will return to normal shortly after patient awakens. Heart rate > 180 beats/min suggests tachyarrhythmia and may be associated with weak or absent pulses. Neurologic causes of syncope typically are associated with normal or elevated BP.

G. **Did patient sustain injury?** Injury suggests that patient had little or no warning prior to losing consciousness, raising a higher concern for cardiac causes of syncope.

H. **How much had patient had to drink on day of episode?** Inadequate fluid intake is often present with neurally mediated syncope. Patients are especially at risk when insensible fluid losses are high (ie, on hot days, following exertion).

I. **Does patient have any underlying medical problems?** Patients with known heart disease are presumed to have cardiac syncope until proven otherwise. History of migraine headaches, seizure disorder, or head trauma makes neurologic etiology more likely.

J. **Does patient take any medications?** Diuretics, antihypertensive medications, and tricyclic antidepressants predispose patients to orthostatic hypotension. Most antiarrhythmic agents actually have proarrhythmia as a significant side effect. Erythromycin, ketoconazole, tricyclic antidepressants, cisapride, and nonsedating antihistamines (terfenadine and astemizole) may predispose patients to corrected QT prolongation and ventricular arrhythmia.

K. **Is there a family history of recurrent syncope, seizures, or unexplained sudden death?** Dominantly inherited cardiac abnormalities such as hypertrophic cardiomyopathy or long QT syndrome are associated with sudden death. Ask about family history of sudden infant death syndrome.

III. **Differential Diagnosis**

A. **Neurally Mediated Syncope.** The most common cause of syncope in children; typically benign and often transient. Prodrome is common, usually following exercise.

1. **Neurocardiogenic syncope (vasovagal or reflex syncope).** Benign; includes vasodepressor type, with marked hypotension; cardioinhibitory type, with marked bradycardia; and mixed type, combination of previous two.

2. **Postural orthostatic tachycardia syndrome.** Upright posture results in exaggerated sinus tachycardia and modest hypotension. Often patients have history of chronic fatigue, palpitations, exercise intolerance, lightheadedness, or cognitive impairment.

3. **Situational syncope.** Specific triggers lead to syncope. Underlying mechanisms: peripheral vasodilation for "shower syncope," vagal stimulation and Valsalva for "micturition syncope," central autonomic activation for emotional stimuli, and hypocapnia-induced cerebral vasoconstriction for hyperventilation and breath-holding spells.

B. Cardiac Syncope

1. Structural heart disease

a. Hypertrophic cardiomyopathy.

b. Dilated cardiomyopathy or myocarditis.

c. Aortic stenosis or other significant left heart obstruction.

d. Mitral valve prolapse.

e. Coronary artery abnormality (anomalous origin or course of coronary artery, coronary ostial stenosis or atresia, Kawasaki disease).

f. Marfan syndrome; patient is at risk for aortic dissection or rupture.

g. Pulmonary hypertension.

2. Arrhythmia

a. **Long QT syndrome.** Associated with torsades de pointes and ventricular fibrillation. Exacerbated by exercise, sudden noise, surprise. Autosomal-dominant inheritance. Corrected QT measures > 450 msec.

b. **Wolff-Parkinson-White syndrome.** Manifests on ECG as delta waves and short PR interval. Atrial fibrillation or flutter can conduct rapidly to ventricles, producing ventricular fibrillation. Most likely to occur during exercise.

c. **Arrhythmogenic right ventricular dysplasia.** Associated with malignant ventricular arrhythmias. Myocardium in the right ventricular outflow tract is partially replaced by fibrous or adipose tissue.

d. **Ventricular tachycardia.** Can occur in patients with corrected or uncorrected congenital heart disease. Rare in children with structurally normal hearts in absence of conditions listed earlier in entries a or c.

e. **Sick sinus syndrome (tachycardia-bradycardia syndrome).** Occurs almost exclusively in pediatric patients who have undergone extensive surgery in atria.

C. Noncardiac Syncope

1. **Neurologic causes.** Seizures, transient ischemic attacks, complex migraine headaches, subarachnoid hemorrhage, subclavian steal syndrome, carotid sinus syndrome.

2. **Psychiatric causes.** Conversion disorder, psychogenic seizures.

3. **Systemic or metabolic causes**

a. Drugs, carbon dioxide exposure.

b. Electrolyte abnormalities or hypoglycemia; most often occurs in association with diabetes, ketotic hypoglycemia, or congenital metabolic abnormalities.

IV. Database. Detailed history, including careful family history, physical exam, and ECG are key elements in evaluation.

   A. Physical Exam Key Points
     1. Vital signs.
     2. Pathologic murmur, gallop, click.
     3. Irregular heart rhythm.
     4. Scar on chest.
     5. Focal neurologic signs.
     6. Evidence of injury sustained during episode.

   B. Laboratory, Radiographic, and Other Studies. Routine evaluation of syncope should include ECG. If history, physical exam, and ECG are typical of neurally mediated syncope, further testing is unnecessary. With atypical history or presence of any red flags (Table I–25), further cardiac or neurologic testing is guided by specific presentation. These further tests should be obtained as part of consultation with a pediatric cardiology or pediatric neurology specialist.

     1. ECG. Excellent screening tool; advisable in all patients who present with syncope.
     2. Echocardiogram. Indicated when red flag is present (see Table I–25).
     3. Cardiopulmonary exercise testing. Indicated if symptoms are consistently associated with exercise.
     4. Head up tilt-table testing. Relatively insensitive test in children and adolescents. May be helpful in patients with recurrent unexplained syncope, recurrent unexplained seizures, recurrent prolonged dizziness, chronic fatigue syndrome, or for evaluation of therapy.
     5. EEG. Consider when seizure or suspected seizure activity is associated with loss of consciousness.

TABLE I–25. RED FLAGS SUGGESTING CARDIAC CAUSE OF SYNCOPE

Syncope during exertion
Syncope provoked by fright, loud noise, or extreme emotional stress
Syncope preceded by palpitations or crushing chest pain
Absence of prodrome
Injury or neurologic sequelae following syncopal episode
Need for CPR
Patient history of exercise intolerance, arrhythmia, or structural heart disease
Family history of sudden death, seizure disorder, arrhythmia, long QT syndrome, or hypertrophic cardiomyopathy
Abnormal cardiac exam or ECG

6. **Twenty-four–hour Holter monitoring.** Rarely helpful unless episodes occur at least once daily.
7. **Transtelephonic event monitoring.** Appropriate for patients with red flag suggesting arrhythmia.
8. **Electrophysiology study.** Indicated if arrhythmia is documented or strongly suspected as cause of episodes, particularly in patients with known structural heart disease.
9. **Cardiac MRI scan.** Useful to identify arrhythmogenic right ventricular dysplasia.

V. Plan. Depends on suspected diagnosis.
   A. Neurally Mediated Syncope. Cornerstones of therapy are reassurance, education, and maintenance of intravascular volume.
   1. **Education.** Teach patients to avoid triggers or abort episode if possible.
   2. **Maintenance of intravascular volume.** Initiate aggressive fluid- and salt-loading regimen to maintain intravascular volume.
   3. **Medications**
      a. **Mineralocorticoids.** Enhance central blood volume by increasing sodium and fluid retention. Fludrocortisone has predominantly mineralocorticoid and minimal glucocorticoid activity.
      b. **β-Blockers.** Reduce cardiac inotropy and mechanoreceptor activation; most commonly used are atenolol, metoprolol, and pindolol.
      c. **α-Agonists.** Promote vasoconstriction; agents include midodrine and methylphenidate.
      d. **Serotonin reuptake inhibitors.** Block serotonin reuptake, which diminishes inhibition of sympathetic nervous system by serotonin; agents include sertraline, fluoxetine, and nefazodone.
   B. Arrhythmias. Treatment measures include radiofrequency ablation, antiarrhythmic therapy, automatic internal defibrillator, and pacemaker.
   C. Structural Heart Disease. Treatment may include surgical intervention, if warranted; and β-blockers for hypertrophic cardiomyopathy or for aortic root dilation in patients with Marfan syndrome.
   D. Noncardiac Syncope. Treat underlying condition as warranted.

VI. Problem Case Diagnosis. The two episodes of syncope in this 14-year-old girl occurred after she played soccer on a hot summer day. Episodes were associated nausea, lightheadedness, and sudden standing (not exertion). Otherwise, patient's present, past, and family histories were unremarkable. Screening ECG was normal. Patient was diagnosed with neurally mediated syncope and managed with reassurance and education.

VII. Teaching Pearl: Question. What heart rate changes are typically seen in children with benign syncope?

VIII. Teaching Pearl: Answer. Initially, tachycardia along with pallor, hyperventilation, nausea, and pupillary dilation may occur from autonomic discharge of both sympathetic and parasympathetic systems. This tachycardia is transient and is replaced by bradycardia and hypotension from arteriole dilation by the cholinergic vasodilator system.

REFERENCES

Johnsrude CL. Current approach to pediatric syncope. *Pediatr Cardiol* 2000; 21:522–531.

Massin MM. Neurocardiogenic syncope in children: Current concepts in diagnosis and management. *Pediatr Drugs* 2003;5:327–334.

McLeod KA. Syncope in childhood. *Arch Dis Child* 2003;88:350–353.

Tanel RE, Walsh EP. Syncope in the pediatric patient. *Cardiol Clin* 1997;15:277–294.

86. TACHYCARDIA

I. Problem. A 6-year-old boy is brought to the emergency department because he has a rapid heartbeat. Heart rate in triage is 225 beats/min.

II. Immediate Questions

A. What are the vital signs? Heart rate and BP are important factors in determining management strategy and differential diagnosis. Significant hypotension from tachydysrhythmia is an indication for immediate cardioversion, especially when related to ventricular tachycardia or fibrillation. Hypotension and tachypnea in infants can result from prolonged tachycardia and congestive heart failure (tachycardia-induced cardiomyopathy). Hypertension and tachycardia can be associated with pheochromocytoma, thyrotoxicosis, drugs, pain, or anxiety.

B. What is past medical history? Family history? Cardiac abnormalities or previous cardiac surgery predispose individuals to various rhythm disorders. Additionally, noncardiac disease (eg, hyperthyroidism), tuberous sclerosis (rhabdomyomas), pheochromocytoma, and renal disease may produce various tachycardias. Some tachycardias are the result of genetic syndromes (long QT, Brugada, arrhythmogenic right ventricular dysplasia) or are familial (atrial fibrillation).

C. Has patient previously experienced rhythm abnormality? Patients with frequent premature atrial beats can develop atrial tachycardia; frequent premature ventricular beats can develop into ventricular tachycardia.

D. Has patient received any medications? Stimulant medications (cold preparations, therapies for attention-deficit/hyperactivity disorder, thyroid replacement therapy) may induce supraventricular tachycardia or produce extreme sinus tachycardia. Other medications may lead to electrolyte disturbances (diuretics) or produce tachydsrhythmias as a side effect (antiarrhythmics, psychotropic medications, some antibiotics).

E. Pertinent Historical Information
  1. If a newborn, what is the prenatal and birth history?
  2. Any history of exposures or ingestions? Ask about possibility that child ingested someone else's medication, and about use of illicit drugs.
  3. Any recent illnesses or surgeries?

III. Differential Diagnosis. Tachycardia is defined as elevation in heart rate above the age-dependent norm. Sinus tachycardia as fast as 220 beats/min has been noted in all age groups. However, tachycardias > 200 beats/min outside of infancy should be strongly considered nonsinus. Rate of tachycardia is generally a poor predictor of its mechanism. Tachycardias are generally classified by mechanism (reentry, automatic-ectopic) and cardiac tissue involved (atrial, ventricular, atrioventricular [AV] nodal). Tachycardias that arise from above the AV node typically have a narrow QRS complex; those originating below the AV node, a wide QRS complex. However, rate-related aberrancy of QRS sometimes occurs, producing wide QRS tachycardia during supraventricular rhythm. Additionally, ventricular tachycardia in infants may have a relatively narrow QRS (~100 msec). Therefore, normal ranges for QRS duration based on age have been established.

A. Narrow-Complex Tachycardias. Any high catecholamine state may produce tachycardia that is sinus or nonsinus in nature. Various factors (eg, fever, pain, exercise, medications, anxiety or stress, sepsis, dehydration, anemia, acidosis, thyrotoxicosis, respiratory disease, and pheochromocytoma), as well as others, may elevate catecholamine levels. Except for atrial fibrillation, P waves are generally associated with each QRS complex (in front or behind). The atrium is said to be associated with the ventricle.

  1. **Sinus tachycardia.** Increased heart rate with a P-wave axis consistent with sinus mechanism (upright in leads I and aVf). Sinus tachycardia is the result of body's response to physiologic derangement or external influence. If perturbation is corrected, sinus tachycardia will resolve.

  2. **AV tachycardia.** One of the common causes of supraventricular tachycardia (SVT). Mechanism involves reentry via an accessory connection between atrium and ventricle. Pathway may be evident on 12-lead ECG as preexcitation (short PR interval and delta wave of Wolff-Parkinson-White syndrome). During tachycardia, a retrograde P wave may be seen following QRS complex early in the T wave, representing conduction up accessory pathway.

3. **AV node reentry tachycardia.** More commonly seen in older children and adolescents. Involves reentry between two sets of inputs to AV node (slow and fast). Atrial tissue acts as connection between inputs. Typically, no P waves are seen during tachycardia, because atrial and ventricular activation occurs simultaneously (QRS hides P wave).

4. **Atrial flutter.** Tachycardia involving reentry within atrial tissue. Most commonly seen in newborn infants and patients with congenital heart disease. Characteristic sawtooth pattern may be observed on ECG. This may be difficult to see in infants whose ventricular rates could reach 200–300 beats/min with 2:1 conduction (atrial rates > 400 beats/min). Ventricular rhythm is generally regular but may vary depending on degree of AV block during tachycardia (2:1, 3:1, 3:2, etc).

5. **Atrial fibrillation.** In pediatric population, this tachycardia typically is seen only in patients with congenital heart disease or familial atrial fibrillation. Ventricular response may be rapid in younger children, presenting as tachycardia that is irregular in rhythm. May also be associated with atrial flutter or result of SVT.

6. **Ectopic atrial tachycardia.** Tachycardia with regular rhythm that has P-wave axis different from sinus rhythm. Rates tend to be slower than most other SVTs, sometimes just slightly faster than intrinsic sinus rate.

7. **Multifocal atrial tachycardia.** Evidence of more than one P-wave morphology during tachycardia. Rhythm is usually irregular, with variable conduction from atrium to ventricle (also known as *chaotic atrial rhythm*). More commonly seen in infants and associated with adrenergic medications (inotropes, β-agonists).

B. **Wide-Complex Tachycardias.** Tachycardias with widened QRS complexes. They may be the result of ventricular focus or bundle branch aberrancy during SVT. Wide-complex tachycardias can also be seen in patients who have baseline bundle branch block following congenital heart surgery and then develop atrial tachycardia. Such patients are difficult to manage given their risk for ventricular and atrial arrhythmias. Comparison of a previous baseline ECG would be beneficial in this circumstance.

1. **Ventricular tachycardia.** Site of origin is predicted by morphology of QRS complex. For example, right bundle branch morphology originates from the left ventricle, and vice versa. Rates are quite variable, ranging from slightly above sinus rate with no symptoms to rapid rates that produce hypotension and shock. Most often distinguishable from SVT with aberrancy because of AV dissociation (QRS complexes with no association to a P wave). Fusion with sinus beats may also be observed. Ventricular tachycardia may be the result of structurally

abnormal myocardium (myocarditis, cardiomyopathy, surgery, hypertrophy, rhabdomyomas), abnormal conductivity (long QT syndrome), or idiopathic (catecholamine-sensitive ventricular tachycardia).

2. **Torsade de pointes.** Translated as "turning about a point," this form of ventricular tachycardia is characterized by widened QRS complexes that change amplitude over several beats in an organized fashion (increases-decreases-increases, etc). This is the typical ventricular tachycardia associated with prolongation of QT interval, either congenital (long QT syndrome), related to medications (antiarrhythmics, antipsychotics, some antibiotics), or as the result of electrolyte disturbances (hypokalemia, hypomagnesemia, hypocalcemia). Torsade de pointes is an inherently unstable rhythm that often resolves spontaneously but is prone to recurrences.

IV. Database
A. Physical Exam Key Points
1. **Vital signs.** Check heart rate and regularity. Assess respiratory rate, BP, and temperature. Perform peripheral pulse oximetry as indicated by exam (respiratory distress, cyanosis) or history (congenital heart disease, respiratory disease).
2. **Heart.** Assess pulses and perfusion. Look for signs of congestive heart failure (liver size, gallop, peripheral edema). Check for murmurs.
3. **Lungs.** Listen for evidence of respiratory illness or congestive heart failure. Assess for presence of pneumothorax.
4. **Skin.** Assess for discoloration of skin consistent with café au lait spots of neurofibromatosis (pheochromocytoma) or ash-leaf spots of tuberous sclerosis (cardiac rhabdomyomas and ventricular tachycardia).
5. **Neck.** Assess for thyromegaly.

B. Laboratory Data.
Not every patient with tachycardia needs a complete laboratory assessment. Patients with routine SVT need little more than an ECG. Unusual presentations or histories warrant further laboratory investigations.
1. **Electrolytes.** Assess levels of potassium, magnesium, and calcium.
2. **ABGs.** Assess for hypoxemia and acidemia in patients with significant respiratory distress, cyanosis, or hypoperfusion.
3. **CBC with differential.** May demonstrate anemia or evidence of infection.
4. **Glucose.** Hyperglycemia or hypoglycemia may cause tachycardia.
5. **Cultures.** Obtain if infection is suspected.
6. **Thyroid profile.** Assess levels of thyroid-stimulating hormone and thyroxine.

7. **Plasma, urine catecholamines.** These tests, which assess levels of circulating catecholamines, are helpful in diagnosis of pheochromocytoma and some forms of autonomic dysfunction.

C. **Radiographic and Other Studies**

1. **Twelve-lead ECG, rhythm strip.** ECG and rhythm strips obtained during tachycardia are the most important studies for diagnosing type of tachycardia. If patient is not experiencing tachycardia when ECG is obtained, assess for delta wave (Wolff-Parkinson-White syndrome) or signs of myopathic changes (hypertrophy, strain, ischemia). If patient has an irregular rhythm, a multilead rhythm strip is important for diagnosing origin of irregularity (premature atrial or ventricular contraction).

2. **Chest x-ray.** Examine for abnormal cardiac size, signs of interstitial lung disease, evidence of mediastinal mass, pneumothorax, or bony abnormalities.

3. **Echocardiogram.** Used to confirm cardiac disease when suspected or to determine presence or absence of cardiac disease in cases less certain. Transthoracic or transesophageal echocardiography is performed in patients with congenital heart disease and atrial flutter or fibrillation because of possibility of clot formation in left atrial appendage.

4. **Other imaging studies.** CT or MRI scanning or ultrasonography of head, chest, or abdomen may be performed if neurologic disease, adrenal abnormalities, or mediastinal abnormalities are suspected.

V. **Plan**

A. **General Management.** Assess patient quickly for level of distress and perform ECG to diagnose rhythm abnormality. Obtain IV access, if necessary. Support airway and circulation, as necessary. If possible, obtain multilead rhythm strips during termination of tachycardia.

B. **Specific Management.** Management of specific tachycardias centers on stabilizing patient by changing rhythm or by making rhythm more tolerable. If patient is hemodynamically unstable due to tachycardia, electrical cardioversion is treatment of choice for any of these dysrhythmias (synchronized unless a pulseless tachycardia). Pay special consideration to patient with congenital heart disease who has atrial flutter or fibrillation because of possibility of clot formation in left atrial appendage and risk of subsequent stroke following cardioversion. Digoxin and calcium channel blockers are contraindicated in patients with Wolff-Parkinson-White syndrome because of risk of rapid conduction down accessory pathway, promoting ventricular fibrillation.

1. **AV and AV-nodal tachycardias.** Generically thought of as SVT, these tachycardias use the AV node as a critical part of

tachycardia circuit. Therefore, blocking the AV node should terminate tachycardia. However, effectively blocking AV-nodal conduction without producing high-grade block is sometimes difficult.

   a. Adenosine. Causes significant AV block for a very transient amount of time; drug is deactivated by enzymes of RBCs and, therefore, has a very short half-life (~9 seconds). SVTs that involve the AV node typically respond to IV adenosine, 100–300 mcg/kg, up to maximum of ~12 mg. Administer as rapid bolus followed by saline push (~10 mL). IV access should be as large and as close to the heart as possible to allow for rapid delivery of drug to myocardium (ie, arm is better than foot). Doses may be repeated incrementally as needed. Effect should be seen within a few seconds after administration. Potential side effects include mild bronchospasm, atrial fibrillation, asystole (dependent on dose relative to size of patient and level of catecholamines), brief hypotension, chest pain, headaches, and flushing.

   b. Vagal maneuvers. May also be tried; among these are bag of ice to face (best as slush), Valsalva, gag, and cough.

   c. Verapamil, procainamide, amiodarone. Other IV agents that have been effective in acute treatment of SVT resistant to adenosine. **Verapamil is contraindicated in infants or patients with Wolff-Parkinson-White syndrome.** Once termination of tachycardia is achieved, oral therapy can be instituted as necessary.

2. Atrial tachycardias

   a. Adenosine. Ectopic atrial tachycardia and atrial flutter or fibrillation do not use AV node as a critical part of their circuit and generally are not responsive to treatment with adenosine. However, adenosine can have a role in management of these tachycardias. Some ectopic atrial foci and flutter circuits use specialized conduction tissue that is adenosine sensitive and will be terminated with administration of adenosine. Adenosine can be used diagnostically to demonstrate that atrial tachycardia persists despite block of AV node. This phenomenon can be observed on a rhythm strip performed with administration of adenosine. P waves will march along at tachycardia rate with loss of AV conduction (atrial rate constant with slowed ventricular rate).

   b. AV-nodal blocking agents. Short-term goal is to control ventricular rate with administration of AV-nodal blocking drugs such as calcium channel blockers (verapamil, diltiazem), β-blockers (esmolol), or digoxin.

   c. Cardioversion. Patients who do not respond to medications or who are hemodynamically unstable should undergo synchronized DC cardioversion. Once rhythm is controlled, more potent oral antiarrhythmic medications can be instituted.

3. **Ventricular tachycardia.** Most wide-complex tachycardias are ventricular in origin, especially if AV dissociation is present.

   a. **Adenosine.** If patient is hemodynamically stable and QRS complexes are associated with P waves, adenosine should be considered due to possibility of terminating SVT with aberrancy. This is especially true in patients with baseline bundle branch block who now have SVT. If the rhythm is ventricular tachycardia, adenosine will produce AV-nodal block and dissociate the P wave from the QRS complex (ventricular rate remains same and atrial rate slows).

   b. **Lidocaine.** May be used in hemodynamically stable patients. Administer IV bolus of 1 mg/kg, followed by infusion of 20–50 mcg/kg/min.

   c. **Amiodarone.** May also be used to treat stable patients. Initial dose is 5 mg/kg over 20 minutes, repeated up to 3 times; with infusion of 7 mcg/kg/min after conversion. Most significant side effect involves α-blockade (hypotension, bradycardia). Be prepared to treat these effects (with volume expanders, temporary pacing) should they occur.

   d. **DC cardioversion.** Use in treatment of hemodynamically unstable VT (synchronized if pulse is present).

4. **Torsades de pointes.** Treatment is directed at electrolyte imbalance if present or withdrawing offending medication. Infusion of magnesium can terminate tachycardia or prevent recurrence even in patients with normal magnesium levels. Unstable patients should undergo DC cardioversion and magnesium therapy. Patients with known long QT syndrome may benefit from infusion of esmolol. Ventricular pacing may also prevent recurrence, because induction of tachycardia usually involves a prolonged pause.

VI. **Problem Case Diagnosis.** The 12-lead ECG in this 6-year-old boy demonstrated a wide-complex tachycardia with no discernible P waves. Patient was awake and talking with no hemodynamic instability. Clinician suspected ventricular tachycardia rather than SVT with aberrancy. (For further discussion, see VII and VIII, below.)

VII. **Teaching Pearl: Question.** Given this patient's current hemodynamic stability, what could be done to both diagnose and possibly treat his rhythm disturbance?

VIII. **Teaching Pearl: Answer.** Administration of adenosine while obtaining a multilead rhythm strip should allow clinician to discriminate ventricular tachycardia from SVT with aberrancy and also treat supraventricular arrhythmia. Children frequently have retrograde AV-nodal conduction during ventricular tachycardia, with activation of atrium and production of P waves within or following the QRS complex. This is also true for AV node reentry tachycardia, because it is the mechanism of tachycardia. These P waves may not be discernible during arrhythmia or, if they are seen, will be associated with the QRS complex. Therefore, in a hemodynamically stable patient, adenosine can be used to block conduction in the AV node and dissociate the P wave from QRS, in the case of ventricular tachycardia, or terminate SVT, at least temporarily. It is of utmost importance that this maneuver be performed during recording of a multilead rhythm strip, because P waves that are demonstrated in other leads may be missed in a single lead. Dissociation of P wave from QRS with no change in tachycardia is diagnostic for ventricular tachycardia. Hemodynamic stability or instability should not be used to differentiate ventricular tachycardia from supraventricular tachycardia with aberrancy.

REFERENCES

Deal BJ. Supraventricular tachycardia mechanisms and natural history. In: Deal BJ, Wolff GS, Gelband H, eds. *Current Concepts in Diagnosis and Management of Arrhythmias in Infants and Children.* Futura, 1998:117–143.

Dick M II, Russell MW. Ventricular tachycardia. In: Deal BJ, Wolff GS, Gelband H, eds. *Current Concepts in Diagnosis and Management of Arrhythmias in Infants and Children.* Futura, 1998:181–222.

Gillette PC, Garson A Jr, eds. *Clinical Pediatric Arrhythmias,* 2nd ed. Saunders, 1999.

87. THROMBOCYTOPENIA

I. **Problem.** A 5-year-old girl is brought to the emergency department because she has had intermittent nosebleeds for several days. She has several large bruises on her legs and back, and her platelet count is 15,000/mcL.

II. **Immediate Questions**

A. **Is there active bleeding?** There is increased risk of spontaneous hemorrhage with platelet counts < 20,000/mcL.

B. **Has patient experienced head trauma?** Intracranial hemorrhage is unusual but can occur with platelet counts < 20,000/mcL.

C. **Is patient febrile?** Presence of fever increases risk of thrombocytopenia due to significant infection or disseminated intravascular coagulation (DIC).

D. **Has patient recently received chemotherapy?** Chemotherapy is a frequent cause of thrombocytopenia.

E. **Is there a past history of low platelet count?** This could be consistent with chronic idiopathic thrombocytopenic purpura (ITP) or an inherited thrombocytopenia.

F. **Does patient take any medication?** Thrombocytopenia is often seen in patients who take valproic acid.

III. **Differential Diagnosis (Table I–26)**

A. **Spurious Thrombocytopenia**

1. **Platelet clumping due to activation during collection.** Review peripheral smear.

2. **Undercounting of macrothrombocytes.** Review peripheral smear and check platelet size.

TABLE I–26. DIFFERENTIAL DIAGNOSIS OF THROMBOCYTOPENIA DURING CHILDHOOD

Decreased Production	Increased Destruction	Sequestration
Hereditary disorders:	**Immune-Mediated:**	**Sequesration:**
Hereditary thrombocy-topenia	ITP	Hypersplenism
TAR syndrome	Autoimmune (SLE)	Hypothermia
Wiskott-Aldrich syndrome	HIV	Burns
May-Hegglin anomaly	Neonatal immune reaction	Portal hypertension
	Drugs	Gaucher disease
	Allergy and anaphylaxis	
	Post-transplant or post-transfusion	
Acquired Disorders:	**Nonimmune:**	
Aplastic anemia	Infection	
Infection	Microangiopathic (HUS, ITP, drugs)	
Marrow infiltration or damage (malignancy)	Congenital heart disease	
Drugs	Kasabach-Merritt syndrome	

AIDS = acquired immunodeficiency syndrome; HIV = human immunodeficiency syndrome; HUS = hemolytic uremic syndrome; ITP = idiopathic thrombocytopenic purpura; SLE = systemic lupus erythematosus; TAR = thrombocytopenia with absent radii.

3. **Pseudothrombocytopenia due to EDTA-dependent antibodies, cold agglutinins, or drugs.** For ethylenediamine tetra-acetic acid (EDTA)–related problems, recheck platelet counts with alternative anticoagulants (eg, heparin).

B. Destructive Thrombocytopenia
   1. Immune thrombocytopenia
      a. **Acute and chronic ITP.** Caused by antiplatelet antibodies. Chronic ITP is defined as lasting longer than 6 months.
      b. **Autoimmune diseases with thrombocytopenia as a manifestation.** Immune thrombocytopenia associated with cancer, systemic lupus erythematosus (SLE), Evans syndrome, antiphospholipid antibody syndrome, cyclic thrombocytopenia (variant of chronic ITP), autoimmune lymphoproliferative syndrome.
      c. **HIV-associated thrombocytopenia.**
      d. **Neonatal immune thrombocytopenia**
         i. **Alloimmune.** Usually due to incompatibility for alloantigen HPA-1a (PL^{A1} or ZW^a).
         ii. **Autoimmune.** In infants of mothers with immune thrombocytopenia related to, for example, ITP or SLE.
      e. Drug-induced immune thrombocytopenia (heparin, gold salts, levodopa, interferon-α, procainamide).
      f. Allergy and anaphylaxis.
      g. Post-transplantation.
      h. Post-transfusion purpura.

   2. Nonimmune thrombocytopenia
      a. Infection. Protozoan, bacteria, fungal, viral (Epstein-Barr virus).
      b. Microangiopathic
         i. Hemolytic uremic syndrome. Patients typically have thrombocytopenia, hemolytic anemia, and renal failure. These symptoms typically occur following diarrheal illness secondary to *E coli* O157:H7.
         ii. Thrombotic thrombocytopenic purpura (TTP). More likely to produce neurologic symptoms than is hemolytic uremic syndrome.
         iii. Post–bone marrow transplantation.
         iv. Drug induced.
      c. Congenital heart disease.
      d. Direct antiplatelet effects of drugs (protamine; ristocetin).
      e. Platelet contact with foreign material.
      f. Type 2B or platelet-type von Willebrand disease.
   3. Combined platelet-fibrinogen consumption syndromes
      a. Kasabach-Merritt syndrome (giant hemangioma associated with thrombocytopenia and microangiopathic anemia).
      b. Virus-associated hemophagocytic syndrome.
      c. DIC.
C. Impaired Platelet Production
   1. Hereditary disorder
      a. Congenital amegakaryocytic thrombocytopenia.
      b. Thrombocytopenia with absent radii (TAR) syndrome.
      c. Wiskott-Aldrich syndrome (X-linked thrombocytopenia).
      d. Thrombocytopenia associated with macrothrombocytes (May-Hegglin anomaly, Sebastian syndrome, Epstein syndrome, Montreal platelet syndrome).
   2. Acquired disorders
      a. Aplastic anemia.
      b. Infection.
      c. Marrow infiltrative processes (leukemia, rhabdomyosarcoma, neuroblastoma, Ewing sarcoma, Langerhans cell histiocytosis, storage diseases).
      d. Secondary to drugs or radiation.
      e. Osteopetrosis.
      f. Paroxysmal nocturnal hemoglobinuria.
      g. Neonatal hypoxia or placental insufficiency.
      h. Nutritional deficiencies (iron, folate, vitamin B_{12}), anorexia nervosa.
      i. Myelodysplastic syndrome.
D. Sequestration
   1. Hypersplenism.
   2. Hypothermia.
   3. Burns.

       4. Portal hypertension.
       5. Gaucher disease.

IV. Database

A. Physical Exam Key Points

1. **Vital signs.** Fever raises concerns of infection, leukemia, and ITP.
2. **Skin and mucous membranes.** Petechiae and mucous membrane bleeding suggest low platelet number or abnormal platelet function, or both.
3. **Lymph nodes.** Enlarged nodes suggest infection or malignancy.
4. **Abdomen.** Enlargement of liver or spleen, or both, can suggest malignancy (leukemia), but splenomegaly can also be seen with hypersplenism, storage diseases, or infection.
5. **Neurologic exam.** Abnormal findings raise concerns regarding TTP.

B. Laboratory Data

1. **Peripheral smear.** Review of smear is important to rule out pseudothrombocytopenia. Large platelets may be seen with destructive thrombocytopenia, especially ITP. RBC abnormalities may be seen in DIC or microangiopathic disease. Blasts may be seen in peripheral smear in leukemia.
2. **Coagulation studies.** Abnormal PT, PTT, and fibrinogen may be consistent with DIC.
3. **HIV test.** Isolated thrombocytopenia may be an early sign of HIV.
4. **ANA.** May be positive in SLE or other collagen vascular diseases.
5. **BUN and creatinine.** Renal failure can be seen in hemolytic uremic syndrome, sepsis, DIC, and TTP.
6. **Immunoglobulins.** IgA deficiency may influence selection of an immunoglobulin product to treat ITP.
7. **Bone marrow biopsy.** May be vital to confirm destructive versus decreased production problem.

C. Radiographic and Other Studies

1. **Chest x-ray.** May reveal pneumonia, mediastinal mass (leukemia, lymphoma), or cardiac abnormalities.
2. **Abdominal ultrasound.** May reveal hepatosplenomegaly.

V. Plan

A. Significant bleeding must be controlled by direct pressure if possible. If platelets are small to normal in size, a production problem may be present. In this situation, platelet transfusion may be necessary.
B. Large platelets on the smear may suggest destructive process, especially ITP. This may respond to intravenous gamma globulin (IVGG) or steroids.
C. If more than one cell line is decreased, a marrow infiltrative process (eg, leukemia) or marrow failure problem may exist. In

this situation, bone marrow evaluation will be important to establish diagnosis. If leukemia is a possibility, obtain chest x-ray to rule out mediastinal mass. Order chemistry panel, including phosphorous and uric acid levels.

D. Plasma therapy (plasmapheresis) is mainstay of treatment of TTP.

VI. Problem Case Diagnosis. The 5-year-old girl has ITP. The peripheral smear showed large platelets without RBC or WBC abnormalities. Results of PT and PTT tests and international normalized ratio (INR) were normal. Platelet number retuned to normal after IVGG was administered.

VII. Teaching Pearl: Question. What is the treatment of choice for neonatal alloimmune thrombocytopenia?

VIII. Teaching Pearl: Answer. Administration of washed, irradiated maternal platelets.

REFERENCES

Butros L, Bussell J. Intracranial hemorrhage in immune thrombocytopenic purpura, a retrospective analysis. *J Pediatr Hematol Oncol* 2003;24:460–464.

Hann IM, Gibson BES, Letsky EA. *Fetal and Neonatal Haematology.* Baillere Tindori, 1991.

Homans A. Thrombocytopenia in the neonate. *Pediatr Clin North Am* 1996;43: 737–756.

Wilson D. Acquired platelet defects. In: Nathan D, Orkins S, Ginsburg D, Look AT, eds. *Nathan & Osti's Hematology of Infancy & Childhood,* 6th ed. Saunders, 2003:1597–1630.

88. TRANSFUSION REACTION

I. Problem. A 14-year-old boy develops fever and rigors during RBC transfusion. He has acute myelogenous leukemia and has been treated with consolidation chemotherapy.

II. Immediate Questions

A. What are the vital signs? The critical first step in response to *any* transfusion reaction is to **stop the transfusion.** Then assess vital signs and cardiovascular status. If hypotension is present, lay patient flat and begin fluid resuscitation with normal saline. Pharmacologic support of BP may be required.

B. Does patient's identity match that of blood tag? Most acute hemolytic transfusion reactions result from human error. Therefore, clinician must check for clerical mistake. If fever complicates RBC transfusion, hemolytic transfusion reaction must be excluded by checking at bedside and in laboratory to ensure that the proper blood component was selected and administered.

C. What is post-transfusion direct antiglobulin test (DAT)? DAT and inspection of patient plasma for free hemoglobin can be performed on a postreaction specimen. If no clerical discrepancy is noted, and laboratory tests on post-transfusion specimens are negative, hemolysis can usually be excluded as cause of reaction.

D. Does patient complain of any symptoms or exhibit signs of hemolysis? In addition to fever, chills, and hypotension, patients experiencing hemolytic transfusion reaction may have nausea or vomiting; pain localizing to flanks, abdomen, groin, chest, head, or infusion site; dyspnea; or hemoglobinuria.

E. What is patient's transfusion history? Always note any previous history of transfusion reaction(s).

III. Differential Diagnosis

A. Comorbid Conditions. Many patients requiring blood transfusion have complex medical or surgical conditions. Therefore, it is not uncommon for such patients to develop fever and chills from infection unrelated to transfusions.

B. Medications. Some medications can cause fever and rigors (eg, amphotericin B). Infusion of such medications around the time of transfusion makes it difficult to determine the specific cause of fever.

C. Hemolytic Transfusion Reaction

  1. Classification. Identified as acute or delayed based on whether reaction occurs within 24 hours of transfusion.

  2. Mechanisms

    a. Antigen-positive RBCs are transfused into recipient who has an alloantibody.

    b. Antibodies of plasma-containing blood components (eg, fresh frozen plasma and platelets) are directed against antigen on recipient RBCs, which, in turn, causes hemolysis.

    c. There is incompatibility between RBCs from one donor and plasma from another donor, which results in hemolysis when admixed in blood of recipient.

D. Bacterial Contamination of Blood Components. Transfusion-associated sepsis should be considered when any patient develops high fever, rigors, or hypotension during or immediately after transfusion. Microorganisms most frequently isolated from platelet units include coagulase-negative staphylococci, *Bacillus* spp, and *Staphylococcus aureus.* Microorganisms commonly implicated in sepsis associated with contaminated RBC units include *Yersinia enterocolitica,* psychrophilic pseudomonads, and *Serratia marcescens.*

E. Transfusion-Related Acute Living Injury (TRALI). Manifests as noncardiogenic pulmonary edema, usually within 6 hours of transfusion. In its full form, TRALI presents as marked respiratory distress with accelerating dyspnea, tachypnea, hypoxemia, fever, chills, cough, and hypotension. Physical exam shows rales and decreased breath sounds. Chest x-ray shows normal cardiac silhouette with bilateral fluffy infiltrates that can progress to complete whiteout of lung fields. Mortality is 5–10%.

IV. Database

A. Physical Exam Key Points

1. **Vital signs.** Absence of fever and presence of cutaneous manifestations (pruritus, urticaria, erythema, flushing, angioedema) distinguish transfusion reactions of anaphylaxis from those due to hemolysis or sepsis. Fever with hypotension raises concerns of acute hemolytic transfusion reaction or septic shock.

2. **Lungs.** Stridor and wheezing with cutaneous manifestations and hypotension are consistent with anaphylaxis. Dyspnea, cyanosis, rales, and hypotension suggest TRALI.

3. **Skin and mucous membranes.** Generalized ecchymoses, petechiae, and bleeding from mucosal surfaces and venipuncture sites suggest disseminated intravascular coagulation (DIC); sepsis and acute hemolytic transfusion reaction should be considered.

B. Laboratory Data

1. **Hemoglobin.** Check for decrease in hemoglobin, which suggests hemolysis secondary to acute hemolytic transfusion reaction or sepsis. Free serum hemoglobin is consistent with hemolysis.

2. **Urinalysis.** Hemoglobinuria suggests hemolysis.

3. **Bilirubin.** Hyperbilirubinemia suggests hemolysis.

4. **DAT.** Positive DAT on a postreaction sample is consistent with hemolysis.

5. **Gram stain and culture.** Of unit associated with reaction and recipient's blood sample.

6. **DIC panel.**

7. **Peripheral smear.** Evaluate for hemolysis

C. Radiographic and Other Studies. Order pulse oximetry and chest x-ray in patients with respiratory distress.

V. Plan

A. Febrile Nonhemolytic Transfusion Reactions. Not typically life-threatening.

1. **Stop transfusion.**

2. Treat with antipyretics.

3. Avoid future reactions by premedication with acetaminophen and use of leukocyte reduction filters.

B. Hemolytic Transfusion Reaction. Severity of reaction is directly related to volume of blood transfused. Thus, early recognition and cessation of transfusions are critical first steps in treatment.

1. Maintain airway.

2. Treat hypotension with IV fluids and vasopressors; increase renal blood flow with IV fluids and diuresis.

3. Monitor for DIC, and administer blood components as needed.

C. Septic Shock. Administer isotonic fluids, vasopressors, and broad-spectrum antibiotics.

D. TRALI. Provide supportive care; reaction typically resolves within 96 hours after onset of symptoms.

VI. Problem Case Diagnosis. The 14-year-old boy has had a febrile nonhemolytic transfusion reaction. Vital signs were stable, and free hemoglobin was absent from urine. He improved after administration of antipyretics. Leukocyte-poor filtered RBCs should be used for future transfusions.

VII. Teaching Pearl: Question. What is the most common infectious complication of blood transfusions?

VIII. Teaching Pearl: Answer. Bacterial sepsis from platelets occurs in 1 in 50,000 transfusions. Other, less common infectious complications include hepatitis B (1:205,000), bacterial sepsis from RBCs (1:500,000), hepatitis C (1:1,935,000), and infection with HIV-1 and -2 (1:2,135,000).

REFERENCES

Brecher ME, ed. *Technical Manual,* 14th ed. American Association of Blood Banks Press, 2002.
Popovsky MA, ed. *Transfusion Reactions,* 2nd ed. American Association of Blood Banks Press, 2001.
Simon TL, ed. *Rossi's Principles of Transfusion Medicine,* 3rd ed. Lippincott Williams & Wilkins, 2002.

89. TRAUMA AND INJURIES

I. Problem. A 6-year-old boy is struck by a car while riding his bike.

II. Immediate Questions

A. What are the circumstances of the collision (eg, speed of car, use of protective gear, whether patient was thrown)? Answers give an idea of how significant injuries might be. If child presents as a passenger in an automobile collision, questions include the following:

1. Was child riding in rear or front seat? Restrained or unrestrained?

2. How are other passengers? Children injured in collisions in which others are killed or seriously injured as well as those involved in accidents in which steering wheel of car has been damaged are more likely to incur significant injury.

B. What was status of patient at scene? Loss of consciousness increases likelihood of intracranial injury. Paramedics on scene may be able to give information about signs of obvious injury.

C. What is status of patient now? Identification of patient's hemodynamic and respiratory status enables prompt preparation of appropriate team members and equipment.

1. Does patient have spontaneous respirations? Pulses?

2. Is cervical spine stabilized?

III. Differential Diagnosis

A. Categorization of Trauma

1. Local versus multiple. May be difficult to know early in evaluation, because injured children often cry and are unable to localize injury.

2. **Blunt versus penetrating.** Blunt trauma is more common in children.

3. **Mild versus severe.** Mild injuries often accompany severe injuries (eg, superficial forehead lacerations with fracture of the femur).

B. **Potential Injuries by System.** The following discussion is not all-inclusive but will help identify problems that can be encountered in trauma patients.

1. **Head.** Scalp laceration, skull fracture, subdural hematoma, epidural hematoma, concussion (mild to severe), intracerebral contusions or hematomas, diffuse axonal injury.

2. **Spine.** Injury can be from atlas (C1) to lumbar spine (eg, Chance fracture, which is a lumbar distraction fracture seen with seat belt injuries), fractures, dislocations, and penetrating neck trauma. Factors associated with high risk of spinal injury include high-speed collisions, unconsciousness, multiple injuries, neurologic deficits, and spinal tenderness.

3. **Thorax.** Pneumothorax, hemothorax, pulmonary contusion, tracheobronchial tree injuries, blunt cardiac injury, aortic disruption, diaphragmatic injury, and penetrating chest wounds are all potentially lethal.

4. **Abdomen.** Diaphragmatic injury, duodenal rupture or hematoma, pancreatic injury, renal injury or hematoma, small bowel injury.

5. **GU.** Injury is more likely in patients with pelvic fracture or disruption. Consider urethral tears, large vessel injury, scrotal and perineal injury.

6. **Orthopedic.** Fractures (open or closed), joint dislocations, amputation, crush injury, and compartment syndrome.

7. **Skin.** Lacerations, contusions, burns.

IV. **Database**

A. **Physical Exam Key Points.** Use systematic approach to all trauma patients to rapidly identify serious threats to life or limb, followed by thorough identification of all potential injuries. Begin cardiac and pulse-oximetry monitoring as survey is initiated.

1. **Vital signs.** Obtain vital signs as part of primary survey. *Do not* wait to obtain vital signs before beginning initial trauma survey and treatment.

2. **Primary survey (ABCs).** Address problems immediately within primary survey. (This survey should be completed within 10 seconds.)

a. **Airway.** Evaluate patency of airway while ensuring immobilization of cervical spine. (All trauma patients are assumed to have cervical spine injury until "cleared.") Perform jaw-thrust or chin-lift maneuver as needed and based on likelihood of cervical spine injury. Remove visible debris and secretions. Significant facial or oral trauma will jeopardize an adequate airway. If patient is not able to maintain airway, secure airway before moving on. (See Section III, Chapter 6, Endotracheal Intubation [Oral and Nasal], p. 497).

   b. **Breathing.** Assess air movement, chest excursion, and respiratory rate. Support clinical impression with data from pulse-oximetry and CO_2 monitors, if available. If air exchange is inadequate, provide oxygen and prepare to secure airway.

   c. **Circulation.** Examine pulses, skin color, and capillary refill time. Palpable peripheral pulse correlates with systolic BP > 80 mm Hg; central pulse correlates with BP of 50–60 mm Hg. Capillary refill time ≤ 2 seconds suggests euvolemia. Obvious bleeding should be stopped with direct pressure, tourniquet, or hemostats to bleeding vessels. If IV lines are not in place, obtain IV access and begin fluid resuscitation.

   d. **Disability.** Perform rapid neurologic assessment, including level of consciousness, and pupillary size and response.

   e. **Exposure.** Undress patient to expose major injuries. Be sure to check body temperature and prevent hypothermia during assessment and resuscitation.

3. **Secondary survey.** Head-to-toe evaluation should begin after primary survey is complete, resuscitative efforts are established, and patient is stable or being stabilized.

   a. **AMPLE History.** Includes **A**llergies, **M**edications, **P**ast history (brief), **L**ast meal, and **E**vents and environment related to injury. Sources include patient, prehospital personnel, and family.

   b. **Head.** Check scalp for lacerations or contusions. Check eyes (pupils, ocular movements, visual acuity); remove contacts. Identify midface fractures. If potential risk for cribriform plate fracture exists, *do not* insert nasogastric tube.

   c. **Cervical spine and neck.** Keep immobilized while assessing, inspecting, palpating, and auscultating neck for lacerations, tenderness, crepitus, or bruits. Be extra cautious when examining children with distracting injuries.

   d. **Chest.** Palpate ribs, clavicles, and sternum; inspect for contusions and hematomas. Listen for breath sounds, especially high anterior (pneumothorax) and at bases (hemothorax). Percussion of chest can help identify pneumothorax. Distant heart sounds raise concerns of cardiac tamponade.

   e. **Abdomen.** Inspect for bruising, and palpate for rigidity and tenderness. If decreased mental status, consider imaging. Perform frequent reevaluations. *Diagnostic peritoneal lavage may still be considered appropriate if patient is unstable, but has been replaced by CT scan as test of choice (see later discussion).*

   f. **GU exam.** Observe for blood at urethral meatus, and perform rectal exam, examining tone and checking for blood.

   g. **Musculoskeletal exam.** Check for function, contusions, and deformities of extremities. Palpate for tenderness as well as instability or bruising over pelvis. Check function, sensation, and pulses to address possibility of compartment syndrome. Inspect and palpate entire spine.
   h. **Skin.** Inspect for lacerations, bruising, and burns.
   i. **Neurologic exam.** Continue to reassess pupillary response and level of consciousness; perform complete neurologic evaluation. Reevaluate as often as possible (at least every 20 minutes), documenting and noting time for all findings. Use Glasgow Coma Scale to obtain quantitative assessment of neurologic status (See Appendix F, p. 765).
B. **Laboratory Data**
   1. **Blood studies.** Obtain hemoglobin and hematocrit; platelets; PT and PTT; and metabolic panel, including electrolytes (baseline), liver enzymes, amylase, lipase, ABGs, type and screen, and crossmatch. Many facilities have a so-called trauma panel that includes all of these tests.
   2. **Urine studies.** Obtain urinalysis for blood (urethral tear is a surgical emergency); perform pregnancy screening for adolescents.
C. **Radiographic and Other Studies**
   1. **Plain x-rays.** Focus on area of injury; consider mechanism and screen for possible injuries. In major trauma, x-rays of cervical spine (AP, lateral, odontoid), chest (AP and lateral), and pelvis should be obtained routinely. Evaluate for fractures and soft tissue swelling on cervical spine. Children may have spinal cord injury without radiographic abnormality (SCIWORA); use caution and "clear" cervical spine with both x-rays and exam. Look for a widened mediastinum and pneumothorax.
   2. **CT scan.** Use clinical judgment; not considered a routine study. Loss of consciousness, abnormal neurologic exam, or significant mechanism will drive decision to obtain head CT scan. Neck CT scan is indicated for patients with poor-quality x-rays or significant mechanism of injury. Altered level of consciousness, physical findings, or mechanism determine whether chest and abdomen CT scans are indicated.

V. Plan. Clinician's approach to evaluation and management of trauma patients should be systematic, as outlined above, and aggressive until possibility of serious life-threatening injury is eliminated. A well-organized trauma team will be able to assess patient thoroughly and efficiently. Once patient has been evaluated and resuscitated, management plan to address injuries is begun. Depending on injuries identified and level of suspicion for serious injury, patient can be observed and discharged to home, admitted to hospital, admitted to ICU, transferred to operating room, or transferred to specialty care location (eg, spinal cord injury center, burn center). Identify patient's family, and notify them of patient's status if patient is unable. In automobile collisions, assault, foul play, and other legal situations, police may be present and asking questions. Clinician should cooperate with police by stating patient's status (eg, stable, critical). Further communication without official subpoena of medical record can put clinician at risk for violating patient's privacy.

A. Initial Assessment and Resuscitation. Perform primary and secondary survey (see earlier discussion at IV, A, 1 and 2).

1. **Airway and breathing.** Stabilize airway and administer oxygen to patient (nasal canula, simple mask, nonrebreather mask). Intubate and provide oxygen if airway is unstable or oxygenation or ventilation is inadequate. In this initial phase, clinician may need to treat tension pneumothorax with needle decompression. Difficult intubation may result in a cricothyrotomy (see Section III, Chapter 5, Cricothyrotomy, p. 495).

2. **Circulation.** Place two large-bore IV lines during initial assessment. If IV access is difficult, place intraosseous line. If appropriate, start isotonic fluid resuscitation using normal saline or Ringer lactate, 20 mL/kg rapid bolus; repeat as needed. Consider type-specific or type O–negative blood if 60 mL/kg of isotonic fluid has been administered and bleeding is suspected.

3. **Disability.** Document brief neurologic exam prior to administration of any sedative or paralytic medications. If intracranial injury is suspected, tailor therapies to minimize increased intracranial pressure (ICP). Use medications for intubation that prevent increased ICP (thiopental, lidocaine). Avoid hypercarbia and hyperthermia. Notify neurosurgery colleagues. If patient exhibits signs of impending herniation (fixed dilated pupil, hypertension, bradycardia) hyperventilate and give mannitol. (For further discussion, see Chapter 56, Increased Intracranial Pressure, p. 258.)

B. Treatment of Injuries

1. **Cervical spine.** Assume cervical spine injury and immobilize patient until x-rays are reviewed and patient can be thoroughly evaluated for neck pain or tenderness.

2. **Head.** See discussion at V, A, 3, earlier.

3. **Chest.** Treat tension pneumothorax immediately with needle decompression (see Chapter 73, Pneumothorax, p. 336). Consider chest tube placement if simple pneumothorax or hemothorax exists. Patients with multiple rib fractures and other severe injury to chest require intubation, if not already performed.

4. **Abdomen.** Patients with significant injury (penetration, free air, splenic rupture, severe liver laceration) require surgical intervention. Many injuries can be observed in the hospital (minor liver lacerations, duodenal hematomas). Diagnosis of abdominal

injuries in children is a process. Injury may not be obvious initially, but rather may develop over time. Children with high likelihood of intra-abdominal injury should undergo abdominal CT scan to diagnose potential serious injury.

5. **GU tract.** If perineal injury is obvious, obtain retrograde urethrogram to rule out urethral tear prior to placement of urinary catheter. Suspect urethral injury if pelvic fracture or hematuria is present.

6. **Musculoskeletal system.** Extremities with obvious deformity must be assessed for neurovascular integrity. Emergency reduction is required if nerve or blood supply is threatened. If perfusion is maintained, reduction of dislocations and displaced fractures can be managed by orthopaedic colleagues. Open fractures are treated in the operating room to ensure thorough debridement and cleaning. Begin IV antibiotics (most commonly, cephazolin) to prevent infection. Splint all extremity fractures for comfort until definitive management is determined. Treat pain as quickly as possible.

VI. **Problem Case Diagnosis.** The 6-year-old boy was not wearing a helmet when he was struck by a car traveling approximately 25 mph. He was thrown 5 feet to an adjacent lawn and lost consciousness for several minutes. When he awoke, he was combative. On arrival in the emergency department, patient had already undergone endotracheal intubation for altered mental state and placement of a splint on the left thigh for an obvious fracture of the femur. After administration of 40 mL/kg of normal saline, he had good perfusion. CT scan of the head showed multiple contusions to frontal lobes, with surrounding areas of edema. Patient had stable vital signs, reactive pupils bilaterally, and was combative. He was placed supine, with head of bed elevated to 30 degrees, and ventilated to maintain normal P_{CO_2}. Neurosurgery department was notified. Hyperventilation and mannitol were considered in the setting of impending herniation. Orthopedic surgery will be deferred until patient is more stable.

VII. **Teaching Pearl: Question.** What is the most common single injury associated with death in injured children?

VIII. **Teaching Pearl: Answer.** Head trauma, alone or in combination with other injuries, is responsible for 80% of trauma deaths. Over half of major injuries have associated injuries of chest, head, and musculoskeletal system. Children should be encouraged to wear protective helmets to reduce these preventable losses.

REFERENCES

Advanced Trauma Life Support Program for Doctors Student Manual, 6th ed. Committee on Trauma, American College of Surgeons, 1997.

Fleisher GR, Ludwig S. *Textbook of Pediatric Emergency Medicine,* 4th ed. Lippincott Williams & Wilkins, 2000.

Stafford PW, Blinman TA, Nance ML. Practical points in evaluation and resuscitation of the injured child. *Surg Clin North Am* 2002;82:273–301.

90. URINARY INCONTINENCE

I. **Problem.** A 4-year-old girl is brought to the pediatrician's office because of daytime and nighttime wetting.

II. **Immediate Questions**
   A. **Does patient have primary or secondary incontinence? Is this condition new or life-long?** Secondary incontinence is more likely to have an organic etiology.
   B. **Is there a history of UTIs (documented or treated)?** A child with a history of UTI is at increased risk for subsequent infections.
   C. **What are the associated symptoms?** Irritative bladder symptoms include dysuria, urgency, and voiding of small volumes. Systemic symptoms include fever, abdominal or flank pain, and vomiting.
   D. **Does patient have symptoms of voiding dysfunction?** These include urinary urgency, frequency, body posturing (avoidance maneuvers such as crossing of legs, holding genitalia, urgency dance, Vincent curtsy), and constipation.
   E. **How severe is incontinence?** Does wetting involve small amount of urine or soaking through?
   F. **What is the pattern of urination?** Does patient have intermittency of urination, short urination, or staccato voiding?
   G. **Pertinent Historical Information**
      1. **Social and developmental history.** Is there evidence of stressful social circumstances that could interfere with toilet training, such as physical or sexual abuse, arrival of new sibling, parental discord or separation, recent move?
      2. **Neurologic history.** Does patient have any difficulty walking or running? Problem with muscular development? Back pain?

III. **Differential Diagnosis**
   A. **Functional Causes**
      1. **Delayed toilet training or immature bladder.**
      2. **Voiding dysfunction.** Incoordination between bladder contractions and external sphincteric relaxation, producing detrusor instability (involuntary contractions).
      3. **Constipation.**
      4. **Infrequent voiding.**
   B. **Anatomic Causes**
      1. **Urinary structural anomalies**
         a. **Ectopic ureter.** Any ureter that ends outside normal trigone region of bladder; drainage may occur in distal urethra, introitus, vestibule, or vagina.
            i. Bilateral ectopic ureters can produce bladder neck incompetence, small bladder capacity, and gross urinary incontinence.

          ii. Ectopic ureters do not usually cause incontinence in boys.
- **b. Prolapsing ectopic ureterocele.**
- **c. Urogenital sinus anomalies.**
- **d. Epispadias.** Bifid clitoris.
- **e. Vaginal pooling.** Urine refluxes into vagina and causes postvoid dribbling.
- **f. Posterior urethral valves and detrusor hypertonicity or dysfunction in boys.**
2. Neurogenic bladder. Spinal cord anomalies.
- **a. Congenital.** Spinal dysraphism (myelomeningocele, cord lipoma, tethered cord).
- **b. Acquired.** Trauma, tumor.

IV. Database
A. Physical Exam Key Points
1. Abdomen. Assess for palpably distended bladder or palpable sigmoid colon (fecal impaction).
2. Genital exam. Assess for anomalies noted earlier, at III, B, 1.
- **a. Dermatitis.** Indicates severe wetting.
- **b. Introital anomalies**
  - **i. Single opening.** Urogenital sinus anomalies.
  - **ii. Prolapsing ureterocele.**
- **c. Ectopic ureter.** Urine pooling in vagina; suspect ectopic ureter rather than vaginal reflux.
3. Back. Look for lumbosacral skin abnormalities (café au lait spots, hemangiomas, fatty appearance, skin dimple or skin tag, tuft of hair, dermal vascular malformation, or subcutaneous lipomas).
4. Anus and rectum. Assess for constipation, fecal impaction, and anal tone.
B. Laboratory Data
1. Urinalysis and urine culture.
2. Voiding diary and defecation log. To include frequency and volume voided; episodes of incontinence.
C. Radiographic and Other Studies
1. Ultrasound of kidney and bladder. Ectopic ureter is evident by identification of duplication anomaly (upper pole hydronephrosis) and dilated ureter. Assess for bladder wall thickening.
2. Voiding cystourethrogram with KUB. To assess constipation and rule out ureteral reflux.
3. Uroflow study and postvoid residual. Basic study to evaluate flow rate and bladder emptying.
4. Urodynamic study. To evaluate functional status of bladder, identify detrusor instability, and assess bladder emptying.
5. Intravenous pyelogram, CT scan, magnetic resonance urogram, and DMSA scan. To evaluate GU anatomy and function.

6. **MRI scan of spine.** To exclude neurologic source of bladder dysfunction.

V. **Plan**
  A. **UTI.** Treat with appropriate antibiotics prior to any investigation (see Chapter 91, Urinary Tract Infections, p. 428).
  B. **Obtain Ultrasound, Voiding Diary, and KUB**
    1. In patients with hydronephrosis and upper pole anomaly, upper pole nephrectomy will cure incontinence.
    2. **Bladder wall thickening.** Consider voiding dysfunction; treatment strategies include:
       a. Encouragement of timed voiding.
       b. Bowel regimen, if constipation is present.
       c. Anticholinergic medication to treat uninhibited bladder contractions.

VI. **Problem Case Diagnosis.** The 4-year-old girl complained of urinary frequency and urgency in addition to wetting. Findings on physical exam were normal, and results of urinalysis and urine culture were negative. Urodynamic evaluation showed detrusor contractions during the filling phase. Diagnosis is detrusor instability with urge incontinence. (For further discussion, see VII and VIII, below.)

VII. **Teaching Pearl: Question.** What medications are used to treat detrusor instability and why?

VIII. **Teaching Pearl: Answer.** Oxybutynin and tolterodine are common anticholinergic medicines used to treated detrusor instability (ie, bladder hyperactivity, overactive bladder, unstable bladder). They work by decreasing detrusor hyperactivity and increasing the threshold volume at which unstable contractions occur, thereby enlarging functional capacity of bladder. These contractions cease as most children develop adult patterns of urinary control.

REFERENCES

Baskin LS, Kogan BA, Duckett JW. *Handbook of Pediatric Urology.* Lippincott-Raven, 1997.

Homsy YL, Austin PF. Dysfunctioning voiding disorders and nocturnal enuresis. In: Belman AB, King LR, Kramer SA, eds. *Clinical Pediatric Urology,* 4th ed. Saunders, 2001:345–370.

Koff SA, Jayanthi VR. Dysfunctional elimination syndromes of childhood. In: Walsh PC, Retik AB, Vaughn ED, Wein AJ, eds. *Campbell's Urology,* 8th ed. Elsevier, 2002:2262–2283.

91. URINARY TRACT INFECTIONS

I. **Problem.** A 6-month-old girl is hospitalized because of fever (temperature of 39°C [102.2°F]), along with decreased oral intake and activity. Findings on physical exam are noncontributory. Laboratory evaluation shows normal electrolytes and renal function. WBC count is 22,000, with 4% bands and 80% segmented WBCs. Results of urinalysis show 10–15 WBCs per high power field, positive leukocyte esterase test, and negative nitrite test.

II. Immediate Questions

A. What are the vital signs? Poor oral intake and fever may cause dehydration, especially in infants. In the preceding patient scenario, clinical suspicion centers on acute pyelonephritis, a condition that impairs renal concentrating ability, increasing patient's fluid losses. Infants up to 2 years of age are at risk of developing bacteremia because of UTIs. Although UTIs are believed to arise by the ascending route following entry of bacteria through the urethra, infants younger than 2 months of age may have UTI as a result of hematogenous spread.

B. Does patient have normal growth parameters? Failure to thrive may indicate presence of chronic condition in an infant suspected of acute pyelonephritis (eg, vesicoureteral reflux [VUR], chronic renal insufficiency).

C. Is there a past medical history of similar episodes? Recurrence of unexplained fever may indicate VUR or other urologic abnormalities causing recurrent episodes of pyelonephritis.

D. What is patient's voiding pattern? Ask about infrequent voiding, straining during urination, or urge incontinence. These symptoms may indicate presence of voiding dysfunction, which may cause UTIs or specific posturing (eg, leg crossing, squatting).

E. Pertinent Historical Information

  1. Inquire about oral intake, abdominal pain, odor and clarity of urine. Does patient have a past history of constipation? Constipation is associated with increased incidence of UTIs.

  2. If a girl, ask about use of bubble bath and manner of wiping genitalia after voiding. Back-to-front wiping may introduce bacteria into urinary tract and cause UTI.

  3. Is there a family history of UTIs or VUR? Approximately 35% of siblings of children with reflux have reflux as well; most are asymptomatic. Risk of a sibling having reflux is independent of severity of reflux or sex of index case. In addition, 50% of offspring of women with VUR have reflux.

III. Differential Diagnosis

A. UTI. Suggested by fever with pyuria. Three basic forms of UTI are cystitis, pyelonephritis, and asymptomatic bacteriuria.

  1. Cystitis. Occurs when bladder is infected; patient presents with dysuria, urgency, frequency, suprapubic pain, and malodorous urine. Some children develop enuresis. Cystitis does not cause fever or result in renal injury.

  2. Pyelonephritis. Occurs when infection involves renal parenchyma. Symptoms include all or any of the following: flank or abdominal pain, nausea, vomiting, diarrhea, and fever. Infants may present with nonspecific symptoms such as jaundice, poor feeding, irritability, lethargy, and weight loss.

3. **Asymptomatic bacteriuria.** Refers to repeat positive urine cultures found in asymptomatic individuals during routine checkup or investigation. Condition is benign and does not cause renal scarring.

B. **Chemical Irritation** (eg, dysuria secondary to bubble bath use).

C. **Vaginitis** (see Chapter 93, Vaginal Discharge, p. 433).

D. **Interstitial Nephritis.** Idiopathic urgency, dysuria, and frequency; bladder of pelvic pain; symptoms relieved by voiding, but without evidence of UTI.

IV. **Database**
A. **Physical Exam Key Points**
1. **Hydration status.** Check for signs of dehydration, including hypotension, loss of skin turgor, depressed anterior fontanel, lack of tears, and prolonged capillary refill time. In patients with fever, tachycardia may occur in the absence of dehydration. Children with pyelonephritis continue to have urine output and wet diapers in the presence of dehydration due to loss of renal concentrating ability.

2. **Abdomen.** Palpate for enlarged kidney(s) (eg, hydronephrosis), distended bladder (eg, posterior urethral valves), and distended bowel due to constipation.

3. **Back and spine.** Inspect for signs of spinal abnormalities, including lipoma, telangiectasia, abnormal pigmentation, spinal dimple, hair patch, gluteal asymmetry, and abnormal gluteal cleft. Inspect spine for curvature (eg, scoliosis), presence of sacrum, and completeness of vertebrae.

4. **Genitalia.** In girls, inspect for separation of urethral opening from vaginal opening, labial adhesions, and epispadias (bifid clitoris). In boys, visualize urethral meatus by gently retracting foreskin in uncircumcised children.

5. **Neurologic exam.** Should include assessment of anocutaneous and bulbocavernous reflexes, gait, muscle mass, and deep tendon reflexes of lower extremities to eliminate spinal dysraphism.

B. **Laboratory Data**
1. **Urine culture.** The gold standard for diagnosis of UTI (Table I–27). Urine specimens may be obtained by suprapubic bladder aspiration, urethral catheterization, or voided midstream technique in toilet-trained child. Cleansing of urethral meatus before collecting urine sample does not have significant effect on rate of urine specimen contamination. Applying adhesive-sealed sterile urine collection bag after cleansing skin of genitals in infants can be helpful, if urine culture is negative. However, this technique has a high rate of false-positive cultures because of contamination by periurethral

TABLE I–27. CRITERIA FOR DIAGNOSIS OF URINARY TRACT INFECTIONS

Method of Collection	Colony Count (pure culture)	Probability of Infection (%)
Suprapubic aspiration	Gram-negative bacilli: any number	>99
	Gram-positive cocci: > few thousand	>99
Catheterization	>10^5 CFU/mL	95
	10^4–10^5 CFU/mL	Infection likely
	10^3–10^4 CFU/mL	Suspicious; repeat
	<10^3 CFU/mL	Infection unlikely
Clean-voided		
Boy	>10^4 CFU/mL	Infection likely
Girl	3 specimens: > 10^5 CFU/mL	95
	2 specimens: > 10^5 CFU/mL	90
	1 specimen: > 10^5 CFU/mL	80
	5×10^4 to 10^5 CFU/mL	Suspicious; repeat
	10^4 to 5×10^4 CFU/mL	Symptomatic; suspicious; repeat
	10^4 to 5×10^4 CFU/mL	Asymptomatic; infection unlikely
	<10^4 CFU/mL	Infection unlikely

CFU = colony-forming units.

flora, especially in girls and uncircumcised boys. Urine sample should be processed immediately. If that is not possible, refrigerate specimen at 4°C (34.6°F) and process within 24 hours. Most common isolated pathogen is *Escherichia coli. Pseudomonas* spp, *Klebsiella* spp, *Enterobacter* spp, *Enterococci, Proteus mirabilis,* and staphylococci may be isolated.

2. **Urinalysis.** Findings on urinalysis are suggestive but not diagnostic of UTI. Pyuria suggests infection; however, UTI may occur in the absence of pyuria. Nitrites and leukocyte esterase are usually positive in infected urine. However, presence of nitrite is dependent on capacity of bacteria to convert nitrate to nitrite. Hence, it is not observed in UTIs due to *Pseudomonas* or gram-positive organisms (eg, *Staphylococcus*). Often hematuria is present in cystitis. Specific gravity may be falsely low in upper tract infections because of loss of concentrating ability.

3. **Blood cultures.** Consider, especially in infants, suspected pyelonephritis, and ill-appearing children.

4. **CBC.** Often demonstrates leukocytosis.

5. **ESR and C-reactive protein.** Elevated in pyelonephritis.

6. **BUN and creatinine.** To assess renal function.

7. **Serum electrolytes.** To assess for hyponatremia, hyperkalemia, and metabolic acidosis (abnormalities often seen in

patients with dehydration or renal insufficiency). Transient hyperkalemic renal tubular acidosis has been reported in patients with pyelonephritis.

C. Radiographic and Other Studies. Goal of imaging studies in children with UTI is to identify anatomic abnormalities. One third of white girls evaluated after documented UTI have VUR, and 10–30% have evidence of cortical filling defects on renal scans. Imaging is indicated in all children with suspected pyelonephritis (febrile UTI), all boys irrespective of presence or absence of fever, all girls 5 years or younger with cystitis, and school-age girls with two or more UTIs.

1. **Renal ultrasound.** Should be obtained to define renal size and structure, and to detect dilation (eg, hydronephrosis). Ultrasound may show focal or generalized enlargement of the pyelonephritic kidney in 30–60% of the cases. Small kidney may indicate renal scarring or chronic infection; however, test cannot detect small scars or VUR. Test can be ordered during the acute phase of infection.

2. **Voiding cystourethrogram (VCUG).** To define presence of VUR and its grade, as well as obstruction. Timing of VCUG is controversial. Some centers delay test for 2–6 weeks to allow inflammation in bladder to resolve. However, this delay does not change incidence of VUR; therefore, some centers recommend performing test before discharge from hospital. Contrast VCUG is indicated in all boys with UTI. It defines anatomy of bladder and urethra and permits grading of VUR. If available, radionuclide VCUG can be used in girls, but it does not provide anatomic definition of bladder or accurately define VUR grade.

3. **Technetium-labeled DMSA or glucoheptonate renal scan.** Useful when diagnosis of acute pyelonephritis is uncertain. Presence of photopenic area indicates acute pyelonephritis or cortical scar due to previous episode of infection.

V. Plan

A. Goals of Management

1. Identify concomitant bacteremia or meningitis, especially in children younger than 2 months of age.

2. Prevent renal scars by eradicating pathogen early (delay in treatment is associated with development of renal scars, which if recurrent, may result in chronic renal failure or hypertension, or both).

3. Relieve symptoms related to infection.

B. In-Patient Management

1. Consider hospitalization in children who are systemically ill, vomiting, and those younger than 2 years of age, who may have a high risk of bacteremia. Children who are not ill and can tolerate oral fluids and antibiotics can be treated as outpatients, provided there is adequate follow-up.

   2. Hydration. Provide maintenance IV fluid; rehydrate as necessary.
   3. Antibiotic therapy. In hospitalized patients, parenteral admin-
      istration of ceftriaxone, 50–75 mg/kg/24 h (not to exceed 2 g)
      or ampicillin, 100 mg/kg/day, with an aminoglycoside such as
      gentamicin, 3–5 mg/kg/day, is recommended. Adjust antibiotic
      regimen once sensitivity panel of pathogen is available.
      Continue parenteral treatment until defervescence occurs.
      Appropriate oral antibiotic can be started and continued for a
      total course of 10–14 days.
   C. Outpatient Management. For patients who can be managed as out-
      patients, a third-generation cephalosporin may be used. Cefdinir,
      14 mg/kg/day (maximum 600 mg/day), or cefixime, 8 mg/kg/day
      (maximum 300 mg/day) are recommended. Trimethoprim-
      sulfamethoxazole (TMP-SMX), 8 mg trimethoprim/kg/day admin-
      istered twice daily, may be used. However, 30% of pathogens are
      resistant to TMP-SMX.
   D. Follow-up. Obtain follow-up urine culture during or immediately
      after treatment.
   E. Prophylaxis. Indicated in patients who have VUR. If VCUG is per-
      formed 2–6 weeks after episode of UTI, patient should be placed
      on prophylaxis until result of test is available. TMP-SMX or
      trimethoprim, 1–2 mg/kg/day, is recommended in children older
      than 2 months of age. For infants younger than 2 months of age,
      amoxicillin, 15 mg/kg/day, may be used.

VI. Problem Case Diagnosis. The 6-month old girl was diagnosed with
   acute pyelonephritis. Urine culture obtained by urethral catheterization grew *E coli*, sensitive to ceftriaxone and TMP-SMX. Patient was
   treated with IV ceftriaxone for 3 days, followed by a course of oral TMP-
   SMX for 7 more days. Prophylaxis with TMP-SMX was prescribed until
   results of VCUG became available. Prophylaxis was continued
   because of presence of VUR.

VII. Teaching Pearl: Question. In the patient scenario described earlier,
   what would explain the negative nitrite test on urinalysis, despite
   urine culture that grew *E coli* (an organism capable of converting
   nitrate to nitrite)?

VIII. Teaching Pearl: Answer. To test positive for nitrite, urine needs
   to dwell in the bladder for at least 4 hours. Because infants void
   constantly, the nitrite test is often negative in this age group.

REFERENCES

Elder J. Urinary tract infections. In: Behrman RE, Kliegman RM, Jenson HB, eds.
   Nelson Textbook of Pediatrics, 17th ed. Saunders, 2004:1785–1790.
Hansson S, Jodal U. Urinary tract infection. In: Avner ED, Harmon WE, Niaudet P,
   eds. *Pediatric Nephrology.* Lippincott Williams & Wilkins, 2004:1007–1026.
Mahant S, To T, Friedman J. Timing of voiding cystourethrogram in the investigation
   of urinary tract infections in children. *J Pediatr* 2001;139:568–571.

Schlager TA. Urinary tract infections in infants and children. *Infect Dis Clin North Am* 2003;17:353–365.

92. VAGINAL BLEEDING

I. **Problem.** A 14-year-old girl comes to the pediatric clinic because of vaginal bleeding.

II. **Immediate Questions**

A. **What is patient's menstrual history?** Has patient had a previous menstrual period? If so, when was the last period? Obtain menstrual history, including usual period interval and duration. This information is critical to assess current episode of bleeding.

B. **How much bleeding has occurred?** Quantifying amount of blood loss may be difficult. Changing pad or tampon more than once per hour, for several hours in a row, or bleeding for more than 8 days constitutes hypermenorrhea.

C. **Does patient have pain?** Identifying presence, timing, location, and intensity of pain aids in determining cause of bleeding.

D. **What is patient's sexual and contraceptive history?** Sexual activity, especially recent, has an immediate impact on possible causes of vaginal bleeding. Use of contraceptives, in particular condoms and hormonal contraceptives, is a factor in patient's risk of pregnancy and STDs.

E. **Does patient have other health problems or currently take medication?** Systemic illnesses (eg, thyroid disease or diabetes) may influence bleeding patterns; emotional stress or acute illness can also affect bleeding pattern.

III. **Differential Diagnosis**

A. **Normal Menstrual Period.** The most likely cause of vaginal bleeding. During first 2 years after menarche, periods may be normal even without precise pattern.

B. **Pregnancy-Related Bleeding**

1. **Implantation.** May produce bleeding that manifests at time of expected menses, but bleeding pattern and duration may be lighter and shorter.

2. **Threatened or spontaneous abortion.** Produces vaginal bleeding ranging from light spotting to heavy flow with clots and tissue. Cramping may be associated with this process.

3. **Ectopic pregnancy.** May produce irregular bleeding associated with abdominal pain that varies in severity from mild cramping to acute abdomen.

4. **Retained placental tissue.** May cause bleeding for many weeks after spontaneous or therapeutic abortion or after a delivery, or recur at a later time.

C. **Hormonal Causes of Irregular Bleeding**

1. **Polycystic ovarian syndrome.** Associated symptoms include androgen excess, obesity, and insulin resistance.

2. **Adrenal androgen excess.** Consider atypical congenital adrenal hyperplasia.
3. **Endocrinopathies.** Hypothyroidism or hyperprolactinemias may cause irregular bleeding. Elevated prolactin more commonly causes amenorrhea.
4. **Medications.** Hormonal contraceptives may cause breakthrough bleeding.
5. **Dysfunctional uterine bleeding.** Hormonal bleeding with no obvious explanation.

D. **Infection.** Includes vulvovaginitis, cervicitis, and pelvic inflammatory disease.
E. **Pelvic Trauma.** May cause bleeding. With penetrating-type trauma, surgical evaluation may be necessary.
F. **Anatomic Abnormalities of Uterus and Vagina.** May be associated with irregular bleeding.
G. **Neoplasms of Genital Tract.** Both benign and malignant.
H. **Coagulopathies.** May present with abnormal vaginal bleeding. Menometrorrhagia at menarche, in particular, should prompt evaluation for a bleeding disorder.

IV. **Database**
A. **Physical Exam Key Points**
1. **Vital signs.** BP and pulse may be markers for profuse blood loss. Elevated temperature may indicate infection. Body mass index indicates degree of obesity.
2. **General appearance.** Examine body habitus, skin, and hair for signs of endocrinopathies. Bruising may be indicative of trauma or of bleeding diathesis.
3. **Abdomen.** Examine for masses and tenderness. Mass may be indicative of pregnancy or tumor. Pattern, location, and intensity of discomfort may be helpful in diagnosing infections or ectopic pregnancy.
4. **Pelvic exam**
   a. Look first at vulva for any signs of lesions or infections.
   b. Inspect vagina for quantity of blood in vault and any lesions.
   c. Evaluate cervix for tenderness, dilation, presence of tissue at os, or other lesions.
   d. Palpate fundus and ovaries bimanually for size and tenderness.

B. **Laboratory Data**
1. **Pregnancy test.** HCG in urine or serum.
2. **CBC with differential.** Important guide to amount of blood loss and possible infection. Low platelet count may indicate bleeding problem.
3. **PT and PTT.** To evaluate coagulopathy.
4. ***Chlamydia* and gonorrhea tests.** Perform in all sexually active patients. Obtain other cultures if indicated.

    5. **Pap test.** May not be possible if bleeding is present.
    6. **Other workup.** As indicated by physical exam (eg, testosterone, DHEAS, thyroid-stimulating hormone, luteinizing hormone, or follicle-stimulating hormone).
  C. **Radiographic and Other Studies.** Pelvic ultrasound is primary means of observing anatomy directly. In the presence of positive pregnancy test, ultrasound may identify intrauterine or ectopic pregnancy. Also helpful in suggesting pelvic inflammatory disease or identifying a pelvic mass.

V. **Plan**
  A. **Normal Menstrual Period.** If most likely explanation, no further workup is needed.
  B. **Pregnancy.** If pregnant and stable, refer routinely to obstetrician. If unstable or if ectopic pregnancy is suspected, refer emergently.
  C. **Pathologic Etiology**
    1. **Sex hormone imbalances.** May best be treated with birth control pills.
    2. **Systemic illnesses or isolated endocrinopathies.** Treat appropriately (eg, thyroid disease and diabetes mellitus).
    3. **Infections.** Treat with appropriate antibiotics (see Chapter 93, Vaginal Discharge, p. 434).
  D. **Marked Blood Loss.** Iron supplementation or transfusion may be necessary.
  E. **Patient Education.** Provide information about normal menstrual pattern in adolescence, and prevention of pregnancy and STDs.

VI. **Problem Case Diagnosis.** The 14-year-old girl is experiencing normal first menses. Physical exam findings are normal. Patient began to develop breast buds about $1^{1}/_{2}$ years ago and is now Tanner stage III.

VII. **Teaching Pearl: Question.** When does menarche usually occur?

VIII. **Teaching Pearl: Answer.** Menarche occurs 18–24 months after appearance of secondary sexual characteristics. Normal age for onset of first menses is as early as $9^{1}/_{2}$ but no later than 16 years of age.

REFERENCES

Breech LL, Carpenter SE. Management quandary. Persistent vaginal bleeding at menarche. *J Pediatr Adolesc Gynecol* 2002;12:53–55.

Levine LJ, Catallozzi M, Schwarz DF. An adolescent with vaginal bleeding. *Pediatr Case Rev* 2003;3:83–90.

Merritt DF. Evaluation of vaginal bleeding in the preadolescent child. *Semin Pediatr Surg* 1998;7:35–42.

Pfeifer SM. Management quandary. Vaginal bleeding and abdominal pain. J *Pediatr Adolesc Gynecol* 2002;15:53–55.

93. VAGINAL DISCHARGE

I. **Problem.** A 5-year-old girl presents with vaginal discharge.

II. **Immediate Questions**
   A. **What color is discharge?**
      1. **Clear to white.** Generally does not represent infection; may be normal, especially as child approaches puberty. Urine may be mistaken for vaginal secretions.
      2. **Yellow.** Indicates infection or inflammation from irritants.
      3. **Green to gray.** Indicates infection.
      4. **Blood tinged or bloody.** Indicates infection, tumor, or trauma. Any bloody discharge in prepubertal girl requires full evaluation to identify cause; may require referral to gynecologist and examination under anesthesia.
   B. **How long has discharge been present?** Chronic discharge may be associated with irritants such as soap, bubble baths, or fabric softeners.
   C. **Does patient have any other genital tract symptoms?**
      1. **Itching.** Consider *Candida.*
      2. **Pain.** May be associated with chronicity or acute trauma.
      3. **Odor.** Consider bacterial infection or foreign bodies.
   D. **Any other non–genital tract symptoms?** Diarrhea may cause breakdown in vaginal hygiene. Dysuria is associated with UTIs. Systemic dermatologic disease may affect inflammation of skin of vulvovaginal area. Bruising or petechiae are signs of trauma or coagulopathy.
   E. **Recurrent problem?** If similar incident has occurred before, its previous course and treatment can be directive. In particular, successful or unsuccessful treatment may guide intervention.
   F. **Is there a history of recent acute or chronic illness?** Illness that occurs simultaneously with, or just prior to, discharge may be related or even etiologic.
   G. **Any trauma?** Trauma includes vaginal or pelvic injury, masturbation, and sexual abuse.

III. **Differential Diagnosis**
   A. **Normal.** Clear, otherwise nonsymptomatic discharge is nonpathologic.
   B. **Irritants.** Includes soaps and bubble bath, laundry detergents or fabric softeners, sand, and tight clothing.
   C. **Infection**
      1. **Bacteria.** Most commonly group A β-hemolytic streptococci, *Staphylococcus aureus,* and *Escherichia coli.*
      2. **Fungi.** Primarily *Candida albicans.*
      3. **Parasites** (eg, pinworms).
      4. **STDs.**
      5. Systemic infections, such as Epstein-Barr virus (mononucleosis).

   D. Foreign Body in Vagina. May cause discharge, irritation, and infection. Discharge may be any color. Nature of foreign body and length of time it has been in vagina influences color. The most common foreign bodies are paper products (eg, toilet tissue).
   E. Dermatologic Diseases. May manifest with vulvovaginal irritation and discharge (eg, eczema, psoriasis, atopic dermatitis, lichen sclerosis).
   F. Neoplasms. Rare cause, but tumors such as sarcoma botryoides should be considered, especially with bloody discharge.

IV. Database
A. Physical Exam Key Points
   1. **Vital signs.** Fever may be indicative of systemic infection. Obesity is associated with intertriginous irritation.
   2. **Skin.** Observe for signs of systemic dermatologic illnesses, allergic reactions, or viral illnesses.
   3. **Abdomen.** Palpate for tenderness or masses. Mass in lower abdomen may indicate pelvic tumor. Tenderness may be present with infections.
   4. **Pelvic exam**
      a. Observe vulva for lesions, erythema, and tenderness.
      b. Examine vagina and obtain sample of discharge for wet mount and laboratory assessment.
      c. Perform rectoabdominal exam if foreign body is suspected. Paper products are rarely palpable.
      d. Intravaginal exam is rarely necessary at first visit.
B. Laboratory Data
   1. **Wet mount evaluation.**
   2. **Cultures.** If bacterial infection or STD is suspected.
   3. **Urinalysis and urine culture.** If indicated.
   4. **CBC with differential.** To check for leukocytosis.
C. Radiographic and Other Studies
   1. **Flat plate of lower abdomen.** May show radiopaque foreign body.
   2. **Pelvic ultrasound.** Helpful if pelvic or abdominal mass is suspected.
   3. **Examination under anesthesia.** May be necessary if adequate examination of child is otherwise not possible. Especially true when bloody discharge is present or foreign body must be removed.

V. Plan
A. Nonpathologic Discharge.
   Provide education and support to patient and caregivers.
B. Irritant or Allergen
   1. Remove source.
   2. Encourage sitz baths followed by air drying (consider using a blow dryer for the latter).

3. Topical steroid cream or ointment (1% hydrocortisone cream if condition is mild; triamcinolone cream or ointment if moderate or severe).
4. Topical estrogen cream for labial adhesions and thinning of vaginal mucosa. Instruct patient to apply fingertip-full nightly for 2 weeks.
5. Topical emollients.

C. **Infection.** Treat according to diagnosis as well as with local care, described earlier.

1. **Candidiasis.** Usually responds to topical antifungal agents (betaconazole, miconazole, terconazole), or to oral fluconazole, 96 mg/kg in one dose to maximum of 150 mg.
2. **Coliform bacteria.** Give amoxicillin, 40 mg/kg/day, to maximum of 500 mg twice daily.
3. **β-Hemolytic group A streptococci.** Usually respond to preceding regimen. In patients with penicillin allergy, use trimethoprim-sulfamethoxazole, azithromycin, or ciprofloxacin.
4. **Pinworms.** Administer mebendazole, 100 mg one time orally.
5. **STDs.** Sexual abuse may lead to trichomonas, chlamydia, gonorrhea, syphilis, herpes simplex I and II, and human papillomavirus infections.

   a. Report any suspicion of sexual abuse to local authorities immediately (see Chapter 15, Child Abuse: Sexual, p. 78).
   b. *Chlamydia*
      i. **For children > 45 kg.** Give azithromycin, 1000 mg PO in a single dose, or doxycycline, 100 mg PO twice daily for 7 days (if child is older than 8 years of age).
      ii. **For children < 45 kg.** Give erythromycin, 50 mg/kg/day four times daily for 14 days.
   c. **Gonorrhea.** Give ceftriaxone, 125 mg IM, or ciprofloxacin, 10 mg/kg PO in single dose. Unless known that child does not have chlamydial infection, give treatment for *Chlamydia* at same time.

D. **Dermatologic Disease.** Treat as per systemic diagnosis.
E. **Foreign Body.** Any foreign body must be removed. An attempt may be made to flush out foreign body with saline, but consider referral.

VI. **Problem Case Diagnosis.** The 5-year-old girl has had yellow vaginal discharge for several weeks. Mother has tried sitz baths without improvement in symptoms. Child had previously been referred to pediatric gynecologist for removal of foreign body. Referral is again indicated.

VII. **Teaching Pearl: Question.** Is candidal vulvovaginitis commonly seen in prepubertal girls?

VIII. **Teaching Pearl: Answer.** Vulvovaginitis due to *Candida* is unusual in prepubertal girls because pH of vaginal secretions is less acidic before than after puberty. Usually such infection is seen only with a predisposing condition (eg, diabetes mellitus) or prior use of systemic antibiotics.

REFERENCES

Emans SJ, Laufer MR, Goldstein DP. *Pediatric and Adolescent Gynecology,* 4th ed. Lippincott-Raven, 1998.
Sanfilippo JS, Muram D, Dewhurst J, Lee P. *Pediatric and Adolescent Gynecology,* 2nd ed. Saunders, 2001.
Workowski KA, Levine WC. Sexually transmitted disease treatment guidelines, 2002. *MMWR Morb Mortal Wkly Rep* 2002;51:RR-6.

94. VOMITING

   I. **Problem.** A 10-year-old girl has had vomiting, diarrhea, and fever for 3 days.

  II. **Immediate Questions**
     A. How old is patient? Diagnostic possibilities should be stratified by child's age, although certain etiologies may be seen in more than one age group (Table I–28).
     B. Is a serious or life-threatening cause of vomiting likely? This decision must be made early in evaluation. Life-threatening causes of vomiting are listed in Table I–29.

TABLE I–28. COMMON CAUSES OF VOMITING IN CHILDREN

Birth to 2 Months	2 Months to 5 Years	6 Years and Older
Allergic colitis	Brain tumor	Adhesions
Anatomic abnormalities of GI tract	Diabetic ketoacidosis	Appendicitis
Gastroesophageal reflux	Foreign body	Cholecystitis
Increased intracranial pressure	Gastroenteritis	Diabetic ketoacidosis
Malrotation with volvulus	Gastroesophageal reflux	Gastroenteritis
Meconium ileus	Head trauma	Head trauma
Necrotizing enterocolitis	Incarcerated hernia	Hepatitis
Overfeeding	Intussusception	Inflammatory bowel disease
Pyloric stenosis	Posttussive	Intoxication
	Pyelonephritis	Migraine headache
		Ovarian torsion
		Pancreatitis
		Peptic ulcer disease
		Posttussive
		Pregnancy
		Pyelonephritis

TABLE I–29. LIFE-THREATENING CAUSES OF VOMITING

Appendicitis with perforated bowel
Diabetic ketoacidosis
Gastroenteritis with hypovolemic shock
GI obstruction
Head trauma with cerebral edema or intracranial hemorrhage
Incarcerated hernia with bowel ischemia
Intoxication
Intussusception with bowel ischemia
Necrotizing enterocolitis
Peritonitis

C. **Is there evidence of GI tract obstruction?** Such evidence includes abdominal pain and distention, bilious emesis, and constipation.
D. **Is there evidence of non-GI tract etiologies?** Most causes of vomiting are associated with abdominal pain; lack of abdominal pain suggests an etiology outside the GI tract. History of headaches, confusion, or diplopia suggests neurologic causes (eg, brain tumor or intracranial hemorrhage). Renal causes might be associated with flank pain, dysuria, or frequency. Adrenal insufficiency, which may be associated with malaise, anorexia, and weight loss, is an uncommon cause of vomiting.
E. **What does vomited material look like?** Mallory-Weiss tear is a common cause of hematemesis, although more serious etiologies (peptic ulcer disease, esophageal varices) must be pursued if large volume of blood is present. Vomiting of undigested food is consistent with pyloric stenosis, gastroenteritis, or gastroesophageal reflux. Yellow or green-tinged emesis may represent gastric acid but also raises concern for intestinal obstruction.

III. **Differential Diagnosis.** An age-based discussion of causes of vomiting in children follows. Conditions that occur in more than one age group are listed for the group in which they would most commonly appear.
   A. **Birth to 2 Months**
      1. **Allergic colitis.** Allergy to cow's milk or soybean-based formulas. Marked by diarrhea, bleeding from rectum, and fussiness.
      2. **Anatomic abnormalities of GI tract.** Congenital anomalies, including stenosis or atresia. Manifests as feeding intolerance in first days of life.
      3. **Gastroesophageal reflux.** Frequent regurgitation of undigested milk soon after feeding. Very common in neonates; clinically important only if condition causes failure to thrive, apnea, or bronchospasm.
      4. **Increased intracranial pressure.** Fussiness or lethargy in absence of abdominal tenderness. Consider birth trauma and shaken baby syndrome.

5. **Malrotation with volvulus.** Eighty percent of cases present in first month of life; most have bilious emesis. Hematochezia suggests bowel necrosis.

6. **Meconium ileus.** Inspissated meconium in distal colon; consider diagnosis of cystic fibrosis.

7. **Necrotizing enterocolitis.** Occurs almost exclusively in premature infants, especially if hypoxic at birth. Presents with irritability or lethargy, distended abdomen, hematochezia.

8. **Overfeeding.** Regurgitation of undigested milk soon after feeding; frequent "wet-burps" in an overweight infant who is given too much volume per feed.

9. **Pyloric stenosis.** Peaks at 3–6 weeks of life. Male-to-female ratio is 5:1, and condition is more common in first-born males. Manifests as progressively worsening, projectile, nonbilious emesis.

B. **2 Months to 5 Years**
1. **Brain tumor.** Consider especially if progressive headaches, vomiting, ataxia, and no abdominal pain.

2. **Diabetic ketoacidosis.** Moderate to severe dehydration; recent history of polydipsia, polyuria, and polyphagia.

3. **Foreign body.** Associated choking episode or abrupt onset of coughing spasm or drooling. Child with an esophageal foreign body may appear to be well.

4. **Gastroenteritis.** Very common; history of sick contacts is common; often associated with diarrhea and fever.

5. **Head trauma.** Inflicted or accidental. Frequent or progressive emesis suggests concussion or intracranial hemorrhage.

6. **Incarcerated hernia.** Abrupt onset of crying, anorexia, and scrotal swelling.

7. **Intussusception.** Peaks at 6–18 months of life; produces spasms of abdominal pain alternating with listlessness. Patient is less likely to have diarrhea or fever than child who has gastroenteritis.

8. **Posttussive.** Frequently, young children will vomit after forceful or repetitive coughing.

9. **Pyelonephritis.** High fever, ill appearance, dysuria or frequency. Patient may have history of prior UTIs.

C. **Age 6 Years and Older**
1. **Adhesions.** Especially after abdominal surgery or peritonitis.

2. **Appendicitis.** Variable clinical presentation and location of pain. Common symptoms include progressively worsening pain that migrates to right lower quadrant, pain preceding vomiting, anorexia, low-grade fever, constipation.

3. **Cholecystitis.** More common in girls, especially with hemolytic disease (eg, sickle cell anemia). Abrupt epigastric or right upper quadrant pain occurs soon after a meal.

4. **Hepatitis.** Especially viral or drug-induced; patient may have history of clay-colored stools or dark urine.

5. **Inflammatory bowel disease.** Associated with diarrhea, hematochezia, abdominal pain. Strictures may cause obstruction.

6. **Intoxication.** More common in toddlers and adolescents. Suspect if history of depression. May present with altered mental status.

7. **Migraine headache.** Severe, incapacitating headache; often preceded by aura, such as scotoma. Patient may have past history of chronic headaches or family history of migraines.

8. **Ovarian torsion.** Abrupt, severe, unilateral, low abdominal or pelvic pain in an adolescent girl.

9. **Pancreatitis.** Risk factors include upper abdominal trauma, recent or concurrent infections, corticosteroid use, alcohol, and cholelithiasis.

10. **Peptic ulcer disease.** Among teenagers, has a 4:1 male-to-female ratio. Chronic or recurrent epigastric pain, often worse at night.

11. **Pregnancy.** Usually in first trimester; recent history of amenorrhea.

IV. Database
A. Physical Exam Key Points

1. **General appearance and vital signs.** Assess to determine degree of dehydration and whether immediately life-threatening or surgical condition exists. Altered mental status raises concern for head injury, intussusception, intoxication, or shock. Somnolence, tachycardia, tachypnea, and orthostatic hypotension suggest shock associated with bowel perforation, diabetic ketoacidosis, or severe gastroenteritis. Stupor, bradycardia, irregular respirations, and hypertension suggest raised intracranial pressure. Fever, of course, indicates infectious etiologies such as gastroenteritis or pyelonephritis.

2. **Abdomen.** Distention suggests obstruction or ileus. Hypoactive bowel sounds are consistent with ileus; hyperactive bowel sounds suggest gastroenteritis. Presence of abdominal tenderness elicited by examiner and its specific location provide important diagnostic clues, as outlined in Table I–30. Signs of peritonitis include increased pain with movement, rebound tenderness, involuntary guarding, and, for child with appendicitis, Rovsing sign (tenderness on right with palpation on left).

3. **Rectal exam.** Performed selectively, but indicated if patient has history of hematochezia or melena or abdominal tenderness on exam. Assess for gross blood, hard stool, or mass.

4. **Neurologic exam.** Perform comprehensive exam to assess for one of several neurologic causes of vomiting.

5. **Suggestive findings.** Certain physical exam findings may be highly suggestive of a specific diagnosis; refer to Table I–31.

TABLE I–30. ETIOLOGIES OF VOMITING AND LOCATION OF ABDOMINAL PAIN OR TENDERNESS

Clinical Condition	Usual Location of Pain or Tenderness
Appendicitis	Right lower quadrant, but is variable
Cholecystitis	Right upper quadrant; also epigastric
Gastroenteritis	Diffuse or periumbilical; often pain without tenderness
Hepatitis	Right upper quadrant
Intussusception	Diffuse; right upper quadrant mass may be palpated
Ovarian torsion	Unilateral lower abdominal or pelvic
Pancreatitis	Epigastric; also back and upper quadrants
Peptic ulcer disease	Diffuse or epigastric
Pyelonephritis	Flank

B. Laboratory Data. Laboratory testing should be guided by patient's history and physical exam findings. Tests that may be helpful include CBC with differential, electrolytes, BUN and creatinine, liver function tests, amylase and lipase, qualitative human chorionic gonadotropin (HCG) in urine, urinalysis, and urine culture.

TABLE I–31. PHYSICAL EXAM FINDINGS SUGGESTIVE OF SPECIFIC DIAGNOSES

Finding	Suggested Diagnosis
Olive-shaped mass just to right of midline in upper quadrant of young infant	Pyloric stenosis
Currant jelly stool on rectal exam	Intussusception
Hard, impacted stool on rectal exam of neonate	Meconium ileus
Swollen, red, tender hemiscrotum	Incarcerated hernia
Characteristic clinical features of drug overdose (toxidrome); see Chapter 74, Poisoning and Overdoses, p. 338	Intoxication
Right lower quadrant tenderness with signs of peritonitis	Appendicitis
Psoas sign (abdominal pain with hip flexion against examiner's hand)	Appendicitis
Obturator sign (abdominal pain with internal rotation of hip)	Appendicitis
Flank tenderness	Pyelonephritis
Kussmaul respirations, ketotic breath, severe dehydration	Diabetic ketoacidosis
Murphy sign (pain with inspiration when examiner palpates deeply in right upper quadrant)	Cholecystitis
Icteric sclera, jaundice, right upper quadrant tenderness, hepatomegaly	Hepatitis
Papilledema	Reflects increased intracranial pressure, one of neurologic causes of vomiting

TABLE I–32. ABDOMINAL RADIOGRAPHIC FINDINGS FOR SPECIFIC DISEASES

Diagnosis	KUB Findings
Appendicitis	Fecalith, localized right lower quadrant ileus, scoliosis concave to right, blurred psoas margins
Cholecystitis	Right upper quadrant calcifications
Foreign body	Opaque esophageal foreign body
Intussusception	Signs of obstruction (see below), right-sided soft tissue mass, paucity of air on right
Malrotation with volvulus	Signs of obstruction (see below); double-bubble: distended stomach and duodenum
Necrotizing enterocolitis	Pneumatosis intestinalis (air within intestinal wall)
Obstruction[a]	Air-fluid levels, dilated loops, paucity of gas distally
Pyloric stenosis	Distended stomach

[a] Includes anatomic abnormalities, meconium ileus, intussusception, adhesions, inflammatory bowel disease.

C. Radiographic and Other Studies

1. **Plain abdominal x-rays.** If obstruction is a concern, order supine and upright or left-lateral decubitus film. If patient may be pregnant, defer KUB until result of HCG test is known. Table I–32 lists radiographic findings that may be seen with certain diseases. In many cases, these findings are helpful or even pathognomonic if present; their absence does not preclude the diagnosis.

2. **Abdominal ultrasound.** Very helpful in establishing diagnosis of pyloric stenosis, intussusception, cholecystitis, or pancreatitis; not as sensitive as CT scan for appendicitis.

3. **Barium or air contrast enema.** Both diagnostic and therapeutic for intussusception.

4. **Upper GI series.** Very helpful in establishing diagnosis of anatomic abnormalities of GI tract (eg, malrotation with volvulus) or gastroesophageal reflux.

5. **Endoscopy.** Very helpful in establishing diagnosis of peptic ulcer disease or inflammatory bowel disease.

6. **Abdominal CT scan.** Study of choice for patient suspected of having appendicitis, with equivocal clinical findings; also useful for abdominal trauma, masses, perforation, and abscesses.

V. Plan.

Differential diagnosis should be focused simply by knowing age of patient. Many conditions such as pyloric stenosis or intussusception appear primarily among children within a narrow age range. Initial history and physical exam must be aimed at identifying serious causes of vomiting. Laboratory data and radiographic studies should serve only to confirm diagnoses that are strongly suspected on clinical grounds.

A. Causes of Vomiting That May Require Emergency Surgery.

These include anatomic abnormalities of GI tract (eg, malrotation with volvulus), necrotizing enterocolitis, pyloric stenosis, incarcerated hernia, intussusception, appendicitis, and ovarian torsion.

    B. Non-GI Causes of Vomiting. These include brain tumor, intracranial hemorrhage, concussion, posttussive, and migraine headache.

VI. Problem Case Diagnosis. The 10-year-old girl with vomiting, diarrhea, and fever had right lower quadrant tenderness with signs of peritonitis. Abdominal CT scan was consistent with an inflamed appendix, which was removed in the operating room.

VII. Teaching Pearl: Question. What is the most likely cause of vomiting in a 14-month-old boy who has a 1-day history of episodes of crying and drawing legs to his chest, alternating with periods of sleepiness? The child does not have fever or diarrhea.

VIII. Teaching Pearl: Answer. Age of patient and nature of pain suggest intussusception as the most likely cause. Plain x-ray may be normal or may demonstrate right-sided soft tissue mass or paucity of air on right. Air (or barium) enema can establish the diagnosis and reduce intussusception nonsurgically using hydrostatic pressure.

REFERENCES

Hulka F, Campbell TJ, Campbell JR, et al. Evolution in the recognition of infantile hypertrophic pyloric stenosis. *Pediatrics* 1997;100:E9.

Paulson EK, Kalady MF, Pappas TN. Suspected appendicitis. *N Engl J Med* 2003;348:236–242.

Stevens MW, Henretig FH. Vomiting. In: Fleisher GR, Ludwig S, eds. *Textbook of Pediatric Emergency Medicine,* 4th ed. Lippincott Williams & Wilkins, 2000:625–633.

95. WHEEZING

    I. Problem. A 15-month-old girl is hospitalized with acute onset of wheezing, retractions, and oxygen saturation of 78%.

    II. Immediate Questions

        A. What are the vital signs? Hyperthermia indicates infection and the body's ability to produce pyrogens. Hypothermia reflects loss of compensatory mechanisms to maintain body temperature and suggests impending cardiorespiratory decompensation. Tachycardia, tachypnea, and hypertension may indicate compensatory mechanisms, whereas bradycardia, bradypnea, and hypotension suggest impending cardiopulmonary arrest.

        B. Is patient cyanotic? Cyanosis is seen with severe hypoxemia and acute respiratory distress.

        C. Is patient able to communicate? Inability to communicate indicates airway obstruction and impending acute respiratory failure.

        D. Does patient have a history of wheezing, pneumonia, or croup? Wheezing can be acute or chronic and intermittent, recurrent, or persistent. Pneumonia can cause airway reactivity, and spasmodic croup may be a manifestation of reactive airway disease of the upper airway.

   E. **Is patient eating and drinking?** Diminished oral intake of food
      and fluids causes dehydration and respiratory compromise.
   F. **Does patient have easy emesis, go to sleep immediately after
      drinking, or, if an infant, drink large quantities (ie, > 32 oz) of
      milk daily?** Gastroesophageal reflux, even when occult, can
      cause wheezing.
   G. **Did patient aspirate a foreign body?** Foreign body aspiration
      can result in wheezing, cough, and acute and chronic respiratory
      distress. It occurs in individuals of all ages but is more frequent
      during toddler years.
   H. **Does patient have systemic illness?** Cystic fibrosis, bron-
      chopulmonary dysplasia, α_1-antitrypsin deficiency, immunodefi-
      ciency, and congenital heart disease can cause wheezing.
      Neurologic deficits and developmental delay can result in aspira-
      tion of saliva and oral feedings, with resultant wheezing.

III. **Differential Diagnosis**
   A. **Reactive Airway Disease and Asthma.** Acute wheezing may be
      a result of exacerbation of chronic airway reactivity. Reactive
      airway disease is a spectrum of airway reactivity resulting from
      irritation or inflammation of airways extending from larynx distally
      to bronchioles. Hoarseness, croup, cough, chest discomfort, inter-
      mittent wheezing, and persistent and chronic wheezing with
      changes in pulmonary function can occur.
   B. **RSV Bronchiolitis.** Bronchiolitis resulting from respiratory syncy-
      tial viral (RSV) infection can be severe in young children with small
      airways and can be associated with respiratory distress, wheez-
      ing, and oxygen desaturation. Normally narrow airways in infants
      readily decrease further in caliber with inflammation and infection.
      Small airway resistance (R) is inversely proportional to airway
      radius (r): $R = 1/r^4$. If an airway is narrowed by 75% with mucus,
      submucosal edema, and bronchospasm, its resistance increases
      256 times. Older children and adults with RSV infection have
      milder wheezing because their airway diameters are relatively
      larger.
   C. **Infections.** Airway inflammation, parenchymal disease, and
      extrinsic airway compression with adenopathy can occur.
      1. **Viral.** Influenza A and B viruses, parainfluenza viruses, aden-
         oviruses, rhinoviruses, coronaviruses, rubeola virus, Epstein-
         Barr virus.
      2. **Bacterial.** *Streptococcus pneumoniae,* group A β-hemolytic strep-
         tococci, *Bordetella pertussis, B parapertussis, Staphylococcus
         aureus, Haemophilus influenzae* type B, *Chlamydia pneu-
         moniae, Legionella pneumophila, Moraxella catarrhalis,
         Corynebacterium diphtheriae.*
      3. **Mycoplasmal.** *Mycoplasma pneumoniae.*
      4. **Mycobacterial.** *Mycobacterium tuberculosis, M bovis,* nontu-
         berculous mycobacteria.

5. Fungal. *Aspergillus* spp, *Histoplasma capsulatum.*

D. Allergens

   1. Types

      a. Inhalants. Cigarette smoke (active, passive), pollens (trees, grasses), dust mites, molds, animal dander, ozone, chemicals (sulfur dioxide, nitrous oxide, formaldehyde, hydrochloric acid), smoke from fires.

      b. Ingestants. Foods (peanuts, shellfish, red dyes), medications (penicillins).

   2. Diseases

      a. Anaphylaxis, angioneurotic edema.

      b. Allergic bronchopulmonary aspergillosis. Wheezing, peripheral eosinophilia (> 1000 eosinophils/mm^3), markedly elevated blood IgE levels, immediate wheal and flare skin test reaction to *Aspergillus fumigatus,* serum IgG precipitins to *Aspergillus* spp, specific IgE antibody to *A fumigatus,* recurrent infiltrates radiographically, and central bronchiectasis occur. Brown plugs and growth of *A fumigatus* in sputum may be present.

E. Aspiration

   1. Foreign body

      a. Airway. Frequent site is right mainstem bronchus, because of its wider diameter and less acute angle with trachea than left mainstem bronchus.

      b. Esophagus. Extrinsic compression on trachea can occur.

   2. Saliva.

   3. Feedings

      a. Gastroesophageal reflux. Gastric acidity in lower esophagus or aspiration of gastric contents causes release of chemical mediators, producing wheezing.

      b. Oral feedings. Aspiration of food or liquids from oropharynx occurs with pharyngeal incoordination; seen in neurologically impaired and even normal children.

      c. Tracheoesophageal fistula, laryngeal cleft.

F. Upper Airway Obstruction. Stridor at rest (spasmodic croup) and with exercise (vocal cord dysfunction) can be accompanied by tracheal wheezing.

G. Airway Wall Abnormalities

   1. Malacia of larynx (laryngomalacia)

      a. Congenital. Anatomic or neuromuscular dysfunction.

      b. Acquired. CNS injury (seizures, anoxia, brainstem dysfunction, toxins, infections).

   2. Malacia of trachea (tracheomalacia) and bronchus (bronchomalacia)

      a. Congenital. Absent or defective cartilage in trachea or bronchus (Williams-Campbell, Mounier-Kuhn, Ehlers-Danlos, and Marfan syndromes).

  b. Acquired. Cartilage weakness, gastroesophageal reflux
    with aspiration, severe coughing and wheezing, tracheoe-
    sophageal fistula, extrinsic compression (tumor, bronchogenic
    cyst, vascular ring), prolonged endotracheal intubation.
H. Congenital Anomalies
  1. Vascular. Vascular ring (double aortic arch, left aortic arch with
    anomalous subclavian or innominate artery), cor triatriatum,
    pulmonary artery sling, enlarged left atrium, congenital heart
    disease with right-to-left shunting of blood.
  2. Other. Bronchogenic cyst, congenital lobar emphysema, con-
    genital cystic lung disease, esophageal duplication, bron-
    chogenic tumor.
I. Immunodeficiency. Humoral (selective IgA deficiency, X-linked
  agammaglobulinemia, common variable immunodeficiency),
  T-lymphocyte (severe combined immunodeficiency disease
  [SCID]), phagocytic (chronic granulomatous disease), hyper IgE
  syndrome.
J. Other Causes. Exercise-induced asthma, emotions (fear, anxiety,
  anger, laughter, fatigue), weather changes (humidity, cold),
  α_1-antitrypsin deficiency, cystic fibrosis, bronchopulmonary dysplasia, sarcoidosis, acute chest syndrome of sickle cell disease,
  immotile cilia syndrome.

IV. Database
A. Physical Exam Key Points
  1. General appearance. Note presence of retractions, nasal flar-
    ing, and grunting, indicating use of accessory muscles and
    severe respiratory distress.
  2. Vital signs. Note whether dyspnea is present while talking.
    Pulsus paradoxus, a reduction in systolic BP > 10 mm Hg
    during inspiration, can occur with severe wheezing.
  3. Skin. Examine for cyanosis. Oxygen desaturation may be pres-
    ent without cyanosis if anemia occurs. Examine for surgical
    scars, which may indicate cardiac surgery or chest tube place-
    ment if on chest wall or fundoplication if on abdomen.
  4. HEENT. Examine for evidence of infection and note whether
    adenopathy (cervical, axillary, epitrochlear) is present.
  5. Chest. Examine for pectus carinatum (may occur after cardiac
    surgery), pectus excavatum (can occur with abnormal rib cage
    contour and prolonged and severe respiratory distress), alter-
    ations in configuration and contour (scoliosis, kyphosis, fused
    ribs), asymmetry (chest bulge or prominence with congenital
    cardiac disease if on left side and pneumothorax if on either
    side) and retractions (unilateral or bilateral; lower intercostal,
    substernal, or supraclavicular). Prolonged expiration suggests
    partial airway obstruction, and hyperresonance to percussion
    reflects increased air.

6. **Lungs.** Note presence of wheezing (inspiratory or expiratory, or both; unilateral or bilateral; localized or diffuse), crackles, rhonchi, and character, clarity, and equality of breath sounds.
7. **Heart.** Note location of apical impulse, regularity of rhythm, quality of heart sounds, and presence and type of murmur.
8. **Abdomen.** Note presence and extent of organomegaly, masses, and tenderness; presence of enteral (gastrostomy or jejunostomy) tube.
9. **Extremities.** Examine peripheral pulses (radial, dorsalis pedis, femoral) and capillary refill time; check for clubbing.
10. **Neurologic exam.** Identify level of consciousness and ability to communicate.

B. **Laboratory Data**
1. **Oxygen saturation by pulse oximetry and ABGs.** Hypoxemia indicates mismatch of ventilation (V) with perfusion (Q), shunting of blood, and hypoventilation. Carbon dioxide is elevated with hypoventilation. Assess respiratory acidosis and respiratory failure with ABGs.
2. **Examine for infection**
   a. **CBC.** Evaluate hemoglobin, WBC count, and differential.
   b. **Cultures.** Obtain specimens from nasopharynx for viruses; throat for streptococci; and sputum, pleural effusion, and bronchoalveolar lavage for bacteria, viruses, mycobacteria, and fungi.
   c. **Rapid antigen studies.** Test for RSV and influenza A and B viruses.
3. **Allergy testing.** Evaluate blood IgE level, skin testing with allergens, and radioallergosorbent testing (RAST) to specific antigens.
4. **Immunologic studies.** Obtain quantitative levels of IgG, IgA, IgM, IgE, and IgG subclasses.
5. **Pulmonary function testing.** Evaluate spirometry and lung volumes, if possible. Obtain diffusing capacity, airflow rates, pre- and post-bronchodilator testing, exercise testing, cold air challenge testing, and methacholine challenge testing, as appropriate.

C. **Radiographic and Other Studies.** Obtain upright views of chest in anteroposterior (AP) and lateral positions.
1. **Chest x-ray.** May show:
   a. Generalized hyperaeration with flattened diaphragms, widened intercostal spaces, horizontal ribs, and increased AP diameter.
   b. Unilateral hyperaeration (airway obstruction).
   c. Contralateral mediastinal and tracheal shift if unilateral hyperaeration is present.
   d. Adenopathy (hilar, perihilar, paratracheal).
   e. Atelectasis.
   f. Infiltrate.

g. Pleural effusion.
h. Cardiomegaly.
i. Right-sided aortic arch.
j. Radiopaque foreign body.
2. **Lateral decubitus x-rays.** May show:
a. Unilateral air trapping; if foreign body is present, expiratory lateral decubitus x-ray may reveal hyperaeration because lung cannot decrease its volume during expiration with partial airway obstruction.
b. Pleural effusion (may be nonmobile).
3. **Other studies**
a. **Bronchoscopy**
i. **Flexible.** Evaluate airway anatomy and function. Identify presence of foreign body. Obtain bronchoalveolar lavage for cultures and stains and lipid-laden macrophages for aspiration of food and fluids.
ii. **Rigid.** Evaluate airway anatomy and presence of foreign body.
b. **ECG and echocardiogram.** Evaluate for cardiac disease.

V. Plan. Goals include identification, treatment, and prevention, if possible, of cause(s) of wheezing and reduction in extent and severity of wheezing.
   A. Patient Education. Teach patient and family to avoid potential inhalant allergens at home, school, and play.
   B. Preventive Measures. Immunizations to prevent respiratory infections (influenza, pertussis, *Haemophilus influenzae,* and pneumococcal vaccines) and administration of prophylactic medications (palivizumab, amantadine, oseltamivir).
   C. Medications to Treat Wheezing
      1. **Bronchodilators**
         a. **β_2-Adrenergic agonists**
            i. **Short-acting.** Albuterol (metered dose inhaler [MDI], nebulized), levalbuterol (nebulized), pirbuterol (inhalation), terbutaline (nebulized, IV), metaproterenol (MDI).
            ii. **Long-acting.** Salmeterol (inhalation powder dispenser), formoterol (inhalation).
         b. **Anticholinergics.** Ipratropium (MDI, nebulized, intranasal)
      2. **Leukotriene receptor antagonists.** Montelukast (PO), zafirlukast (PO).
      3. **Mast cell inhibitors.** Cromolyn (MDI, nebulized).
      4. **Corticosteroids.** Budesonide (inhalation), fluticasone (MDI, inhalation powder dispenser), flunisolide (MDI), triamcinolone (MDI), beclomethasone (MDI), mometasone (intranasal), prednisolone (PO, IV), prednisone (PO). Inhaled steroids are beneficial in prevention of future attacks, with minimal adverse effects (minimal systemic absorption).

     5. Theophylline (PO, IV). Reserved for children who do not respond to above therapeutics. Must monitor serum levels.

D. Medications to Treat Acute Wheezing and Status Asthmaticus

    1. Nebulized β₂-adrenergic agonist (albuterol). Administer continuously or every 1–2 hours.

    2. Corticosteroid. Beneficial to initiate early in disease.

    3. Nebulized anticholinergic. Usefulness is controversial; reserve for sicker patients.

    4. IV terbutaline. Useful in severe cases.

    5. Heliox inhalation. Heliox contains 80% helium and 20% oxygen; has one third the density of air and less resistance than an air-oxygen mixture or 100% oxygen. Readily traverses narrowed airways and facilitates deposition of aerosol particles in small airways. Airway resistance and work of breathing are reduced during initial phases of acute wheezing treated with heliox.

E. Chronic Wheezing With Acute Exacerbations. Types, dosing, and frequency of medications vary according to acuity and severity of wheezing. Guidelines from National Institutes of Health are helpful in determining plan of treatment.

    1. β₂-Adrenergic agonist (inhaled, nebulized).

    2. Corticosteroid (inhaled, nebulized, oral).

    3. Anticholinergic (inhaled, nebulized).

    4. Theophylline (oral); rarely used. Reserve for severe cases.

F. Treatment of Gastroesophageal Reflux

    1. Feeding and positioning

      a. Thicken feedings for infants.

      b. Position upright during and following feedings.

      c. Avoid feeding prior to sleep.

    2. Medications. Antacids, prokinetics, proton pump inhibitors.

VI. Problem Case Diagnosis. The 15-month-old girl had a history of rhinorrhea and cough with low-grade fever for several days. Her chest x-ray revealed hyperinflated lungs with bilateral patchy infiltrates. Her WBC count was normal. Diagnosis is wheezing secondary to RSV bronchiolitis.

VII. Teaching Pearl: Question. What is the most frequent cause of wheezing in childhood?

VIII. Teaching Pearl: Answer. Respiratory viral infections.

REFERENCES

Busse WW, Lemanske RF Jr. Asthma. *N Engl J Med* 2001;344:350–362.

Cifuentes L, Caussade S, Villagrán C, et al. Risk factors for recurrent wheezing following acute bronchiolitis: A 12-month follow-up. *Pediatr Pulmonol* 2003;36: 316–321.

Martinez FD, Wright AL, Taussig LM, et al. Asthma and wheezing in the first six years of life. *N Engl J Med* 1995;332:133–138.

National Asthma Education and Prevention Program. Expert panel report: Guidelines for the diagnosis and management of asthma update on selected topics—2002. *J Allergy Clin Immunol* 2002;110:S141–219.

II. Laboratory Tests and Their Interpretation

Note: Reference ranges for each laboratory may vary from the values given in this section; therefore, clinician should interpret results of a patient's laboratory value in light of an individual facility's range.

■ ACID-FAST STAIN
Positive: Mycobacterium species (tuberculosis and atypical mycobacteria such as *M avium-intracellulare*) and *Nocardia*.

■ ACTH (ADRENOCORTICOTROPIC HORMONE) STIMULATION TEST
Used to help diagnose adrenal insufficiency. Cosyntropin (Cortrosyn), an ACTH analogue, is given at a dose of 0.25 mg IM or IV. Collect blood at times 0, 30, and 60 minutes for cortisol.

Normal Response: Basal cortisol of at least 5 mcg/dL, an increase of at least 7 mcg/dL, and a final cortisol of 16 mcg/dL at 30 minutes or 18 mcg/dL at 60 minutes.

Subnormal or Abnormal Response: Addison disease (primary adrenal insufficiency) and secondary adrenal insufficiency. Secondary insufficiency is caused by pituitary insufficiency or suppression by exogenous steroids. ACTH level and pituitary stimulation tests can be used to differentiate primary from secondary adrenal insufficiency.

■ ALBUMIN, SERUM
Newborn, term: 3.2–4.8 g/dL.
1 month to 1 year: 2.1–5.7 g/dL.
1–5 years: 2.0–5.8 g/dL.
5–19 years: 3.2–5.0 g/dL.

Decreased: Malnutrition, nephrotic syndrome, cystic fibrosis, multiple myeloma, Hodgkin disease, leukemia, protein-losing enteropathies, chronic glomerulonephritis, cirrhosis, inflammatory bowel disease, collagen-vascular diseases, hyperthyroidism.

■ ALBUMIN, URINE
Normal: < 30 mg/day.
Microalbuminuria (30–300 mg/day) is a sign of early renal damage in diabetes mellitus, hypertension, and other diseases affecting the kidney.

Microalbuminuria can be detected by determining the albumin-to-creatinine ratio (obtained from a spot urine for albumin and creatinine). Urinary protein-to-urinary creatinine ratio ($U_{Pr}:U_{Cr}$) is < 0.5 in first few months of life and < 0.2 in older children. $U_{Pr}:U_{Cr}$ > 1.0 is considered nephrotic proteinuria range. Confirm ratio with 24-hour urine collection.

Note: Microalbuminuria can be seen with prolonged exercise, hematuria, fever, or prolonged upright posture. Nephrotic proteinuria > 40 $mg/m^2/h$.

■ ALKALINE PHOSPHATASE

Infant: 150–420 units/L.
2–10 years: 100–320 units/L.
Adolescent male: 100–390 units/L.
Adolescent female: 100–320 units/L.
Adult: 30–120 units/L.

γ-Glutamyltransferase (GGT) level is often useful to differentiate whether elevated alkaline phosphatase originates from bone or liver. Normal GGT level suggests bone origin.

Increased: Increased calcium deposition in bone (hyperparathyroidism), osteomalacia, pregnancy, childhood, liver disease, and hyperthyroidism.

Decreased: Malnutrition, excess vitamin D ingestion.

■ ALT (ALANINE AMINOTRANSFERASE) (SGPT: SERUM GLUTAMIC-PYRUVIC TRANSFERASE)

Neonate and infant: 13–45 units/L.
Adolescent male: 10–40 units/L.
Adolescent female: 7–35 units/L.

Increased: Liver disease, biliary obstruction, liver congestion, hepatitis (ALT is more elevated than AST in viral hepatitis).

■ AMMONIA

Newborn: 79–150 mcg/dL.
> 1 month: 29–70 mcg/dL.
Adult: 0–50 mcg/dL.

Increased: Hepatic encephalopathy, Reye syndrome.

■ AMYLASE

Newborn: 5–65 units/L.
Adult: 25–125 units/L.

Increased: Acute pancreatitis, pancreatic duct obstruction (stones, stricture, tumor), mumps, parotiditis, renal disease, cholecystitis, peptic ulcers, intestinal obstruction, diabetic ketoacidosis, ruptured ectopic pregnancy.

Decreased: Pancreatic destruction (pancreatitis, cystic fibrosis), liver disease.

■ ANION GAP

Normal: 8–12 mmol/L.

Note: Anion gap is a calculated estimate of unmeasured anions and is used to help differentiate cause of metabolic acidosis.

$$\text{Anion gap} = (\text{Na}^+) - (\,([\text{Cl}^-] + [\text{HCO}_3^-])\,)$$

Increased (High; > 12 mmol/L): Lactic acidosis, ketoacidosis (diabetic, starvation), uremia, toxins (salicylates, methanol, ethylene glycol, paraldehyde); in addition, dehydration, alkalosis, use of certain penicillins (carbenicillin), and salts of strong acids such as sodium citrate (used as a preservative in packed RBCs) can cause a mild increase in anion gap.

Decreased (Low; < 8 mmol/L): Seen with bromide ingestion, hypercalcemia, hypermagnesemia, multiple myeloma, and hypoalbuminemia.

■ ANTINEUTROPHIL CYTOPLASMIC ANTIBODIES (ANCA)

Negative: < 10 units/mL.
Equivocal: 10–20 units/mL.
Positive: > 20 units/mL.
Antibodies to cytoplasmic components of neutrophils, seen in vasculitides. Two types:

1. **C-ANCA (cytoplasmic-staining ANCA).** Present in ~90% of patients with generalized Wegener granulomatosis; also seen in rapidly progressive glomerulonephritis and a type of polyarteritis nodosa (microscopic). C-ANCA may be used to follow disease activity; it is also especially useful in distinguishing active disease from an infectious complication. C-ANCA is not present in other collagen-vascular diseases.

2. **P-ANCA (perinuclear-staining ANCA).** Seen in a variety of collagen-vascular diseases such as limited Wegener granulomatosis, polyarteritis nodosa, Goodpasture syndrome, other vasculitides, and inflammatory bowel disease (Crohn disease). It is also seen in several types of glomerulonephritides.

■ ANTINUCLEAR ANTIBODIES (ANA)

Useful screening test in patients with symptoms suggesting collagen-vascular disease. A titer of > 1:320 is likely significant.

Positive: Systemic lupus erythematosus (SLE), drug-induced lupus (procainamide, hydralazine, isoniazid, etc), scleroderma, mixed connective tissue disease (MCTD), rheumatoid arthritis, polymyositis, juvenile rheumatoid arthritis (5–20%). Low titers are also seen in patients with non–collagen-vascular disease and in those without any disease.

Specific Immunofluorescent ANA Patterns and Clinical Correlation

1. **ANA Patterns**
   - **Homogeneous:** Nonspecific, from antibodies to deoxyribonucleoproteins (DNP) and native double-stranded deoxyribonucleic acid (DNA); seen in SLE and a variety of other diseases. Antihistone is consistent with drug-induced lupus.
   - **Speckled:** Pattern seen in many connective tissue disorders. From antibodies to extractable nuclear antigens (ENA), including antiribonucleoproteins (anti-RNP), anti-Sm, anti-PM-1, and anti-SS. Anti-RNP is positive in MCTD and SLE. Anti-Sm is found in SLE. Anti-SS-A and anti-SS-B are seen in Sjögren syndrome and subacute cutaneous lupus. The speckled pattern is also seen with scleroderma.
   - **Peripheral RIM pattern:** From antibodies to native double-stranded DNA and DNP. Seen in SLE.
   - **Nucleolar pattern:** From antibodies to nucleolar ribonucleic acid (RNA). Positive in Sjögren syndrome and scleroderma.
2. **Other Autoantibodies**
   - **Antimitochondrial:** Primary biliary cirrhosis.
   - **Anti–smooth muscle:** Low titers are seen in a variety of illnesses; high titers (> 1:100) are suggestive of chronic active hepatitis.
   - **Antimicrosomal:** Hashimoto thyroiditis.

■ ANTIPHOSPHOLIPID ANTIBODIES

Note: There are two basic categories of antiphospholipid antibody—anticardiolipin and lupus anticoagulant. Both are associated with recurrent arterial or venous thrombosis or fetal demise.

Anticardiolipin Antibody

Two forms: IgG, IgM.
IgG normal: < 23 units.
IgM normal: < 11 units.

Lupus Anticoagulant

Negative: Normal.
Positive: Presence.
Should be suspected in patients with isolated elevated PTT and no other likely cause.

■ AST (ASPARTATE AMINOTRANSFERASE) (SGOT: SERUM GLUTAMIC-OXALOACETIC TRANSFERASE)

Newborn: 25–75 units/L.
1–9 years: 15–60 units/L.

10–19 years: 10–45 units/L.
Adult: 8–20 units/L.
Generally parallels changes in ALT in liver disease.

Increased: Liver disease, muscle trauma and injection, pancreatitis, intestinal injury or surgery, factitious increase (erythromycin, opiates), burns, brain damage.

Decreased: Beri-beri, diabetes mellitus with ketoacidosis, chronic liver disease.

■ BASE EXCESS/DEFICIT
See Tables II–1 and II–2, p. 454 and p. 455. A decrease in base (bicarbonate) is termed *base deficit;* an increase in base is termed *base excess.*

Excess: Metabolic alkalosis (see Section I, Chapter 5, Alkalosis, p. 23), respiratory acidosis (see Section I, Chapter 3, Acidosis, p. 13).

Deficit: Metabolic acidosis (see Section I, Chapter 3, Acidosis, p. 13), respiratory alkalosis (see Section I, Chapter 5, Alkalosis, p. 23).

■ BICARBONATE (SERUM HCO_3^-)
See Tables II–2 and II–3, p. 455.
Normal: 22–28 mmol/L.
Note: Newborn and infant values may be slightly lower, 17–24 mmol/L.

Increased: Metabolic alkalosis, compensation for respiratory acidosis. See Section I, Chapter 3, Acidosis, p. 13; and Section I, Chapter 5, Alkalosis, p. 23.

Decreased: Metabolic acidosis, compensation for respiratory alkalosis. See Section I, Chapter 3, Acidosis, p. 13; and Section I, Chapter 5, Alkalosis, p. 23.

■ BILIRUBIN
Total:

0–1 day: < 8.7 mg/dL or < 149 micromoles/L.
1–2 days: < 11.5 mg/dL or < 197 micromoles/L.
3–5 days: < 12 mg/dL or < 205 micromoles/L.
Older infant: < 1.1 mg/dL or < 21 micromoles/L.
Adult: 0.3–1.2 mg/dL or 5–21 micromoles/L.
Note: Values are for term infant.

TABLE II-1. BASIC APPROACH TO DIAGNOSIS OF ACID-BASE DISORDERS

Step 1. Obtain arterial blood gas (ABG; for normal values, see Table II-2, p. 455)

Step 2. Look at pH:
1. If pH < 7.35, there is **acidosis**
2. If pH > 7.45, there is **alkalosis**
3. If 7.35 < pH < 7.45, there is:
   No acid-base disorder, or
   Compensated disorder, or
   Mixed disorder

Step 3. Look at Pco_2:
1. If pH < 7.35 and $Paco_2$ > 45, it is **respiratory acidosis**
2. If pH < 7.35 and $Paco_2$ < 35, it is **metabolic acidosis**
3. If pH > 7.45 and $Paco_2$ < 35, it is **respiratory alkalosis**
4. If pH > 7.45 and $Paco_2$ > 45, it is **metabolic alkalosis**

Step 4.
1. If **respiratory acidosis,** look at increase in HCO_3 for each 10-mm increase in $Paco_2$:
   If 1.0–1.2, it is **acute respiratory acidosis**
   If 1.3–3.0, it is **partially compensated**
   If 3.1–4.0, it is **fully compensated**
2. If **pure metabolic acidosis:**
   $Paco_2 = (1.5 \times HCO_3) = 8 \pm 2$
   $Paco_2 = HCO_3 + 15$ if $HCO_3 > 10$
3. If **respiratory alkalosis,** look at fall of HCO_3 for each 10-mm fall of $Paco_2$:
   If 2.5, it is **acute respiratory alkalosis**
   If 5.0, it is **chronic respiratory alkalosis**
4. If **respiratory alkalosis,** look at rise in pH for 10-mm fall of $Paco_2$:
   If 0.08, it is **acute respiratory alkalosis**
   If 0.03, it is **chronic respiratory alkalosis**
5. If **metabolic alkalosis:**
   $Paco_2 = 0.7 \times HCO_3 + 20 \pm 1.5$

Limits of compensation
1. In acute respiratory acidosis HCO_3 cannot rise above 30
2. In chronic respiratory acidosis HCO_3 can rise above 55
3. In respiratory alkalosis $Paco_2$ cannot fall below 16 mm Hg
4. In metabolic acidosis $Paco_2$ cannot fall below 10 mm Hg
5. In metabolic alkalosis $Paco_2$ cannot rise above 55
6. If values deviate from the above it is a mixed disorder
7. There is never overcompensation

From Lefor AT, ed. Critical Care On Call. McGraw-Hill. Copyright © 2002.

Direct:

Neonate: < 0.6 mg/dL or < 10 micromoles/L.
Infant through adult: < 0.2 mg/dL or < 3.4 micromoles/L.

Increased Total (Direct Plus Indirect): Hepatic damage (hepatitis, toxins, cirrhosis), biliary obstruction (gallstone or tumor), hemolysis, fasting.

TABLE II-2. NORMAL BLOOD GAS VALUES

Measurement	Arterial	Mixed Venous[a]	Venous
pH (range)	7.40 (7.35–7.45)	7.36 (7.31–7.41)	7.36 (7.31–7.41)
P_{O_2} (decreases with age)	80–100 mm Hg	35–40 mm Hg	30–50 mm Hg
P_{CO_2}	35–45 mm Hg	41–51 mm Hg	40–52 mm Hg
O_2 saturation (decreases with age)	> 95%	60–80%	60–80%
HCO_3	22–26 mEq/L	22–26 mEq/L	22–28 mEq/L
Base difference (deficit/excess)	−2 to +2	−2 to +2	−2 to +2

[a] From right atrium.
Modified and reproduced with permission from Gomella LG, Haist SA, eds. Clinician's Pocket Reference, 10th ed. McGraw-Hill. Copyright © 2004.

Increased Direct (Conjugated): See Section I, Chapter 37, Hyperbilirubinemia, Direct (Conjugated), p. 180.

Increased Indirect (Unconjugated): See Section I, Chapter 38, Hyperbilirubinemia, Indirect (Unconjugated), p. 185.

■ BLEEDING TIME
Duke, Ivy: < 6 minutes.
Template: < 10 minutes.

Increased: Thrombocytopenia, thrombocytopenic purpura, von Willebrand disease, defective platelet function (aspirin, NSAIDs, uremia).

TABLE II-3. ACID-BASE DISORDERS WITH APPROPRIATE COMPENSATION

Disorder	Changes in Normal Values		
	pH	HCO_3^-	P_{CO_2}
Metabolic acidosis	↓	↓↓	↓
Metabolic alkalosis	↑	↑↑	↑
Acute respiratory acidosis	↓	Slight ↑	↑↑
Chronic respiratory acidosis	Slight ↓	↑	↑↑
Acute respiratory alkalosis	↑	Slight ↓	↓↓
Chronic respiratory alkalosis	Slight ↑	↓	↓↓

From Haist SA, Robbins JB, eds. Internal Medicine On Call, 3rd ed. McGraw-Hill. Copyright © 2002.

■ BLOOD GAS

See Tables II–2 and II–3, p. 455.

Arterial: pH 7.36–7.44; PaO_2 80–100 mm Hg; $PaCO_2$ 35–45 mm Hg; HCO_3^- 22–26 mEq/L.

Note: Newborn PaO_2 may be lower, 70 mm Hg.

Venous: PCO_2 averages 6–8 mm Hg higher than arterial PO_2 and pH is slightly lower. Venous blood gas should not be used to assess oxygenation.

Capillary: Blood gases correlate best with arterial pH; $PaCO_2$ correlates fairly well.

For acid–base disorders, see Section I, Chapter 3, Acidosis, p. 13; and Chapter 5, Alkalosis, p. 23.

■ BLOOD UREA NITROGEN (BUN)

Normal: 7–18 mg/dL or 1.2–3.0 mmol urea/L.

Increased: Renal failure, prerenal azotemia (decreased renal perfusion secondary to congestive heart failure, shock, volume depletion), postrenal obstruction, GI bleeding, hypercatabolic states.

Decreased: Starvation, malnutrition, liver failure (hepatitis, drugs), pregnancy, infancy, nephrotic syndrome, overhydration.

■ BLOOD UREA NITROGEN/CREATININE RATIO

Normal: Between 10 and 20:1.

Elevated Ratio (> 20:1): Congestive heart failure, dehydration, GI bleeding, increased protein intake, drugs such as tetracycline and steroids, infection (sepsis), high fevers, burns, cachexia.

Decreased Ratio (< 10:1): Acute tubular necrosis, low-protein diet, starvation, malnutrition, liver disease, syndrome of inappropriate antidiuretic hormone (SIADH), pregnancy, rhabdomyolysis.

Note: Ratio may not be accurate if patient is in diabetic ketoacidosis or receiving drugs such as cephalosporin. Ratio can be altered by interferences in the chemical methods used to measure creatinine or BUN, resulting in spurious results. The presence of ketones may seriously elevate serum creatinine level. Drugs such as cephalosporins, ascorbic acid, and barbiturates may also interfere with serum creatinine measurement.

■ CALCIUM, SERUM

Total:

Newborn, preterm: 6.2–11 mg/dL or 1.6–2.8 mmol/L.
Newborn, term < 10 days: 7.6–10.9 mg/dL or 1.9–2.6 mmol/L.
10 days to 24 months: 9.0–11.0 mg/dL or 2.3–2.8 mmol/L.
2–12 years: 8.8–10.8 mg/dL or 2.2–2.7 mmol/L.
Adult: 8.6–10.2 mg/dL or 2.1–2.5 mmol/L.

Ionized:

Newborn, < 36 hours: 4.2–5.48 mg/dL or 1.05-1.37 mmol/L.
Newborn, 36–84 hours: 4.40–5.68 mg/dL or 1.10–1.42 mmol/L.
1–18 years: 4.8–5.52 mg/dL or 1.20–1.38 mmol/L.
Adult: 4.64–5.28 mg/dL or 1.16–1.32 mmol/L.
Note: To interpret total calcium value, you must know the albumin level. If albumin is not within normal limits, a corrected calcium level can be roughly calculated with the following formula. Values for ionized calcium need no special correction.

Corrected total Ca = 0.8 (Normal albumin − Measured albumin)
+ Reported Ca

Increased: See Section I, Chapter 39, Hypercalcemia, p. 189.

Decreased: See Section I, Chapter 46, Hypocalcemia, p. 218.

■ CARBOXYHEMOGLOBIN (% OF TOTAL HEMOGLOBIN)

Nonsmoker: < 2%.
Smoker: < 6%.
Toxic: > 15%.
Lethal: > 50%.

Increased: Smoking, smoke inhalation; exposure to automobile exhaust; faulty heating units with inadequate ventilation.

■ CATECHOLAMINES, SERUM

See Table II–4.

Increased: Pheochromocytoma, neural crest tumors (neuroblastoma).

■ CATECHOLAMINES, URINE

Dopamine: 100–440 mcg.
Epinephrine: < 15 mcg.

TABLE II-4. SERUM CATECHOLAMINES

Catecholamine	Supine (mcg)	Sitting (mcg)
Dopamine	<87	<87
Epinephrine	<50	<60
Norepinephrine	110–410	120–680

Norepinephrine: 15–86 mcg.
Homovanillic acid (HVA): 0–10 mg.
Vanillylmandelic acid (VMA): 2–10 mg.
Metanephrine: < 0.4 mg.
Normetanephrine: < 0.9 mg.

Increased: Pheochromocytoma, neural crest tumors (neuroblastoma).

■ CBC (COMPLETE BLOOD COUNT, HEMOGRAM)
For normal values, see Appendix A, Blood Cell Indices, p. 752. For differential, see specific tests.

■ CHLORIDE, SERUM
Normal: 98–106 mEq/L.
Note: Newborn levels may be slightly higher, 98–113 mEq/L.

Increased: Metabolic nongap acidosis such as diarrhea, renal tubular acidosis, mineralocorticoid deficiency, hyperalimentation, medications (acetazolamide, ammonium chloride).

Decreased: Vomiting, diabetes mellitus with ketoacidosis, mineralocorticoid excess, renal disease with sodium loss.

■ CHOLESTEROL, TOTAL
Child, desirable level: < 170 mg/dL; high, > 200 mg/dL.
Adult, desirable level: < 200 mg/dL; high, > 240 mg/dL.

Increased: Primary hypercholesterolemia, elevated triglycerides, biliary obstruction, nephrosis, hypothyroidism, diabetes mellitus.

Decreased: Chronic liver disease, hyperthyroidism, malnutrition (cancer, starvation), myeloproliferative disorders, steroid therapy, lipoproteinemias.

High-Density Lipoprotein (HDL) Cholesterol

Normal: < 45 mg/dL.

Note: HDL highly correlates with development of coronary artery disease; decreased HDL leads to an increased risk, and increased HDL is associated with a decreased risk.

Increased: Estrogen (females), exercise, ethanol.

Decreased: Male gender, anabolic steroids, uremia, obesity, diabetes, liver disease, β-blockers.

Low-Density Lipoprotein (LDL) Cholesterol

Child, desirable: < 110 mg/dL; high, > 130 mg/dL.
Adult, desirable: < 130 mg/dL; high, > 160 mg/dL.

Increased: Excess dietary saturated fats, hyperlipoproteinemia, biliary cirrhosis, endocrine disease (diabetes, hypothyroidism), myocardial infarction.

Decreased: Malabsorption, severe liver disease, abetalipoproteinemia.

Triglycerides

Term newborn to 5 years: male, 0–86 mg/dL; female, 32–99 mg/dL.
6–11 years: male, 31–108 mg/dL; female, 35–114 mg/dL.
12–15 years: male, 36–138 mg/dL; female, 41–138 mg/dL.
Adult: male, 40–160 mg/dL; female, 35–135 mg/dL.

Increased: Hyperlipoproteinemias, hypothyroidism, liver diseases, diabetes mellitus, pancreatitis, nephrotic syndrome.

Decreased: Malnutrition, congenital abetalipoproteinemia.

■ COLD AGGLUTININS

Normal: < 1:32.

Increased: *Mycoplasma* pneumonia, viral infections (especially mononucleosis, measles, mumps), some parasitic infections.

■ COMPLEMENT C3

Noeonate: 53–130 mg/dL.
Infant (< 1 year): 62–180 mg/dL.
Child: 77–195 mg/dL.
Adult: 80–155 mg/dL.
Note: Normal values may vary greatly depending on assay used.

Increased: Rheumatic fever, neoplasms.

Decreased: Systemic lupus erythematosus, glomerulonephritis (poststreptococcal and membranoproliferative), vasculitis, severe hepatic failure.

Variable: Rheumatoid arthritis.

■ COMPLEMENT C4

Neonate: 7–27 mg/dL.
Infant and child: 7–40 mg/dL.
Adult: 20–50 mg/dL.

Increased: Neoplasia (GI, lung, others).

Decreased: Systemic lupus erythematosus, chronic active hepatitis, cirrhosis, glomerulonephritis, hereditary angioedema.

Variable: Rheumatoid arthritis.

■ COMPLEMENT CH50 (TOTAL)

Tests for complement deficiency in the classic pathway.
Normal: 30–75 mg/mL.

Increased: Acute-phase reactants (eg, tissue injury, infections).

Decreased: Hereditary complement deficiencies, any cause of deficiency of individual complement components. See Complement C3 and Complement C4, earlier.

■ COOMBS TEST, DIRECT

Uses patient's erythrocytes; tests for presence of antibody or complement on patient's RBCs.

Positive: Autoimmune hemolytic anemia (leukemia, lymphoma, collagen-vascular diseases [eg, systemic lupus erythematosus]), hemolytic transfusion reaction, sensitization to some drugs (methyldopa, levodopa, penicillins, cephalosporins).

■ COOMBS TEST, INDIRECT

More useful for RBC typing. Uses serum that contains antibody from the patient.

Positive: Isoimmunization from previous transfusion; incompatible blood as a result of improper cross-matching.

■ CORTISOL

Serum:

Pre-ACTH or 8 AM: 5.0–23.0 mcg/dL.
1 hour post-ACTH: 16–36 mcg/dL.

Urine:

Prepubertal child: 3-9 mcg/day.
Adult: 10–100 mcg/day.

Increased: Adrenal adenoma, adrenal carcinoma, Cushing disease, non-pituitary ACTH-producing tumor, steroid therapy.

Decreased: Primary adrenal insufficiency (Addison disease), Waterhouse-Friderichsen syndrome, ACTH deficiency.

■ CORTROSYN STIMULATION TEST
See ACTH Stimulation Test, p. 449.

■ C-PEPTIDE
Fasting: ≤ 4.0 g/mL or = 4.0 mcg/L.
Female: 1.4–5.5 g/mL or 1.4–5.5 mcg/L.

Decreased: Diabetes mellitus (type 1), insulin administration, hypoglycemia.

Increased: Insulinoma. Test is useful to differentiate insulinoma from surreptitious use of insulin as a cause of hypoglycemia.

■ C-REACTIVE PROTEIN (CRP)
An acute-phase reactant with a relatively short half-life.
Normal: < 8 mg/L.

Increased: Infections (increase in bacterial infections > increase in viral infections), inflammatory disorders, tissue injury or necrosis (malignant disease, organ rejection following transplantation). With certain inflammatory disorders, such as systemic lupus erythematosus, scleroderma, and Crohn disease, CRP will not be elevated as much as one would expect for the degree of inflammation; therefore, ESR may be a better marker of inflammation in these disorders.

■ CREATINE PHOSPHOKINASE (CK)
Newborn: 100–200 units/L.
Adult: 25–145 units/L.

Increased: Cardiac muscle (acute myocardial infarction, myocarditis, defibrillation), skeletal muscle (intramuscular injection, hypothyroidism, rhabdomyolysis, polymyositis, muscular dystrophy), cerebral infarction, cardiac muscle.

■ CREATININE, SERUM

Newborn: 0.3–1.0 mg/dL.
Infant: 0.2–0.4 mg/dL.
Child: 0.3–0.7 mg/dL.
Adolescent: 0.5–1.0 mg/dL.
Adult male: 0.7–1.3 mg/dL.
Adult female: 0.6–1.1 mg/dL.

Increased: Renal failure (prerenal, renal, or postrenal), large body mass. Falsely elevated with ketones and certain cephalosporins, depending on assay.

■ FERRITIN

Newborn: 25–200 ng/mL.
1 month: 200–600 ng/mL.
2–5 months: 50–200 ng/mL.
6 months to 15 years: 7–140 ng/mL.
Adult male: 15–200 ng/mL.
Adult female: 12–150 ng/mL.

Increased: Any inflammatory process (acute-phase reactant), hemochromatosis, hemosiderosis, sideroblastic anemia.

Decreased: Iron deficiency, severe liver disease.

■ FIBRIN DEGRADATION PRODUCTS (FDP)

Normal: < 10 mcg/mL.

Increased: Any thromboembolic condition (deep venous thrombosis, myocardial infarction, pulmonary embolus); disseminated intravascular coagulation; hepatic dysfunction.

■ FIBRINOGEN

Newborn: 125–300 mg/dL.
Adult: 150–450 mg/dL.

Increased: Inflammatory processes (acute-phase reactant).

Decreased: Congenital, disseminated intravascular coagulation, burns, neoplastic and hematologic malignancies, acute severe bleeding, snake bite.

■ FOLATE RED BLOOD CELL

Newborn: 150–200 ng/mL.
Infant: 75–1000 ng/mL.

2–16 years: > 160 ng/mL.
Adult: 160–640 ng/mL.
Note: More sensitive for detecting folate deficiency from malnourishment if patient has started proper nutrition before serum folate is measured (even one well-balanced hospital meal can increase serum folate to normal levels).

Increased: See Folic Acid (Serum Folate), below.

Decreased: See Folic Acid (Serum Folate), below.

■ FOLIC ACID (SERUM FOLATE)
Newborn: 5–65 ng/mL.
Infant: 15–55 ng/mL.
2–16 years: 5–21 ng/mL.
Adult: 2–14 ng/mL.

Increased: Folic acid administration.

Decreased: Malnutrition, malabsorption, massive cellular growth (cancer), hemolytic anemia, pregnancy.

■ FTA-ABS (FLUORESCENT TREPONEMAL ANTIBODY ABSORBED)
Normal: Nonreactive.

Positive: Syphilis (test of choice to confirm diagnosis). Test may be negative in early primary syphilis; may remain positive after adequate treatment.

■ GALACTOSE
Newborn: 0–20 mg/dL.
> 28 days: < 5 mg/dL.

Increased: Galactosemia, galactokinase deficiency.

■ γ-GLUTAMYLTRANSFERASE (GGT)
Infant, 0–3 weeks: 0–130 units/L.
3 weeks to 3 months: 4–120 units/L.
3–12 months: male, 5–65 units/L; female, 5–35 units/L.
1–15 years: 0–23 units/L.
Adult male: 9–50 units/L.
Adult female: 8–40 units/L.
Note: Generally parallels changes in serum alkaline phosphatase and 5′-nucleotidase in liver disease.

Increased: Liver disease (hepatitis, cirrhosis, obstructive jaundice), pancreatitis.

■ GLUCOSE

Newborn, < 24 hours: 40–60 mg/dL.
Newborn, > 24 hours: 50–80 mg/dL.
Child: 60–100 mg/dL.
Adult: 70–105 mg/dL.

Increased: See Section I, Chapter 40, Hyperglycemia, p. 194.

Decreased: See Section I, Chapter 47, Hypoglycemia, p. 223.

■ GRAM STAIN
Rapid Technique

Spread a thin layer of specimen onto glass slide and allow it to dry. Fix with heat. Apply Gentian violet (15–20 seconds); follow with iodine (15–20 seconds), then alcohol (just a few seconds until effluent is barely decolorized). Rinse with water and counterstain with safranin (15–20 seconds). Examine under oil immersion lens: gram-positive bacteria are dark blue and gram-negatives are red.

Gram-Positive Cocci: Staphylococcus, Streptococcus, Enterococcus, Micrococcus, Peptococcus (anaerobic), and *Peptostreptococcus* (anaerobic) species.

Gram-Positive Rods: Clostridium (anaerobic), *Corynebacterium, Listeria,* and *Bacillus.*

Gram-Negative Cocci: Neisseria, Branhamella, Moraxella, and *Acinetobacter* species.

Gram-Negative Coccoid Rods: Haemophilus, Pasteurella, Brucella, Francisella, Yersinia, and *Bordetella* species.

Gram-Negative Straight Rods: Acinetobacter (Mima, Herellea), Aeromonas, Bacteroides (anaerobic), *Campylobacter* (comma-shaped) species, *Eikenella, Enterobacter, Escherichia, Fusobacterium* (anaerobic), *Helicobacter, Klebsiella, Legionella* (small, pleomorphic; weakly staining), *Proteus, Providencia, Pseudomonas, Salmonella, Serratia, Shigella, Vibrio, Yersinia.*

■ HAPTOGLOBIN

Newborn: 5–48 mg/dL.
> 1 month: 26–185 mg/dL.

Increased: Obstructive liver disease, any inflammatory process.

Decreased: Hemolysis (eg, transfusion reaction), severe liver disease.

■ HEMATOCRIT
For normal values, see Appendix A, Blood Cell Indices, p. 758.

Increased: Dehydration.

Decreased: See Section I, Chapter 8, Anemia, p. 39.

■ HEMOGLOBIN
For normal values, see Appendix A, Blood Cell Indices, p. 758.

Increased Dehydration.

Decreased: See Section I, Chapter 8, Anemia, p. 39.

■ HEMOGLOBIN A$_{1C}$
Normal: 4.0–6.0%.

Increased Poorly controlled diabetes mellitus.

■ HEPATITIS TESTS
See Table II–5, p. 466.

- **Anti-HAV Tot:** Total antibody to hepatitis A virus, *both IgG and IgM.* Confirms previous exposure to hepatitis A virus and is also positive with acute infection.
- **Anti-HAV IgM:** IgM antibody to hepatitis A virus. Indicates acute infection with hepatitis A virus.
- **HBsAg:** Hepatitis B surface antigen. Indicates either chronic or acute infection with hepatitis B. Used by blood banks to screen donors and part of routine hepatitis panel for evaluation of liver injury.
- **Total Anti-HBc:** IgG and IgM antibody to hepatitis B core antigen. Confirms either previous exposure to hepatitis B virus (HBV) or ongoing infection. Used by blood banks to screen donors.
- **Anti-HBc IgM:** IgM antibody to hepatitis B core antigen. Early and best indicator of acute infection with hepatitis B.
- **HBeAg:** Hepatitis B$_e$ antigen. When present, indicates high degree of infectiousness. Order *only* when evaluating a patient with *chronic* HBV infection.
- **Anti-HBe:** Antibody to hepatitis B$_e$ antigen. Order with HBeAg. Presence is associated with resolution of active viral proliferation, but often means virus is integrated into host DNA, especially if host remains HBsAg-positive.
- **Anti-HBs:** Antibody to hepatitis B surface antigen. Typically indicates immunity associated with clinical recovery from an HBV infection or previous immunization with hepatitis B vaccine. Order *only* to assess effectiveness of vaccine, and results will often be reported as a titer.

TABLE II-5. HEPATITIS PANEL TESTING

Profile Name	Test	Purpose
Screening		
Admission: High-risk patients (homosexuals, IV drug users, dialysis patients)	HBsAg Anti-HCV	To screen for chronic or active infection
All pregnant women	HBsAg	To screen for chronic or active infection
Percutaneous inoculation	HBsAg Anti-HCV	Test serum of patient (if known) for possible infectivity; start hepatitis B vaccination if health care worker not previously immunized
	Anti-HBs	Determine if vaccinated health care worker is immune and protected
Pre-HBV vaccine in high-risk patients	HbsAg Anti-HBc	To determine if an individual is infected or already has antibodies and is immune
Diagnosis		
Differential diagnosis of acute hepatitis	Anti-HAV IgM HBsAg Anti-HBc IgM Anti-HCV	To differentiate among hepatitis A, hepatitis B, and hepatitis C (anti-HCV may take 4–8 wk to become positive)
Differential diagnosis of chronic hepatitis (abnormal liver function tests [LFTs])	HBsAg Anti-HCV (and RIBA or HCV RNA if anti-HCV is positive)	To rule out chronic hepatitis B or C as a cause of chronically elevated LFTs
Monitoring		
Chronic hepatitis B	LFTs HBsAg HBeAg/Anti-HBe Anti-HDV IgM α-Fetoprotein HBV DNA	To test for activity, late seroconversion, or disease latency in known hepatitis B carrier, superinfection with HDV, development of hepatoma, or resolution of infection after therapy or spontaneously
Chronic hepatitis C	LFTs HCV RNA α-Fetoprotein	To test for activity of hepatitis likelihood of response to interferon, or development of hepatoma
Postvaccination screening	Anti-HBs	To ensure immunity after vaccination
Sexual contact	HBsAg	To monitor sexual partners with acute or chronic hepatitis B

From Haist SA, Robbins JB, eds. Internal Medicine On Call, 3rd ed. McGraw-Hill. Copyright © 2002.

- **HBV-DNA:** Detects presence of viral DNA in serum (pg/mL) quantitatively to confirm infection and assess therapy with antiviral agents such as lamivudine and adefovir. Relatively expensive assay.
- **Anti-HDV:** Antibody to delta-agent hepatitis. Order *only* in patients with known chronic HBV infection who have flare of transaminase elevation.

- **Anti-HCV:** Antibody against hepatitis C. Order to evaluate both acute and chronic hepatitis. Has a low false-positive rate. Used by blood banks to screen donors and part of routine hepatitis panel for evaluation of liver injury.
- **Anti-HCV RIBA:** Measures antibody to four separate HCV antigens. However, no longer used to confirm positive anti-HCV test.
- **HCV-RNA:** Detects presence of virus either qualitatively by sensitive RT-PCR or quantitatively by one of a number of tests with varying sensitivities and dynamic ranges. The qualitative test is used to confirm that the HCV-Ab represents an active infection; it is also used to assess the end-of-treatment response and "sustained viral response" (RNA negative at 24 weeks after therapy and likely cured) to interferon and ribavirin antiviral therapies. The quantitative test (viral load, in International Units) is obtained only before instituting antiviral therapy and at 12 weeks into therapy. This is to determine whether there has been an "early viral response" to therapy defined as $\geq$ 100-fold drop in IU or undetectable virus. Therapy is not continued beyond 12 weeks without an early viral response. HCV viral load does *not* correlate with amount of liver injury.
- **HCV-Genotype:** Important for determining likelihood of HCV infection responding to antiviral therapy with interferon and ribavirin. Genotype 1 patients with quantitative RNA values > 850,000 IU are less likely to respond to therapy than genotypes 2 and 3 patients. Genotype 1 patients usually require 48 weeks of therapy to achieve a 40–50% chance of cure; genotypes 2 and 3 patients require only 24 weeks of therapy to achieve a 70–80% chance of cure.

■ HUMAN CHORIONIC GONADOTROPIN, SERUM (HCG β-SUBUNIT)

Normal: < 3.0 mIU/mL.

Pregnancy: 7–10 days postconception, > 3 mIU/mL; 30 days, 100–5000 mIU/mL; 10 weeks, 50,000–140,000 mIU/mL; > 16 weeks, 10,000–50,000 mIU/mL; thereafter levels slowly decline.

Increased: Pregnancy, testicular tumors, trophoblastic disease (hydatidiform mole, choriocarcinoma levels usually > 100,000 mIU/mL).

■ HUMAN IMMUNODEFICIENCY VIRUS (HIV) ANTIBODY TEST

Negative: Used in diagnosis of acquired immunodeficiency syndrome (AIDS) and HIV infection and to screen blood for use in transfusion. May be negative in early HIV infection.

ELISA (Enzyme-Linked Immunosorbent Assay)

Used to detect HIV antibody. A positive test is usually repeated and then confirmed by Western blot analysis.

Positive: AIDS, asymptomatic HIV infection, false-positive test.

Western Blot

The technique is used as the reference procedure for confirming presence or absence of HIV antibody, usually after a positive HIV antibody by ELISA determination.

Positive: AIDS, asymptomatic HIV infection.

Note: Polymerase chain reaction is a very useful tool for detection of HIV virus. It is especially useful in very early infection, when antibody may not be present.

■ INTERNATIONAL NORMALIZED RATIO (INR)

See Table II–6, p. 469. See also Prothrombin Time, p. 474.
Normal: 1.0.
INR is used to standardize prothrombin results in patients taking anticoagulants. An INR of 2–3 is considered therapeutic for most indications. However, INR therapeutic goal ranges may vary for particular diseases.

■ IRON

Newborn: 100–250 mcg/dL.
Infant: 40–100 mcg/dL.
Child: 50–120 mcg/dL.
Adult male: 65–175 mcg/dL.
Adult female: 50–170 mcg/dL.

Increased: Hemochromatosis, hemosiderosis caused by excessive iron intake, excess destruction or decreased production of erythrocytes, liver necrosis.

Decreased: Iron deficiency anemia, nephrosis (loss of iron-binding proteins), anemia of chronic disease.

■ IRON-BINDING CAPACITY, TOTAL (TIBC)

Infant: 100–400 mcg/dL.
Adult: 250–450 mcg/dL.
Normal iron-to-TIBC ratio is 20–50%; < 15% is characteristic of iron deficiency anemia.

Increased: Acute and chronic blood loss, iron deficiency anemia, hepatitis.

Decreased: Anemia of chronic disease, nephrosis, hemochromatosis, cirrhosis.

■ KETONES, SERUM

Normal: 0.5–3.0 mg/dL.

Increased: Starvation, diabetic ketoacidosis, uncontrolled diabetes.

TABLE II–6. SELECTED AGE-SPECIFIC COAGULATION VALUES

Selected Coagulation Tests and Inhibitors	Preterm Infant, 30–36 Weeks, Day of Life #1	Term Infant, Day of Life #1	1–5 Years	6–10 Years	11–16 Years	Adult
Selected Coagulation Tests						
PT(s)	15.4 (14.6–16.9)	13.0 (10.1–15.9)	11 (10.6–11.4)	11.1 (10.1–12.1)	11.2 (10.2–12.0)	12 (11.0–14.0)
INR	—	—	1.0 (0.96–1.04)	1.0 (0.91–1.11)	1.02 (0.93–1.10)	1.10 (1.0–1.3)
APTT(s)	108 (80–168)	42.9 (31.3–54.3)	30 (24–36)	31 (26–36)	32 (26–37)	33 (27–40)
Fibrinogen (g/L)	2.43 (1.50–3.73)	2.83 (1.67–3.09)	2.76 (1.70–4.05)	2.79 (1.57–4.0)	3.0 (1.54–4.48)	2.78 (1.56–4.0)
Bleeding time (min)	—	—	6 (2.5–10)	7 (2.5–13)	5 (3–8)	4 (1–7)
Thrombin time(s)	14 (11–17)	12 (10–16)	—	—	—	10
II (units/mL)	0.45 (0.20–0.77)	0.48 (0.26–0.70)	0.94 (0.71–1.16)	0.88 (0.67–1.07)	0.83 (0.61–1.04)	1.08 (0.70–1.46)
V (units/mL)	0.88 (0.41–1.44)	0.72 (0.43–1.08)	1.03 (0.79–1.27)	0.90 (0.63–1.16)	0.77 (0.55–0.99)	1.06 (0.62–1.50)
VII (units/mL)	0.67 (0.21–1.13)	0.66 (0.28–1.04)	0.82 (0.55–1.16)	0.85 (0.52–1.20)	0.83 (0.58–1.15)	1.05 (0.67–1.43)
VIII (units/mL)	1.11 (0.50–2.13)	1.00 (0.50–1.78)	0.90 (0.59–1.42)	0.95 (0.58–1.32)	0.92 (0.53–1.31)	0.99 (0.50–1.49)
VWF (units/mL)	1.36 (0.78–2.10)	1.53 (0.50–2.87)	0.82 (0.47–1.04)	0.95 (0.44–1.44)	1.00 (0.46–1.53)	0.92 (0.50–1.58)
IX (units/mL)	0.35 (0.19–0.65)	0.53 (0.15–0.91)	0.73 (0.47–1.04)	0.75 (0.63–0.89)	0.87 (0.59–1.22)	1.09 (0.55–1.63)
X (units/mL)	0.41 (0.11–0.71)	0.40 (0.12–0.68)	0.88 (0.58–1.16)	0.75 (0.55–1.01)	0.79 (0.50–1.17)	1.06 (0.70–1.52)
XI (units/mL)	0.30 (0.08–0.52)	0.38 (0.10–0.66)	0.97 (0.56–1.50)	0.86 (0.52–1.20)	0.74 (0.50–0.97)	0.97 (0.67–1.27)
XII (units/mL)	0.38 (0.10–0.66)	0.53 (0.13–0.93)	0.93 (0.64–1.29)	0.92 (0.60–1.40)	0.81 (0.34–1.37)	1.08 (0.52–1.64)
D-Dimer	—	—	—	—	—	Positive titer ≥ 1:8
FDPs	—	—	—	—	—	Borderline titer = 1:25–1:50 Positive titer > 1:50
Selected Coagulation Inhibitors						
Protein C (units/mL)	0.28 (0.12–0.44)	0.35 (0.17–0.53)	0.66 (0.40–0.92)	0.69 (0.45–0.93)	0.83 (0.55–1.11)	0.96 (0.64–1.28)
Protein S (units/mL)	0.26 (0.14–0.38)	0.36 (0.12–0.60)	0.86 (0.54–1.18)	0.78 (0.41–1.14)	0.72 (0.52–0.92)	0.81 (0.60–1.13)

APTT = activated partial thromboplastin time; FDPs = fibrin degradation products; INR = international normalized ratio; PT = prothrombin time; vWF = von Willebrand factor.

Modified from Gunn, VL, Nechyba C. The Harriet Lane Handbook: A Manual for Pediatric House Officers, 16th ed. Mosby, 2002:296–297.

■ KOH PREP
Normal: Negative.

Positive: Superficial mycoses (*Candida, Trichophyton, Microsporum, Epidermophyton, Keratinomyces*).

■ LACTATE
Newborn: < 27 mg/dL.
Child and adult (venous): 4.5–19.8 mg/dL; arterial values are typically lower, 5–14 mg/dL.

Increased: In hypoxia, hemorrhage, circulatory collapse, sepsis, cirrhosis, with exercise.

■ LACTATE DEHYDROGENASE (LDH)
Newborn, 0–4 days: 290–775 units/L.
4–10 days: 545–2000 units/L.
10 days to 2 years: 180–430 units/L.
2–12 years: 110–295 units/L.
> 12 years: 100–190 units/L.

Increased: Acute myocardial infarction, cardiac surgery, hepatitis, pernicious anemia, malignant tumors, pulmonary embolus, hemolysis, renal infarction, prognostic factor in HIV patients with *pneumocystis carinii* pneumonia.

■ LIGASE CHAIN REACTION FOR *NEISSERIA GONORRHOEAE* AND *CHLAMYDIA TRACHOMATIS* FOR URINE
Normal: Not detected.
Useful screening test for infections by these agents in populations in which there is high prevalence; patient should not have voided 2 hours before providing specimen.

■ LIPASE
Variable, depending on method:
Infant, 0–3 months: 10–85 units/L.
3–12 months: 9–128 units/L.
1–11 years: 10–150 units/L.
Adult: 10–220 units/L.

Increased: Acute pancreatitis, pancreatic duct obstruction (stone, stricture, tumor). Usually normal in mumps.

■ MAGNESIUM
Normal: 1.2–2.6 mg/dL.

Increased: See Section I, Chapter 42, Hypermagnesemia, p. 201.

Decreased: See Section I, Chapter 49, Hypomagnesemia, p. 229.

■ MONOSPOT
Normal: Negative.

Positive: Mononucleosis.

■ MYOGLOBIN, URINE
Normal: Qualitative negative.

Positive: Disorders affecting skeletal muscle (crush injury, rhabdomyolysis, electrical burns, seizures, surgery), fever, malignant hyperthermia, some metabolic disorders. Can be positive with influenza.

■ OSMOLALITY, SERUM
Normal: 275–295 mOsm/kg.
Note: A rough estimation of osmolality is [2(Na) + BUN/2.8 + glucose/18]). The calculation will not be accurate if foreign substances that increase osmolality (eg, mannitol) are present. If foreign substances are suspected, osmolality should be measured directly.

Increased: Hyperglycemia, alcohol or ethylene glycol ingestion, increased sodium resulting from water loss (diabetes insipidus, hypercalcemia, diuresis), mannitol.

Decreased: Low serum sodium, diuretics, Addison disease, hypothyroidism, syndrome of inappropriate antidiuretic hormone (SIADH), iatrogenic causes (poor fluid balance).

■ OSMOLALITY, URINE
Spot: 50–1400 mOsm/kg; > 850 mOsm/kg after 12 hours of fluid restriction. Loss of ability to concentrate urine, especially during fluid restriction, is an early indicator of impaired renal function.

■ PARTIAL THROMBOPLASTIN TIME (PTT)
Normal: 27–38 seconds.
Note: Newborns may have slightly higher values, up to 42 seconds.

Prolonged: Heparin and any defect in the intrinsic clotting mechanism, such as severe liver disease or disseminated intravascular coagulation (includes factors I, II, V, VIII, IX, X, XI, and XII); prolonged use of tourniquet before drawing a blood sample; hemophilia A and B; lupus anticoagulant; liver disease. Also, elevated in the presence of lupus anticoagulant. See Section I, Chapter 16, Coagulopathy, p. 80.

■ PH, ARTERIAL
See Tables II–2 and II–3, p. 455.

Increased: Metabolic and respiratory alkalosis. See Section I, Chapter 5, Alkalosis, p. 23.

Decreased: Metabolic and respiratory acidosis. See Section I, Chapter 3, Acidosis, p. 13.

■ PHOSPHORUS
Newborn, 0–5 days: 4.8–8.2 mg/dL.
1–3 years: 3.8–6.5 mg/dL.
4–11 years: 3.7–5.6 mg/dL.
12–15 years: 2.9–5.4 mg/dL.
16–19 years: 2.7–4.7 mg/dL.

Increased: See Section I, Chapter 44, Hyperphosphatemia, p. 209.

Decreased: See Section I, Chapter 51, Hypophosphatemia, p. 236.

■ PLATELETS
For normal values, see Appendix A, Blood Cell Indices, p. 758.
Note: Platelet counts may be normal in number, but abnormal in function (eg, aspirin therapy). Platelet function with a normal platelet count can be assessed by measuring bleeding time. Bleeding time is normally < 6–10 minutes, depending on the laboratory.

Increased: Primary thrombocytosis; secondary thrombocytosis (collagen-vascular diseases, chronic infection [osteomyelitis, tuberculosis], sarcoidosis, hemolytic anemia, iron deficiency anemia, recovery from vitamin B_{12} deficiency, solid tumors and lymphomas; after surgery, especially post-splenectomy; Kawasaki disease).

Decreased: See Section I, Chapter 87, Thrombocytopenia, p. 408.

■ POTASSIUM, SERUM
Newborn: 3.7–5.9 mEq/L.
Infant: 4.1–5.3 mEq/L.
Child: 3.4-4.7 mEq/L.
Adult: 3.5–5.1 mEq/L.

Increased: See Section I, Chapter 41, Hyperkalemia, p. 196.

Decreased: See Section I, Chapter 48, Hypokalemia, p. 226.

■ PROTEIN, SERUM (TOTAL)
Newborn: 4.6–7.4 g/dL.
1–7 years: 6.1–7.9 g/dL.
8–12 years: 6.4–8.1 g/dL.
Adult: 6.0–7.8 g/dL.

Increased: Chronic inflammatory disease, lymphoma, multiple myeloma.

Decreased: Any cause of decreased albumin or any cause of hypogammaglobulinemia.

■ PROTEIN, URINE
See also Albumin, Urine, pp. 449–450.
Full term: 32 (range: 15–68) mg/24-h urine.
2–12 months: 38 (17–85) mg/24-h urine.
2–4 years: 49 (20–121) mg/24-h urine.
4–10 years: 71 (26–194) mg/24-h urine.
10–16 years: 83 (29–238) mg/24-h urine.
Adults: < 100 mg/24-h urine.
Spot: < 10 mg/dL (< 20 mg/dL if early-morning collection).
Dipstick: Negative.

Increased: Nephrotic syndrome, glomerulonephritis, lupus nephritis, renal vein thrombosis, postural proteinuria, polycystic kidney disease, diabetic nephropathy, radiation nephritis, malignant hypertension, multiple myeloma.

False-Positive: Gross hematuria, very concentrated urine, phenazopyridine hydrochloride (Pyridium), very alkaline urine.

■ PROTEIN C, PLASMA
See Table II–6, p. 469.

Decreased: Hypercoagulable states resulting in recurrent venous thrombosis, chronic liver disease, disseminated intravascular coagulation, postoperatively, neoplastic disease and autosomal-recessive deficiency.

■ PROTEIN S, PLASMA
See Table II–6, p. 469.

Decreased: See Protein C, Plasma, above. Protein S is a cofactor of protein C; should be ordered along with protein C.

■ PROTHROMBIN TIME (PT)

See International Normalized Ratio (INR), p. 468. See also Table II–6, p. 469. Evaluates extrinsic clotting mechanism (factors I, II, V, VII, and X).

Prolonged: Drugs such as sodium warfarin (Coumadin), decreased vitamin K, fat malabsorption, liver disease, prolonged use of a tourniquet before drawing a blood sample, disseminated intravascular coagulation, lupus anticoagulant (usually selectively increased PTT). See Section I, Chapter 16, Coagulopathy, p. 80.

■ QUANTITATIVE IMMUNOGLOBULINS

See Table II–7, p. 475.

Increased: Bacterial and viral infections, liver disease, sarcoidosis, amyloidosis, myeloproliferative disorders, lymphoma.

Decreased: Hereditary immunodeficiency, leukemia, lymphoma, nephrotic syndrome, protein-losing enteropathy, malnutrition.

■ RAPID PLASMA REAGIN (RPR)

See VDRL, p. 484.

■ RED BLOOD CELL COUNT (RBC)

For normal values, see Appendix A, Blood Cell Indices, p. 758. See also Hematocrit, p. 465.

■ RED BLOOD CELL INDICES

For normal values, see Appendix A, Blood Cell Indices, p. 758.

MCV (Mean Cell Volume)

Increased: Megaloblastic anemia (vitamin B_{12}, folate deficiency), reticulocytosis, chronic liver disease, hypothyroidism, aplastic anemia.

Decreased: Iron deficiency, thalassemia, some cases of lead poisoning, hereditary spherocytosis, sideroblastic anemia.

MCH (Mean Cellular Hemoglobin)

Increased: Macrocytosis (megaloblastic anemias, high reticulocyte counts).

Decreased: Microcytosis (iron deficiency).

MCHC (Mean Cellular Hemoglobin Concentration)

Increased: Severe and prolonged dehydration; spherocytosis.

TABLE II–7. SERUM IMMUNOGLOBULIN LEVELS[a]

Age	IgG (mg/dL)	IgM (mg/dL)	IgA (mg/dL)	IgE (IU/mL)
Cord blood (term)	1121 (636–1606)	13 (6.3–25)	2.3 (1.4–3.6)	0.22 (0.04–1.28)
1 mo	503 (251–906)	45 (20–87)	13 (1.3–53)	—
6 wk	—	—	—	0.69 (0.08–6.12)
2 mo	365 (206–601)	46 (17–105)	15 (2.8–47)	—
3 mo	334 (176–581)	49 (24–89)	17 (4.6–46)	0.82 (0.18–3.76)
4 mo	343 (196–558)	55 (27–101)	23 (4.4–73)	—
5 mo	403 (172–814)	62 (33–108)	31 (8.1–84)	—
6 mo	407 (215–704)	62 (35–102)	25 (8.1–68)	2.68 (0.44–16.3)
7–9 mo	475 (217–904)	80 (34–126)	36 (11–90)	2.36 (0.76–7.31)
10–12 mo	594 (294–1069)	82 (41–149)	40 (16–84)	—
1 y	679 (345–1213)	93 (43–173)	44 (14–106)	3.49 (0.80–15.2)
2 y	685 (424–1051)	95 (48–168)	47 (14–123)	3.03 (0.31–29.5)
3 y	728 (441–1135)	104 (47–200)	66 (22–159)	1.80 (0.19–16.9)
4–5 y	780 (463–1236)	99 (43–196)	68 (25–154)	8.58 (1.07–68.9)[b]
6–8 y	915 (633–1280)	107 (48–207)	90 (33–202)	12.89 (1.03–161.3)[c]
9–10 y	1007 (608–1572)	121 (52–242)	113 (45–236)	23.6 (0.98–570.6)[d]
14 y	—	—	—	20.07 (2.06–195.2)
Adult	994 (639–1349)	156 (56–352)	171 (70–312)	13.2 (1.53–114)

[a]Numbers in parentheses are 95% confidence intervals (CIs).
[b]IgE data for 4 years.
[c]IgE data for 7 years.
[d]IgE data for 10 years.

From Kjellman NM, Johansson SG, Roth A. Clin Allergy 1976;6:51–59; Joliff CR, et al. Clin Chem 1982;28:126–128; and Zetterström O, Johansson SG. Allergy 1981;36(8):537–547 (Blackwell Publishing). In Gunn VL, Nechyba C. The Harriet Lane Handbook: A Manual for Pediatric House Officers, 16th ed. Mosby. 2002:312, with permission from Elsevier.

Decreased: Iron deficiency anemia, overhydration, thalassemia, sidero-blastic anemia.

RDW (Red Cell Distribution Width)

Measure of degree of homogeneity of RBC size.

Increased: Suggests two different populations of RBCs, such as a combination of macrocytic and microcytic anemia or recovery from iron deficiency anemia (microcytosis plus reticulocytosis).

■ RED BLOOD CELL MORPHOLOGY
- **Poikilocytosis:** Irregular RBC shape (sickle, burr).
- **Anisocytosis:** Irregular RBC size (microcytes, macrocytes).
- **Basophilic stippling:** Lead, heavy metal poisoning, thalassemia.
- **Howell-Jolly bodies:** Seen after splenectomy and in some severe anemias.
- **Sickling:** Sickle cell disease and trait.
- **Nucleated RBCs:** Severe bone marrow stress (hemorrhage, hemolysis), marrow replacement by tumor, extramedullary hematopoiesis.
- **Target cells:** Thalassemia, hemoglobinopathies (sickle cell disease), obstructive jaundice, any hypochromic anemia, after splenectomy.
- **Spherocytes:** Hereditary spherocytosis, immune or microangiopathic hemolysis.
- **Helmet cells (schistocytes):** Microangiopathic hemolysis, hemolytic transfusion reaction, other hemolytic anemias.
- **Burr cells (acanthocytes):** Severe liver disease; high levels of bile, fatty acids, or toxins.
- **Polychromasia:** Appearance of a bluish-gray RBC on routine Wright stain suggests reticulocytes.

■ RETICULOCYTE COUNT
Normal: 0.5–1.5%.
See also Appendix A, Blood Cell Indices, p. 758.
If the hematocrit is abnormal, a corrected reticulocyte count should be calculated as follows:

$$\text{Corrected reticulocyte count} = \frac{\% \text{ Reticulocytes} \times \text{Patient's Hct}}{4 \%}$$

Increased: Hemolysis, acute hemorrhage, therapeutic response to treatment for iron, vitamin B_{12}, or folate deficiency.

Decreased: Infiltration of bone marrow (leukemia, lymphoma); marrow aplasia; chronic infections such as osteomyelitis; toxins; drugs (> 100 reported); many anemias.

■ RHEUMATOID FACTOR (RA LATEX TEST)
Normal: < 15 IU by microscan kit or < 1:40.

Increased: Rheumatoid arthritis, systemic lupus erythematosus, Sjögren syndrome, scleroderma, dermatomyositis, polymyositis, syphilis, chronic inflammation, subacute bacterial endocarditis, hepatitis, sarcoidosis, interstitial pulmonary fibrosis.

■ SEDIMENTATION RATE (ESR)
Neonate, term: 0–4 mm/h.
Child: 4–20 mm/h.
Adult male: 1–15 mm/h.
Adult female: 4–25 mm/h.

Increased: Infection, inflammation, rheumatic fever, endocarditis, neoplasm, acute myocardial infarction. Anemia may falsely elevate some ESR scales. Obesity, renal disease, pregnancy, and heparin may also falsely elevate values.

■ SGGT (SERUM γ-GLUTAMYLTRANSFERASE)
See γ-Glutamyltransferase (GGT), p. 463.

■ SGOT (SERUM GLUTAMIC-OXALOACETIC TRANSFERASE) OR AST (SERUM ASPARTATE AMINOTRANSFERASE)
See AST, pp. 452–453.

■ SGPT (SERUM GLUTAMIC-PYRUVIC TRANSFERASE) OR ALT (SERUM ALANINE AMINOTRANSFERASE)
See ALT, p. 450.

■ SODIUM, SERUM
Normal: 136–146 mEq/L.

Increased: See Section I, Chapter 43, Hypernatremia, p. 203.

Decreased: See Section I, Chapter 50, Hyponatremia, p. 232.

■ STOOL FOR OCCULT BLOOD (HEMOCCULT TEST)
Normal: Negative.

Positive: Swallowed blood, ingestion of red meat, any GI tract lesion, bacterial enteritis (*Salmonella, Shigella, Campylobacter, Yersinia,* enteropathogenic *E coli* [O157:H7]), large doses of vitamin C (> 500 mg/day).

■ STOOL FOR WHITE BLOOD CELLS (WBCS)
Normal: Occasional WBCs, usually polymorphonuclear neutrophils.

Increased: Shigella, Salmonella, enteropathogenic E coli, pseudomembranous colitis (*Clostridium difficile*), ulcerative colitis.

■ T$_3$ (TRIIODOTHYRONINE) RADIOIMMUNOASSAY
Newborn: 99–380 ng/dL.
1 month to 5 years: 102–269 ng/dL.
6–10 years: 94–241 ng/dL.
≥ 11 through adolescence: 80–213 ng/dL.
Adult: 70–204 ng/dL.

■ T$_4$ (THYROXINE), FREE
Infants, 1–10 days: 0.6–2.0 ng/dL.
> 10 days: 0.7–1.7 ng/dL.
See also Table II–8.

Increased: Hyperthyroidism, exogenous thyroid hormone, any cause of increased thyroid-binding globulin (eg, estrogens, pregnancy, or hepatitis), euthyroid sick state.

Decreased: Hypothyroidism, euthyroid sick state, any cause of decreased thyroid-binding globulin (eg, malnutrition).

■ THROMBIN TIME
See Table II–6, p. 469.

TABLE II-8. THYROID FUNCTION TESTS: INTERPRETATION

Condition	TSH	T$_4$	Free T$_4$
Primary hyperthyroidism	L	H	High N to H
Primary hypothyroidism	H	L	L
Hypothalamic/pituitary hypothyroidism	L, N, H[a]	L	L
TBG deficiency	N	L	N
Euthyroid sick syndrome	L, N, H[a]	L	L to low N
TSH adenoma or pituitary resistance	N to H	H	H
Compensated hypothyroidism[b]	H	N	N

H = high; L = low; N = normal; T$_4$ = thyroxine; TBG = thyroid-binding globulin; TSH = thyroid-stimulating hormone.
[a] Can be normal, slightly low, or slightly high.
[b] Treatment may not be necessary.
From Gunn VL, Nechyba C. The Harriet Lane Handbook: A Manual for Pediatric House Officers, 16th ed. Mosby, 2002:217.

Increased: Heparin, disseminated intravascular coagulation, elevated fibrin degradation products, fibrinogen deficiency, congenitally abnormal fibrinogen molecules. See Section I, Chapter 16, Coagulopathy, p. 80.

■ THYROID-BINDING GLOBULIN (TBG)
1–4 weeks: 0.5–4.5 mg/dL.
1–12 months: 1.6–3.6 mg/dL.
> 1 year: 1.2–2.8 mg/dL.

Increased: Hypothyroidism, pregnancy, medications (oral contraceptives, estrogens), hepatitis, acute porphyria, familial.

Decreased: Hyperthyroidism, medications (androgens, anabolic steroids, corticosteroids, phenytoin), nephrotic syndrome, severe illness, liver failure, malnutrition.

■ THYROID-STIMULATING HORMONE (TSH)
1–3 days: < 2.5–13.3 milliunits/mL.
1–4 weeks: 0.6–10.0 milliunits/mL.
1–15 years: 0.6–6.3 milliunits/mL.
> 15 years: 0.2–7.6 milliunits/mL.
See also Table II–8, p. 478.
Note: Newer sensitive assays are excellent screening tests for hyperthyroidism as well as hypothyroidism; they allow clinician to distinguish between a low normal and a decreased TSH.

Increased: Hypothyroidism.

Decreased: Hyperthyroidism. A few cases of hypothyroidism result from pituitary or hypothalamic disease that causes a decreased TSH.

■ TRANSFERRIN
Newborn: 130–275 mg/dL.
3 months to 10 years: 203–360 mg/dL.
Adult: 220–400 mg/dL.

Increased: Acute and chronic blood loss, iron deficiency anemia, hepatitis, oral contraceptives.

Decreased: Anemia of chronic disease, cirrhosis, malnutrition nephrosis, hemochromatosis.

■ TRYPTASE
Normal: 5.6–13.5 mcg/L.

Increased: Diseases of mast cell activation such as anaphylaxis or mastocytosis.

Note: Released in a slower manner than histamine and more stable so that it can be detected for a longer period of time than histamine. In anaphylaxis, histamine peaks in 5 minutes and returns to normal in < 1 hour. Tryptase peaks in 1–2 hours and returns to normal after a few hours.

■ URIC ACID

Term newborn to 2 years: 2.4–6.4 mg/dL.
2–12 years: 2.4–5.9 mg/dL.
12–14 years: 2.4–6.4 mg/dL.
Adult male: 4.5–8.2 mg/dL.
Adult female: 3.0–6.5 mg/dL.

Increased: Destruction of massive amounts of nucleoproteins (tumor lysis after chemotherapy), drugs (especially diuretics), hypothyroidism, polycystic kidney disease, parathyroid diseases, renal failure.

Decreased: Uricosuric drugs (salicylates, probenecid, allopurinol), Wilson disease, Fanconi syndrome.

■ URINALYSIS, ROUTINE
Appearance

- **Normal:** Yellow, clear, straw-colored.
- **Pink/red:** Blood, hemoglobin, myoglobin, food coloring, beets.
- **Orange:** Pyridium, rifampin, bile pigments.
- **Brown/black:** Myoglobin, bile pigments, melanin, cascara bark, iron, nitrofurantoin, metronidazole, sickle cell crisis.
- **Blue:** Methylene blue, *Pseudomonas* UTI (rare), hereditary tryptophan metabolic disorders.
- **Cloudy:** UTI (pyuria), blood, myoglobin, chyluria, mucus (normal in ileal loop specimens), phosphate salts (normal in alkaline urine), urates (normal in acidic urine), hyperoxaluria.
- **Foamy:** Proteinuria, bile salts.

pH

Normal: 4.6–8.0.

Acidic: High-protein diet, acidosis, ketoacidosis (starvation, diabetic), diarrhea, dehydration.

Basic: UTI involving *Proteus;* renal tubular acidosis; diet (high vegetable, milk, immediately postprandial); sodium bicarbonate or acetazolamide therapy; vomiting; metabolic alkalosis; chronic renal failure.

Specific Gravity

Normal: 1.001–1.035.

Increased: Volume depletion, congestive heart failure, adrenal insufficiency, diabetes mellitus, SIADH, increased proteins (nephrosis). If markedly increased (1.040–1.050), suspect artifact, excretion of radiographic contrast medium, or some other osmotic agent.

Decreased: Diabetes insipidus, pyelonephritis, glomerulonephritis, water load with normal renal function.

Bilirubin

Normal: Negative dipstick.

Positive: Obstructive jaundice, hepatitis, cirrhosis, congestive heart failure with hepatic congestion, congenital hyperbilirubinemia (Dubin-Johnson syndrome).

Blood (Hemoglobin)

Normal: Negative dipstick.

Positive: Hematuria (See Section I, Chapter 35, Hematuria, p. 172); free hemoglobin (from trauma, transfusion reaction, or lysis of red blood cells); or myoglobin (crush injury, burn, or tissue ischemia).

Glucose

Normal: Negative dipstick.

Positive: Diabetes mellitus, other endocrine disorders (pheochromocytoma, hyperthyroidism, Cushing syndrome, hyperadrenalism); stress states (sepsis, burns), pancreatitis, renal tubular disease, medications (corticosteroids, thiazides, birth control pills), false-positive with vitamin C ingestion.

Ketones

Normal: Negative dipstick.

Positive: Starvation, high-fat diet, diabetic ketoacidosis, vomiting, diarrhea, hyperthyroidism, febrile states, pregnancy.

Leukocyte Esterase

Normal: Negative dipstick.

Positive: Infection (test detects 5 or more WBCs per high-power field (HPF) or lysed WBCs).

Microscopy

Note: Many laboratories no longer perform urine microscopy on a routine basis when dipstick is negative and gross appearance is normal.

- **RBCs:** (Normal: 0–2/HPF.) Trauma, UTI, golmerulonephritis, nephrolithiasis, genitourinary tuberculosis.
- **WBCs:** (Normal: 0–4/HPF.) Infection anywhere in urinary tract, acute glomerulonephritis, radiation damage, interstitial nephritis (analgesic abuse), genitourinary tuberculosis. (Glitter cells represent WBCs lysed in hypotonic solution.)
- **Epithelial cells:** (Normal: Occasional.) Acute tubular necrosis.
- **Parasites:** (Normal: None.) *Trichomonas vaginalis, Schistosoma haematobium.*
- **Crystals:** (Normal: *Acid urine:* Calcium oxalate (small square crystals with a central cross), uric acid. *Alkaline urine:* Calcium carbonate, triple phosphate (resemble coffin lids.) Abnormal: Cystine, sulfonamide, leucine, tyrosine, cholesterol, or excessive amounts of crystals noted earlier.
- **Contaminants:** Cotton threads, hair, wood fibers, amorphous substances (all usually unimportant).
- **Mucus:** (Normal: Small amounts.) Large amounts suggest urethral disease.
- **Hyaline cast:** (Normal: Occasional.) Benign hypertension, nephrotic syndrome.
- **RBC cast:** (Normal: None.) Acute glomerulonephritis, lupus nephritis, subacute bacterial endocarditis, Goodpasture disease, vasculitis, malignant hypertension.
- **WBC cast:** (Normal: None.) Pyelonephritis or interstitial nephritis.
- **Epithelial cast:** (Normal: Occasional.) Tubular damage, nephrotoxin, viral infections.
- **Granular cast:** (Normal: None.) Results from breakdown of cellular casts, leads to waxy casts.
- **Waxy cast:** (Normal: None.) End stage of a granular cast; evidence of severe chronic renal disease.
- **Fatty cast:** (Normal: None.) Nephrotic syndrome, diabetes mellitus, damaged renal tubular epithelial cells.
- **Broad cast:** (Normal: None.) Chronic renal disease.

Nitrite

Normal: Negative dipstick.

Positive: Bacterial infection (negative test does not rule out infection).

Protein

See also Albumin, Urine, pp. 449–450.
Normal: Negative dipstick.

Positive: See Protein, Urine, p. 473.

Reducing Substance

Normal: Negative dipstick.

Positive: Glucose, fructose, galactose.

False-Positives: Vitamin C, antibiotics.

Urobilinogen

Normal: Negative dipstick.

Positive: Bile duct obstruction, suppression of gut flora with antibiotics.

■ URINARY ELECTROLYTES

These "spot urines" are of limited value because of large variations in daily fluid and salt intake. Results are usually indeterminate if a diuretic has been given. Sodium is most useful in the differentiation of volume depletion, oliguria, or hyponatremia. Chloride is useful in the diagnosis and treatment of metabolic alkalosis. Urinary potassium levels are often used in the evaluation of hypokalemia.

- **Chloride < 10 mmol/L:** Chloride-sensitive metabolic alkalosis. See Section I, Chapter 5, Alkalosis, p. 23.
- **Chloride > 20 mmol/L:** Chloride-resistant metabolic alkalosis. See Section I, Chapter 5, Alkalosis, p. 23.
- **Potassium < 10 mmol/L:** Hypokalemia, from extrarenal losses.
- **Potassium > 10 mmol/L:** Renal potassium wasting (diuretics, brisk urinary output).
- **Sodium < 20 mmol/L:** Volume depletion, hyponatremic states, prerenal azotemia (congestive heart failure, shock, others), hepatorenal syndrome, edematous states.
- **Sodium > 40 mmol/L:** Acute tubular necrosis, adrenal insufficiency, renal salt wasting, SIADH.
- **Sodium > 20–40 mmol/L:** Indeterminate.

■ URINARY INDICES

The indices in Table II–9 are used in determining the cause of oliguria. See Section I, Chapter 78, Renal Failure, Acute, p. 360.

■ VANILLYLMANDELIC ACID (VMA), URINE

See Catecholamines, Urine, pp. 457–458. VMA is urinary metabolite of both epinephrine and norepinephrine.

Increased: Pheochromocytoma; neural crest tumors (neuroblastoma, ganglioneuroma). False-positive with methyldopa, chocolate, vanilla, others.

TABLE II-9. URINARY INDICES IN ACUTE RENAL FAILURE ACCOMPANIED BY OLIGURIA: DIFFERENTIAL DIAGNOSIS OF OLIGURIA

Index	Prerenal	Renal (ATN)
Urine osmolality	>500	<350
Urinary sodium	<10–20	>30–40
Urine/serum creatinine	>40	<20
Fractional excreted sodium[a]	<1	>1
Renal failure index[b]	<1	>1

ATN = acute tubular necrosis.

[a] Fractional excreted sodium $= \dfrac{\text{(Urine/serum sodium)}}{\text{(Urine/serum creatinine)}} \times 100$.

[b] Renal failure index $= \dfrac{\text{(Urine sodium} \times \text{serum creatinine)}}{\text{(Urine creatinine)}}$.

Modified and reproduced with permission from Gomella LG, Haist SA, eds. Clinician's Pocket Reference, 10th ed. McGraw-Hill. Copyright © 2004.

■ VDRL TEST (VENEREAL DISEASE RESEARCH LABORATORY) OR RAPID PLASMA REAGIN (RPR)

Normal: Nonreactive.

Useful for screening syphilis. Almost always positive in secondary syphilis, but frequently becomes negative in late syphilis. Also, in some patients with HIV infection, VDRL can be negative in primary and secondary syphilis.

Positive (Reactive): Syphilis, systemic lupus erythematosus, pregnancy, and drug addiction. If reactive, confirm with FTA-ABS (false-positives may occur with bacterial or viral illnesses.

■ WHITE BLOOD CELL COUNT

For normal values, see Appendix A, Blood Cell Indices, p. 758.

Increased: See Section I, Chapter 62, Leukocytosis, p. 282.

Decreased: See Section I, Chapter 63, Leukopenia and Neutropenia, p. 287.

■ WHITE BLOOD CELL DIFFERENTIAL

See Table II–10, p. 485. Many hospitals now perform differentials on automated machines. The newer automated differentials can differentiate neutrophils, lymphocytes, monocytes, eosinophils, and basophils. A manual differential must be done to differentiate segmented and banded neutrophils.

Neutrophils

Normal: 40–70% segmented neutrophils, 5–10% banded neutrophils.

TABLE II–10. AGE-SPECIFIC LEUKOCYTE DIFFERENTIAL

Age	Total Leukocytes[a] Mean (range)	Neutrophils[b] Mean (range)	%	Lymphocytes Mean (range)	%	Monocytes Mean	%	Eosinophils Mean	%
Birth	18.1 (9–30)	11 (6–26)	61	5.5 (2–11)	31	1.1	6	0.4	2
12 h	22.8 (13–38)	15.5 (6–28)	68	5.5 (2–11)	24	1.2	5	0.5	2
24 h	18.9 (9.4–34)	11.5 (5–21)	61	5.8 (2–11.5)	31	1.1	6	0.5	2
1 wk	12.2 (5–21)	5.5 (1.5–10)	45	5.0 (2–17)	41	1.1	9	0.5	4
2 wk	11.4 (5–20)	4.5 (1–9.5)	40	5.5 (2–17)	48	1.0	9	0.4	3
1 mo	10.8 (5–19.5)	3.8 (1–8.5)	35	6.0 (2.5–16.5)	56	0.7	7	0.3	3
6 mo	11.9 (6–17.5)	3.8 (1–8.5)	32	7.3 (4–13.5)	61	0.6	5	0.3	3
1 y	11.4 (6–17.5)	3.5 (1.5–8.5)	31	7.0 (4–10.5)	61	0.6	5	0.3	3
2 y	10.6 (6–17)	3.5 (1.5–8.5)	33	6.3 (3–9.5)	59	0.5	5	0.3	3
4 y	9.1 (5.5–15.5)	3.8 (1.5–8.5)	42	4.5 (2–8)	50	0.5	5	0.3	3
6 y	8.5 (5–14.5)	4.3 (1.5–8)	51	3.5 (1.5–7)	42	0.4	5	0.2	3
8 y	8.3 (4.5–13.5)	4.4 (1.5–8)	53	3.3 (1.5–6.8)	39	0.4	4	0.2	2
10 y	8.1 (4.5–13.5)	4.4 (1.5–8.5)	54	3.1 (1.5–6.5)	38	0.4	4	0.2	3
16 y	7.8 (4.5–13.0)	4.4 (1.8–8)	57	2.8 (1.2–5.2)	35	0.4	5	0.2	2
21 y	7.4 (4.5–11.0)	4.4 (1.8–7.7)	59	2.5 (1–4.8)	34	0.3	4	0.2	3

[a]Numbers of leukocytes are × 10³/mm³; ranges are estimates of 95% confidence limits; percents refer to differential count.
[b]Neutrophils include band cells at all ages and a small number of metamyelocytes and myelocytes in the first few days of life.
From Dallman PR. In: Rudolph AM, ed. Pediatrics. 20th ed. New York: McGraw-Hill, 1996.

Increased: Exercise, pain, stress, infection, burns, drugs, thyrotoxicosis, steroids, malignancy, chronic inflammatory disease (vasculitis, collagen-vascular disease, colitis), lithium, epinephrine, asplenia, idiopathic.

Decreased: Congenital, immune-mediated, drug-induced, infectious (viral, rickettsial, parasitic).

Lymphocytes

Normal: 24–44%.

Increased: Measles, German measles (rubeola), mumps, whooping cough (*Bordetella pertussis*), smallpox, chickenpox (varicella), influenza, viral hepatitis, infectious mononucleosis (Epstein-Barr virus), virtually any viral infection, leukemia.

Decreased: Following stress, burns, trauma; normal finding in 22% of population; uremia; some viral infections (including HIV).

Lymphocytes, Atypical

Normal: 0–3%.

> *20%:* Infectious mononucleosis (Epstein-Barr virus), cytomegalovirus infection, viral hepatitis, toxoplasmosis.

3–20%: Viral infections (mumps, rubeola, varicella), rickettsial infections, tuberculosis.

Monocytes

Normal: 3–7%.

Increased: Subacute bacterial endocarditis, brucellosis (*Brucella*), typhoid fever (*Salmonella typhi*), kala-azar (visceral leishmaniasis), trypanosomiasis (*Trypanosoma*), rickettsial infection, ulcerative colitis, sarcoidosis, Hodgkin disease, monocytic leukemias, collagen-vascular diseases.

Decreased: Myelodysplasia, aplastic anemia, hairy cell leukemia, cyclic neutropenia, thermal injuries, collagen-vascular diseases.

Eosinophils

Normal: 0–3%.

Increased: Allergies, parasites, skin diseases, malignancy, drugs, asthma, Addison disease, collagen-vascular diseases. (A handy mnemonic is **NAACP: N**eoplasm, **A**llergy, **A**ddison disease, **C**ollagen-vascular diseases, **P**arasites).

Decreased: After steroids; ACTH; after stress (infection, trauma, burns); Cushing syndrome.

Basophils

Normal: 0–1%.

Increased: Chronic myeloid leukemia; rarely, in recovery from infection and from hypothyroidism.

Decreased: Acute rheumatic fever, lobar pneumonia, after steroid therapy, thyrotoxicosis, stress.

■ WHITE BLOOD CELL MORPHOLOGY
- **Auer rod:** Acute myelogenous leukemias.
- **Döhle bodies:** Severe infection, burns, malignancy, pregnancy.
- **Hypersegmentation:** Megaloblastic anemias, iron deficiency, myeloproliferative disorders, drug induced.
- **Toxic granulation:** Severe illness (sepsis, burns, high temperature).

■ ZINC
Normal: 60–130 mcg/dL or 9–20 micromoles/L.

Increased: Atherosclerosis, coronary artery disease.

Decreased: Inadequate dietary intake (parenteral nutrition, alcoholism); malabsorption; increased needs such as pregnancy or wound healing; acrodermatitis enteropathica.

REFERENCES

Burtis CA, Ashwood ER. *Tietz's Textbook of Clinical Chemistry,* 3rd ed. Saunders, 1999.

Coudrey L. The troponins. *Arch Intern Med* 1998;158:1173.

Gunn VL, Nechyba C. *The Harriet Lane Handbook: A Manual for Pediatric House Officers,* 16th ed. Mosby, 2002.

Henry JB, ed. *Clinical Diagnosis and Management by Laboratory Methods,* 20th ed. Saunders, 2001.

Jurado R, Mattix H. The decreased serum urea nitrogen-creatinine ratio. *Arch Intern Med* 1998;115:2509.

Lefor AT, ed. *Critical Care On Call.* McGraw-Hill, 2002.

Pettijohn TL, Doyle T, Spiekerman AM, et al: Usefulness of positive troponin-T and negative creatine kinase levels in identifying high-risk patients with unstable angina pectoris. *Am J Cardiol* 1997;80:510.

III. Bedside Procedures

Note: Before a procedure is performed, properly identify child and wash hands. Consent should be discussed with parent or legal guardian before a nonemergency procedure is performed.

1. ARTERIAL LINE PLACEMENT

Indications

1. Frequent sampling of arterial blood.
2. Blood gas determination.
3. Hemodynamic monitoring when continuous BP readings are needed (eg, child who is receiving vasopressor medication).

Contraindications

1. Poor collateral circulation.
2. Skin infection near planned puncture site.
3. Bleeding disorders or thrombolytic therapy (relative contraindication).

Materials: 22-gauge (or smaller), 1.5–2-inch catheter-over-needle assembly (Angiocath) or similar size prepackaged arterial line set; 25-gauge needle; arterial line setup per ICU routine (transducer, tubing, and pressure bag with heparinized saline); armboard; sterile gloves; mask; adhesive tape; gauze; sterile dressing; 3-0 silk suture; 1% lidocaine.

Procedure

1. The radial artery is most frequently used; this approach is described here. Other less preferable sites include dorsalis pedis, femoral, and axillary arteries. Axillary arteries are infrequently used; catheters in these arteries should be placed by an intensivist or anesthesiologist.
2. Verify patency of collateral circulation between radial and ulnar arteries using the **Allen test.** Clench child's hand while simultaneously compressing the ulnar and radial arteries. The hand will blanch. Release pressure from the ulnar artery and observe the flushing response. If the ulnar-brachial arterial arch is patent, the entire hand should flush within seconds.
3. Secure child's hand to a short armboard. A roll of gauze behind the wrist may be used to elevate the wrist and bring the radial and brachial arteries closer to the surface. Leave the fingers exposed to observe any color change. Prepare the wrist with sterile technique and drape with sterile towels. Operator should wear gloves and mask.
4. Raise a very small skin wheal at the puncture site with 1% lidocaine using a 25-gauge needle. Carefully palpate the artery and choose the puncture site where it appears most superficial.

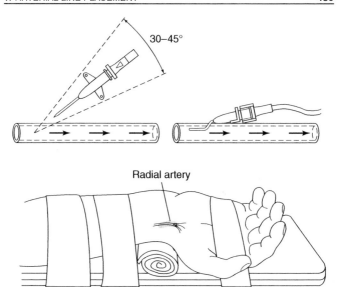

Figure III–1. Technique of radial artery catheterization. (*Reproduced with permission from Gomella TL, ed. Arterial access. In: Neonatology: Management, Procedures, On-Call Problems, Diseases, and Drugs, 5th ed. Originally published by Appleton & Lange. Copyright © 2004 by The McGraw-Hill Companies, Inc.*)

5. While palpating the path of the artery with the nondominant hand, advance the 22-gauge (or smaller) catheter-over-needle assembly into the artery at a 30-degree angle to the skin with the needle bevel up (Figure III–1).

6. Once a "flash" of blood is seen in the hub, hold the needle steady and advance the entire unit by 1–2 mm so that the needle and catheter are in the artery. If blood flow in the hub stops, carefully pull the entire unit back until flow is reestablished.

7. Hold the needle steady and advance the catheter over the needle into the artery.

8. Remove the needle while briefly occluding the artery with manual pressure, and connect the pressure tubing.

9. Pressure tubing should be preflushed to clear all air bubbles before connection.

10. Suture the line in place with a 3-0 silk and apply a sterile dressing.

11. When using the femoral artery, remember the mnemonic **NAVEL** to aid in locating the important structures in the groin. Palpate the femoral artery just below the inguinal ligament. From lateral to medial, the structures are **N**erve, **A**rtery, **V**ein, **E**mpty space, **L**ymphatic.

Prepackaged Technique: Kits are available with a needle and guide wire, which allow the Seldinger technique to be used (see Chapter 14, Percutaneous Central Venous Catheterization, p. 514. The entry needle is placed at a 30-degree angle to the skin site and is inserted until there is a "flash" of blood in the catheter. The guide wire is inserted in the vessel and the catheter is advanced. The wire is removed, and the catheter is connected to pressure tubing.

Complications: Infection, hemorrhage, thrombosis, hematoma, arterial embolism, arterial spasm, pseudoaneurysm formation.

REFERENCE

Haist SA, Robbins JB. Arterial line placement. In: *Internal Medicine On Call,* 3rd ed. McGraw-Hill, 2002:390–391.

2. ARTERIAL PUNCTURE

Indications

1. Blood gas determination.
2. Arterial blood sampling to determine blood chemistries.

Contraindications

1. Poor collateral circulation.
2. Skin infection near planned puncture site.
3. Bleeding disorders, including thrombocytopenia, systemic fibrinolytic states, and thrombolytic therapy (relative contraindications).

Materials: Blood gas sampling kit or 3–5-mL syringe, 1 mL heparin (1000 units/mL), alcohol or povidone-iodine swabs, and a cup of ice; use a 23–25-gauge needle (20–22 gauge for femoral artery); sterile gloves; gauze; sterile dressing; adhesive tape.

Procedure

1. Use a heparinized syringe for blood gas and a nonheparinized syringe for chemistry determinations. Obtain a blood gas kit (containing a preheparinized syringe), or a small syringe (3–5 mL) with a small-gauge needle (23- or 25-gauge for radial artery, 20- or 22–gauge is acceptable for femoral artery). Heparinize the syringe (if not preheparinized) by drawing up about 0.5–1 mL of heparin, pulling the plunger all the way back, and discarding the heparin.
2. The radial artery is the most frequently used site for arterial blood gas sampling. Other sites include dorsalis pedis, posterior tibial, and femoral arteries. If using the radial artery, perform the **Allen test** to verify collateral flow from the ulnar artery. (For a description of this test, see Chapter 1, Arterial Line Placement, p. 488.)

3. It may be helpful to secure the dorsum of the wrist and place gauze behind the wrist to hyperextend the joint. Elevating the wrist will often bring the radial and brachial arteries closer to the surface. (See Chapter 1, Arterial Line Placement, p. 489.) If using the femoral artery, the mnemonic **NAVEL** will aid in locating the important structures in the groin (see earlier procedure, p. 489).

4. Prepare the area with either a povidone-iodine solution or an alcohol swab. Hold the syringe like a pencil with the needle bevel up and enter the skin at a 60- to 90-degree angle. Maintain slight negative pressure on the syringe.

5. Aspirate very slowly. A good arterial sample requires only minimal backpressure. If a glass or blood-gas syringe is used, the barrel will usually rise spontaneously. If the vessel cannot be located, redirect the needle without taking it out of the skin.

6. Obtain about 2–3 mL of blood.

7. To avoid a hematoma, withdraw the needle quickly and apply *firm* pressure at the site for at least 5–10 minutes, even if the sample was not obtained. Apply a sterile dressing.

8. If the sample is for a blood gas, expel any air from the syringe, mix the contents thoroughly by twirling the syringe between your fingers, and make the syringe airtight with a cap. Place the syringe on ice before the sample is taken to the laboratory.

Complications: Localized bleeding; thrombosis of the artery, which may lead to arterial insufficiency; infection.

REFERENCE

Haist SA, Robbins JB. Arterial puncture. In: *Internal Medicine On Call,* 3rd ed. McGraw-Hill, 2002:391–392.

3. BLADDER CATHETERIZATION

Indications

1. Collection of a sterile specimen for culture.
2. Relief of urinary retention.
3. Evaluation for postvoid residuals.
4. Certain radiology studies, such as voiding cystourethrogram.
5. Monitoring of urine output.

Contraindications

1. Urethral injury due to trauma (typically indicated by blood at the urethral meatus).
2. Perineal hematoma.
3. High-riding prostate.

Materials: Prepackaged Foley catheter kit, appropriate catheter size (typically 8 Fr for infants, 10 Fr for young children, and 12 Fr for older children), sterile gloves.

Procedure

1. Position child supine on a flat surface. It is helpful to have an assistant to help hold child's legs during the procedure. A frog-leg position in girls aids in identifying the urethral opening.
2. Open the catheter kit, put on sterile gloves, and soak sterile cotton balls in the cleansing solution. Apply lubricating jelly to the end of the catheter.
3. Inflate and deflate the balloon of the catheter with 5–10 mL of saline to be sure it is functioning appropriately (only necessary if the catheter is being left in place).
4. In girls, use one gloved hand to separate and hold the labia. With the other gloved hand, clean the area with the cotton balls by wiping the vaginal area from front to back.
5. In boys, use one gloved hand to hold the penis. With the same hand gently retract the foreskin in uncircumcised boys, if possible, to help identify the urethral opening. With the other gloved hand, clean the area with the cotton balls.
6. Insert the catheter into the urethra. Be sure that the hand used to hold the labia or penis does not touch the catheter, as it is no longer sterile.
7. In girls, it is often helpful to identify the vaginal opening and then move superiorly to find the urethral opening. Insert the catheter until urine is obtained. In boys, hold the penis stretched and upright, perpendicular to the child's body, to pass the catheter. Insert the catheter until urine is obtained. If the foreskin is retracted in uncircumcised boys, be sure to pull it back over the glans when the catheterization is complete.
8. When the catheter is to be left in place for an extended period of time, blow up the balloon with 5–10 mL of normal saline after it is fully inserted. Then gently pull back the catheter until resistance is met, indicating the balloon is resting against the bladder neck.
9. Tape the catheter to the child's leg.

Complications: Bleeding, infection, a false tract, paraphimosis.

REFERENCE

Boenning DA, Henretig FM. Bladder catheterization. In: Henretig FM, King C, eds. *Textbook of Pediatric Emergency Procedures.* Williams & Wilkins, 1997:991–998.

4. CHEST TUBE INSERTION

Indications

1. Pneumothorax (simple or tension).
2. Hemothorax.
3. Chylothorax.
4. Empyema.

Contraindication: Coagulopathy problem (relative).

Materials: Chest tube (28–36 Fr for older adolescents; 18–28 Fr for children), 14-gauge needle, water-seal drainage system (Pleur-Evac, etc) with connecting tubing, minor procedure tray and instrument tray, silk suture (0 or 2-0), Vaseline and sterile gauze, sterile gloves and drapes, povidone-iodine or other skin cleansing agent, syringe and needle, 1% lidocaine, scalpel, 4 × 4 gauze squares or Tegaderm, and adhesive tape.

Procedure

1. Choose a high anterior site, such as the second or third intercostal space, midclavicular line, or subaxillary (more cosmetic) position for a pneumothorax. Place a low lateral chest tube in the fifth intercostal space in the midaxillary line and directed posteriorly for fluid removal. In most children, this location corresponds to the inframammary crease. For a traumatic pneumothorax, use a low lateral tube because this condition usually is associated with bleeding. Use a smaller (24–28 Fr) tube for pneumothorax and a larger (36 Fr) tube for fluid removal.

2. Sedation should be used whenever possible. Prepare the area with antiseptic and drape it with towels. Use 1% lidocaine (with or without epinephrine) to anesthetize the skin and periosteum of the rib; start at the center of the rib and gently work over the top to avoid the neurovascular bundle (Figure III–2). Pull back on the syringe before injecting the lidocaine to ensure a blood vessel is not penetrated.

3. Make a 1–2 cm transverse incision over the center of the rib. Use a hemostat to bluntly dissect over the top of the rib and create a subcutaneous tunnel. Injection of additional lidocaine into the muscle may help ease the discomfort.

4. Puncture the parietal pleura with the hemostat and spread the opening. Insert a gloved finger into the pleural cavity to gently clear any clots or adhesions and to make certain the lung is not accidentally punctured by the tube.

5. Carefully insert the tube superiorly into desired position with a hemostat or gloved finger. Be sure all holes in the tube are in the chest cavity. Rotating the tube away from the child's body while it is being inserted will assist in posterior placement. Attach the end of the tube to a water-seal or Pleur-Evac suction system.

6. Suture the tube in place. Place a heavy silk (0 or 2-0) suture through the incision next to the tube. Tie the incision together, and then tie the ends around the chest tube. Alternatively, a purse-string suture can be placed. Be sure all of the suction holes are beneath the skin before the tube is secured. An alternative technique is to secure the tube with tape and suture the tape to the skin. This approach is most useful for smaller chest tubes used in infants and children (see Figure III–2).

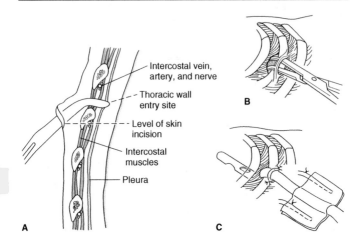

Figure III–2. Procedures of chest tube insertion. **(A)** Level of skin incision and thoracic wall entry site in relation to rib and the neurovascular bundle. **(B)** Opened hemostat, through which chest tube is inserted. **(C)** Chest tube is then secured to skin with silk sutures. (*Reproduced with permission from Gomella TL, ed. Chest tube placement. In: Neonatology, Management, Procedures, On-Call Problems, Diseases, and Drugs, 5th ed. Originally published by Appleton & Lange. Copyright © 2004 by The McGraw-Hill Companies, Inc.*)

7. Wrap the tube with Vaseline gauze and cover with plain gauze. Make the dressing as airtight as possible with tape.
8. Start suction (usually 220 cm in older adolescents; 216 cm in children) and obtain a chest x-ray immediately to check the placement of the tube and to evaluate for residual pneumothorax or fluid. Exercise great caution in children with large pleural fluid collections. Rapid evacuation of large amounts of fluid can be fatal because of hypotension caused by volume shifts.
9. When a child manifests signs of a tension pneumothorax (acute shortness of breath, hypotension, distended neck veins, tachypnea, tracheal deviation) before a chest tube is placed, urgent treatment is needed. Insert a 14-gauge needle into the chest in the second intercostal space in the midclavicular line to rapidly decompress tension pneumothorax and proceed with chest tube insertion.
10. To remove a chest tube, be sure pneumothorax or hemothorax is cleared. Check for an air leak by having child cough; observe water-seal system for bubbling that indicates either a system (tubing leak) or a persistent pleural air leak.
11. Take the tube off suction but not off water seal, and cut the retention suture. Have child perform the Valsalva maneuver while clinician applies pressure with Vaseline gauze and 4 × 4 gauze squares or

Tegaderm. Pull the tube rapidly and make an airtight seal with tape. Obtain an upright chest x-ray to evaluate for pneumothorax.

Complications: Infection, bleeding, lung damage, subcutaneous emphysema, persistent pneumothorax or fluid collection, poor tube placement, liver injury, splenic injury, postprocedure shock.

REFERENCES

Etoch SW, Bar-Natan MF, Miller FB, Richardson JD. Tube thoracostomy. Factors relating to complications. *Arch Surg* 1995;130:521–525.

Lefor AT, ed. Chest tube insertion. In: *Critical Care On Call*. McGraw-Hill, 2002:328–331.

Milikan JS, Moore EE, Steiner E, et al. Complications of tube thoracostomy for acute trauma. *Am J Surg* 1980;140:738–741.

5. CRICOTHYROTOMY

Indications: This procedure is lifesaving for individuals *in extremis* and at risk of hypoxic brain injury and or death. "Percutaneous tracheotomy" is often being performed at the bedside for older adolescents in the ICU setting.

1. Cyanotic, critically ill patient with signs of acute airway obstruction (eg, stridor, apnea, absent breath sounds) who has failed essential airway management techniques.
2. Patient with major trauma (especially facial trauma) who has failed intubation.

Contraindications: (All relative.)

1. Morbidly obese children or adolescents with short and rounded neck tissues are poor candidates.
2. Children younger than 10 years of age have a much higher degree of injury to internal organs (trachea, esophagus, recurrent laryngeal nerves) because their cartilage lacks calcium and is quite soft.
3. Infants and toddlers younger than 2 years possess very supple cricoid and laryngeal cartilage, which combines with adjacent pleural cavities that extend higher into the neck. Surgical invasion into the neck must be reserved for life-threatening circumstances because of its high risk for injury.
4. Pneumothorax.

Materials

1. **Needle procedure:** Sterile, sharp, pointed 18-gauge (or larger) catheter-over-needle assembly (Angiocath), 3–8-inch diameter roll blanket or pillow, 5-mL syringe with sterile water or saline (optional), sterile gloves.

2. **Surgical open procedure:** Surgical blade (No. 15 or 20) and surgical knife handle; 3–8-inch diameter roll blanket or pillow; endotracheal tube (3 mm or larger) or appropriate size tracheotomy tube; gauze squares (4 × 4) or suction (Fraser No. 5 or 7); pointed, curved hemostats; suture material (eg, 3-0 silk or Vicryl on a cutting needle); sterile gloves.

Procedure: The needle procedure is simpler and more straightforward than surgical cricothyrotomy and can often be performed before proceeding to the surgical version. A successful needle procedure may afford time to transport child to a more stable medical environment such as the emergency department or operating room suite. If the needle procedure is unsuccessful, physician or designee must proceed to the surgical open procedure within 4–8 minutes.

Needle Procedure

1. Place child in a supine position and on a firm ground or table. (A soft bed or mattress is not conducive to surgical approaches to the anterior neck.)
2. Place an appropriately sized roll under child's shoulders and shoulder blades; extend the neck, with neck and chin held midline in the sagittal plane; and stabilize the occiput.
3. The right-handed physician generally kneels or stands toward child's right shoulder and side of neck; left-handed physician to the left side.
4. Palpate the neck for the surgical site, the cricothyroid membrane. It is the soft depression between the notch of the thyroid lamina (or Adam's apple) and the cricoid laminar ring (about 2–4 inches inferior to the thyroid lamina).
5. With the left hand, stabilize the thyroid cartilage, so that the cricothyroid membrane is between and just below the thumb and index finger of the left hand.
6. Attach the 18-gauge (or larger) needle to the syringe and enter perpendicular to the skin and soft tissue in the exact midline, advancing through the skin and subcutaneous fat and into the cricothyroid membrane.
7. Gently pull back the plunger of the syringe until air enters the water within the syringe and the needle has sufficiently penetrated the tracheal wall. Then advance the needle about 3 mm, pointing inferiorly at 45 degrees.
8. Secure the needle by hand and insufflate with atmospheric air. Attach the needle or catheter to an oxygen source, if available. The larger the bore of the needle (eg > 14 gauge), the more effective and sustained will be the ventilation to the child.
9. Avoid positive pressure ventilation to reduce the chance of pneumothorax or pneumomediastinum.

Surgical Open Procedure

1. Follow the same sequence described for the needle procedure, steps 1–5.

2. Insert a No. 15 surgical blade perpendicularly to the skin on a horizontal angle, and cut the soft tissue in the exact midline about 1 inch in length.
3. Advance the blade deeper through the subcutaneous fat, staying in the midline, and make an incision into the cricothyroid membrane about 1/2 inch in width. Blood and air should bubble and be visible.
4. Gently advance the handle of the blade or hemostat. As air enters the surgical field, the tracheal lumen will be visible.
5. Using the hemostat or the top end of the surgical handle, penetrate the anterior tracheal wall.
6. Advance the surgical knife handle about 3 mm, pointing inferiorly at 45 degrees, and pry open the cricoid and thyroid cartilages and the cricothyroid membrane.
7. Place the tracheotomy tube or the endotracheal tube into the trachea, secure by tape or hand, and insufflate with atmospheric air. Attach the needle or catheter to an oxygen source, if available. The larger the endotracheal tube or tracheotomy tube, the more effective and sustained will be the ventilation to child.
8. Confirm breath sounds by auscultation of the chest.
9. Positive pressure ventilation can be undertaken at pressures low enough to reduce the chance of pneumothorax or pneumomediastinum.
10. Secure the airway with conversion to a tracheotomy.

Complications: Bleeding, tracheal tear or laryngeal tracheal separation, pneumothorax, pneumomediastinum, esophageal laceration, recurrent laryngeal nerve injury, infection.

REFERENCES

Buckels N, Khan ZH, Irwin ST, Gibbons JR. Post-operative sputum retention treated by minitracheostomy—a ward procedure? *Br J Clin Pract* 1990;44:169–171.

Cote C, Eavey R, Jones RD, et al. Cricothyroid membrane puncture: Oxygenation and ventilation in a dog model using and intravenous catheter. *Crit Care Med* 1988;16:615–619.

Hughes RK. Needle tracheostomy. *Arch Surg* 1966;93:834–837.

Oppenheimer P. Needle tracheostomy. *Otorhinolaryngol Digest* 1977;39:9.

6. ENDOTRACHEAL INTUBATION (ORAL AND NASAL)

Indications

1. Airway management during cardiopulmonary resuscitation.
2. Acute hypoxemic respiratory failure.
3. Prolonged ventilatory support.
4. Patient with altered mental status at risk for aspiration.
5. Presence of overwhelming secretions or massive hemoptysis.

TABLE III-1. RECOMMENDED ENDOTRACHEAL TUBE SIZES

Age	Internal Diameter (mm)
Premature infant	2.5–3.0 (uncuffed)
Newborn infant	3.5 (uncuffed)
13–12 mo	4.0 (uncuffed)
1–8 y	4.0–6.0 (uncuffed)[a]
8–16 y	6.0–7.0 (cuffed)
Adult	7.0–9.0 (cuffed)

[a]Rough estimate is to measure child's little finger.
Modified from Lefor AT, ed. Critical Care On Call. McGraw-Hill. Copyright © 2004.

Contraindications

1. Massive maxillofacial trauma, fractured larynx, suspected cervical spinal cord injury (all relative).
2. Nasotracheal intubation is contraindicated in suspected basilar skull fractures. Fiberoptic intubation or tracheotomy may be indicated in these instances.

Materials: Sterile gloves, protective eye wear, endotracheal tube (ET tube; for sizes, see Table III-1), laryngoscope handle and blade (straight or curved; No. 3 for adults, Nos. 1–1.5 for small children), 10-mL syringe, adhesive tape, suction equipment, water-soluble lubricant, bag-valve mask, malleable stylet (optional), oximeter and end-tidal CO_2 monitoring (if available).

Procedure: Orotracheal intubation is most commonly used and is described here. It should be performed with great care in any child with possible trauma to the cervical spine.

1. If child is hypoxic or apneic, use a bag and mask with 100% O_2 prior to and during intubation procedure. The risk of hypoxemia during intubation can be minimized by preoxygenation with 100% O_2 at high flow rates for 3–4 minutes and by avoiding prolonged periods without ventilation. Monitor O_2 saturation throughout procedure if possible.
2. Prepare equipment. Extend the laryngoscope blade to 90 degrees to verify that the light is working. Inflate cuff, if used, to ensure competency. Apply water-soluble lubricant to the tube. Enlist a respiratory therapist to maintain oxygenation and assist in airway control during the procedure.
3. Position child in the "sniffing position" (neck flexed and head slightly extended) by placing a rolled towel under child's lower neck and upper shoulders. Avoid if cervical spine injury is suspected.

4. IV sedation may be required in children who are agitated, uncooperative, or combative. (See Section I, Chapter 81, Sedation and Analgesia, p. 377).
5. Open child's mouth by placing the thumb and index finger of the right hand on the lower and upper incisors, respectively, and spreading the thumb and finger with a scissor-like motion.
6. Grip the laryngoscope with the left hand. Insert the extended blade into the right side of the mouth. Use the blade to push the tongue to the left while keeping the tongue anterior to the blade. Advance carefully toward the midline until the epiglottis is seen (Figure III–3).
7. Pass the straight (Miller) laryngoscope blade posterior and inferior to the epiglottis. When using the curved (MacIntosh) blade, pass it anterior and superior to the epiglottis. Thrust the left arm upward at

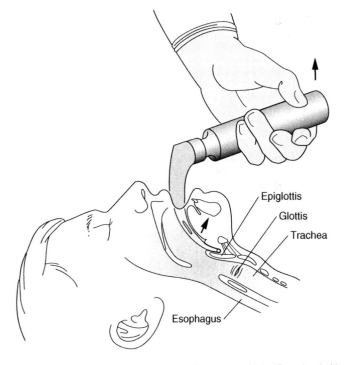

Figure III–3. Endotracheal intubation using a curved laryngoscope blade. (*Reproduced with permission from Gomella LG, Haist SA, eds. Clinicians Pocket Reference, 10th ed. McGraw-Hill. Copyright © 2004.*)

a 45-degree angle from the horizontal and visualize the vocal cords. Avoid using the maxillary teeth as a fulcrum by keeping the wrist rigid and lifting only with the arm and shoulder. If the cords are not visualized, the straight blade may have progressed too far posterior and inferior into the esophagus. In that case, slowly retract the laryngoscope while watching for the cords to appear. With either type of blade, application of cricoid pressure by an assistant may be a useful adjunct while attempting cord visualization.

8. While maintaining visualization of the cords, grasp the ET tube in the right hand, pass it into the right corner of the mouth, and advance the cuff beyond the cords. With more difficult intubations, a malleable stylet can be used to direct the tube. In average-sized children, the incisors should be at the 23-cm mark for boys and 21-cm mark for girls.

9. Gently inflate the cuff with air until an adequate seal is obtained (about 5 mL). Auscultate over the epigastrium (with ventilation, loud gurgling over the epigastrium suggests a gastric intubation), then auscultate over the left and right anterior and midaxillary chest. If the left side lacks breath sounds, a right mainstem bronchus intubation is likely. In that case, deflate cuff, retract ET tube 1–2 cm, reinflate cuff, and reassess breath sounds. Auscultation and end-tidal CO_2 monitoring will confirm tracheal intubation. Confirm proper positioning with a chest x-ray. The end of the ET tube should be 3–4 cm superior to the carina.

10. Secure tube position with tape. Record the centimeter mark at the incisors. Consider inserting an oropharyngeal airway to prevent child from biting the ET tube.

Complications: Oropharyngeal trauma, aspiration, improper tube positioning (esophageal or right mainstem bronchus intubation). Complications associated with a prolonged intubation attempt include cardiac arrest, seizures, and gastric distention. Right mainstem bronchus intubation has adverse consequences, including pneumothorax and left lung atelectasis. Prolonged intubation (greater than 10–14 days) can lead to tracheal stenosis.

REFERENCES

Kaur S, Heard SO. Airway management and endotracheal intubation. In: Irwin RS, Rippe JM, Cerra FB et al, eds. *Procedures and Techniques in Intensive Care Medicine,* 2nd ed. Lippincott Williams & Wilkins, 1999:3–16.

Pingleton SK. Management of complications of acute respiratory failure. In: Bone RC, ed. *Pulmonary and Critical Care Medicine,* 6th ed. Mosby, 1998:R11–16.

7. GASTROINTESTINAL TUBE INSERTION

Indications

1. GI decompression for ileus or obstruction.
2. Gastric lavage for GI bleeding or drug overdose.

    3. Obtunded or heavily sedated patient at risk of aspiration. (Consider endotracheal intubation for airway protection as well.)

    4. Feeding a patient who is unable to take oral feedings or supplementation of feeding in a patient who is unable to meet caloric needs with oral feeding alone.

Contraindications

    1. Nasal fracture.

    2. Severely enlarged or edematous nasal turbinates.

    3. Basilar skull fracture.

    4. Esophageal perforation.

Materials: Appropriate GI tube (see below), water-soluble lubricant, adhesive tape, catheter tip syringe, stethoscope, glass or bottle of water, sterile gloves.

    1. Nasogastric (NG) tubes

        a. For decompression: Salem sump (double-lumen tube with an air vent [leave vent open]); can be used for continuous suction. Levine (single-lumen tube); must be placed on intermittent suction. Repogle (use in neonates).

        b. For lavage: Ewald (large-bore [18–36 Fr] single-lumen tube); usually placed by orogastric route.

        c. For feeding: Corpak, Keogh (soft with weighted-tips [usually tungsten, so acceptable for use in MRI scanners]); can use stylet for placement.

        d. For tamponade: Sengstaken-Blakemore tube (triple-lumen tube used exclusively for tamponade of esophageal bleeding sources, usually esophageal varices, for temporary control of bleeding). One lumen is for aspiration, one for the gastric balloon (to anchor it in place), and the third for the esophageal balloon (for tamponade). The esophageal balloon can be inflated only for a short period and not above 15 mm Hg pressure to avoid esophageal ischemia. These tubes should not remain in place longer than 48 hours. Surgical consultation should be obtained in any child who requires a Sengstaken-Blakemore tube.

    2. Gastrostomy tubes: Can be placed surgically, endoscopically (percutaneous endoscopic gastrostomy), or fluoroscopically.

        a. G-tubes: Various tubes are available, including Ross, Mic, and Corpak. Most are silicone with an internal (gastric) bolster that is a dome or crossbar. Tubes may be removed by traction, by cutting at skin level and allowing the internal bolster to pass, or by endoscopic removal of the internal bolster after cutting the tube.

        b. Low-profile gastrostomy tubes (button G-tubes): Mic-Key, Ross, and Corpak; these tubes have a balloon that is water-filled as the internal bolster and can therefore be removed and replaced easily. Because they are not as visible as regular G-tubes, they are also more appealing.

c. **Gastrostomy–jejunostomy (G-J) tubes:** These tubes generally use a gastrostomy site for threading a double-lumen tube under fluoroscopic guidance; one port is gastric, the other, jejunal. G-J tubes are useful in children who already have a gastrostomy, avoiding the necessity of another surgical procedure. There is no jejunal bolster, so the tube is prone to displacement from migration, usually into the stomach.

Procedure

1. Inform both parent and child of the nature of the procedure and encourage them to cooperate.
2. Choose the nasal passage that is most patent by occluding one nostril and having child sniff.
3. Measure the length of tube needed by placing tip at the subxiphoid region of child's abdominal wall and then extending the tube up toward nose and around ear. Mark the tube at the point where it meets the earlobe.
4. Lubricate distal 2–3 inches of the tube with water-soluble lubricant and insert tube gently along the floor of the nasal passage. Maintain gentle pressure that will allow the tube to pass into the nasopharynx.
5. When child can feel the tip of the tube in the back of the throat, ask him or her to swallow as the tube is slowly advanced. This may not be possible in an infant or toddler; in those situations, usually the tube can be advanced as the child pauses during crying.
6. Once the tube has been inserted so that the mark is at the nostril, attach a 10-mL syringe to the tube tip and inject 10 mL of air while listening over the area of the stomach with the stethoscope. A "pop" or "gurgle" (representing air in the stomach) should be audible. To check placement of the tube, attempt to aspirate gastric contents. Tape the tube securely without putting pressure on the nasal ala to avoid ischemic necrosis.
7. Obtain a chest x-ray to verify placement before starting feedings.

Complications: Inadvertent passage into the trachea; coiling of tube in the mouth or pharynx; bleeding from the nose, pharynx, or stomach; sinusitis; inability to place the tube.

REFERENCES

Campos ACL, Marchesini JB. Recent advances in the placement of tubes for enteral nutrition. *Curr Opin Clin Nutr Metab Care* 1999;2:265–269.

Chait PG, Weinberg J, Connolly BL, et al. Retrograde percutaneous gastrostomy and gastrojejunostomy in 505 children: A 4 1/2-year experience. *Radiology* 1996;201: 691–695.

8. GYNECOLOGIC EVALUATION

Indications

1. Gynecologic problem at any age.
2. Abnormal pubertal development.
3. Sexually active adolescent at any age, and by 4 years postmenarche if no problems.

Contraindication: Severe emotional distress with the procedure, when scheduled at parent's request and not otherwise indicated.

Materials: Proper table with stirrups, appropriate focused light source (ie, head lamp or otoscope), specula of varying sizes (0.5–3.0 cm in width) and shapes (ie, Huffman and Petersen), vaginoscope (if warranted), sterile nonbacteriostatic saline, cotton-tipped applicators, Calgiswabs, Nitrazine paper, Pap test supplies, appropriate specimen containers for cultures (as per local laboratory), magnifying source, sterile gloves.

Procedure

Adolescent Patient

1. Have appropriate testing material close at hand.
2. Examine the abdomen for tenderness and lower abdominal masses.
3. Place patient in the dorsolithotomy position.
4. Examine the vulva, and separate and palpate labia majora and minora.
5. Place a single gloved, minimally lubricated finger in the vagina to identify hymenal elasticity, vaginal direction, and size.
6. Choose an appropriately sized speculum. It may be helpful to place the speculum into the vagina over the finger that is gradually being simultaneously removed from the vagina.
7. Visualize the upper vaginal vault and cervix, looking for discharge and cervical lesions.
8. Obtain test specimens.
   a. If a Pap test is to be performed, collect this specimen first. Then obtain cultures and wet mount, if indicated.
   b. To perform a wet mount, collect vaginal discharge with a cotton-tipped applicator. Mix with a small quantity of sterile nonbacteriostatic saline by either directly placing both on a microscope slide or first mixing the two in a small test tube. Mixture is used for microscopic evaluation.
9. Remove the speculum.
10. Proceed with bimanual exam.

Prepubertal Patient

1. Approach slowly, explaining to both parent and child what will occur.
2. Examine abdomen, as previously described for adolescent patient (step 2).

3. An internal vaginal exam is rarely necessary in this age group.
4. Position for exam may vary, based on child's size and comfort. If child is tall enough to fit the gynecologic stirrups without discomfort, the dorsolithotomy position may be used. Other positions include supine frog-leg (heels and feet together and knees in maximum abduction) or prone knee-chest (head and chest down on table, hips and knees flexed, and buttocks up in the air). Frog-leg is better as a starting position and for obtaining any specimens needed. Knee-chest allows a better view of the anus and the anterior vagina.
5. Examine the vulva and vaginal vestibule.

    a. With child in the frog-leg position, place one finger at the base of each labia majorum and push gently and simultaneously in a posterior and lateral direction.
    b. Another approach in the frog-leg position is to gently grasp the base of the labia majora and pull out toward examiner.
    c. The use of a magnifying device may improve the evaluation of this area.

6. Techniques for obtaining specimens.

    a. Calgiswabs may be placed more easily in the vagina than cotton-tipped applicators, because they are thinner and may be able to be placed without touching the hymenal ring.
    b. The tubing from a butterfly needle with needle end removed or a small feeding tube may be inserted in the vagina and specimens obtained by suction with or without insertion of sterile nonbacteriostatic saline.
    c. In cases where insertion of any object into the vagina is problematic, specimens may be obtained by flushing sterile nonbacteriostatic saline through the vagina and collecting the runoff on cotton-tipped applicators placed directly on the lower vulvar surface.

Complications: Postexamination bleeding or spotting, short-term discomfort, emotional distress (all rare).

REFERENCES

Eman SJ. Office evaluation of the child and adolescent. In: Emans SJ, Laufer MR, Goldstein DP, eds. *Pediatric and Adolescent Gynecology,* 4th ed. Lippincott-Raven, 1998:1–48.

Pokorny SF. Genital examination of pre-pubertal and peri-pubertal females. In: Sanfilippo JS, Muram D, Dewhurst J, Lee P, eds. *Pediatric and Adolescent Gynecology,* 2nd ed. Saunders, 2001:182–198.

9. HEELSTICK (CAPILLARY BLOOD SAMPLING)

Indication: Collection of blood from neonates and infants.

Contraindications
1. Edematous skin puncture site.
2. Children older than 1 year of age

Materials: Sterile gauze, alcohol wipe, heel warmer, automatic lancet device, appropriate microtainers for blood sample, adhesive bandage, sterile gloves.

Procedure
1. Warm infant's heel for approximately 5 minutes. With gloved hands, cleanse the area with the alcohol wipe. Hold the foot firmly with the leg in a tucked-flexed position.
2. Grasp infant's heel in a moderately firm grip, with the forefinger at the arch of the foot and the thumb below the puncture site at the ankle.
3. Puncture the heel on the most medial or lateral portions of the plantar surface of the heel (medial to a line drawn posteriorly from the mid-great toe to the heel, or lateral to a line drawn posteriorly between the fourth and fifth toes to the heel).
4. Wipe away the first drop of blood with sterile gauze. If blood is not free flowing, use gentle massage to produce a rounded drop of blood. Gentle pressure should be eased and reapplied as drops of blood flow into containers.
5. After blood has been collected, elevate infant's foot above the rest of the body and press sterile gauze against the puncture site until bleeding stops. Cover the site with an adhesive bandage.

Complications: Necrotizing osteochondritis, infection or abscess of the heel.

REFERENCES

Clinical Laboratory Specimen Collection Manual. Alfred I duPont Hospital for Children, 2002:7–8.
Wong D, Hockenberry MJ. *Nursing Care of Infants and Children,* 7th ed. Mosby, 2003:1147–1148.

10. INTRAOSSEOUS CANNULATION

Indications
1. Administration of drugs, fluid, and blood during pediatric resuscitation.
2. Treatment of severe shock.

Contraindications

1. Fractured bone.
2. Bone in which an intraosseous (IO) cannulation has been previously attempted and infiltrated.

Materials: IO needle, antiseptic solution, 10-mL syringe, saline, adhesive tape, bulky dressing, sterile gloves.

Procedure

1. Put on gloves and select site. Optimal sites include distal tibia, proximal tibia, and distal femur. The anteromedial aspect of the tibia, 1–3 cm below the tibial tuberosity, is the preferred site for children. Using aseptic technique, cleanse the site with antiseptic solution.
2. Support child's leg on a firm surface.
3. Identify the tibial tuberosity by palpation. Feel for the flat surface of the tibia approximately 1 fingerbreadth below and medial to the tuberosity. With the nondominant hand, grasp the medial and lateral edges of the tibia. *Do not* let any part of the hand rest behind child's leg.
4. Insert the IO needle through the skin, using a gentle, but firm, twisting motion. Direct the needle at a 90-degree angle or slightly toward the toes. Avoid the growth plate (epiphysial) by directing the needle away from the joint. If the IO needle has threads, turn the needle in a clockwise motion.
5. Stop advancing the needle when a decrease in resistance is felt on forward motion.
6. Remove the stylet and confirm placement by attaching an empty 10-mL syringe and aspirating blood and bone marrow.
7. If aspiration is successful, flush the needle with 10 mL of saline. If aspiration is not successful and needle is thought to be in the bone marrow, attempt to flush with 10 mL of saline. If needle is not thought to be in the bone marrow, it may need to be advanced further.
8. If insertion is successful and there are no signs of swelling of the extremity, stabilize the needle with tape and support with bulky dressing. Connect to IV tubing and infuse fluids or medications as indicated.

Complications: Fracture of the tibia, lower extremity compartment syndrome, severe extravasation of drugs, osteomyelitis.

REFERENCES

Hankins J, Waldman Lonsway RA, Hedrick C, Perdue MB. *Infusion Therapy in Clinical Practice.* Saunders, 2001.
Hazinski MF, Zartsky AL. *Pediatric Advanced Life Support Provider Manual.* American Heart Association, 2002:350.
Infusion Nurses Society. *Policies and Practice for Infusion Nursing,* 2nd ed. Infusion Nurses Society, 2002:96–98.

11. KNEE ARTHROCENTESIS

Indications

1. **Diagnostic**
   a. Removal of fluid for culture if suspicious of septic joint.
   b. Removal of fluid if suspicious of hemarthrosis or traumatic joint injury.

2. **Therapeutic**
   a. Relief of discomfort caused by intra-articular pressure and distention of joint capsule and ligaments by accumulating fluid.
   b. Drainage of pus to decrease the damaging effects of bacteria, WBCs, and inflammatory response on joint space.
   c. Injection of medications, such as glucocorticoids (one of the modalities of treatment in noninfectious inflammatory arthritis, such as juvenile rheumatoid arthritis).

Contraindications

1. Hemophilia.
2. Overlying skin infection or cellulitis.
3. Bacteremia.
4. Anatomic inaccessibility.

Materials: Sterile drapes; sterile gloves; 3 povidone-iodine swabs; sterile 2 × 2 gauze squares; 25-gauge, 1.5-inch needle (to administer lidocaine); 21-gauge, 1.5-inch needle (to draw up lidocaine); 18-gauge, 1.5-inch needle (to enter joint capsule); 5-, 10-, or 20-mL syringes (depending on size of effusion); 1% lidocaine; sterile container for joint fluid; hemostat; adhesive bandage.

Procedure: The knee joint is the most easily aspirated joint. Other joints that may need aspiration should be evaluated by examiners with more experience (eg, orthopedic specialists) to avoid damage to cartilage and growth plates.

1. Locate landmarks as part of a careful physical exam, with child's knee in full extension. Palpate the posterior edge of the patella medially or laterally. The patella should be easily mobile and the quadriceps muscle relaxed to ensure easy aspiration.
2. There are two approaches, as follows:
   a. **Medial (rheumatologic) approach:** Preferred with small effusions. Target area is under the midpoint of the patella. Remember to allow 1–2 cm posterior to the medial edge of the patella to avoid the gliding surface.
   b. **Lateral (orthopedic) approach:** Easier with large effusion. Target area is directly into the center of the bulging suprapatellar pouch, at the level of the cephalad border of the patella (Figure III–4).

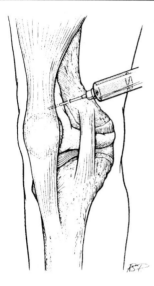

Figure III–4. Lateral (orthopedic) approach for knee arthrocentesis. (*Reproduced, with permission, from Haist SA, Robbins JB, eds. Internal Medicine On Call, 3rd ed. Originally published by Appleton & Lange. Copyright © 2002 by the McGraw-Hill Companies, Inc.*)

3. If needed, conscious sedation may be administered at this time.
4. Clean the knee liberally with povidone-iodine, including the medial and lateral aspects of the joint over the patella (> 180 degrees).
5. Prepare and drape the joint in a sterile fashion.
6. Anesthetize the aspiration site and subcutaneous tissue with 1% lidocaine using the 25-gauge, 1.5-inch needle. Lidocaine may be mixed with sodium bicarbonate at a ratio of 9-mL lidocaine to 1-mL bicarbonate to minimize stinging (1–2 mL lidocaine, total, infused).
7. Approach will be lateral (orthopedic approach) or medial (rheumatologic approach) with an 18-gauge, 1.5-inch needle attached to a 10-mL or 20-mL syringe.
8. Aspiration of joint fluid confirms correct placement. Pressure on the opposite side of the injection site may enhance the suprapatellar pouch, and thus facilitate removal of fluid when using the lateral approach. With the medial approach, squeezing the pouch may facilitate fluid flow.
9. Remove only as much fluid as flows freely.
10. Remove the needle, use sterile 2 × 2 gauze squares to cover the injection site, and apply gentle pressure.
11. Cover the injection site with an adhesive bandage and remove excess povidone-iodine.
12. Send joint fluid to the laboratory for analysis.

Complications: Infection, bleeding, damage to the articular cartilage.

REFERENCES

Koopman WJ. *Arthritis and Allied Conditions—A Textbook of Rheumatology,* 13th ed. Williams & Wilkins, 1997.

Lefor AT, Gomella LG. *Surgery On Call,* 3rd ed. McGraw-Hill, 2001.

Scott N. *Procedures in Practice.* BMJ publishing Group, 1994.

Siberry G, Iannone R. *The Harriet Lane Handbook.* Mosby, 2000.

12. LUMBAR PUNCTURE

Indications

1. Evaluation of CSF for cells, protein, glucose, and bacteria.
2. Measurement of CSF pressure (opening and closing).
3. Injection of therapeutic agents (chemotherapy).

Contraindications

1. Increased intracranial pressure associated with a mass or obstruction.
2. Infection near procedure site.
3. Cardiopulmonary instability.
4. Coagulopathy (relative).

Materials: Sterile lumbar puncture kit (adult, pediatric, or infant kit depending on age and size of patient), manometer if pressure measurement desired or indicated, spinal needles (22-gauge for children, 20–21-gauge for older adolescents; length of needle depends on size of patient), sterile specimen tubes, sterile gloves.

Procedure

1. Ophthalmologic exam should be performed to evaluate for papilledema. Obtain and review CT scan of the head if there is a possibility of increased intracranial pressure or underlying intracranial mass or obstruction.
2. If lumbar puncture does not need to be performed urgently, consider placing EMLA cream over the L4-5 interspace area.
3. Place patient in the lateral decubitus position close to the edge of the bed or table. Patient's body should be in the flexed position with head toward chest and knees drawn up to abdomen. (In younger children and infants, it is helpful to have an assistant hold patient). Occasionally, depending on patient habitus or physician bias, it may be helpful to place patient in a flexed and seated position. Pressure measurements should be obtained with patient as relaxed as possible.
4. Identify landmarks (L4-5 interspace). Find the top of the iliac crests. An imaginary line between them intersects the spine at the L4 vertebrae and the space just below it is the L4-5 interspace.
5. Once patient is positioned and landmarks have been identified, open the sterile procedure tray and put on sterile gloves. Clean the area with povidone-iodine using a circular motion and covering several

TABLE III–2. DIFFERENTIAL DIAGNOSIS OF CEREBROSPINAL FLUID

Condition	Color	Opening Pressure (mm H_2O)	Protein (mg/100 mL)	Glucose (mg/100 mL)	Cells (No./mL)
Adult (normal)	Clear	70–180	15–45	45–80	0–5 lymphs
Newborn (normal)	Clear	70–180	20–120	2/3 serum glucose	40–60 lymphs
Viral infection	Clear or opalescent	Normal or slightly ↑	Normal or slightly ↑	Normal	10–500 lymphs (polys early)
Bacterial infection	Opalescent or yellow, may clot		50–1500	↓, usually < 20	25–10,000 polys
Granulomatous (TB, fungal)	Clear or opalescent	Often ↑	↑, but usually < 500	↓, usually < 20–40	10–500 lymphs
Subarachnoid hemorrhage	Bloody or xanthochromic after 2–8 h	Usually ↑	↑	Normal	WBC:RBC ratio same as blood

↓ = decreased; ↑ = increased; lymphs = lymphocytes; polys = polymorphonuclear lymphocyte; RBC = red blood cell; TB = tuberculosis; WBC = white blood cell. *Reproduced with permission from Lefor AT, ed. Critical Care On Call. McGraw-Hill. Copyright © 2002.*

interspaces. Place appropriate drapes over patient, with the circular opening placed just over the L4-5 interspace.

6. Using a sterile 25-gauge needle and 1% lidocaine solution, create a wheal over the L4-5 interspace. Then inject the lidocaine to anesthetize deeper structures using a sterile 22-gauge needle.

7. After inspecting for any defects, insert the spinal needle with a stylet into the skin wheal through the L4-5 interspace. The needle should be parallel to the bed and directed at a 30–45 degree angle toward patient's head. Keep the bevel of the needle parallel to the long axis of the body to decrease shearing of the dural fibers. Continue through the major structures until a "pop" is felt, indicating passage through the dura into the subarachnoid space. Remove the stylet and look for fluid to come through. If no fluid returns, it may help to gently rotate the needle.

8. Once fluid return is obtained, if a pressure reading is required, attach a manometer with a stopcock and measure the opening pressure.

9. Collect 0.5–2.0 mL of fluid in each tube and send to the laboratory for analysis: Gram stain and cultures (routine, fungal, acid-fast bacilli), glucose and protein, cell count and differential (some clinicians may opt to send first and last tubes for cell count to help differentiate between subarachnoid hemorrhage and traumatic tap), and other special studies (eg, viral culture, polymerase chain reaction, India ink) (Table III-2).

Complications: Spinal headache (most common), CSF leak, bleeding, introduction of infection.

REFERENCE

Lefor AT, ed. Lumbar puncture. In: *Critical Care On Call.* McGraw-Hill, 2002:343–345.

13. PARACENTESIS

Indications

1. **Diagnostic:** Evaluation of new onset of ascites, exclusion of peritonitis, assessment of clinical deterioration in known cirrhotic patients.

2. **Therapeutic:** Decompression of tense ascites in symptomatic patients (dyspnea, abdominal discomfort, early satiety).

Contraindications: (All relative.)

1. Coagulopathy (consider platelet transfusion for platelet count < 50,000 and fresh frozen plasma for international normalized ratio (INR) > 1.5; use a small needle).

2. Uncooperative child (consider sedation).
3. Multiple surgical operations (consider surgical consultation).

Materials: Minor procedure tray, 18–22-gauge, 1.5-inch catheter-over-needle assembly (Angiocath), syringe (10–30 mL for infants and small children, 20–60 mL for older children and adolescents), sterile specimen containers, blood culture bottles, povidone-iodine solution, pressure dressing, sterile gloves.

Procedure

1. Verify that child's bladder is empty. Place child in supine position.
2. If there is doubt about the presence or position of ascites, or if the amount of ascites is small, abdominal ultrasound can be helpful in locating ascites during the procedure.
3. The entry site is usually the midline, 2 cm below the umbilicus. Alternatively, a site in the right or left lower quadrant, lateral to the rectus sheath, and 2–3 cm above the superior iliac spine in the midline can be used. Avoid the upper abdomen, collateral vessels, and surgical scars (bowel may adhere to the abdominal wall).
4. Prepare child's skin with povidone-iodine solution and apply sterile drapes. Use sterile technique throughout procedure. Raise a skin wheal with 1% lidocaine over the entry site.
5. With the catheter-over-needle assembly mounted on the syringe, advance the needle into the anesthetized area carefully while gently aspirating. Angling the needle slightly to one side once the skin has been entered minimizes leaking (Z track). Some resistance will be felt at the fascia. Once return of fluid is obtained, leave the catheter in place, remove needle, reattach syringe, and aspirate. It may be necessary to reposition the catheter because of abutting omentum or bowel wall.
6. Aspirate the amount of fluid needed for testing (10–30 mL). Bedside inoculation of blood culture bottles with ascitic fluid increases sensitivity of cultures.
7. For a therapeutic tap, leave the catheter in place. In older children and adolescents, the catheter can be connected to a suction bottle with tubing. In infants and children, manually remove the fluid with a syringe and 3-way stopcock. In adults, a large volume of paracentesis (5–10 L) can be safely removed over 60–90 minutes. Infants and small children often benefit from simultaneous administration of a colloid solution, such as albumin or fresh frozen plasma, during fluid removal. Watch vital signs carefully during and following the procedure.
8. Remove the needle quickly and apply a pressure dressing.
9. Depending on the clinical picture, send samples for the following studies: albumin, total protein, amylase, lipase, glucose, LDH, urea

TABLE III–3. LABORATORY CLUES IN ASCITIC FLUID

Laboratory Test	Finding
Albumin (ALB) gradient	$ALB_{Serum} - ALB_{Ascites} = x$ If $x > 1.1$ g/dL: Consider either portal hypertension (liver disease, veno-occlusive disease, Budd-Chiari syndrome, portal vein thrombosis, hepatic metastasis), cardiac disease, or fluid overload secondary to dialysis If $x < 1.1$ g/dL: Portal hypertension unlikely; consider peritoneal inflammation or neoplasm, nephrotic syndrome, protein-losing enteropathy, pancreatitis, biliary disease
Amylase/Lipase	Elevated in pancreatitis
Bacterial culture	Blood culture bottles: 85% sensitivity Routine cultures: 50% sensitivity
Cell count	Absolute neutrophil count > 250/mcL: Presume bacterial infection
Cytology	Bizarre cells with large nuclei may represent reactive mesothelial cells and not malignancy; malignant cells suggest tumor
Food fibers	Found in most cases of perforated viscus
Total protein	< 1.0 g/dL: High risk for spontaneous bacterial peritonitis
Urea and creatinine	Can be elevated in uro-ascites

and creatinine, CBC and differential, bacterial culture, acid-fast bacilli, fungal smears and culture, and cytology. Table III–3 summarizes laboratory clues in ascitic fluid.

Complications: Peritonitis, bowel perforation, intra-abdominal hemorrhage, abdominal wall hematoma, abdominal wall abscess, perforation of the bladder, persistent leaking of ascitic fluid.

REFERENCES

Colletti RB, Krawitt EL. Ascites. In: Wyllie R, Hyams JS, eds. *Pediatric Gastrointestinal Disease*, 2nd ed. Saunders, 1999:104–115.

Wasserman D. Ascites. In: Altschuler SM, Liacouras CA, eds. *Clinical Pediatric Gastroenterology.* Churchill Livingston, 1998:323–330.

14. PERCUTANEOUS CENTRAL VENOUS CATHETERIZATION

Indications

1. Administration of fluids and medications when peripheral administration is impossible, inappropriate, or unreliable.
2. Hemodynamic monitoring.

Contraindication: Coagulopathy dictates use of the femoral or median basilic vein approach to avoid bleeding complications.

Materials: Sterile gown, mask, head covering, sterile gloves, sterile towels, appropriate skin preparation solution (povidone-iodine), 2 × 2 sterile gauze squares, saline flush, heparin flush (10 units/mL), sterile syringes, appropriate-sized catheter kit (4 or 5 Fr; single versus double versus triple lumen), 1% lidocaine, sutures, sterile transparent dressing.

Procedure

Seldinger Technique for Catheter Placement: Especially useful in establishing vascular access in children.

1. Put on head cover and mask. Open supplies, prepare sterile field, and draw up saline and heparin flushes. Put on sterile gown and gloves.
2. Sterilize the site with povidone-iodine and drape with sterile towels.
3. Administer lidocaine to provide local anesthesia in the area to be explored.
4. Obtain initial entry through the skin into the vessel of choice (femoral, internal jugular, subclavian), using a small-gauge needle or a catheter-over-needle assembly (Angiocath). A syringe is attached to the end of the needle.
5. Apply constant negative pressure while the needle is advanced. Once free flow of nonpulsating venous blood is achieved, detach the syringe and pass a small-gauge wire through the needle or catheter into the vein. (For subclavian and internal jugular approaches, place a finger over the hub of the needle when disconnecting syringe to prevent entrainment and embolism of air.)
6. Slide the needle or catheter out of the vessel and over the wire while making sure to hold onto the wire.
7. With a scalpel, make a small skin incision at the point of insertion to allow for passage of the catheter.
8. Slide a dilator over the wire and into the vessel, again making sure to hold onto the wire. Advance the dilator using a pushing and twisting motion.
9. Remove the dilator while continuing to hold onto the wire to avoid dislodging it.
10. Slide a catheter or catheter-introducing sheath over the guide wire into the vein and withdraw the guide wire. If using a catheter-introducing sheath, insert the catheter through the sheath and remove the sheath by pulling slowly apart and out from under the skin.

11. Check all lumens of the catheter for blood return, and flush with saline.
12. Secure the wings of the catheter to the skin using sutures. Apply a sterile transparent dressing over the insertion site; 2 × 2 sterile gauze may be used under the transparent dressing to wick away any blood drainage.
13. Obtain a chest x-ray to verify position of the line and identify complications, such as pneumothorax for internal jugular and subclavian approaches.

Central Venous Access Sites and Approaches

1. Femoral Vein

a. Immobilize the leg of choice with slight external rotation of the leg.
b. Place a small diaper or towel under the buttocks of an infant to flatten the inguinal area.
c. Identify the femoral artery by palpation. If the pulses are not palpated, find the midpoint between the anterior superior iliac spine and the pubis symphysis.
d. Guard the artery with the fingers of one hand. The point of entry is medial to the operator's fingers and femoral artery.
e. Follow steps 1 and 2 of the Seldinger technique, described earlier, for insertion.

2. Internal jugular Vein

a. Position child's head 30 degrees down and turned away from the side to be used. The right internal jugular vein is preferable.
b. Identify the sternocleidomastoid muscle and clavicle. Three different sites may be used to cannulate the internal jugular vein: anterior, middle, and posterior. The middle approach is the most commonly used and has the advantage of well-defined landmarks.
c. Percutaneous entry should be made at the apex of the triangle formed by the two heads of the sternocleidomastoid muscle and the clavicle. Direct the needle slightly laterally toward the ipsilateral breast, keeping as superficial as possible. Often a notch can be palpated on the posterior surface of the clavicle, which helps locate the vein in the lateral or medial plane, as the vein lies deep in the shallow notch.
d. Follow steps 1 and 2 of the Seldinger technique, described earlier, for insertion (Figure III–5).

3. Subclavian Vein

a. Place a small rolled-up towel between child's shoulder blades.
b. Place child in Trendelenburg position (15–30 degrees head down). Turn child's head away from the side to be punctured. The right side is preferred for insertion.

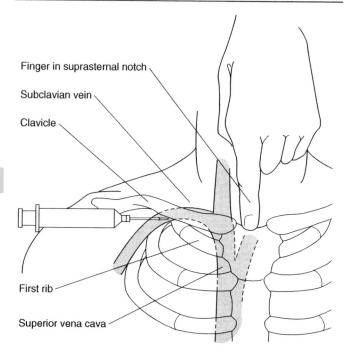

Finger in suprasternal notch

Subclavian vein

Clavicle

First rib

Superior vena cava

Figure III–5. Technique for subclavian vein catheterization. (*Reproduced, with permission, from Gomella LG, Haist SA, eds. Clinician's Pocket Reference, 10th ed. McGraw-Hill. Copyright © 2004.*)

   c. Auscultate and document bilateral breath sounds before beginning the procedure. Percutaneous entry is made caudal to the midclavicle and directed toward the suprasternal notch.
   d. Identify the junction of the middle and medial thirds of the clavicle. Introduce the needle under the clavicle, keeping near the clavicle to avoid the pleura, and direct it toward a fingertip placed in the suprasternal notch (Figure III–6).

Complications: Arterial puncture, laceration of the thoracic duct, pneumothorax, hemothorax, air embolism, sepsis, deep vein thrombosis.

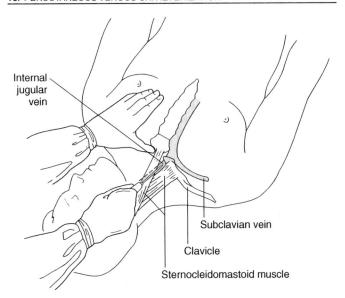

Figure III–6. Technique for internal jugular vein catheterization, central approach. (*Reproduced, with permission, from Gomella LG, Haist SA eds. Clinician's Pocket Reference, 10th ed. McGraw-Hill. Copyright © 2004.*)

REFERENCES

Haziniski MF, Zartsky AL. *Pediatric Advanced Life Support Provider Manual.* American Heart Association, 2002.
Lefor AT, ed. Central venous catheterization. In: *Critical Care On Call.* McGraw-Hill, 2002:323–328.

15. PERCUTANEOUS VENOUS CATHETERIZATION

Indications

1. Administration of fluids, medications, or blood products.
2. Administration of peripheral parenteral nutrition.

Contraindications

1. An extremity with an arteriovenous fistula or graft.
2. History of previous surgery of an extremity.
3. Previous complications associated with vascular access placement that would contraindicate future catheter placement.

Materials: Appropriate size and type of IV catheter (24-, 22-, 20-gauge) for insertion, alcohol wipes, tourniquet, T-connector, 3- or 5-mL syringe, saline flush, adhesive tape, sterile transparent dressing, 2 × 2 gauze squares, gloves, armboard, sterile gloves.

Procedure

1. Assemble equipment. Make strips of tape and flush the air out of the T-connector with saline before beginning the procedure. Secure and comfort child (eg, use blanket around infant as a "mummy" wrap).
2. Wrap extremities in warm compresses before performing the venipuncture to assist in vein dilation. Apply tourniquet 2–6 inches above the intended insertion site. Start with the most distal site on the extremity and work upward for future insertions.
3. Put on gloves, clean insertion site with alcohol wipes or appropriate antiseptic, and apply friction for 30 seconds.
4. Inspect the bevel of the IV catheter for product integrity.
5. Apply traction to the side of the insertion site with the free hand to prevent the vein from rolling and the child from moving.
6. With the bevel up, hold the catheter at a 10–20-degree angle as it penetrates the skin.
7. Check the flashback chamber for blood return. When blood return is obtained, decrease the angle of the needle and advance the catheter an additional 1/16 inch.
8. Using the same hand that performed the venipuncture, gently advance the catheter as the stylet is withdrawn. Once the catheter is advanced into the vein, remove the tourniquet.
9. Carefully activate the needle safety feature on the device while stabilizing the catheter. It may be helpful to place a piece of adhesive tape across the hub of the catheter onto the skin at this point.
10. Apply pressure over the vein just proximal to the insertion site to decrease blood loss while attaching a saline flush to the T-connector with the catheter. Flush with saline to check patency of the vein, and observe for signs of induration or swelling.
11. Secure the catheter to the skin using sterile transparent dressing, tape, and an armboard. Stockinette and gauze wrap are additional items used to prevent pediatric patients from dislodging the intravascular device.

Complications: Mechanical failure (tourniquet not released; catheter kinked or bent), ecchymosis, hematoma, infiltration, extravasation, phlebitis, site infection, sepsis.

REFERENCE

Hankins J, Waldman Lonsway RA, Hedrick C, Perdue MB. *Infusion Therapy in Clinical Practice.* Saunders, 2001.

16. SKIN BIOPSY

Indications

1. Identification or differentiation of skin diseases.
2. Identification of an underlying medical condition (eg, inborn errors of metabolism).

Contraindications

1. Underlying palpable pulse.
2. Site above the temporal, angular, or supraorbital arteries of the face.
3. History of a bleeding disorder (relative).
4. Thrombocytopenia (especially < 10,000 platelets).
5. Suspicion of melanoma (must be excised widely and deeply).

Materials: Alcohol, 1% lidocaine or alternative anesthetic agent (see below); syringe with 30-gauge needle; disposable No. 15 scalpel (shave biopsy); smooth-tipped forceps, skin punch, and sharp scissors (punch biopsy); probe-pointed scissors (scissors excision); 4 × 4 gauze squares; adhesive bandage; suture (3-0, 4-0 nonabsorbable); electrocautery device; specimen container with appropriate preservative; sterile gloves.

Procedure: A better biopsy specimen is obtained if a "fresh" lesion is sampled (the most recent lesion available that is typical of others seen).

1. Clean the wound with alcohol before administering anesthetic agent and again before beginning biopsy excision. Use of a broader spectrum agent, such as povidone-iodine, is not indicated because it might stain the specimen or kill an active infectious agent.
2. Inject 1% lidocaine around and under the lesion but not into the biopsy area itself. Use a very small needle (30-gauge if available) and a very long injection time to minimize pain from anesthesia. Pinching the area prior to injection or applying an ice pack for 5 minutes helps to decrease initial pain from anesthesia. Bacteriostatic saline with benzoyl alcohol can be injected in the same manner in children with lidocaine allergies, but pain relief is brief (not recommended in newborns). EMLA cream (lidocaine and prilocaine in an oil emulsion) is effective if the biopsy incision is not very deep. A drawback of topical cream is the need to apply to skin 1 hour before the procedure, which may increase child's anxiety.
3. Obtain skin biopsy specimen using one of the following approaches.
   a. **Punch biopsy:** Used for superficial inflammatory and bullous lesions. Sterilize and anesthetize the area, as described in steps 1 and 2, above. Stretch the skin with the thumb and index finger of the free hand. With the other hand, hold the skin punch perpendicular to the skin between these two fingers. Rotate the punch, while pushing firmly into the skin. Unlike the dermis, the subcutaneous tissue does not resist the effort to biopsy. Obtain

a 2–6-mm punch specimen, including the entire lesion if possible. Withdraw the punch from the skin. Pull up gently on the biopsy specimen with loosely held, smooth-tipped forceps, and cut deeply with sharp scissors to include subcutaneous material. Immediately place the biopsy specimen in the preservative appropriate for the test to be performed. Apply firm pressure on the wound for at least 3 minutes.

b. **Shave biopsy:** Used for nevi and other elevated lesions in which sampling of subcutaneous tissue is not relevant. Inject 1% lidocaine into the area to elevate the lesion. Stretch the skin with the thumb and index finger of the free hand. With the other hand, lay the flat surface of a disposable No. 15 scalpel against the skin and remove the lesion using a smooth, back-and-forth sawing technique. Scissors may be used at the end to remove the last piece. Close the lesion with electrocautery or a single suture.

c. **Simple scissors excision:** Similar to use of the scalpel in the shave biopsy, described above. Using probe-pointed scissors and cutting with only the very tip, advance the tip very slowly toward the center of the lesion. Close the subsequent gap in the skin with electrocautery or a single suture.

4. Adequate control of bleeding can be achieved in most cases by simple pressure with gauze pads and coverage with a regular adhesive bandage. If bleeding persists, electrocautery, a simple suture, or two sutures parallel to the lines of the skin are indicated. Remove sutures within 3–4 days (face) or 7–8 days (rest of the body).

Complications: Poor healing of the wound, formation of a lumpy scar (keloid), bleeding, infection.

REFERENCES

Habif TE. *Clinical Dermatology, A Color Guide to Diagnosis and Therapy,* 3rd ed. Mosby-Year Book, 1996.
Rakel RE. *Textbook of Family Practice,* 6th ed. Saunders, 2002.

17. SPLINTING

Note: Casts and splints are methods of immobilization. Because casting consists of circumferential fiberglass or plaster, which does not allow space for swelling, caution should be taken when applying casts in the setting of acute injury. Splinting is the preferred method of immobilization for these injuries and is discussed here. For fractures that require an immediate orthopaedic consultation and management, a temporary splint (board with gauze wrap) should be applied loosely for stabilization until orthopedic consultation is obtained.

Indications

1. Acute management of nondisplaced, closed fractures for at least the first 24–48 hours.
2. Definitive treatment or support of sprains in adolescents with closed growth plates.
3. Stabilization of injury with pain near an open growth plate (Salter-Harris type I fracture).
4. Immobilization to allow for healing of sutured wounds or burns over joints.

Contraindications

1. Neurovascular compromise.
2. Open fractures.
3. Fractures of the elbow or femur.
4. Fractures with angulation > 30 degree.
5. Fractures through the physis (Salter-Harris types III, IV, and V).

Materials

1. **Preformed splint (commercially available):** Includes stockinette, padding, and fiberglass or plaster in one unit; tape measure; elastic bandages to secure splint.
2. **Custom splint:** Stockinette, soft cotton rolls, plaster or fiberglass sheets, tape measure, elastic bandages. (Fiberglass is often preferred because it is durable, lightweight, and easier to work with than plaster.)

Procedure

1. Review x-rays to determine fracture type, growth plate involvement, and angulation of bone fragments.
2. Choose the appropriate type of splint and identify an assistant. To place most splints on children, 4 hands are usually needed. Figures III–7 through III–15 illustrate different types of splints with their indications.
3. Measure materials using a tape measure on the uninjured extremity. Cut out notches in the splint to bend around joints without excessive folding.
4. If making a custom splint, begin with stockinette and then cotton roll. Smooth out uneven areas and prevent bunching or folding of the material, especially in flexor surfaces, to prevent cuts or abrasions of the skin beneath the splint. If using preformed splint material, extra padding with cotton material may be needed over joints or bony prominences.
5. Position child comfortably to maximize ease of splint application. If child is fearful, restrain or have child sit on a parent's lap.
6. Wet the plaster or fiberglass with cool or tepid water. Using too much water will increase the time needed for splint material to

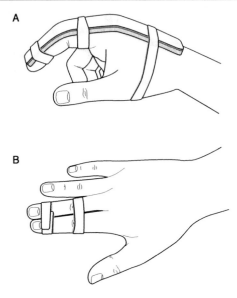

Figure III-7. A. Finger splint. **B.** Buddy taping. Indications: Fractures, lacerations, and sprains of fingers. (*Redrawn with permission from Dieckmann RA, Fiser DH, Selbst SM, eds. Illustrated Textbook of Pediatric Emergency & Critical Care Procedures. Mosby, 1997.*)

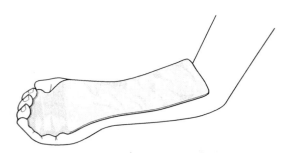

Figure III-8. Volar splint. Indications: Fractures of distal forearm and wrist, wrist sprains. (*Redrawn with permission from Dieckmann RA, Fiser DH, Selbst SM, eds. Illustrated Textbook of Pediatric Emergency & Critical Care Procedures. Mosby, 1997.*)

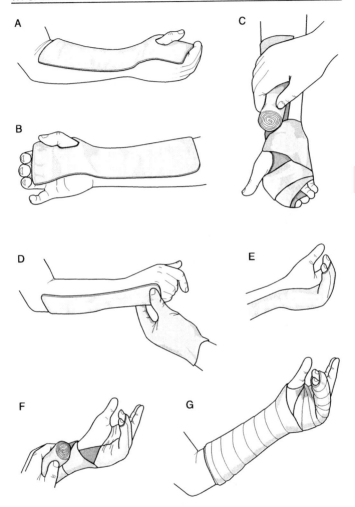

Figure III–9. Gutter splint. **A–C.** Radial gutter splint. **D–G.** Ulnar gutter splint. Indications: Radial gutter (second or third metacarpal or phalangeal fractures), ulnar gutter (fourth or fifth metacarpal or phalangeal fractures). (*Redrawn with permission from Dieckmann RA, Fiser DH, Selbst SM, eds. Illustrated Textbook of Pediatric Emergency & Critical Care Procedures. Mosby, 1997.*)

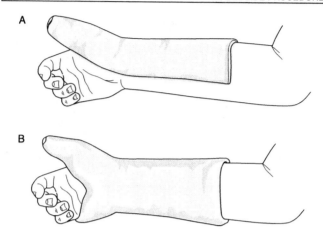

Figure III–10. A, B. Thumb spica splint. Indications: Navicular or scaphoid fractures, thumb dislocations and fractures, ulnar collateral ligament injuries (gamekeeper thumb). (*Redrawn with permission from Dieckmann RA, Fiser DH, Selbst SM, eds. Illustrated Textbook of Pediatric Emergency & Critical Care Procedures. Mosby, 1997.*)

harden; using hot water will add heat to the exothermic reaction and can burn the skin.

7. Place the splint material in position and begin initial shaping.
8. Secure the splint with the elastic bandage at a large distal joint. Overwrap the splint from distal to proximal (to reduce swelling) with the elastic bandage.

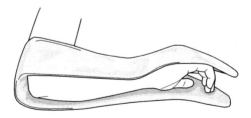

Figure III–11. Sugar tong arm splint. Indications: Fracture of distal forearm. (*Redrawn with permission from Dieckmann RA, Fiser DH, Selbst SM, eds. Illustrated Textbook of Pediatric Emergency & Critical Care Procedures. Mosby, 1997.*)

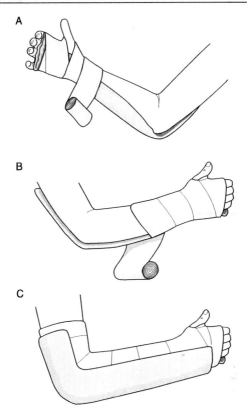

Figure III-12. A–C. Posterior arm splint. Indications: Elbow fractures and sprains, stable supracondylar fractures. (*Redrawn with permission from Dieckmann RA, Fiser DH, Selbst SM, eds. Illustrated Textbook of Pediatric Emergency & Critical Care Procedures. Mosby, 1997.*)

9. Maintain the splint's positioning for approximately 15 minutes until it hardens.

10. Discharge instructions should include the following: advice to child, parent, or caregiver to elevate and apply ice, and keep the splint dry; pain management guidelines; splint care instructions (advise to check for perfusion, sensation, and function distal to the splint and return immediately for alterations if changes are noted); and information about orthopedic follow-up.

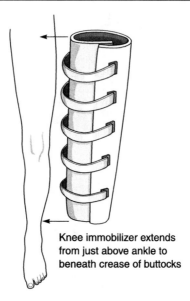

**Knee immobilizer extends
from just above ankle to
beneath crease of buttocks**

Figure III–13. Long leg and knee immobilizer splint. Indications Injuries to soft tissue or ligament of knee, fracture of distal femur, fracture of proximal tibia, and fibula. (*Redrawn with permission from Dieckmann RA, Fiser DH, Selbst SM, eds. Illustrated Textbook of Pediatric Emergency & Critical Care Procedures. Mosby, 1997.*)

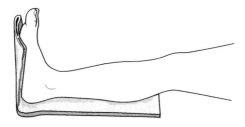

Figure III–14. Posterior short leg splint. Indications: Fractures of distal tibia and fibula, ankle sprains, tarsal and metatarsal fractures. (*Redrawn with permission from Dieckmann RA, Fiser DH, Selbst SM, eds. Illustrated Textbook of Pediatric Emergency & Critical Care Procedures. Mosby, 1997.*)

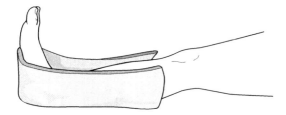

Figure III–15. Sugar tong and stirrup splint. Indications: Fractures of distal tibia and fibula, ankle sprains. (*Redrawn with permission from Dieckmann RA, Fiser DH, Selbst SM, eds. Illustrated Textbook of Pediatric Emergency & Critical Care Procedures. Mosby, 1997.*)

11. Always check the splint prior to discharge for continued proper positioning and fit and neurovascular integrity distal to the splint. Document proper splint fit.

Complications: Compromised perfusion caused by swelling during first 24–48 hours following injury (to avoid, do not fully encircle injury or overwrap too tightly; include instruction to elevate limb in discharge information); skin abrasions from folding and bunching of the cushioning material beneath the splint; contact dermatitis from the splinting material; joint stiffness from prolonged immobilization.

REFERENCES

Dieckmann RA, Fiser DH, Selbst SM, eds. *Illustrated Textbook of Pediatric Emergency & Critical Care Procedures.* Mosby, 1997.
Henretig FM, King C, eds. *Textbook of Pediatric Emergency Procedures.* Williams & Wilkins, 1997.

18. THORACENTESIS

Indications
1. Determination of type of pleural effusion (transudate, exudate, cultures).
2. Therapeutic removal of fluid.
3. Instillation of sclerosing compounds or lytic agents into pleural space.

Contraindications
1. Pneumothorax, hemothorax, or respiratory impairment on the contralateral side.

2. Coagulopathy (relative).
3. Patient who is receiving positive pressure ventilation (relative).

Materials: Prepackaged thoracentesis kit or minor procedure tray, 20–50-mL syringe, 20- or 22-gauge needle, 3-way stopcock, 1% lidocaine, specimen containers, bandage, sterile gloves.

Procedure

1. Consider procedural sedation (See Section I, Chapter 81, Sedation and Analgesia, p. 377).
2. The site of thoracentesis in children (posterior back or midaxillary line) is dependent on child's clinical situation. If child is able to sit and lean forward on pillows or over a chair, the procedure can be accomplished by entering the pleural space from the posterolateral aspect of the back, several centimeters lateral to the spine. If child is not able to sit, the effusion may drained by placing child in a decubitus position or supine with the head of the bed elevated.
3. To select the entry site, percuss out the fluid level. In general, the entry point is one intercostal space below the point where percussion becomes dull. If percussion is not possible, use a chest x-ray and count ribs. Consider using an ultrasound-guided technique for high-risk patients, a loculated collection of fluid, or a small fluid collection.
4. Use sterile technique.
5. Enter the skin superior to the rib to avoid arteries, veins, and nerves that traverse the inferior aspect of the ribs. To avoid injury to the spleen or liver, do not attempt thoracentesis below the eighth intercostal space.
6. Anesthetize the skin, periosteum of the rib, and parietal pleura using a small-bore needle and 1% lidocaine. Make a skin wheal over the proposed site. Infiltrate up and over the rib and anesthetize by repeated injection and aspiration of small amounts of anesthetic agent. Withdraw the needle once fluid is aspirated.
7. Introduce a 22- or 20-gauge needle attached to a 20–50-mL syringe with a 3-way stopcock into the previously anesthetized track to the same depth with constant aspiration until pleural fluid is obtained.
8. Continue gentle aspiration until the syringe is filled or no fluid is aspirated. A 3-way stopcock inserted between the hub of the needle and the syringe is used to repeatedly aspirate large volumes of fluid. Withdraw the needle as child exhales or performs a Valsalva to increase intrathoracic pressure and decrease the chance of pneumothorax. Bandage the site.
9. Obtain a chest x-ray to evaluate the fluid level and to rule out pneumothorax.
10. Send samples of pleural fluid for the following studies: pH, specific gravity, protein, LDH, glucose, CBC and differential, Gram

TABLE III–4. CONDITIONS COMMONLY ASSOCIATED WITH PLEURAL EFFUSIONS IN CHILDREN

Type of Effusion	Associated Condition
Exudative	Collagen vascular disease (eg, rheumatoid arthritis, systemic lupus erythematosus)
	Idiopathic
	Infectious (especially parapneumonic process, typically bacteria or other infections, including viral, fungal, mycobacteria, mycoplasma)
	Intra-abdominal disease (eg, pancreatitis, hepatitis)
	Neoplastic (eg, lymphoma or leukemia)
	Other (chylothorax, hemothorax, drug-induced pleural disease, radiation therapy, postmyocardial infarction)
	Renal (eg, uremia)
Transudative	Cardiac (eg, congestive heart disease, superior vena cava obstruction, pericarditis)
	Hepatic (eg, cirrhosis with ascites, low albumin)
	Iatrogenic (eg, catheter extravasation from subclavian or internal jugular line)
	Idiopathic
	Pulmonary (eg, acute atelectasis)
	Renal (eg, nephrotic syndrome, peritoneal dialysis)

stain, and bacterial cultures. Consider evaluating the fluid for cytology, fungal and acid-fast bacilli smears and culture, amylase (if effusion secondary to pancreatitis is suspected), and triglycerides (if chylothorax is suspected). Table III–4 lists conditions commonly associated with pleural effusions.

Complications: Pneumothorax, hemothorax, infection, pulmonary laceration, hypoxemia, vasovagal response, reexpansion pulmonary edema, laceration of spleen or liver. Removal of large amounts of pulmonary fluid may cause a potentially fatal syndrome of reexpansion pulmonary edema.

REFERENCE

Haist SA, Robbins JB, eds. *Internal Medicine On Call,* 3rd ed. McGraw-Hill, 2002:431–434.

19. TYMPANOCENTESIS

Indication: Collection of fluid from the middle ear for culture.

Contraindications

1. Prior middle ear or mastoid surgery.
2. Coagulopathy (relative).

Materials: Topical anesthetic (depending on age of child); papoose; operating microscope or magnified open-head otoscope; aural speculum; 25-gauge, 1.5-inch or spinal needle; isopropyl alcohol; suction tubing with No. 5 ear suction; aerobic and anaerobic culturettes; sterile gloves.

Procedure

1. Younger, uncooperative children may require restraint or general anesthesia. Older children will tolerate tympanocentesis as an office procedure.
2. Prepare the ear canal and lateral surface of the tympanic membrane (TM) by instilling isopropyl alcohol (at body temperature to prevent a caloric effect) and then suctioning it from the canal with No. 5 ear suction.
3. Topical anesthesia may be obtained by instilling topical anesthetic drops or cream and waiting 5–10 minutes for this to take effect. Alternately, a small cotton swab may be used to place a drop of phenol on the surface of the TM. Commercial kits for myringotomy contain a prepackaged phenol applicator. Advise child that he or she will feel a brief burning sensation. Place the topical anesthetic on the anteroinferior quadrant of the TM (from the 6 o'clock to the 9 o'clock position).
4. Bend the 25-gauge needle slightly at the hub, so that the syringe and physician's hand will not block the point of view. The hand should always be kept leaning against child's head, so that any sudden or unexpected movement of the head will not result in injury to the canal, TM, or middle ear structure.
5. Pass the needle through the TM at the anteroinferior quadrant (away from the ossicular chain, round window, and facial nerve), and aspirate the fluid.
6. Inject the aspirated fluid into the culturettes.
7. Topical drops are not required after the procedure; however, child should refrain from allowing water to pass directly onto the TM for several days until the site of tympanocentesis has healed.

Complications: Bleeding, infection, hearing loss.

REFERENCE

Bluestone CD, Klein JO. Otitis media and eustachian tube dysfunction. In: Bluestone CD, Stool SE, Alper CM, et al, eds. *Pediatric Otolaryngology,* 4th ed. Saunders, 2003:634–635.

20. UMBILICAL VEIN CATHETERIZATION

Indications

1. Emergency administration of medications and fluids in the delivery room or neonatal intensive care unit.
2. Blood sampling.

Contraindications

1. Omphalitis.
2. Necrotizing enterocolitis.

Materials: 3.5 Fr or 5 Fr umbilical catheter, heparinized saline (0.5–1 unit/mL), 3-way stopcock, syringes, 10% povidone-iodine preparation, sutures, adhesive tape, sterile cutdown tray, sterile gloves, mask, protective eyewear.

Procedure

1. Put on mask, protective eyewear, and sterile gloves. Use aseptic technique and observe standard precautions throughout procedure.
2. Flush a 3.5 Fr or 5 Fr radiopaque umbilical catheter with heparinized saline (0.5–1 unit/mL) attached to a 3-way stopcock.
3. Prepare the umbilical cord. Clean the umbilical clamp, stump, and a wide area of the surrounding abdominal skin with 10% povidone-iodine preparation. Allow to dry.
4. Holding the umbilical cord firmly with an encircling tie to prevent bleeding, cut it with a scalpel blade 1 cm above the skin attachment.
5. The umbilical vein is identified as a single, large, thin-walled oval vessel. It is distinguishable from the two umbilical arteries, which are smaller, thick-walled round vessels that are often constricted and extend above the cut surface of the cord (Figure III–16).

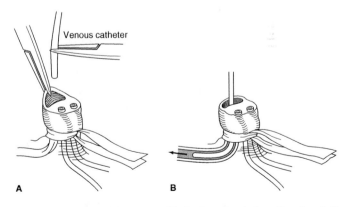

Figure III-16. A, B. Technique for umbilical vein catheterization. *(From Gomella TL. Neonatology, 5th ed. Originally published by Appleton & Lange. Copyright (c) 2004 by The McGraw-Hill Companies, Inc.)*

6. Flush the umbilical catheter with heparinized saline and evacuate any air bubbles to avoid the possible complication of air embolus to the central circulation.
7. Place the catheter in the inferior vena cava above the level of the hepatic veins and the ductus venosus. Initially insert the umbilical catheter upward toward the liver, so that the tip is just below the skin and blood can be readily aspirated.
8. Then guide the catheter tip to a depth of 1–4 cm to avoid the portal vessel.
9. Stabilize the catheter with suture, tape, or both.
10. Assess lower extremities and buttocks for blanching or sudden cyanosis caused by vascular spasm or embolism.
11. Confirm correct placement of catheter tip radiographically.

Complications: Vascular compromise, hemorrhage, air embolism, infection, thrombosis, vascular perforation.

REFERENCES

Gomella TL. *Neonatology,* 4th ed. McGraw-Hill, 1999:187.
Hankins J, Waldman Lonsway RA, Hedrick C, Perdue MB. *Infusion Therapy in Clinical Practice.* Saunders, 2001:587.
Hazinski MF, Zartsky AL. *Pediatric Advanced Life Support Provider Manual.* American Heart Association, 2002:350.
Infusion Nurses Society. *Policies and Practice for Infusion Nursing,* 2nd ed. Infusion Nurses Society, 2002:96–98.

21. VENIPUNCTURE (PHLEBOTOMY)

Indication: Collection of blood from a vein for diagnostic examination.

Contraindications

1. Extremity with an arteriovenous fistula or graft.
2. Site proximal to an existing and infusing IV site.
3. Site with evidence of infection, vascular injury, or hematoma.

Materials: Tourniquet, towel roll, sterile gloves, gauze, alcohol wipes, butterfly needle (25 or 23 gauge), Vacutainer holder, 3-mL syringe(s), appropriate color-coded blood collection tubes, bandage, biohazard bag, labels for laboratory tubes.

Procedure

1. Gather equipment and check expiration dates on laboratory tubes. For small infants or small-volume specimens, microtainer tubes are sometimes used.

2. Put on gloves and clean the site with alcohol wipes. As a general rule, arm veins are the best source from which to obtain blood.
3. Apply tourniquet midway between the elbow and shoulder. Place a towel roll under the elbow to stabilize arm and decrease movement of young child.
4. Place the thumb of the free hand just below the needle insertion site and press down on the arm while pulling skin taut. With the bevel of the needle up, pinch the wings of the butterfly needle together and puncture the skin.
5. If using a syringe for blood collection, withdraw the plunger of the syringe gently to avoid collapsing the vein. If using a Vacutainer, place tube in the holder and push until the needle punctures the rubber top of the tube. If multiple tubes are necessary, remove one and insert another. Gently rotate each tube as it is removed.
6. Release tourniquet as soon as blood flow is adequate, and always before withdrawing the needle. Remove the last tube from the holder before withdrawing the needle from the vein.
7. Keep child's arm extended, while applying gentle pressure with sterile gauze to the puncture site until bleeding has stopped. Cover puncture site with a bandage.
8. Label all tubes with patient identification information and place in biohazard bag.

Complications: Hematoma, inadvertent arterial puncture.

REFERENCES

Clinical Laboratory Specimen Collection Manual. Alfred I duPont Hospital for Children, 2002:2–5.
Intravenous Nurses Society. Blood drawing. In: *Infusion Nursing Standards of Practice.* Infusion Nurses Society, 2000:66–67.
Wong D, Hockenberry MJ. *Nursing Care of Infants and Children,* 7th ed. Mosby, 2003:1147–1148.

22. WOUND CARE AND SUTURING

Indications
1. Restoration of function and structural integrity of the skin.
2. Prevention of infection.
3. Promotion of cosmetically appealing healing.

Contraindications: (All relative, to avoid infection.)

1. Contaminated wounds and crush injuries, especially those with poor blood supply (lower extremity), should be repaired within 6 hours.

Clean wounds and those on face and scalp (high blood supply, low risk of infection) may be repaired up to 12–24 hours after injury.
2. Puncture wounds and those with high risk of infection (bite wounds, contaminated) are at risk for infection if closed.
3. Immunocompromised patients (diabetic, HIV infected, malignancy) are at risk.
4. Complicated wounds with nerve, tendon, or muscle layer repair and those that would be better served by repair under anesthesia by a plastic surgeon should be referred.

Materials: Sterile gloves, iodophor or chlorhexidine-based solution (povidone-iodine), sterile saline, 20–60-mL syringe for irrigation, splashguard or needle-over-catheter assembly (Angiocath) to direct spray, small-gauge (27- or 30-gauge) needle, 1% lidocaine, sterile drapes, gauze sponges, needle driver, scissors, tissue forceps, scalpel (for debridement if necessary), suture material (Table III–5), local anesthetic, bright lighting, antibiotic ointment, bandage or tape.

Procedure

1. Prepare child and family for the procedure. Inform parents that every effort will be made to keep child comfortable. Warn child of pain.
2. Prepare the wound. Anesthetize the wound with local infiltration of an anesthetic (eg, lidocaine). Use a small-gauge needle (27 or 30 gauge). Confirm whether lidocaine on hand contains epinephrine. Epinephrine is a vasoconstrictor, which can help with hemostasis, but cannot be used on areas of distal perfusion (fingers, toes, penis,

TABLE III–5. SUTURE CHOICE[a]

SUTURE TYPE	ADVANTAGES	DISADVANTAGES	USES
Natural absorbable (gut, chromic)	Dissolve rapidly (within days)	Increased risk of inflammatory reaction	Intraoral, facial
Synthetic absorbable *(Vicryl)*	Less reactivity, greater tensile strength	Foreign body reaction if not absorbed rapidly enough	Subcuticular layers
Nylon *(Ethilon, Prolene)*	Nonreactive Prolene is blue	Must be removed Prolene is stiff to use	Outer layer repair, facial, Prolene in eyebrows or hair for ease of removal
Silk	High tensile strength	High inflammatory reaction	Anchoring of central lines

[a]Use the smallest possible size on an appropriately sized cutting needle; range, 3.0–6.0 (small number = large material). For face, 6.0 or 5.0; high tension (joints), 4.0 or 3.0; scalp, 3.0 or staples; buried sutures, 5.0 or 4.0 if high tension.

ears, nose) or on the vermillion border of the lip during its repair. Dose of lidocaine is 7 mg/kg, or 0.7 mL/kg of 1% solution (5 mg/kg if solution contains epinephrine). Buffer the lidocaine with sodium bicarbonate (1 mL lidocaine to 9 mL bicarbonate) to reduce the burn felt on injection. If desired, place LET (lidocaine, epinephrine, tetracaine) or TAC (tetracaine, adrenaline, cocaine) on the wound 30 minutes before beginning wound care. This sometimes provides sufficient anesthesia to accomplish the repair. If additional local medication is needed, it is more comfortable if the skin is anesthetized first. The same guidelines for distal perfusion apply to the topical anesthetics containing vasoconstrictors.

3. Explore the wound carefully for presence of foreign bodies. If a radiopaque foreign body might be present, obtain an x-ray prior to repair of the wound. If the wound is on an extremity, explore for function distal to the wound.

4. Debride devitalized or heavily contaminated tissue. Accomplish this by excising the area around the wound to make a smooth ellipse for cleaner closure. If excising the wound, be sure there is enough excess tissue to avoid undue tension (Figure III–17).

5. Irrigate the wound vigorously with sterile saline under high pressure using the splashguard or catheter-over-needle assembly (Angiocath) to direct the spray. If desired, a few drops of povidone-iodine may be mixed with saline to irrigate dirty wounds. Using antiseptic solutions

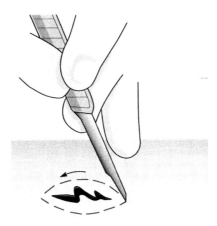

Figure III–17. Elliptical incision for debridement of a jagged laceration.(*Redrawn with permission from Henretig FM, King C, eds. Textbook of Pediatric Emergency Procedures. Williams & Wilkins, 1997.*)

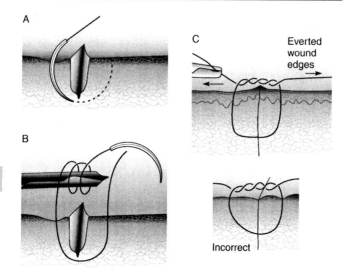

Figure III–18. A–C. Technique for placement of simple interrupted skin sutures with eversion of wound edges. Used for most wound repair in children. (*Redrawn with permission from Henretig FM, King C, eds. Textbook of Pediatric Emergency Procedures. Williams & Wilkins, 1997.*)

    directly on the wound can impede healing. A volume of 1 mL per centimeter of wound should be used for proper cleansing.

6. Apply sutures, following the general principles outlined below. (Refer to Figures III–18 through III–22 for suture techniques.)

    a. Evert the edges by using proper technique.

    b. Match the layers of tissue.

    c. Use the smallest amount of suture material (foreign body) possible for a good closure.

    d. Approximate the tissue rather than closing it tightly, because tight sutures strangulate the skin.

    e. Reduce tension on the sutures by placing them equidistant from each other and from the wound edge. Place deep layers to approximate the skin better and reduce tension.

    f. Approach the wound by dividing it with a central stitch or from one end; either way, avoid forming a "dog ear" with extra tissue.

7. Apply antibiotic ointment and a clean dressing.

8. Postsuture care is important and should always address tetanus prophylaxis (see Appendix L, p. 771), measures to reduce infection and

A

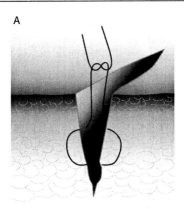

B

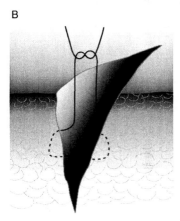

Figure III–19. A, B. Buried subcutaneous suture. Used to close deeper layers of tissue, muscle, and so forth. Limits tension on skin sutures and prevents formation of subcutaneous fluid collection, which can be a potential source of infection. (*Redrawn with permission from Henretig FM, King C, eds. Textbook of Pediatric Emergency Procedures. Williams & Wilkins, 1997.*)

A

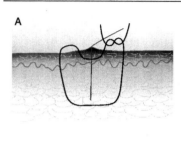

B

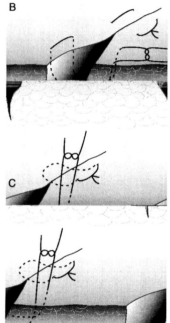

C

Figure III–20. A–C. Mattress sutures (vertical, horizontal, and half-buried horizontal). Useful for eversion of wound edges. Will limit stress on the skin during closure of wounds with high amount of tension. (*Redrawn with permission from Henretig FM, King C, eds. Textbook of Pediatric Emergency Procedures. Williams & Wilkins, 1997.*)

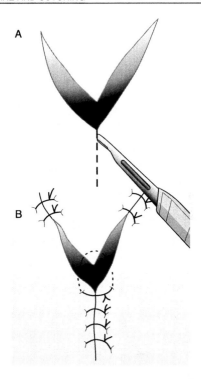

Figure III–21. A, B. Corner stitch or {ss}V–Y flap. An advanced technique, used to secure a flap with a modified half-buried mattress suture. Extension of the apex of the {ss}V to form a {ss}Y will release some of the tension on the corner. (*Redrawn with permission from Henretig FM, King C, eds. Textbook of Pediatric Emergency Procedures. Williams & Wilkins, 1997.*)

scar formation, and plan for removal of sutures (Table III–6). A dry bandage should be placed for the first 1–2 days to prevent bacterial contamination and promote epithelialization. After this time wounds can be washed and patted dry. On some wounds, a bulky dressing may also help with immobilization.

Complications: Infection, formation of a lumpy scar (keloid), retained foreign body, continued loss of function due to injury to deep structures.

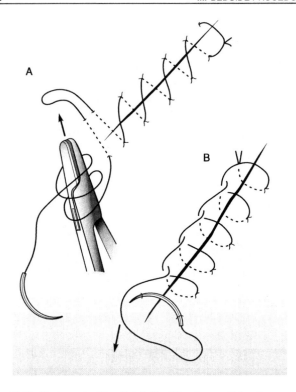

Figure III–22. Simple running **(A)** and interlocking **(B)** continuous stitches. These are useful for saving time, but have the disadvantage of unraveling upon breakage at one point in the stitch. There is a problem with ischemia of the wound edges and also difficulty in releasing part of a wound for drainage of infection. Only to be considered in older children (less risk of breakage) with clean straight wounds. (*Redrawn with permission from Henretig FM, King C, eds. Textbook of Pediatric Emergency Procedures. Williams & Wilkins, 1997.*)

Alternatives to Sutures

1. **Staples:** Often used on scalp lacerations. Remember to send family home with a staple remover, as these are not routinely stocked in offices for follow-up.
2. **Skin glue:** Newer method of skin closure, with limited usage. It cannot be used on lacerations that have tension, are gaping, involve

TABLE III–6. OPTIMAL TIME FOR SUTURE REMOVAL

Location	Days
Face	3–5
Scalp	5–7
Chest	6–8
Back	10–12
Forearm	6–8
Fingers	8–10
Hand	6–8
Lower extremity	6–10
Joint	
Extensor surface	8–10
Flexor surface	6–8
Foot	8–10

Modified from Capellan O, Hollander JE. Management of lacerations in the emergency department. Emerg Med Clin North Am 2003;21:1–22.

hair, are near the eyes, or are at high risk for infection. It is also not advisable to use skin glue on the hands, as it will loosen with water exposure.

3. **Wound tapes:** Also an option, alone or to support sutures.

REFERENCES

Capellan O, Hollander JE. Management of lacerations in the emergency department. *Emerg Med Clin North Am* 2003;21:1–22.

Fleisher GR, Ludwig S. *Textbook of Pediatric Emergency Medicine.* Lippincott Williams & Wilkins, 2000.

Henretig FM, King C, eds. *Textbook of Pediatric Emergency Procedures.* Williams & Wilkins, 1997.

IV. Fluids and Electrolytes

1. MAINTENANCE FLUIDS AND ELECTROLYTES

Fluid and electrolyte therapy during health and disease includes three categories of hydration: maintenance, deficit, and replacement therapy. Fluid and electrolyte homeostatic balance depends on normal renal, pulmonary, endocrine, GI, and CNS function.

Provision of fluids and electrolytes to replace daily losses expended during normal physiologic activities, such as breathing, excreting renal solute, and regulating body temperature, is termed *maintenance needs*. Historically, daily maintenance water needs are estimated based on energy expenditure; for every kilocalorie (kcal) of energy used per day, 1 mL of water must be provided. These requirements are met using the guidelines in Table IV–1, based on the **Holliday-Segar method.** This method is not suitable for neonates younger than 14 days of age, because it overestimates their fluid needs.

The **body surface area method** for fluid and electrolyte therapy is based on the assumption that caloric expenditure is proportional to surface area. It should not be used in children who weigh less than 10 kg. Table IV–2 summarizes these requirements.

Maintenance water losses occur from insensible sources (almost exclusively evaporative and respiratory losses; equivalent to 40 mL H_2O per 100 kcal) and from urine output (up to 75 mL H_2O per 100 kcal). With the generation of 15 mL H_2O for every 100 kcal of energy produced, net water balance is maintained.

Clinical conditions can have a profound impact on water and electrolyte losses. Fever increases insensible water losses by 12% for every degree Celsius increase in temperature above 37°C (98.6°F). Insensible water losses are increased by 25–300% in premature infants (due to their increased surface area), and with use of radiant warmers and phototherapy. These considerations should be taken into account when writing fluid orders.

Estimates for maintenance electrolyte therapy are based on metabolic demands and hence water requirements (see Tables IV–1 and IV–2). Although there can be significant GI or cutaneous losses (under pathologic conditions), most of the electrolyte losses occur in urine under normal conditions.

Glucose also should be added, at a low percentage (5%), because the child's fat stores should compensate for temporary lack of nutrients. Based on the preceding guidelines, these requirements are closely approximated by 5% dextrose $\frac{1}{4}$ isotonic saline (3.9 mEq/100 mL) to which potassium chloride (2 mEq/100 mL) is added.

Total Body Water, Osmolality, and Tonicity

Water homeostasis is crucial in maintaining stable serum osmolality. The major contributing factors to serum osmolality are serum sodium (Na^+),

TABLE IV-1. DAILY FLUID AND ELECTROLYTE REQUIREMENTS BASED ON ENERGY
EXPENDITURE

Weight (kg)	Water Requirement	Electrolyte Requirement (mEq/100 mL H_2O)
2.5–10	100 mL/kg	Sodium (Na^+) 2–3
10–20	1000 mL + 50 mL/kg over 10 kg	Potassium (K^+) 1–2
>20	1500 mL + 20 mL/kg over 20 kg	Chloride (Cl^-) 3–5

BUN, and serum glucose. In most situations, contributions of the latter two
are small. Serum osmolality is assayed by measuring the depression of
the freezing point in serum. It is estimated by the following equation:

$$\text{Serum osmolality} = 2 \times [Na^+]\ (\text{mEq/L}) + \text{Serum glucose (mg/dL)}/1.8$$

$$+ \text{BUN (mg/dL)}/2.8$$

Water is the most abundant body component, accounting for 50–60% of
the weight in older children and adolescents, 65–70% in infants and toddlers, and 70–75% in full-term neonates. Obese individuals and women
have less total body water. It is distributed in two major compartments:
intracellular (two thirds of total body water) and extracellular (one third of
total body water). Na^+ is the major extracellular ion (140 mEq/L), whereas
potassium (K^+) is the major intracellular ion (150 mEq/L). Because the cellular membrane is permeable to water, the distribution of water between
these spaces reflects osmotic, oncotic, and hydrostatic forces. Plasma proteins are effective at maintaining water intravascularly, while hydrostatic
pressure maintains water extravascularly. Na^+ serves as an interstitial
osmole (extracellular), whereas K^+ serves as an intracellular osmole. An
increase in serum Na^+ concentration (which does not freely cross the cell
membrane) affects a shift of water from the intracellular to the extracellular compartment. A rise in BUN, which freely crosses the cell membranes,
does not result in fluid shifts. Hence hyperosmolality (BUN and Na^+) is not
synonymous with hypertonicity (Na^+).

Not All Patients Are Created Equal

Fluid and electrolytes requirements are adjusted according to clinical
needs. Table IV–3 summarizes some of the conditions encountered in
hospitalized children.

TABLE IV-2. DAILY FLUID AND ELECTROLYTE REQUIREMENTS BASED ON BODY SURFACE
AREA

Component	Requirement
Water	1500 mL/m^2/day
Sodium (Na^+)	30—50 mEq/m^2/day
Potassium (K^+)	20—40 mEq/m^2/day

TABLE IV–3. CONDITIONS THAT ALTER DAILY FLUID AND ELECTROLYTE REQUIREMENTS

Clinical Situation	Average Water Requirement (mL H_2O/100 kcal/day)
Normal	100
Anuria	40 (replace insensible water loss with minimum electrolytes)
Fever (40°C [104°F])	115
High humidity	80–100
Hyperventilation (no humidity)	120–200
Diabetes insipidus	Up to 400
Syndrome of inappropriate antidiuretic hormone secretion	40–60

2. DEFICIT REPLACEMENT

The patient's fluid deficit can be estimated by subtracting the illness weight from the preillness weight. If the preillness weight is not available, the degree of dehydration based on clinical signs and symptoms is used. For example, if the degree of dehydration in a 10-kg infant is estimated to be 10%, then

$$\frac{9}{\text{Preillness weight}} = \frac{90}{100}$$

$$\text{Preillness weight} = 10 \text{ kg}$$

$$\text{Deficit} = 1 \text{ kg, which is equivalent to 1000 mL}$$

In isonatremic dehydration, electrolyte deficits are calculated using the following rule: *For every 100 mL of replacement fluid, add 8 mEq of Na^+, 6 mEq of K^+, and 6 mEq of Cl^-.*

For hyponatremic and hypernatremic dehydration, refer to Section I, Chapters 50 (Hyponatremia) and 43 (Hypernatremia), respectively.

There are three phases to deficit replacement therapy.

1. **Rapid phase.** This phase aims to restore circulation and stabilize vital signs. Normal saline, 20 mL/kg, is infused over 20–60 minutes, depending on clinical presentation. This may be repeated as dictated by clinical response. If patient is in severe shock, consider 5% albumin, 10–20 mL/kg over 30 minutes, irrespective of type of dehydration.
2. **Second phase.** During this phase, extracellular fluid losses are replaced and acid-base disturbances are corrected. Half of the estimated fluid and electrolyte are replaced over 8 hours. The initial boluses from the "rapid phase" are subtracted from this volume.
3. **Recovery phase.** This phase aims to restore the body's potassium stores and correct the remaining deficits. The remaining half of the estimated fluid and electrolyte deficits are replaced over the next 18 hours.

In addition to deficit replacement, the patient's maintenance fluids and electrolytes are added to the hourly fluid rate. If there are ongoing losses, they are replaced volume for volume with a fluid containing the appropriate solute concentration, as shown in Tables IV–4 and IV–5.

TABLE IV–4. COMPOSITION AND DAILY PRODUCTION OF BODY FLUIDS

	Electrolytes (mEq/L)				Average Daily
Fluid	Na$^+$	Cl$^-$	K$^+$	HCO$_3^-$	Production (mL)
Sweat	50	40	5	0	Varies
Saliva	60	15	26	50	1500
Gastric juices	60–100	100	10	0	1500–2500
Duodenum	130	90	5	0–10	300–2000
Bile	145	100	5	15	100–300
Pancreatic juice	140	75	5	115	100–800
Ileum	140	100	2–8	30	100–9000
Diarrhea	120	90	25	45	—

Modified and reproduced with permission from Gomella LG, Haist SA, eds. Clinician's Pocket Reference, 10th ed. McGraw-Hill. Copyright © 2002.

TABLE IV–5. COMPOSITION OF COMMONLY USED CRYSTALLOID SOLUTIONS

	Electrolytes (mEq/L)						
Fluid	Glucose (g/L)	Na$^+$	Cl$^-$	K$^+$	Ca$^+$	HCO$_3^-$	kcal/L
D$_5$W (5% dextrose in water)	50	—	—	—	—	—	170
D$_{10}$W (10% dextrose in water)	100	—	—	—	—	—	340
D$_{20}$W (20% dextrose in water)	200	—	—	—	—	—	680
D$_{50}$W (50% dextrose in water)	500	—	—	—	—	—	1700
½ NS (0.45% NaCl)	—	77	77	—	—	—	—
NS (0.9% NS)	—	154	154	—	—	—	—
3% NS	—	513	513	—	—	—	—
D$_5$¼NS	50	38	38	—	—	—	170
D$_5$½ NS (0.45% NaCl)	50	77	77	—	—	—	170
D$_5$% NS (0.9% NaCl)	50	154	154	—	—	—	170
D$_5$LR (5% dextrose in LR)	50	130	110	4	3	27	180
LR	—	130	110	4	3	27	<10

NS = normal saline; LR = lactated Ringer.
Modified and reproduced with permission from Gomella LG, Haist SA, eds. Clinician's Pocket Reference, 10th ed. McGraw-Hill. Copyright © 2004.

Patients receiving fluid and electrolyte replacement therapy should be closely monitored. Accurate recording of intake and output, and weight; monitoring of blood chemistries; and assessment of vital signs and clinical status are important to prevent over- or underhydration.

REFERENCES

Boineau FG, Lewy JE. Estimation of parenteral fluid requirements. *Pediatr Clin North Am* 1990;37:257–264.

Greenbaum LA. Pathophysiology of body fluids and fluid therapy. In: Behrman RE, Kliegman RM, Jenson HB, eds. *Nelson Textbook of Pediatrics,* 17th ed. Saunders, 2004:190.

Haist SA, Robbins JB. *Internal Medicine On Call,* 3rd ed. McGraw-Hill, 2002.

Hill LL. Body composition, normal electrolyte concentrations, and the maintenance of normal volume, tonicity, and acid-base metabolism. *Pediatr Clin North Am* 1990;37:241–256.

Jospe N, Forbes G. Fluids and electrolytes—Clinical aspects. *Pediatr Rev* 1996;17:395–403.

Kallen RJ, Lonergan JM. Fluid resuscitation of acute hypovolemic hypoperfusion states in pediatrics. *Pediatr Clin North Am* 1990;37:287–294.

V. Blood Component Therapy

1. BLOOD COMPONENTS AND THEIR USES IN PEDIATRICS

Many blood products are available in the United States (Table V–1). These products have never been safer, but they can transmit disease. For this reason, children should only receive blood products when conservative measures (eg, crystalloid infusions for acute blood loss) have failed.

Safe Blood Transfusions

In the United States, RBCs, most often received from donors, are carefully screened to prevent transmission of infectious agents. Platelets are often derived from apheresis, either stored by the recipient or by a person well known to him or her. Plasma and other plasma-derived blood factors (clotting factor concentrates, immune globulins, and protein-containing plasma volume expanders) are derived from paid donors, with pooled blood fractionated to remove impurities and infectious agents. Of note, pooled plasma derivatives are more likely to cause an infection than are whole blood–derived products.

General historical questioning, specific individual questioning, laboratory screening, and purification techniques maintain blood safety (Table V–2). Infectious diseases and agents that can be transmitted through blood products are listed in Table V–3.

Safety can be maintained only with strict adherence to blood product transfusion pathways. Before injection of any blood product, at least two people should check the blood bag and patient to be sure that the right blood product is being administered to the patient.

2. TRANSFUSION REACTIONS

All blood products, especially multidonor plasma and cryoprecipitate, may result in transfusion reactions. These reactions include urticaria (hives), fever, nausea, headaches, and pruritus (itching). Rarely, anaphylaxis occurs. Antihistamines, antipyretics, and epinephrine should be available at the bedside for any patient receiving a blood product transfusion.

Two significant post-transfusion reactions can occur with blood products, especially with gamma globulins.

1. **Inflammatory reaction.** This reaction can occur hours to a day after transfusion and consists of severe headache and ague (fever and chills), lethargy, and nausea. Inflammatory reaction is most common in repeated transfusions and will disappear once transfusion is discontinued.

2. **Anaphylactoid reaction.** This reaction results from complement activation and consists of flushing, hypotension, dyspnea, ague, nausea, and back pain.

TABLE V–1. BLOOD PRODUCTS AND INDICATIONS FOR TRANSFUSION

Blood Product	Type	Indications
Red blood cells (RBCs)	Whole blood (rarely used) Packed RBCs (whole blood less 70% of plasma; most commonly used in US) or acute, severe, traumatic blood loss) Leukocyte-poor RBCs (for patients with history of febrile reactions to blood products or who will receive many transfusions) Washed RBCs (to prevent host-versus-graft disease in IgA-deficient recipients and others) CMV-free RBCs (for potential transplantation patients) Frozen, stored RBCs (for presurgical self-transfusion)	Severe anemia (Hgb usually < 7 g%) or acute, severe, traumatic blood loss)
Platelets[a]	—	Potential clotting disorder due to thrombocytopenia (platelets < 10,000 or < 20,000 if surgery planned) or clinically significant quantitative platelet defect
Plasma[b,c]	Available products include: Fresh-frozen plasma (FFP); may not supply clotting factors V and VIII Single-donor plasma; safer than FFP but otherwise same problems	Intravascular fluid depletion, not responsive to crystalloid, or bleeding due to depletion of clotting factors
Clotting factor concentrates	Cryoprecipitate has high levels of VIII, von Willebrand factor, and fibrinogen Genetically engineered factor VIII concentrates only for factor VIII deficiency Vitamin K–dependent factor concentrate has factors II, VII, IX, X, and proteins C and S; associated with hepatitis and thrombus formation	Factor deficiencies or acute liver failure (eg, Wilson disease)
Immune globulins	Nonspecific gamma globulin and intravenous gamma-globulin (IVIG) Specific gamma globulins for rabies (RIG), hepatitis (HBIG), varicella (VZIG), and other uses RhoGAM	Guillain-Barré, Kawasaki, and other autoimmune diseases (eg, ITP) Prevention after exposure to specific diseases Prevention of Rh sensitization and treatment of ITP
Protein-containing volume expanders	—	Intravascular fluid depletion

CMV = cytomegalovirus; Hgb = hemoglobin; ITP = idiopathic thrombocytopenic purpura.
[a]In platelet dysfunction, DDAVP (desmopressin acetate) may alleviate clotting disorder without transfusion.
[b]Single-donor plasma is safer than multidonor products (cryoprecipitate).
[c]If thrombocytopenia is due to autoantibodies or other consumptive problems, transfusions are rarely effective.

TABLE V–2. METHODS USED TO MAINTAIN BLOOD SAFETY

Screening Technique	Description

General history	Interview-style questions:
	  Has donor ever had blood donation refused?
	  Current or chronic illnesses?
	  Presence of fever?

Individual history	Interview-style questions:
	  Any high-risk sexual behaviors in donor or donor's partner(s)?
	  Any injected drug use in donor or donor's partner(s)?
	  Any overseas travel or history of past infection with HIV, HBV,
	    HCV, or parasites?

Laboratory screening	Detection of HIV-1 and -2, HBV, HCV, HTLV-1 and -2, syphilis
Purification techniques	Heat, fractionation, or chemical treatment consistent with maintaining activity of agent

HBV = hepatitis B virus; HCV = hepatitis C virus; HIV = human immunodeficiency virus; HTLV = human T-lymphotropic virus.

   a. If patient develops these symptoms, immediately discontinue
       transfusion and administer the following agents.
       i. Diphenhydramine (Benadryl), 0.25–1.0 mg/kg per dose PO
           or IV q2–6h.
       ii. Steroids, 2 mg/kg/dose, to maximum of 60 mg.
       iii. Epinephrine, 1:1000 0.01 mL/kg per dose SQ, to maximum of
           0.5 mL.
   b. Vasopressors. Administer if the preceding agents do not raise
       BP to a safe level.

TABLE V–3. INFECTIOUS AGENTS THAT CAN BE TRANSMITTED THROUGH BLOOD PRODUCTS

Category	Agents and Diseases
Bacteria	*Staphylococcus* (all types), *Streptococcus* (all types), occasional gram-negative organisms
Parasites	Malaria, Chagas disease
Prions	Jakob-Creutzfeldt disease, mad cow disease
Tick-borne agents	*Babesia, Rickettsia, Borrelia, Ehrlichia*
Viruses	Tested agents: HIV-1 and -2, HBV, HCV, HTLV-1 and -2 Not currently tested: CMV, parvovirus B19, HAV, HGV, transfusion- transmitted virus, SEN virus, human herpesvirus-8, West Nile virus

CMV = cytomegalovirus; HAV = hepatitis A virus; HBV = hepatitis B virus; HCV = hepatitis C virus; HGV = hepatitis G virus; HIV = human immunodeficiency virus; HTLV = human T-lymphotrophic virus.

REFERENCES

Ambruso DR, Hays T, Lane PL, Nuss R. Hematologic disorders. In: Hay WW Jr, Levin MJ, Sondheimer JM, Deterding RR, eds. *Current Pediatric Diagnosis & Treatment,* 17th ed. McGraw-Hill, 2005:855–910.

Pickering LK, ed. *Red Book 2003 Report of the Committee on Infectious Diseases,* 26th ed. American Academy of Pediatrics, 2003.

Strauss RG. Risk of blood component transfusions. In: Behrman RE, Kliegman RM, Jenson HB, eds. *Nelson's Pediatrics,* 17th ed. Saunders, 2003:1646–1650.

Truman JT. Complications of blood transfusions. In: Burg FD, Ingelfinger JR, Poplin RA, Gershon AA, eds. *Gellis & Kagan's Current Pediatric Therapy,* 17th ed. Saunders, 2002:675–676.

VI. Ventilator Management

1. INDICATIONS FOR VENTILATORY SUPPORT

Respiratory failure can be divided into two categories: hypoxemic (type I) respiratory failure and hypoventilatory (type II) respiratory failure. Although hypoxemic respiratory failure is more common, both varieties of respiratory failure are seen in pediatric patients. Ventilatory support is indicated when adequate gas exchange cannot be independently achieved or maintained.

I. **Hypoxemic Respiratory Failure.** Inability to oxygenate is an important indication for ventilatory support. Oxygenation can be determined by measurement of pulse oximetry (SpO_2) or the partial pressure of oxygen in arterial blood (PaO_2). By evaluating PaO_2 in the context of the fraction of inspired oxygen (FiO_2) employed, objective criteria for hypoxemic respiratory failure can be established. A PaO_2/FiO_2 (P/F) ratio < 200 is consistent with acute respiratory distress syndrome (ARDS), whereas a ratio between 200 and 300 is consistent with acute lung injury. Patients with a P/F ratio < 300 or SpO_2 < 90–93% (in the absence of cyanotic heart disease) require additional support, especially if they demonstrate signs of inadequate oxygen delivery, such as tachycardia, metabolic acidosis, or end-organ dysfunction. Although these patients may be managed initially with high oxygen delivery systems, their disease may progress to a point at which ventilatory support is required. Because of their physiologic instability and potential need for advanced therapies, these patients should be closely monitored in a pediatric intensive care unit.

II. **Hypoventilatory Respiratory Failure.** Carbon dioxide clearance is the main function of ventilation. The adequacy of ventilation can be monitored by either end-tidal carbon dioxide ($ETCO_2$) measurement or measurement of the partial pressure of carbon dioxide ($PaCO_2$) in arterial blood. Although a $PaCO_2$ above the normal range for age is consistent with hypoventilatory respiratory failure, it must be considered in the context of the clinical situation. A patient with status asthmaticus may have maximized his or her minute ventilation and have a $PaCO_2$ rise into the normal range as a result of hypoventilatory respiratory failure. Conversely, a patient with bronchopulmonary dysplasia may have developed a metabolic compensation such that the arterial pH is in the normal range despite chronic ventilatory failure. Evaluation of physical exam findings, pH, and $PaCO_2$ are all required to determine the need for ventilatory assistance. Respiratory acidosis with rapidly falling pH or pH < 7.25, rapidly rising $PaCO_2$, and deteriorating mental status secondary to CO_2 "narcosis" are all indications for ventilatory support. The factors involved in determining the need for ventilatory support can be evaluated in the following manner.

A. **Respiratory Drive.** Does patient have the drive to breathe? Breathing control issues are not uncommon in pediatric patients. Premature infants have immature respiratory drive centers that place them at risk for central apnea. This risk is heightened by intercurrent electrolyte imbalances, hypothermia, and infections. The immature respiratory center is also more sensitive to the respiratory depressant effects of anesthetics, narcotics, and sedatives until 48–52 weeks' gestational age. Older children are also at risk for respiratory drive dysregulation secondary to metabolic derangements, central sleep apnea, intoxication, primary CNS infection or disease, or traumatic brain injury.

B. **Respiratory Muscle Strength.** Does patient have the strength to breathe? Anatomic differences in infants and small children result in a greater breathing workload. Airway resistance is higher than in older children and adults due to smaller airway caliber, greater chest wall compliance, relative weakness of the intercostal muscles, and greater fatigability of the diaphragm. The intercurrent disease state may accentuate these anatomic and physiologic conditions, tipping the balance of the strength/workload relationship.

   The combination of insufficient respiratory drive and inadequate muscle strength for workload results in failure of the so-called respiratory pump, leading to type II (hypoventilatory) respiratory failure.

C. **Extrathoracic Airway.** Is obstruction present? The tissues of the extrathoracic airway may be subject to infection or inflammation, intrinsic masses or compression from extrinsic masses, or malacia. In addition to fixed anatomic obstruction, there may be functional obstruction as a result of obstructive sleep apnea or pharyngeal hypotonia that is exacerbated by sedative and analgesic medications.

D. **Intrathoracic Airways and Gas-Exchanging Units.** Is there dysfunction at this level? The smaller size of the intrathoracic airways and alveoli, absence of collateral alveolar ventilation, and similarity between alveolar closing capacity and functional residual capacity in infants and small children increases the likelihood of ventilation-perfusion (V/Q) imbalance secondary to atelectasis. Primary lung injury (eg, from infection or traumatic injury) or secondary lung injury due to the release of inflammatory cytokines may also lead to respiratory failure.

   The combination of extrathoracic airway obstruction and dysfunction of the intrathoracic airways and gas-exchanging units results in the failure of the lung, leading to type I (hypoxemic) respiratory failure.

E. **Other Concerns.** Is there a concurrent medical condition for which intubation and ventilation would be beneficial? The practitioner may want to maintain airway and ventilatory control in a patient whose condition does not directly affect ventilatory adequacy, or provide specific therapies that are best facilitated while patient is intubated and ventilated.

2. VENTILATION OPTIONS AND CLASSIFICATION

I. **Ventilation Options**
   A. **Negative Pressure Ventilation**
      1. **Description.** Negative pressure ventilation is performed by placing patient into a chamber or body suit device, within which negative pressure can be generated. Creation of negative pressure around the thorax results in a pressure gradient that favors gas flow from the atmosphere, through the natural airway, and into the lungs. Exhalation occurs when negative pressure is discontinued and the natural elastic recoil of the pulmonary system promotes lung emptying. Negative pressures up to –30 cm H_2O may be used, cycled at varying rates and inspiratory times as needed to optimize gas exchange. Supplemental oxygen may be introduced to patient's natural airway.
      2. **Advantages.** The advantage to negative pressure ventilation is that it avoids tracheal intubation and may allow patients to be free from ventilatory support for intermittent periods, as tolerated. For patients with "passive" pulmonary **circulation**, negative pressure ventilation also augments pulmonary blood flow.
      3. **Disadvantages.** The disadvantages of negative pressure ventilation include the relative inaccessibility to patient and limitations in patient positioning while in the negative pressure device, the relative inefficiency of ventilation compared with positive pressure techniques, the absence of an artifical airway should the natural airway become obstructed or secretion clearance become suboptimal, and the risk of skin breakdown around seal points. These problems and the use of other ventilatory modalities have made negative pressure ventilation relatively uncommon.
   B. **Positive Pressure Ventilation by Mask**
      1. **Description.** Both continuous positive airway pressure and bilevel positive airway pressure may be delivered by a mask device. Mask devices may cover either the nose or both nose and mouth. Nasal masks may be more comfortable and provide more ready access to the oropharynx for suctioning but may be less efficient secondary to air leak from the mouth than a full face mask device. A properly fitting mask with minimal leakage is essential to success. Mask ventilation is generally well tolerated, although reassurance and the occasional judicious use of sedation may be necessary.
         a. **Continuous positive airway pressure (CPAP).** CPAP may recruit alveoli, restore functional residual capacity, and diminish pulmonary edema, improving oxygenation and pulmonary mechanics. Airway pressures of 3–12 cm H_2O are commonly tolerated, but achieving pressures above these levels may be difficult with a mask system. (See also later discussion, pp. 558, 563.)

      b. Bilevel positive airway pressure (BiPAP). BiPAP may provide significant ventilatory support during both acute and chronic respiratory failure, although not as efficiently as positive pressure ventilation via a tracheal tube. BiPAP may be delivered by three different modes: a spontaneous mode, in which each patient-initiated breath is supported; a timed mode, in which a predetermined number of breaths is delivered per minute independent of patient effort; and a timed-spontaneous mode, which combines the attributes of these two modes. Settings to be manipulated include inspiratory positive airway pressure (IPAP), expiratory positive airway pressure (EPAP), and inspiratory time and mechanical breath rate (when timed or timed-spontaneous modes are employed). Supplemental oxygen can be added into the system as needed. When initiated, low IPAP and EPAP levels are used to allow patient acclimation to the device, and subsequently increased as tolerated. An initial IPAP/EPAP setting of 6/3 cm H_2O may be used, and this can be increased to as high as 20–30/10–12 cm H_2O. Pressures higher than this may be hard to maintain and suggest that another ventilatory modality may be needed.

    2. Advantages. As with negative pressure ventilation, the advantages of mask ventilation include avoidance of tracheal intubation and the opportunity to allow patients to be free of ventilatory support for periods of time as tolerated.

    3. Disadvantages. Potential complications of mask ventilation include gastric distention and aspiration, although this has not been reported in pediatric case series; the relative contraindication to oral or nasogastric tube feedings during therapy; and the risk of skin breakdown due to pressure from the mask. The lack of airway protection with mask ventilation also limits its use in patients with diminished or absent airway protective reflexes.

C. Positive Pressure Ventilation via Tracheal Tube. Mechanical ventilatory support via tracheal tube is the most efficient and most common ventilation method employed. Tracheal tubes include translaryngeal tubes placed via nose or mouth and tubes placed via tracheostomy. A wide variety of modes for providing positive pressure ventilation through a tracheal tube are available.

II. Ventilator Classification. Ventilators can be classified in various ways based on their mechanical characteristics and the means by which they deliver gas to patients. The most common variables used to classify ventilators are initiation, mode, and cycle control.

A. Initiation. The inspiratory cycle may be initiated by time (ie, a breath is initiated after a certain time period has elapsed); by pressure (ie, a breath is initiated after a certain amount of negative pressure is generated by patient's spontaneous respiratory effort); or by flow (ie, a breath is initiated after a certain amount of gas flow is generated by patient's spontaneous respiratory effort). These initiating factors may also be used together.

B. Mode. The amount of gas delivered during inspiration is determined by the mode. The two modes of ventilation are pressure control, in which gas is delivered to a predetermined amount of pressure, and volume control, in which gas is delivered to a predetermined amount of volume.

C. Cycle Control. Cycle control refers to the parameter that terminates inspiration. The four methods of cycle control are time cycled, in which inspiration continues for a predetermined amount of time; volume cycled, in which inspiration continues until a predetermined volume of gas is delivered; flow cycled, in which inspiration continues until a certain gas flow is achieved; and pressure cycled, in which inspiration continues until a predetermined pressure is achieved.

D. Variations. Ventilator classifications can include such variations as time-initiated, pressure-control, flow-cycled ventilation; pressure-initiated, volume-control, time-cycled ventilation; and so forth. In pediatric patients, initiation may be time, pressure, or flow dependent; pressure and volume control modes are both used; and time and flow cycle control are most commonly employed.

3. VENTILATOR SETUP

I. The Ventilator. Today's ventilators provide a variety of ventilatory modality options to practitioners at the bedside. Despite this, some basic concepts apply to any mode chosen. In general, a mode of ventilation that will achieve the practitioner's goals for oxygenation and ventilation with the least amount of toxicity should be chosen. High concentrations of supplemental oxygen can directly injure the lung and the immature retina. A focus on strategies to reduce the FiO_2 to $<$ 50–60% in a timely manner is warranted. Exposure of the lung to excessive inflating pressures and volumes may directly injure the lung and initiate an inflammatory response that may result in secondary lung injury. Recent research suggests that limiting tidal volumes to 5–8 mL/kg may be protective against these effects in patients with acute respiratory distress syndrome (ARDS).

II. Ventilatory Modes. Keeping in mind that a variety of choices for ventilatory support exist, all involve one of two modes or limits: volume or pressure. The amount of gas delivered during inspiration will be determined either by the amount of pressure or by the amount of volume preset by the practitioner. Volume control modes of ventilation offer the advantage of consistently applied minute ventilation despite changes in compliance of the respiratory system. The potential danger of this approach is that excessive peak inspiratory pressures may be achieved should compliance decrease, leading to the risk of barotrauma. Pressure control modes of ventilation allow for control of the peak inspiratory pressure, but minute ventilation may vary as compliance changes occur. With this in mind, volume or pressure control (preset) ventilation can be performed in a variety of ways, depending on patient needs and practitioner preferences.

A. Control Mode Ventilation. This mode of ventilation is time initiated; volume or pressure controlled; and volume, pressure, or time cycled. It is insensitive to patient effort or response. As a result, no support to spontaneous respiratory efforts is provided. Control mode ventilation is appropriate in the operating room or for patients in the pediatric intensive care unit who are sedated and neuromuscularly blocked, and is infrequently used.

B. Assist-Control Ventilation. This mode is pressure, time, or flow initiated; volume or pressure controlled; and volume, pressure, time, or flow cycled. The ventilator senses a sub-baseline pressure or flow when patient makes an adequate respiratory effort, initiating a mechanical breath. The sub-baseline pressure or flow needed to trigger a ventilator breath is determined by the sensitivity that is set on the ventilator. A control rate is initiated when patient effort is inadequate or absent, providing safety should the patient become hypopneic or apneic. Thus, assist-control ventilation allows spontaneous breathing with the safety of a backup mechanical ventilatory rate. All breaths are fully supported by preset ventilator parameters. As a result, the preset volume or pressure must be decreased during the process of weaning from mechanical ventilatory support when this mode is used.

C. Intermittent Mandatory Ventilation. This mode is time initiated; volume or pressure controlled; and volume, pressure, time or flow cycled. A continuous gas flow system is also present on most ventilators that provide this mode of ventilation. Positive pressure breaths are delivered independent of patient effort. The continuous gas flow system allows breathing of a fresh gas source during spontaneous respiratory effort by the patient. As a result, intermittent mandatory ventilation allows for spontaneous breathing of fresh gas with the safety of a backup rate, but the lack of coordination between mechanical breaths and patient efforts may result in ventilator-patient dyssynchrony and is not generally well tolerated. As a result, this method of ventilation is not commonly used.

D. Synchronized Intermittent Mandatory Ventilation. This mode is pressure, time, or flow initiated; volume or pressure controlled; and volume, pressure, time, or flow cycled. Mechanical ventilatory breaths up to the number prescribed by the practitioner are synchronized with patient respiratory effort as sensed by patient's development of a negative inspiratory pressure or flow that exceeds the limit set by the ventilator's sensitivity setting. As a result, full ventilatory support can be provided by setting the ventilator to provide enough breaths to deliver adequate minute ventilation.

Furthermore, partial support can be provided by decreasing the preset mechanical breath rate, allowing patient to contribute to minute ventilation by spontaneous respirations. Patient-ventilator synchrony occurs, making this method of ventilation more comfortable for patient. A demand flow system provides a fresh gas source to patient during spontaneous respiration if patient generates a sufficient negative inspiratory force to open the demand valve. The volume of gas provided is proportional to patient effort and is usually small unless it is augmented by the addition of pressure support. This is in contrast to assist-control ventilation, in which all breaths receive the full amount of preset support. As a result, overventilation and development of respiratory alkalosis are less likely with synchronized intermittent mandatory ventilation as compared with assist-control ventilation. Also, with synchronized intermittent mandatory ventilation, a mechanical breath can be maintained at full tidal volume or inspiratory pressure during the process of ventilator weaning, decreasing the potential for development of atelectasis that may occur with assist-control ventilation (for which the tidal volume or inspiratory pressure must be decreased during the weaning process). For both synchronized intermittent mandatory ventilation and assist-control ventilation, patient's work of breathing is determined by trigger sensitivity, response time of the ventilator, and inspiratory flow rate of the gas provided.

E. **Pressure Support Ventilation.** This mode of ventilation is pressure or flow initiated; pressure controlled; and flow or time cycled. As patient makes a spontaneous respiratory effort, a sub-baseline pressure or flow is detected by the ventilator, activating ventilator gas flow to achieve a preset inspiratory airway pressure. This inspiratory pressure is maintained until either the inspiratory flow generated by patient decreases to a preset level below the maximum flow rate (commonly 75–90%) or the time cycle is complete. The amount of volume delivered depends on the preset level of pressure support, patient effort, and compliance of the pulmonary system. Pressure support ventilation can provide full ventilatory support when a high enough preset pressure level is selected, partial support, or only enough support to overcome the resistance to gas flow imposed by the endotracheal tube (ETT), ventilator tubing, and ventilator demand valves. It may also be combined with other ventilatory support modes (eg, synchronized intermittent mandatory ventilation or continuous positive airway pressure [CPAP]). Pressure support ventilation usually involves minimal work of breathing and is comfortable for patients. Because there is no control element to this form of ventilatory support, care must be taken when using it in patients who may become hypopneic or apneic.

F. **CPAP.** In this mode, continuous positive airway pressure is maintained in spontaneously breathing patients. No mechanical breaths are provided. CPAP may be used independently in patients who only require distending pressure to maintain functional residual capacity or for stenting of airways when malacia is present. It may also be used during spontaneous breathing trials as part of the process of weaning a patient from mechanical ventilatory support. CPAP may be combined with pressure support ventilation during weaning trials.

III. Ventilator Settings

A. **Primary Controls.** Initial ventilator settings should be determined based on patient pathophysiology and goals of the bedside clinician. The primary controls that need to be set initially include the mode of ventilation (as previously discussed), tidal volume (when a volume mode is used) or peak inspiratory pressure (when a pressure mode is used), positive end-expiratory pressure, mechanical breath rate, inspiratory time and resultant inspiratory-to-expiratory (I:E) ratio, and Fio_2.

B. **Tidal Volume (V_T).** V_T is chosen based on body weight. Commonly a V_T of 7–10 mL/kg is chosen. Recent studies in adult patients with ARDS suggest that a low V_T strategy of ventilation, whereby 4–8 mL/kg V_T is employed, is associated with less morbidity and mortality in patients with this condition. This strategy is thought to limit stretch injury to diseased alveoli and reduce secondary lung injury. An adequate V_T should result in good chest rise and air entry bilaterally and generate positive inspiratory pressure < 30–35 cm H_2O.

C. **Peak Inspiratory Pressure (PIP).** PIP is chosen to provide effective support at the minimal pressure possible. In children with normal lung compliance (eg, postsurgical procedure), PIP of 20–25 cm H_2O is often adequate. In small or premature infants, a lower PIP can often be used. In patients with disease processes that worsen compliance or require high minute ventilation, a higher PIP is necessary. PIPs > 30–35 cm H_2O are avoided, if possible, because the risk of barotrauma increases above these levels.

D. **Positive End-Expiratory Pressure (PEEP).** PEEP provides CPAP throughout the expiratory phase. For patients breathing through their natural airway, glottic closure at the end of expiration will generate PEEP of 3–5 cm H_2O. The passage of a tracheal tube through the glottis prevents this process from occurring. Therefore, a "physiologic" amount of PEEP is commonly used for all intubated patients. PEEP helps to maintain expiratory airway patency, restoring functional residual capacity and decreasing closing volume. Atelectasis may be prevented and alveoli that have already become collapsed may be recruited. As a result, total respiratory system compliance decreases and the distribution of pulmonary blood flow to better ventilated lung units is improved. The major effect seen with use of PEEP is an improvement in oxygenation. Excessive amounts of PEEP, however, will worsen oxygenation as alveolar capillaries are collapsed. Thus, it may be necessary to provide a trial using varying levels of PEEP to determine the "best PEEP" for patient's pathophysiology. Other potential adverse effects of PEEP include a decrease in cardiac output secondary to decreased pulmonary venous return (preload) and increased pulmonary vascular resistance, a decrease in cerebral perfusion pressure secondary to decreased cardiac output and decreased cerebral venous drainage, alveolar overdistention and resultant air-leak phenomenon, and potential fluid retention and a decrease in urine output related to a complex interaction of neurohumoral and cardiovascular responses.

E. **Mechanical Breath Rate.** The mechanical rate of ventilation is usually selected based on the physiologic or age-appropriate rate for the patient with normal minute ventilation requirements. If the underlying disease requires increased minute ventilation, the ventilator rate may be increased as needed. However, consideration must be given to the effect of rate on inspiratory and expiratory times. As rates are increased, less cycle time is available for expiration. If expiratory time is decreased excessively, patient's expiration may not be allowed to complete, leading to decreased minute ventilation and air trapping with resultant worsening of the ventilation-perfusion (V/Q) relationship. Conversely, patients with conditions that decrease gas flow on expiration may require a decrease in the mechanical ventilator rate to allow enough expiratory time for completion of expiration.

F. **Inspiratory Time.** When the mode of ventilation includes a time cycle, the inspiratory time is set directly or by setting an I:E ratio. Inspiratory times and I:E ratio are commonly set to physiologic and age-appropriate levels in patients with normal or minimally altered pulmonary physiology. In patients with impaired oxygenation, increasing the inspiratory time will favor additional alveolar recruitment. In patients with ARDS, a strategy of so-called inverse I:E ratio ventilation, in which inspiratory time exceeds expiratory time, may be employed in an attempt to optimize alveolar recruitment. The impact on ventilation due to a decreased expiratory time and hemodynamic complications related to an increase in intrathoracic pressure must be considered. Conversely, patients with airway obstruction (eg, those with status asthmaticus) may benefit from a decreased inspiratory time to increase the time available for expiration.

G. **Fio$_2$.** Upon initiation of mechanical ventilatory support, it is common to begin with an Fio$_2$ setting of 100% until patient is stabilized. Subsequently, there should be rapid efforts to decrease Fio$_2$ based on Spo$_2$ or ABG measurements. The lowest Fio$_2$ that achieves adequate oxygenation should be employed. Generally, FiO_2 of 60% is considered nontoxic, although this will be influenced by amount and duration of exposure, atmospheric pressure, underlying disease state, and individual variation.

IV. Further Considerations

A. Sedation and Analgesia. Provide sedation and analgesia adequate to manage the stress and discomfort associated with an in situ ETT, mechanical ventilation, and underlying disease process. These pharmacologic adjuncts will also blunt the patient's ability to displace the ETT.

B. Safety. Soft physical restraint of the hands may be required in addition to pharmacologic measures for patient safety. Uncontrolled dislodgement of the ETT can have disastrous consequences.

C. Gastric Care

1. Perform gastric decompression with a nasogastric or orogastric tube in all intubated patients unless there are contraindications.
2. Consider gastric buffering for prevention of gastric ulceration, using nasogastric feedings or pharmacologic agents, when the course of ventilation is prolonged or the underlying disease state or treatments increase the risk of ulcer disease.

D. Pulmonary Care. Apply pulmonary toilet. The presence of an ETT and the use of sedative medications will blunt the normal bronchociliary mechanisms and cough reflexes for secretion clearance. Additional therapies may be needed to address the underlying pulmonary pathophysiology.

E. Skin Care. Meticulous skin care to prevent skin breakdown is essential.

F. Nutrition. Provide adequate nutritional support in a timely manner to meet the needs of the growing child recovering from an acute illness. Enteral feedings are always preferred when possible.

G. Electrolyte and Acid-Base Balance. Normalization of electrolyte and acid-base imbalances is needed to optimize patient strength and respiratory drive prior to attempts to decrease mechanical ventilatory support.

4. MODIFICATION OF VENTILATOR SETTINGS

After initiation of ventilatory support, ongoing attention is needed to optimize ventilatory strategy as the patient's pathophysiologic condition evolves. Multiple sources of data are available for analysis of patient condition; however, the cornerstone of this process remains the physical exam. Evaluation of adequacy of chest rise, quality of breath sounds, patient's color and perfusion, respiratory rate and work of breathing, and quality of other end-organ functions will tell volumes about the adequacy of mechanical ventilatory support being provided. Additional information is provided by continuous pulse oximeter (SpO_2) and end-tidal carbon dioxide ($ETCO_2$) measurements, intermittent ABG analysis and chest x-ray interpretation, and review of mechanical ventilator parameters, such as peak inspiratory pressure (PIP), exhaled tidal volume (V_T), and spontaneous minute ventilation. Above all, remember to treat the patient and not the ventilator.

I. **Adjustments to Oxygenation.** Generally, in patients without cyanotic heart disease, $SpO_2 \geq 93\%$ or $PaO_2 > 60$ torr is acceptable.

  A. **To Decrease PaO_2**

   1. FiO_2 can most easily be decreased based on SpO_2 measurement. Once FiO_2 is $\leq 60\%$, further decreases may be achieved in 5–10% increments. In patients with normal ventilation-perfusion (V/Q) relationships, PaO_2 will decrease by 7 mm Hg for each 1% decrease in FiO_2.

   2. If positive end-expiratory pressure (PEEP) is above so-called physiologic levels (3–5 cm H_2O) and FiO_2 has been reduced to $\leq 40\%$, then decreases in PEEP in increments of 1–2 cm H_2O may be performed until physiologic levels are reached.

  B. **To Increase PaO_2**

   1. FiO_2 may be increased in response to a low PaO_2 or SpO_2; however, it is preferable to maintain FiO_2 at $\leq 60\%$. Should this not resolve the problem, other strategies should be pursued.

   2. PEEP can be added in increments of 2–4 cm H_2O to improve oxygenation by improved alveolar recruitment, functional residual capacity, and V/Q matching. The effects of increased PEEP are not immediate and may not be apparent for 1 hour or more. If PEEP levels of 12–15 cm H_2O are not effective, other strategies should be pursued.

   3. Increasing the inspiratory time and performing inverse inspiratory-to-expiratory (I:E) ratio ventilation will have an impact on oxygenation by increasing mean airway pressure and the time over which alveoli are distended. It can be used in conjunction with other measures.

   4. Increasing ventilation will have some impact on oxygenation (as shown by the alveolar gas equation at the end of this section), although this is commonly minimal.

II. **Adjustments to Ventilation.** Maintaining $PaCO_2$ or $ETCO_2$ of 35–45 torr with a normal pH is commonly the goal of ventilation. However, if excessive amounts of ventilation are required to achieve this, so-called permissive hypercapnia ventilation may be performed, in which CO_2 levels are allowed to increase as long as pH can be maintained at ≥ 7.20–7.25 by metabolic compensation or the use of exogenous buffer. This allows mechanical ventilatory support to be decreased to potentially less toxic levels.

  A. **To Decrease $PaCO_2$**

   1. Increase mechanical breath rate.

   2. Increase V_T or PIP.

   3. Check for system leaks.

   4. Optimize patient-ventilator synchrony.

B. To Increase Paco$_2$

1. Decrease mechanical breath rate.
2. Decrease V_T or PIP.
3. If an assist-control mode of ventilation is being used, consider changing to synchronized intermittent mandatory ventilation. Recall that with assist-control, all breaths receive full mechanical ventilatory support.
4. Determine whether patient's spontaneous effort is producing the hyperventilation, and determine the cause. Possible causes include hypoxemia, pain, anxiety, fever, metabolic acidosis, and CNS injury. Treat the underlying problem.
5. Rule out mechanical problems that may be increasing the mechanical ventilatory rate (eg, autocycling related to a low trigger sensitivity).

III. Weaning

A. Criteria. Decreasing the amount of mechanical ventilatory support applied to a patient in preparation for discontinuation of ventilation is termed *weaning*. An aggressive approach to weaning is commonly warranted, because an unnecessary extension of the period of time during which mechanical ventilatory support is applied increases the chances for associated morbidities. Several criteria should be considered as ventilator weaning is entertained.

1. The original indication for the application of mechanical ventilatory support should be resolving or no longer existent.
2. There should be no new indication for mechanical ventilatory support.
3. Other organ systems should be functioning adequately. Hemodynamics should be acceptable. Neurologic function should be such that an appropriate drive to breathe and airway protective reflexes are present when extubation is being considered. The amount of tracheal secretions and the frequency of suctioning should be considered.
4. Oxygenation, ventilation, and acid-base balance should be adequate.
5. Patient should have the strength to breathe and not have excessive work of breathing. Patient's physical exam should be notable for absence of excessive tachypnea, retractions, nasal flaring, or accessory respiratory muscle use while maintaining adequate oxygenation and ventilation. Vital capacity (VC) and maximum negative inspiratory force (NIF) measurements can be performed at the bedside. VC of $> 10–15$ mL/kg and NIF > -20 cm H_2O generally correlate with adequate strength for spontaneous breathing.
6. Prior to extubation, patency of the extrathoracic airway should be considered. The presence of a leak with deflation of the ETT cuff, or with inspiratory pressures of < 30 cm H_2O with an uncuffed ETT, suggests adequate airway patency.

B. Weaning Techniques

1. Synchronized Intermittent Mandatory Ventilation (SIMV)

a. Description. In this mode of ventilation, the number of fully supported breaths provided by the ventilator is determined by the set rate, while patient may breathe spontaneously from a fresh gas source. In addition, pressure support is often added to decrease the work of spontaneous breathing secondary to the resistance of the demand valves and circuit. Weaning is performed by decreasing the set mechanical breath rate, thus allowing patient's spontaneous effort to provide an increasing amount of the minute ventilation. If patient does well at a minimum set rate, extubation may proceed, or a brief testing period using continuous positive airway pressure (CPAP) or a T-piece may be used.

b. Considerations. The advantages to this approach include the presence of a backup rate and alarms should patient become apneic, a graded assumption of the work of breathing, and complete inspiration with set breaths to help decrease the chance of atelectasis development.

2. Pressure Support Ventilation (PSV)

a. Description. This mode of ventilation also allows the application of a variable amount of support to patient's spontaneous breathing effort. Weaning is performed by decreasing the level of pressure support from one that may provide full or partial ventilation to one that only overcomes the resistance of the ventilator and endotracheal tube (ETT). It may also be used in combination with SIMV or CPAP.

b. Considerations. The advantage of this approach is that the level of mechanical ventilatory support can be gradually decreased as patient improves, allowing patient to set his or her own rate, inspiratory time, and expiratory time. The disadvantage of this approach is the lack of a backup rate should patient become fatigued or apneic.

3. CPAP

a. Description. CPAP allows for spontaneous breathing with the application of a continuous distending pressure. It may also be combined with PSV. As patient improves, he or she is weaned by switching from an assisted or controlled mode of ventilation to CPAP for trial periods of spontaneous ventilation with no mechanical ventilatory support.

b. Considerations. Prolonged periods of CPAP are not commonly used because patient may become fatigued secondary to resistance created by the ETT and ventilator circuit. The absence of a safety backup rate must also be considered.

4. T-Piece

a. Description. Patient may be removed completely from ventilatory support and allowed to breathe spontaneously through the ETT, which is connected to a constant flow of fresh gas. The weaning process involves increasing the time patient uses the T-piece.

b. Considerations. This method is not generally used in pediatric patients because of the high resistance to gas flow through smaller pediatric ETTs and the associated excessive work of breathing necessary for spontaneously ventilation. Also, no ventilator alarms are available, creating a safety issue.

5. SPECIAL MODES OF VENTILATION

I. **Inverse Ratio Ventilation.** In patients with inadequate oxygenation, increasing the inspiratory time so that it equals or exceeds the expiratory time will increase the mean airway pressure without increasing peak inspiratory pressures (PIPs) and will increase the time over which noncompliant alveoli may be recruited (see Ventilator Settings, III, F, p. 559). As a result, oxygenation is usually improved. However, there have been no studies that demonstrate an improved outcome in patients with hypoxemic respiratory failure when inverse ratio ventilation is used versus other modalities. Ventilation may be impaired as the time for expiration is decreased. The long inspiratory times are uncomfortable for patients, such that deep sedation or anesthesia and neuromuscular blockade are needed.

II. **Pressure-Regulated Volume Control (PRVC) Ventilation.** PRVC is a hybrid mode of ventilation, combining aspects of volume and pressure control ventilation. Originally, PRVC provided only controlled ventilation. Newer ventilator products now include PRVC with pressure support to assist spontaneous respiratory effort. With PRVC, a tidal volume (V_T) and minute ventilation goal is set by the practitioner. Decelerating inspiratory flow pattens are adjusted by the ventilator to deliver the set V_T at the lowest PIP possible. With changes in pulmonary compliance, however, PIPs are allowed to change by only 3 cm H_2O per breath. As a result, the prescribed V_T may not be delivered during these breaths. In patients with poor pulmonary compliance, PRVC may be useful for providing a goal minute ventilation with minimalization of PIP and resultant barotrauma.

III. **Airway Pressure Release Ventilation (APRV).** With this mode of ventilation, there is an intermittent decrease, or release, of continuous positive airway pressure from a preset high level to a preset low level. Patient may breathe spontaneously from a fresh gas source at either pressure level. Thus, deep sedation can be minimized and neuromuscular blockade avoided. In patients with acute lung injury, atelectatic alveoli can be recruited and stabilized without excessive PIPs while allowing spontaneous ventilation augmented by transient releases of airway pressure. Pediatric experience with APRV is minimal.

IV. **High-Frequency Oscillatory Ventilation (HFOV).** Of the several methods of high-frequency ventilation, HFOV is the most commonly used in pediatrics. Tidal volumes at or below dead space volume are introduced into the airway at a rate of 180–900 times per minute. Inspiration and expiration are both active. The result is the generation of a high mean airway pressure with minimal variation of airway pressure amplitudes around the mean as oscillation occurs. This strategy helps to recruit atelectatic alveoli without overstretching the gas-exchanging units, minimizing volutrauma. HFOV has been found to be effective in the management of children with acute respiratory distress syndrome and pulmonary air leak syndromes. Disadvantages of HFOV include the need to minimize tracheal suctioning, because with every circuit disconnection, alveolar recruitment is lost and must be reacquired over 1–2 hours; potential hemodynamic decompensation due to decreased preload from high intrathoracic pressure; and the common need for deep sedation or anesthesia and neuromuscular blockade.

6. EQUATIONS

I. Metabolic Acidosis

$$\text{Expected } Pa_{CO_2} = 1.5 \times [HCO_3] + 8 \ (\pm 2)$$

II. Metabolic Alkalosis

$$\text{Expected } Pa_{CO_2} = 0.7 \times [HCO_3] + 21 \ (\pm 2)$$

III. Respiratory Acidosis or Alkalosis
A. **Bicarbonate.** For every 10 torr change in Pa_{CO_2}, HCO_3 changes by 2 if acute, 4 (± 1) if chronic.
B. **pH**
1. **Acute change.** For every 10 torr change in Pa_{CO_2}, pH changes by 0.08.
2. **Chronic change.** For every 10 torr change in Pa_{CO_2}, pH changes by 0.03.

IV. Alveolar Gas Equation (Simplified)

$$PA_{O_2} = [Fi_{O_2} \times (P_B - PH_2O)] - Pa_{CO_2}/RQ$$

In which PA_{O_2} = alveolar oxygen tension; P_B = barometric pressure (760 torr at 1 atm); PH_2O = water pressure (47 torr); and RQ = respiratory quotient (0.8 with mixed fuel).

V. Arterial Oxygen Content (Ca_{O_2})

$$Ca_{O_2} = (Hgb \times 1.36 \times Sa_{O_2}) + (Pa_{O_2} \times 0.003)$$

VI. Oxygen Delivery (Do_2)

$$Do_2 = Cao_2 \times CO \times IO$$

$$CO \text{ (cardiac output)} = \text{Heart rate} \times \text{Stroke volume}$$

VII. P/F Ratio

$$\text{P/F ratio} = Pao_2/Fio_2$$

Pao_2 is in mm Hg, and $Fio_2 = 50\% = 0.5$).

VIII. Oxygenation Index (OI)

$$OI = [(MAP \times Fio_2)/Pao_2] \times 100$$

In which MAP = mean arterial pressure.

REFERENCES

Arnold JH, Hanson JH, Toro-Figuero LO, et al. Prospective, randomized comparison of high-frequency oscillatory ventilation and conventional mechanical ventilation in pediatric respiratory failure. *Crit Care Med* 1994;22:1530–1539.

Dreyfuss D, Saumon G. Ventilator-induced lung injury. *Am J Crit Care Med* 1998;157:294–323.

Padman R, Lawless ST, Kettrick RG. Noninvasive ventilation via bilevel positive airway pressure support in pediatric practice. *Crit Care Med* 1998;26:169–173.

Rodgers MC, ed. *Textbook of Pediatric Intensive Care,* 3rd ed. Williams & Wilkins, 1996.

VII. Preoperative Management

1. PREOPERATIVE ASSESSMENT

All children undergoing surgery should have a preoperative assessment and preparation prior to the surgical procedure. Goals of the evaluation are twofold: (1) to identify and optimize management of the surgical condition as well as any coexisting diseases, and (2) to introduce patient, family, and other caretakers to the perioperative process. The anesthesiologist and surgeon usually decide the anesthetic plan. The pediatric consultant can assist with their ascertainment of complete and correct patient information, including patient's baseline physiologic and mental status, current medication, and pertinent psychosocial issues. Table VII–1 outlines common issues that may lead to perioperative pediatric consultation.

I. **Key Considerations in Perioperative Consultation**
   A. **Patient Condition That Requires Surgical Treatment.** As a medical consultant, the pediatrician usually is not being asked to provide an opinion as to the need for surgery or to select among various surgical options; however, a good understanding of the planned intervention allows him or her to better contribute to patient care. Surgical interventions that produce large degrees of tissue trauma and blood loss are generally more likely to require an understanding of baseline metabolic and hematologic laboratory values than are less-extensive procedures. Long procedures, even when they cause relatively minor tissue trauma, may demand intraoperative dosing of chronic medications or other considerations.
   B. **Presence of Coexisting Conditions.** This consideration is particularly important for children with complicated medical conditions. Clarify and clearly document the specific diagnosis, degree of physiologic compromise, and routine management of these conditions, and address any needed modifications to the surgical and anesthetic plan. Use the American Society of Anesthesiologists (ASA) classification system to communicate effectively (see later discussion and Table VII–3).
   C. **Patient Medication Use.** NPO status pre- and postoperatively, length of time intraoperative, degree of fluid or blood loss and replacement, and extent of tissue trauma may modify drug distribution and metabolism. Clarify drug dosage and intervals, appropriate drug levels, alternative medications for periods when enteral intake is prohibited, and need for intraoperative administration of maintenance medications. In general, preoperative "NPO orders" do not preclude oral medications. Advise patients to take their routine oral medications on the morning of surgery with a few sips of

TABLE VII-1. COMMON ISSUES THAT MAY LEAD TO PERIOPERATIVE PEDIATRIC CONSULTATION

System and Condition	Implications for Surgery and Anesthesia	Pediatric Consultant's Potential Contribution to Perioperative Preparation and Management	Comments
Respiratory System			
Acute upper respiratory infection	Patients have an increased incidence of laryngospasm, bronchospasm, secretion occlusion of tracheal tube	Help ascertain if patient's signs and symptoms represent acute or chronic condition. Recommend perioperative medications and dosages if needed (antibiotic, β-agonists, steroid)	Elective surgery and anesthesia during acute illness is not advisable, but suspected upper respiratory infection is so common during young childhood that an overly conservative posture regarding this issue will result in frequent and unnecessary cancellation of needed surgery. Parents' stated perception that their "child is ill" was best predictor of perioperative laryngospasm in several recent studies
Apnea of prematurity	Postanesthetic apnea may occur in young infants, particularly those with history of prematurity	Help make best estimate of infant's postconceptual age	Etiology of postanesthetic apnea is unclear, but maturity of respiratory control center and history of premature birth seem to be independent risk factors; we have adopted practice of requiring automatic hospital admission for postoperative overnight monitoring for infants younger than 52 wk postconception
Bronchopulmonary dysplasia	Postoperative respiratory failure due to interaction of patient's respiratory disease with:	Provide accurate diagnosis and characterization of severity of pulmonary condition	

	1. Instrumentation of airway 2. Fluid administration 3. Compromise of respiratory mechanics after abdominal or thoracic surgery 4. Respiratory depression associated with intraoperative anesthetics and postoperative analgesics	Recommend management and medications to optimize pulmonary function preoperatively Help with postoperative management and weaning of support
Cardiovascular System		
Heart murmur	Stress of surgery may increase catecholamines, cause tachycardia or other abnormal rhythms, place increase demand on cardiac output Some surgeries are associated with transient bacteremia and risk of endocarditis Anesthetic agents are variable myocardial depressants and arrhythmogenic	Help determine if murmur represents pathology Provide estimation of myocardial reserve Recommend prophylactic antibiotics for susceptible patients
History of previous congenital heart disease and repair	Same as above Central and peripheral vascular anatomy may be abnormal	Help provide precise diagnosis and description of current patient's anatomy Same as first two entries above
CNS		
Seizure disorder	Seizures in perioperative period	Provide accurate description of seizures

(Continued)

TABLE VII–1. COMMON ISSUES THAT MAY LEAD TO PERIOPERATIVE PEDIATRIC CONSULTATION (CONTINUED)

System and Condition	Implications for Surgery and Anesthesia	Pediatric Consultant's Potential Contribution to Perioperative Preparation and Management	Comments
	Anticonvulsant treatments may be altered by preoperative preparation requirements and length of intraoperative period. Anticonvulsant drugs may have interactions with other agents. Anticonvulsants may cause hepatic or coagulation abnormalities	Recommend if and what alternative anticonvulsant regimen is best in perioperative period	
Cerebral palsy	Chronic upper motor neuron lesion associated with: 1. Altered response to neuromuscular blocking agents 2. Thoracic dystrophy 3. Generalized spasticity Patients often have associated seizure disorder, feeding dysfunction, other GI problems, and receive multiple medications Patients have increased intraoperative bleeding	Provide complete listing of diagnoses, medications, and care needs Help prioritize medications that are necessary and those that can be stopped temporarily Help chronically ill patient and family cope with acute surgical event and facilitate multiple subspecialist physicians' interactions with surgeon and anesthesiology team	
Muscular dystrophy	Possible risk of malignant hyperthermia Cardiomyopathy Airway and respiratory insufficiency Patients have increased intraoperative bleeding	Characterize degree of respiratory and circulatory dysfunction Participate in preoperative preparation and postoperative titration of respirator and circulatory medications and other treatments	

GI and Hepatic System

Gastroesophageal reflux

Risk of aspiration, associated respiratory disease

Characterize severity of reflux and respiratory dysfunction
Recommend treatment and dosage of antireflux medications and respiratory treatments if necessary

Hepatic failure

Altered drug metabolism and volume of distribution
Altered relationship of body weight to intravascular volume
Coagulation abnormalities

Characterize degree of liver dysfunction
Help with assessment of intravascular volume

Hematologic System

Anemia

Inadequate oxygen carrying capacity in response to surgical stress and trauma
Hypovolemia

Help confirm cause of anemia
Discuss timing and targets for hemoglobin value and strategies to achieve these targets

Clinically important anemia is difficult to define and varies with patient age, disease, and acuteness or chronicity of condition
Without significant clinical suspicion, patient hemoglobin value is rarely checked prior to surgery
When observed, anemia to hemoglobin value > 7.0 g/dL is regularly accepted without transfusion for procedures that are brief and without expected large blood loss
Alternatively, for long, stressful procedures or surgery with large expected blood loss hemoglobin level of 10 g/dL is usually desired

(Continued)

571

TABLE VII–1. COMMON ISSUES THAT MAY LEAD TO PERIOPERATIVE PEDIATRIC CONSULTATION (*CONTINUED*)

System and Condition	Implications for Surgery and Anesthesia	Pediatric Consultant's Potential Contribution to Perioperative Preparation and Management	Comments
Coagulopathy	Inadequate hemostasis, intraoperatively and postoperatively	Help confirm cause of coagulopathy Discuss timing and targets for coagulation profile values, and strategies to achieve (eg, for hemophiliacs, factor transfusion to achieve 100% correction is usually necessary for intraoperative period and several day postoperatively unless surgery is without significant incision)	Similar to anemia, coagulation profile is infrequently checked in healthy children preoperatively History of frequent nosebleeds or easy bruising may suggest von Willebrand disease Patients with mild cases may need only DDAVP, but more commonly hematology consultation and recommendations for cryoprecipitate are required
Sickle cell disease	Inadequate oxygen carrying capacity Promotion of sickling and tissue infarction in response to hypovolemia, hypoxemia, acidemia, or local factors such as use of a tourniquet during extremity surgery	Help prepare patient and family for surgery Discuss alternatives to reduce percentage of sickle hemoglobin: Simple transfusion, chronic transfusion of several weeks, exchange transfusion (erythropheresis)	When percentage of sickle hemoglobin (S or C) is <30%, there is little risk of significant sickling If surgery is necessary during an acute crisis, consider erythropheresis to acutely lower percentage of sickle hemoglobin For planned procedures when the patient is in a state of good general healthimple transfusion to achieve hemoglobin level of ≥ 10 g/dL has been demonstrated to have similarly good results when compared with more aggressive treatment
Oncologic Process			
Child with cancer	Tolerant of usual dosages of analgesics and sedatives	Ascertain history of chemotherapy, and cardiac or pulmonary	Patients and families have often experienced repeated painful events and prolonged

	High expectation that procedures be as stress free as possible	hospitalization; as a result, children often become physiologically tolerant of usual dosages of analgesics and sedatives and may need what at first appear to be unsafe amounts of narcotics and benzodiazepines
	Some chemotherapeutic agents can lead to pulmonary, myocardial, and renal dysfunction	Anthracyclines (doxorubicin, daunorubicin) at doses > 400 mg/m² have a high incidence of causing myocardial dysfunction
		function studies	Pulmonary fibrosis can result from treatment with bleomycin, busulfan and BCNU
	Obtain history of recent reactions to sedation and analgesia	

Endocrinologic System

Diabete	Intraoperative and postoperative hypoglycemia and hyperglycemia	It is most convenient if insulin-dependent diabetic patient is scheduled as "first" case of the day so that NPO preoperative preparation is accomplished during usual overnight fasting period
	Recommend strategy for treatment with insulin	Once access for IV glucose is established, 5% dextrose solution is begun and half the usual AM insulin is provided
		Blood glucose levels are regularly obtained intraoperatively, and IV insulin infused if glucose rises above 200 mg/dL
Acquired adrenal insufficiency	Intraoperative adrenal crisis	Stress of surgery and surgical disease often requires that hypophyseal-pituitary axis (HPA) increase production of adrenal steroids
	Help determine if adrenal steroid supplementation is needed	

(Continued)

TABLE VII-1. COMMON ISSUES THAT MAY LEAD TO PERIOPERATIVE PEDIATRIC CONSULTATION (CONTINUED)

System and Condition	Implications for Surgery and Anesthesia	Pediatric Consultant's Potential Contribution to Perioperative Preparation and Management	Comments
		Recommend steroid replacement dosing, as follows: 1. For simple procedures, 50 mg/m^2 as one-time dose 2. For complex procedures or large blood loss, 50 mg/m^2 initial dose followed by 100 mg/m^2/day	Physiologic output of adrenal steroids approximates 12.5 mg/m^2/day of hydrocortisone. Patients who have received a course of treatment with supraphysiologic dosages (> 15 mg/m^2/day) are likely to have suppression of HPA and be unable to respond to stress of surgery; these patients need replacement therapy. Recovery of HPA is variable but in patients with history of short course of treatment (< 2–4 wk), recovery is likely to occur within 2–4 wk; in children with more prolonged treatment, recovery may take as long as 6–9 mo

BCNU = bis-chloroethyl-nitrosourea; DDAVP = desmopressin acetate.

water; if in doubt, contact the anesthesiologist or surgeon. Address patient or family statements related to medication allergy.

D. Other Diagnoses or Treatments That Might Compromise Respiratory, Circulatory, or Other Vital Functions. Describe the patient in qualitative terms (mild, moderate, or severe) and provide an evaluation of current condition relative to past history.

E. Special Considerations

1. **Vascular access.** All but the briefest of surgical procedures will require that vascular access be obtained. Identify the need for vascular access in the postoperative period and beyond. The intraoperative period is a convenient time to address this issue. Alternatively, some chronically hospitalized patients have a history of vascular loss or thrombosis, and some children are dependent on limited central venous structures (eg, children with Fontan-type palliation of congenital heart disease). Ensure that surgical team is aware of inaccessible or prohibited vascular sites.

2. **Neurobehavioral status.** Large proportions of children in need of surgical procedures have congenital or acquired neurologic injuries. These neurologic abnormalities are associated with abnormalities in the neurologic exam, developmental or behavioral alterations, and seizures. It is important to know the physical exam findings, have a description of ictal state, and ensure proper medical control. Similarly, an understanding of patient's behavior and any limitations in ability to cooperate will be valuable when choosing among options for induction of anesthesia and postoperative care. Many of these children receive medications to manage these problems, including anticonvulsant, antispasmodic, and other behavior-modifying medications. Chronic treatment with these agents alters metabolism of most commonly used anesthetic agents and affects postoperative analgesic requirements. Coagulation and hepatic function tests may also be affected. Most agents used to produce general anesthesia are potent anticonvulsants, so intraoperative seizures are rare. However, because of the combined effect of altered enteral intake in the preoperative period, expected or unanticipated delay in reinstituting treatment postoperatively, and low drug levels associated with blood and body fluid losses and replacement during surgery, increased frequency of seizures in the postoperative period is common.

3. **Social history.** The need for surgical intervention, choice of the best surgical solution, obtaining informed consent, and cooperation with immediate and later postoperative care are all influenced by patient's social and family environment. The pediatrician may have the insight, interest, skills, and access to other tools needed to address these issues more effectively than clinicians who are focused on surgical management.

II. **Participation of Other Clinical Specialists.** Particularly in the case of children with chronic disease and frequent hospitalizations, there are often many clinical specialists involved in care. Patient or family invariably assume, and expect, these clinicians to be in contact with each other or be willing to communicate with each other.

III. **Anesthetic Management Plan.** The pediatric consultant will provide a valuable consultation if some basic principles related to anesthesia care are understood.

   A. **Goals of Anesthesia Management**
      1. To render patient tolerant to the pain and stress of surgery.
      2. To, when necessary, spare patient awareness or memory of the surgical event.
      3. To identify patient conditions (lack of movement and body positioning or exposure) that might complicate the procedure.
      4. To oversee or maintain physical and physiologic safety of patient during intraoperative and immediate postoperative period.

   B. **Anesthesia Methods.** In children, the anesthesiologist frequently needs to induce a state of general anesthesia or provide general anesthetic combined with regional anesthetic technique (eg, neuroaxial block or specific nerve blocks). On occasion, and usually with older children, regional techniques may be used without general anesthesia. General anesthesia can be achieved with a variety of methods. Most commonly, a potent inhaled anesthetic agent (halothane, isoflurane, sevoflurane) is combined with IV sedatives (midazolam, propofol), narcotics (morphine, fentanyl), and paralytics (vecuronium, rocuronium) to create a state in which child is unconscious, unmoving, and has little or no adrenergic response to noxious stimuli of the procedure. As patient enters this state, control of airway, breathing, and circulation (ABCs) is compromised to varying degrees, depending on patient's presurgical disease or condition and anesthetic technique used.

   C. **Effects and Cautions.** Anesthesia results in loss of airway reflexes and increases patient's risk for aspiration of gastric contents. Routinely, enteral intake is restricted preoperatively to reduce the chance of this occurrence (Table VII–2). To counter these effects, patient is usually intubated and mechanical ventilation provided intraoperatively. General anesthetic agents may contribute to compromised circulation because of their vasodilating and myocardial depressing qualities, intraoperative blood loss, direct and indirect (stress) effects of the surgery, and patient's underlying condition. Therefore, respiratory and cardiovascular function should be monitored during surgery. Transfusion of blood components, inotropic support, and extracorporeal support (eg, cardiac surgery) may be required on a regular basis for certain procedures.

TABLE VII–2. PREOPERATIVE FEEDING RESTRICTION GUIDELINES[a]

Time Interval[b]	Patient Group	Allowable Enteral Intake
2 h	Any patient	Clear liquids[c]
4 h	Infants younger than 1 year	Breast milk
6 h	Infants younger than 1 year	Milk formula, solids
8 h	Children 1 year or older	Milk or solid food

[a] Preoperative feeding guidelines are listed here. This guide is based on the consensus of experts and incomplete evidence from a few small controlled trials. It can be remembered easily as the 2, 4, 6, 8 plan.
[b] Refers to last intake prior to hospital arrival for surgery.
[c] Defined as anything that one can "see through"; includes water, juices, and gelatin dessert.

    D. ASA Classification. The ASA physical status score allows anesthesiologists to communicate patient's physical condition, independent of the planned operation. Physical status serves as a common language among different practitioners and institutions for subsequent analysis reporting of morbidity and mortality. Although ASA status is not intended to give an estimation of risk, it is a patient-centered classification that is useful for communicating potential morbidity related to a patient's preexisting disease processes (Table VII–3).

IV. Physical Exam Key Points. These points include, but are not limited to, a thorough evaluation of airway (including teeth and the potential for airway obstruction), respiratory function, and cardiovascular function.

V. Laboratory, Radiographic, and Other Studies
    A. ASA Classes 1 and 2. No routine laboratory or imaging study has been found to be helpful in judging preoperative risk. Therefore, usually no studies are necessary in ASA class 1 and class 2 patients.
    B. ASA Class 3. For patients identified as ASA class 3 or greater, preoperative evaluation laboratory studies and imaging are obtained on a case-by-case basis. Blood chemistries, hematologic and coagulation studies, chest x-rays, ABGs, respiratory studies, or even other specialist consultation (eg, cardiology, pulmonology) may all be of value. If levels of anticonvulsant drugs are used to guide treatment, knowledge of the most recent values and targets are helpful. Patient's values prior to surgery should be measured. If surgery and anesthesia will prevent intake or absorption of enterally administered anticonvulsants, dose modification for IV administration and an alternative drug for IV administration should be recommended.

TABLE VII–3. ASA PHYSICAL STATUS CLASSIFICATION

Classification	Definition	Example
P1 (ASA 1)	Normal healthy patient	Previously healthy 15-year-old who is scheduled to undergo surgery for appendicitis
P2 (ASA 2)	Patient with mild systemic disease	Well infant with chronic otitis media and history of recurrent wheezing, who is undergoing surgery to insert bilateral myringotomy tubes
P3 (ASA 3)	Patient with severe systemic disease	10-year-old boy with cerebral palsy, who is hospitalized for pneumonia and will undergo surgery for central line placement.
P4 (ASA 4)	Patient with severe systemic disease that is a constant threat to life	Premature infant with cardiorespiratory failure who requires surgery to repair patent ductus arteriosus
P5 (ASA 5)	Moribund patient who is not expected to survive without the operation	Child bicyclist who was hit by an automobile, causing acute epidural hematoma, cerebral contusion, and coma, and will undergo surgery for evacuation and debridement of hematoma
P6 (ASA 6)	Patient who has been declared brain dead and whose organs are being removed for donation	2-year-old boy who was declared brain dead after drowning in a swimming pool

ASA = American Society of Anesthesiologists.

2. POSTOPERATIVE CARE

Duration of "postoperative care" may range from discharge within 1 hour of completion of surgery to inpatient hospitalization in a pediatric intensive care unit for many days. For children to be discharged to home on the day of surgery (50–80% of patients in most pediatric surgical programs), tolerance of reintroduced oral intake of fluids, nutrition, and analgesic medications are primary management issues. Postoperative nausea and vomiting has an overall occurrence of 10–45%, (depending on definition) and is common after procedures such as tonsillectomy and eye surgery. Knowledge of the postoperative plan allows the pediatrician to provide effective involvement perioperatively.

REFERENCES

Cote CJ. Preoperative preparation and premedication. *Br J Anesth* 1999;83:16–28.

Evaluation and preparation of pediatric patients undergoing anesthesia. American Academy of Pediatrics Section on Anesthesiology. *Pediatrics* 1996;98 (pt 1): 502–508.

Krane EJ, Davis PJ, Smith RM. Preoperative preparation. In: Motoyama EK, Davis PJ, eds. *Smith's Anesthesia for Infants and Children*, 6th ed. Mosby, 1996: 213–228.

Means LJ. Preoperative evaluation. In: Badgewell JM, ed. *Clinical Pediatric Anesthesia*. Lippincott-Raven, 1997:1–13.

Steward DJ. Screening tests before surgery in children. *Can J Anaesth* 1991; 38:693–695.

VIII. Commonly Used Medications

1. Classes of Generic Drugs, Minerals, and Vitamins

2. Generic Drugs: Indications, Actions, Dosage, Supplied, and Notes

3. Minerals: Indications/Effects, RDA/Dosage, Signs/Symptoms of Deficiency and Toxicity, and Notes

4. Vitamins: Indications/Effects, RDA/Dosage, Signs/Symptoms of Deficiency and Toxicity, and Notes

5. Tables:
   VIII–1. Insulins
   VIII–2. Comparison of Glucocorticoids
   VIII–3. First-Generation Cephalosporins
   VIII–4. Second-Generation Cephalosporins
   VIII–5. Third- and Fourth-Generation Cephalosporins
   VIII–6. Ophthalmic Agents

This section is designed to serve as a quick reference to commonly used medications. You should be familiar with all of the indications, contraindications, side effects, and drug interactions of any medications that you prescribe. Such detailed information is beyond the scope of this manual and can be found in the package insert, or in the *Pediatric Dosage Handbook* by Lexi-Comp. Complete neonatal dosing is not included for all drugs and may be found in Neofax.

Drugs in this section are listed in alphabetical order by generic names. Some of the more common trade names are listed for each medication.

Drugs under the control of the Drug Enforcement Agency (Schedule II–V controlled substances) are indicated by the symbol [C]. Over-the-counter (OTC) medications are marked with an asterisk (*) after the name or strength available without a prescription.

1. CLASSES OF GENERIC DRUGS, MINERALS, AND VITAMINS

Analgesic, Anti-Inflammatory, and Antipyretic Agents

Acetaminophen
Acetaminophen with codeine
Aspirin
Codeine
Fentanyl
Hydrocodone and acetaminophen
Hydromorphone

Ibuprofen
Indomethacin
Ketorolac
Meperidine
Methadone
Morphine sulfate
Nalbuphine
Naproxen
Oxycodone
Oxycodone and acetaminophen
Tolmetin

Anesthetics

Bupivacaine
Cocaine
Ketamine
Lidocaine
Lidocaine and prilocaine
Pramoxine
Pramoxine and hydrocortisone

Antacids and Antigas Agents

Aluminum hydroxide and magnesium hydroxide
Aluminum hydroxide, magnesium hydroxide, and simethicone
Calcium carbonate
Magnesium hydroxide

Antianxiety Agents

Diazepam
Lorazepam
Hydroxyzine

Antiarrhythmics

Class IA
Procainamide
Class IB
Lidocaine
Phenytoin
Class II
Esmolol
Propranolol
Class III
Amiodarone
Bretylium

Class IV
Verapamil
Miscellaneous
Adenosine
Digoxin

Antiasthmatic Agents

Cromolyn
Montelukast
Nedocromil
Zafirlukast

Antibiotics

Amikacin
Amoxicillin
Amoxicillin and clavulanic acid
Ampicillin
Ampicillin and sulbactam
Azithromycin
Aztreonam
Bacitracin
Bacitracin and polymyxin B
Bacitracin, neomycin, and polymyxin B
Cefaclor
Cefadroxil
Cefazolin
Cefdinir
Cefepime
Cefixime
Cefotaxime
Cefoxitin
Cefpodoxime
Cefprozil
Ceftazidime
Ceftriaxone
Cefuroxime
Cephalexin
Chloramphenicol
Ciprofloxacin
Clarithromycin
Clindamycin
Dicloxacillin
Doxycycline
Erythromycin
Ethambutol
Gentamicin

Imipenem and cilastatin
Isoniazid
Levofloxacin
Linezolid
Meropenem
Metronidazole
Mupirocin
Nafcillin
Neomycin sulfate
Neomycin and polymyxin B
Nitrofurantoin
Oxacillin
Penicillin G aqueous
Penicillin G benzathine
Penicillin G procaine
Penicillin V potassium
Pentamidine
Piperacillin
Piperacillin and tazobactam
Pyrazinamide
Quinupristin and dalfopristin
Rifampin
Silver sulfadiazine
Tetracycline
Ticarcillin
Ticarcillin and potassium clavulanate
Tobramycin
Trimethoprim-sulfamethoxazole
Vancomycin

Anticholinergic Agents

Atropine
Glycopyrrolate
Hyoscyamine
Hyoscyamine, atropine, scopolamine, and phenobarbital

Anticoagulant, Thrombolytic, and Related Agents

Alteplase, recombinant (TPA)
Aminocaproic acid
Antihemophilic factor (factor VIII)
Aspirin
Desmopressin (DDAVP)
Enoxaparin
Heparin
Urokinase
Warfarin

Anticonvulsants

Carbamazepine
Clonazepam
Clorazepate
Diazepam
Ethosuximide
Felbamate
Fosphenytoin
Gabapentin
Lamotrigine
Levetiracetam
Lorazepam
Oxcarbazepine
Pentobarbital
Phenobarbital
Phenytoin
Primidone
Tiagabine
Topiramate
Valproic acid
Zonisamide

Antidepressants

Amitriptyline
Fluoxetine
Imipramine
Lithium carbonate
Nortriptyline
Paroxetine
Sertraline
Trazodone

Antidiabetic Agents

Insulin
Metformin

Antidiarrheal Agents

Bismuth subsalicylate
Diphenoxylate and atropine
Kaolin and pectin
Lactobacillus acidophilus and *Lactobacillus bulgaricus*
Loperamide
Octreotide
Paregoric

Antidotes

Acetylcysteine
Charcoal
Digoxin immune FaB
Edrophonium
Flumazenil
Ipecac syrup
Mesna
Naloxone
Physostigmine
Protamine
Sodium polystyrene sulfonate

Antiemetics

Chlorpromazine
Droperidol
Granisetron
Metoclopramide
Ondansetron
Prochlorperazine
Promethazine

Antifungal Agents

Amphotericin B
Amphotericin B lipid complex
Amphotericin B liposomal
Clotrimazole
Fluconazole
Flucytosine
Griseofulvin
Itraconazole
Ketoconazole
Miconazole
Nystatin
Tolnaftate
Voriconazole

Antigout Agent

Allopurinol

Antihistamines

Cetirizine
Chlorpheniramine

Cyproheptadine
Dimenhydrinate
Diphenhydramine
Hydroxyzine
Loratadine

Antihyperlipidemic

Cholestyramine resin

Antihypertensives

Amlodipine
Atenolol
Captopril
Clonidine
Diazoxide
Diltiazem
Enalapril and enalaprilat
Hydralazine
Labetalol
Minoxidil
Nifedipine
Nitroglycerin
Nitroprusside
Prazosin
Propranolol
Verapamil

Antineoplastics

Asparaginase
Bleomycin
Busulfan
Carboplatin
Chlorambucil
Cisplatin
Cyclophosphamide
Cytarabine
Dactinomycin
Daunorubicin
Doxorubicin
Etoposide
Hydroxyurea
Idarubicin
Ifosfamide
Melphalan

Mercaptopurine
Methotrexate
Thioguanine
Thiotepa

Antiparkinsonism Agents

Amantadine
Benztropine

Antiprotozoal Agents

Atovaquone
Dapsone

Antipsychotic Agents

Haloperidol
Lithium carbonate
Prochlorperazine

Antitussives, Decongestants, and Expectorants

Brompheniramine and pseudoephedrine
Codeine
Dextromethorphan
Guaifenesin
Guaifenesin and codeine
Guaifenesin and dextromethorphan
Pseudoephedrine
Triprolidine and pseudoephedrine

Antiviral Agents

Acyclovir
Amantadine
Didanosine
Foscarnet
Ganciclovir
Indinavir
Lamivudine
Nelfinavir
Oseltamivir
Ribavirin
Rimantadine
Ritonavir
Trifluridine
Zalcitabine

Zidovudine
Zidovudine and lamivudine

Bronchodilators

Albuterol
Aminophylline
Epinephrine
Flunisolide
Ipratropium
Salmeterol
Terbutaline
Theophylline

Cardiovascular Agents

Atenolol
Atropine
Digoxin
Diltiazem
Dobutamine
Dopamine
Epinephrine
Esmolol
Inamrinone
Isoproterenol
Milrinone
Minoxidil
Nifedipine
Nitroglycerin
Nitroprusside
Norepinephrine
Phenylephrine
Propranolol
Verapamil

Cathartics and Laxatives

Bisacodyl
Docusate sodium
Glycerin
Kaolin and pectin
Lactulose
Magnesium hydroxide
Mineral oil
Polyethylene glycol–electrolyte solution
Psyllium

Central Nervous System Stimulants

Caffeine
Dextroamphetamine
Dextroamphetamine and amphetamine
Methylphenidate

Corticosteroids

Beclomethasone
Betamethasone
Budesonide
Corticotropin
Dexamethasone
Fludrocortisone
Flunisolide
Fluticasone
Hydrocortisone
Methylprednisolone
Prednisolone
Prednisone
Triamcinolone

Dermatologic Agents

Bacitracin
Bacitracin and polymyxin B
Clotrimazole
Hydrocortisone
Ketoconazole
Lactic acid and ammonium hydroxide
Lindane
Neomycin
Neomycin and polymyxin B
Neomycin, bacitracin, and polymyxin B
Neomycin, bacitracin, polymyxin B, and hydrocortisone
Nystatin
Permethrin
Silver nitrate
Silver sulfadiazine
Tolnaftate
Tretinoin

Diuretics

Acetazolamide
Amiloride

Bumetanide
Chlorothiazide
Ethacrynic acid
Furosemide
Hydrochlorothiazide
Mannitol
Metolazone
Spironolactone

Electrolyte Supplements

Calcium acetate
Calcium carbonate
Calcium glubionate
Calcium gluconate
Calcium chloride
Magnesium oxide
Magnesium sulfate
Potassium chloride
Potassium phosphate
Sodium chloride
Sodium phosphate

Gallstone Dissolution Agent

Ursodiol

Gastrointestinal Agents

Dicyclomine
Famotidine
Hyoscyamine
Infliximab
Lansoprazole
Mesalamine
Metoclopramide
Neomycin sulfate
Octreotide
Omeprazole
Pancrelipase
Pantoprazole
Ranitidine
Simethicone
Sucralfate
Sulfasalazine
Vasopressin

Hormones and Synthetic Substitutes (Also see Thyroid and Antithyroid Agents)

Calcitonin
Desmopressin
Drotrecogin alfa
Epoetin alfa (Erythropoietin)
Etanercept
Filgrastim (G-CSF)
Glucagon
Insulin
Megestrol acetate
Pancrelipase
Vasopressin

Immunosuppressive Agents

Antithymocyte globulin
Azathioprine
Basiliximab
Cyclosporine
Daclizumab
Muromonab-CD3 (OKT-3)
Mycophenolate mofetil
Sirolimus
Tacrolimus (FK-506)

Lung Surfactants

Beractant
Calfactant
Colfosceril

Mineral Supplements

Calcium
Chromium
Copper
Ferrous sulfate
Iron dextran
Iron sucrose
Manganese
Selenium
Zinc

Mucolytics

Acetylcysteine
Dornase alfa

Muscle Relaxants

Baclofen
Dantrolene
Diazepam
Dicyclomine

Neuromuscular Blocking Agents

Atracurium
Cisatracurium
Pancuronium
Rocuronium
Succinylcholine
Vecuronium

Nutritional Supplements (Also see Mineral Supplements)

d-Alpha Tocopherol (vitamin E)
Ascorbic acid (vitamin C)
Calcitriol
Carnitine
Cyanocobalamin (vitamin B_{12})
Ergocalciferol (vitamin D_2)
Fluoride
Folate
Niacin (vitamin B_3)
Phytonadione (vitamin K)
Pyridoxine (vitamin B_6)
Riboflavin (vitamin B_2)
Thiamine (vitamin B_1)
Vitamin A

Ophthalmic Agents

Artificial tears
Brimonidine
Ciprofloxacin
Cyclopentolate
Dexamethasone
Erythromycin
Fluorometholone
Gentamicin

Gentamicin and prednisolone
Phenylephrine
Pilocarpine
Prednisolone
Sulfacetamide
Sulfacetamide and prednisolone
Tobramycin
Tobramycin and dexamethasone
Trifluridine

Otic Agents

Benzocaine and antipyrine
Ciprofloxacin HC
Neomycin, (bacitracin), polymyxin B, and hydrocortisone
Neomycin, polymyxin B, and prednisolone

Plasma Volume Expanders

Albumin
Hetastarch

Progestin

Medroxyprogesterone

Prostaglandin

Alprostadil

Sedative-Hypnotics

Chloral hydrate
Clorazepate
Diazepam
Diphenhydramine
Lorazepam
Midazolam
Hydroxyzine
Propofol

Thyroid and Antithyroid Agents

Levothyroxine
Potassium iodide
Propylthiouracil

Toxoids, Vaccines, Immune Globulins, and Monoclonal Antibodies

Cytomegalovirus immune globulin
Diphtheria, tetanus toxoid, acellular pertussis vaccine
Diphtheria and tetanus toxoid
Haemophilus influenzae type b conjugate vaccine
Hepatitis A vaccine
Hepatitis B immune globulin
Hepatitis B vaccine
Immune globulin intravenous
Infliximab
Influenza vaccine
Palivizumab
Pneumococcal conjugate vaccine (7-valent)
Pneumococcal polysaccharide vaccine (23-valent)
Poliovirus vaccine (inactivated)
Respiratory syncytial virus immune globulin
Tetanus immune globulin
Tetanus toxoid
Varicella vaccine

Urinary (and Genitourinary) Tract Agents

Ammonium aluminum sulfate
Belladonna and opium
Bethanechol
Citrate and citric acid
Hyoscyamine
Hyoscyamine, atropine, scopolamine, and phenobarbital
Oxybutynin
Phenazopyridine
Potassium citrate and citric acid
Sodium bicarbonate

2. GENERIC DRUGS: INDICATIONS, ACTIONS, DOSAGE, SUPPLIED, AND NOTES

ACETAMINOPHEN (TYLENOL, FEVERALL)*

Indications: Mild pain; headache; fever.

Actions: Non-narcotic analgesic; inhibits synthesis of prostaglandins in the CNS and inhibits the hypothalamic heat-regulating center.

Dosage: 10–15 mg/kg per dose PO or 10–20 mg/kg per dose PR q4–6h; *do not* exceed 5 doses or 4 g/24 h.

Supplied: Chewable tablets 80 mg, 160 mg; tablets 160 mg, 325 mg, 500 mg, 650 mg; oral drops 100 mg/mL; suspension 160 mg/5 mL; suppositories 80 mg, 120 mg, 325 mg, 650 mg.

Notes: Overdose causes hepatotoxicity, which is treated with *N*-acetylcysteine. Has no anti-inflammatory or platelet-inhibiting action. Chewable products contain aspartame, which is metabolized to phenylalanine; avoid in phenylketonurics.

ACETAMINOPHEN WITH CODEINE (TYLENOL WITH CODEINE, CAPITAL WITH CODEINE) [C]

Indications: Mild to moderate pain.

Actions: Combined effects of acetaminophen and a narcotic analgesic.

Dosage: 0.5–1 mg codeine per kg per dose PO q4–6h prn or 0.4 mL/kg per dose liquid PO q4–6h prn (max dose of acetaminophen = 4 g/day).

Supplied: Tablets Tylenol No. 2, No. 3, and No. 4 contain 300 mg acetaminophen and 15 mg, 30 mg, and 60 mg codeine, respectively; liquid contains acetaminophen 120 mg and codeine 12 mg per 5 mL.

Notes: Use with caution in patients with hypersensitivity to morphine or derivatives.

ACETAZOLAMIDE (DIAMOX)

Indications: Diuresis; glaucoma; hydrocephalus; refractory epilepsy.

Actions: Carbonic anhydrase inhibitor; decreases renal excretion of hydrogen ions and increases renal excretion of sodium, potassium, bicarbonate, and water.

Dosage: *Diuretic:* 5 mg/kg per dose PO or IV q24h.
   Glaucoma: 8–30 mg/kg/day PO divided q8h or 20–40 mg/kg/day IV divided q6h, not to exceed 1 g/day.
   Hydrocephalus: 5 mg/kg per dose PO or IV q6h, max 100 mg/kg/day.
   Epilepsy: 4–16 mg/kg/day PO in 1–4 divided doses, not to exceed 30 mg/kg/day or 1 g/day.

Supplied: Tablets 125 mg, 250 mg; sustained-release capsules 500 mg; injection 500 mg per vial.

Notes: Contraindicated in hepatic failure and sulfa hypersensitivity. Follow sodium and potassium; watch for metabolic acidosis. Sustained-release dosage forms are not recommended for use in epilepsy. Reduce dosage in patients with renal impairment.
Acetylcysteine (Mucomyst, Acetadote)

Indications: Mucolytic agent as adjuvant therapy of chronic bronchopulmonary diseases and cystic fibrosis; as antidote to acetaminophen hepatotoxicity within 24 hours of ingestion.

Actions: Splits disulfide linkages between mucoprotein molecular complexes; protects liver by restoring glutathione levels in acetaminophen overdose.

Dosage: Inhalation: 3–5 mL 20% solution diluted with equal volume of NS administered via nebulizer 3–4 times daily.
  Antidote: Oral or nasogastric: 140 mg/kg loading dose, then 70 mg/kg q4h for 17 doses; dilute 1:3 in carbonated beverage or orange juice.

Supplied: Solution 10%, 20%.

Notes: Watch for bronchospasm when used by inhalation in asthmatics. For acetaminophen ingestion, therapy should continue until all doses are administered even though acetaminophen plasma level has dropped below therapeutic range; repeat dose if emesis occurs within 1 hour.

ACYCLOVIR (ZOVIRAX)

Indications: Herpes simplex and herpes zoster viral infections.

Actions: Interferes with viral DNA synthesis.

Dosage: Oral:

- *Initial genital herpes:* 200 mg PO q4h while awake, for total of 5 caps/day for 10 days or 400 mg PO 3 times daily for 7–10 days, max dose in children 80 mg/kg/day.
- *Chronic suppression:* 400–500 mg PO twice daily, max dose in children 80 mg/kg/day.
- *Intermittent therapy:* Same as for initial treatment, except treat for 5 days, or 800 mg PO twice daily, initiated at earliest prodrome.
- *Herpes zoster in immunocompetent host:* 800 mg PO 5 times daily for 7–10 days, max dose in children 80 mg/kg/day.
- *Herpes zoster in immunocompromised host: Children:* 250–600 mg/m^2 per dose PO 5 times daily for 7–10 days; *Adults:* 800 mg PO 5 times daily for 7–10 days.
- *Varicella zoster in immunocompetent host:* 80 mg/kg/day PO 4 times daily for 5 days; max 3200 mg/day.

Intravenous: 10–20 mg/kg per dose IV q8h.
Topical initial herpes genitalis: Apply q3h (6 times daily) for 7 days.

Supplied: Capsule 200 mg; tablets 400 mg, 800 mg; suspension 200 mg/ 5 mL; injection 500 or 1000 mg per vial; ointment 5%.

Notes: Adjust dose in patients with renal insufficiency. Maintain adequate hydration and urine output for first 2 hours post–IV infusion to minimize nephrotoxicity.

ADENOSINE (ADENOCARD)

Indications: Paroxysmal supraventricular tachycardia (PSVT) in ACLS and PALS algorithms.

Actions: Class IV antiarrhythmic; slows conduction time through AV node.

Dosage: Children < 50 kg: 0.05–0.1 mg/kg rapid IV bolus, may repeat in 1–2 min to max single dose of 0.3 mg/kg or until termination of PSVT; *Children > 50 kg and adults:* 6 mg rapid IV, may repeat in 1–2 min, max single dose 12 mg.
   PALS dose for SVT: 0.1 mg/kg rapid IV or IO, max dose 6 mg; if not effective, give 0.2 mg/kg, max dose 12 mg.

Supplied: Injection 6 mg/2 mL.

Notes: Doses > 12 mg are not recommended. Caffeine and theophylline antagonize effects of adenosine.

ALBUMIN (ALBUMINAR, BUMINATE, ALBUTEIN, OTHERS)

Indications: Plasma volume expansion for shock resulting from burns, surgery, hemorrhage, or other trauma.

Actions: Maintenance of plasma colloid oncotic pressure.

Dosage: 0.5–1 g/kg per dose (10–20 mL/kg per dose of 5% albumin), may repeat as needed; max dose 6 g/kg/day (120 mL/kg/day of 5% albumin).

Supplied: Solution 5% (50 mg/mL), 25% (250 mg/mL).

Notes: Contains 130–160 mEq Na$^+$/L. Too-rapid infusion may result in vascular overload.

ALBUTEROL (PROVENTIL, VENTOLIN)

Indications: Treatment of bronchospasm in reversible obstructive airway disease; prevention of exercise-induced bronchospasm.

Actions: β-Adrenergic sympathomimetic bronchodilator; relaxes bronchial smooth muscle.

Dosage: Acute asthma exacerbation (NIH guidelines):
- *Metered-dose inhaler:* 4–8 puffs q20min for 3 doses, then q1–4h.
- *Nebulization:* 0.15 mg/kg, minimum dose 2.5 mg q20min for 3 doses, then 0.15–0.3 mg/kg; max dose 10 mg q1–4h prn or 0.5 mg/kg/h by continuous nebulization.

Maintenance therapy (nonacute):

- *Oral: Children 2–6 years:* 0.1–0.2 mg/kg per dose PO 3 times daily, max 12 mg/day; *6–12 years:* 2 mg PO 3–4 times daily, max 24 mg/day; *> 12 years:* 2–4 mg PO 3–4 times daily, max 32 mg/day.
- *Metered-dose inhaler:* 1–2 puffs q4–6h.
- *Nebulization:* 0.15–0.25 mg/kg, max dose 1 mL of 0.5% solution in 2–3 mL NS q4–6h.

Supplied: Tablets 2 mg, 4 mg; extended-release tablets 4 mg, 8 mg; syrup 2 mg/5 mL; metered-dose inhaler 90 mcg per dose; solution for nebulization 0.083%, 0.5%.

Notes: Inhaled albuterol can cause paradoxical bronchospasm; discontinue therapy immediately if this occurs. May cause hypokalemia.

ALLOPURINOL (ZYLOPRIM, ALOPRIM)

Indications: Gout; hyperuricemia of malignancy; recurrent calcium oxalate calculi.

Actions: Xanthine oxidase inhibitor, which decreases production of uric acid.

Dosage: *Hyperuricemia of malignancy:*

- *Children < 10 years: Oral:* 10 mg/kg/day in 2–3 divided doses or 200–300 mg/m^2/day in 2–4 divided doses, max 800 mg/day; *Intravenous:* 200 mg/m^2/day in 1–3 divided doses, max 600 mg/day.
- *Children > 10 years: Oral:* 600–800 mg/day in 2–3 divided doses; *Intravenous:* 200–400 mg/m^2/day in 1–3 divided doses, max 600 mg/day.
 Gout: 200–600 mg PO once daily.
 Recurrent calcium oxalate calculi: 200–300 mg/day PO in 1–2 divided doses.

Supplied: Tablets 100, 300 mg; injection 500 mg/30 mL.

Notes: Aggravates acute gouty attack; *do not* begin until acute attack resolves. Should be taken after meals. IV administration of 6 mg/mL final concentration can be given as single daily infusion or divided at 6-, 8-, or 12-hour intervals. Adjust dose in patients with renal impairment.

ALPROSTADIL (PROSTIN)

Indications: Temporary maintenance of patency of ductus arteriosus.

Actions: Direct vasodilation of vascular and ductus arteriosus smooth muscle.

Dosage: 0.05–0.4 mcg/kg/min continuous IV infusion.

Supplied: 500 mcg/mL injection.

Notes: Gradually reduce rate to lowest effective dosage; maximum concentration for infusion 20 mcg/mL.

ALTEPLASE, RECOMBINANT [T-PA] (ACTIVASE, CATHFLO ACTIVASE)

Indications: Systemic thromboses and occluded central venous catheters.

Actions: Tissue plasminogen activator, resulting in thrombolysis; inhibits local fibrinolysis by binding to fibrin in thrombus.

Dosage: Occluded IV catheter (dose per lumen): Children 10–30 kg: Using 1 mg/1 mL concentration, instill volume equal to 110% of internal volume of catheter, dwell 2 hours; may repeat dose if catheter remains occluded, max dose 2 mg/2 mL; *Children > 30 kg:* 2 mg in 2 mL.
   Systemic thromboses: 0.1 mg/kg/h IV infusion for 6 hours; if no response increase infusion by 0.1 mg/kg/h at 6-hour intervals to max of 0.5 mg/kg/h.
   Low-dose (local) infusion for occluded catheter: 0.01 mg/kg/h IV infusion for 6 hours; if no response increase infusion by 0.01 mg/kg/h at 6-hour intervals to max of 0.05 mg/kg/h.

Supplied: Powder for injection 2 mg, 50 mg, 100 mg.

Notes: May cause bleeding; for systemic thromboses maintain fibrinogen > 100 mg/dL.

ALUMINUM HYDROXIDE WITH MAGNESIUM HYDROXIDE (MAALOX)*

Indications: Stomach upset with hyperacidity.

Actions: Neutralizes gastric acid.

Dosage: Infants: 1–2 mL/kg per dose PO 4 times daily; *Children:* 5–15 mL per dose PO 4 times daily; *Adults:* 15–45 mL PO 4 times daily.

Supplied: Tablets; suspension.

Notes: Doses 4 times daily are best given after meals and at bedtime. May cause hypermagnesemia in patients with renal insufficiency.

ALUMINUM HYDROXIDE WITH MAGNESIUM HYDROXIDE AND SIMETHICONE (MYLANTA, MYLANTA II, MAALOX PLUS)*

Indications: Hyperacidity with bloating.

Actions: Neutralizes gastric acid.

Dosage: *Infants:* 1–2 mL/kg per dose PO 4 times daily; *Children:* 5–15 mL per dose PO 4 times daily; *Adults:* 15–45 mL PO 4 times daily.

Supplied: Tablets; suspension.

Notes: May cause hypermagnesemia in patients with renal insufficiency. Mylanta II contains twice the amount of aluminum and magnesium hydroxide as Mylanta; use half the volume of the stated dose.

AMANTADINE (SYMMETREL)

Indications: Treatment or prophylaxis of influenza A viral infections; parkinsonism.

Actions: Prevents release of infectious viral nucleic acid into host cell; releases dopamine from intact dopaminergic terminals.

Dosage: *Influenza A:* 5 mg/kg/day PO in 1–2 divided doses, max 200 mg/day. *Parkinsonism:* 100 mg PO twice daily.

Supplied: Capsule 100 mg; tablet 100 mg; solution 50 mg/5 mL.

Notes: Reduce dose in patients with renal insufficiency.

AMIKACIN (AMIKIN)

Indications: Serious infections caused by gram-negative bacteria and mycobacterial infections.

Actions: Aminoglycoside antibiotic; inhibits protein synthesis.

Dosage: *Infants and children:* 15–30 mg/kg/day divided q8h. *Adults:* 15 mg/kg/day divided q8–12h; max 1.5 g/day.

Supplied: Injection 100 mg/2 mL, 500 mg/2 mL.

Notes: May be effective against gram-negative bacteria resistant to gentamicin and tobramycin. Monitor renal function carefully for dosage adjustments. Monitor serum levels (peak 20–30 mcg/mL; trough < 10 mcg/mL).

AMILORIDE (MIDAMOR)

Indications: Management of edema associated with congestive heart failure.

Actions: Potassium-sparing diuretic; interferes with potassium-sodium exchange in distal tubules.

Dosage: *Children 6–20 kg:* 0.625 mg/kg/day PO once daily; *Children > 20 kg:* 5–10 mg PO once daily, max 20 mg/day.

Supplied: Tablet 5 mg.

Notes: Hyperkalemia may occur; monitor serum potassium levels.

AMINOCAPROIC ACID (AMICAR)

Indications: Excessive bleeding resulting from systemic hyperfibrinolysis and urinary fibrinolysis.

Actions: Inhibits fibrinolysis via inhibition of plasminogen activator substances.

Dosage: 100–200 mg/kg PO or IV loading dose followed by 100 mg/kg per dose q6h, max 30 g/day.

Supplied: Tablet 500 mg; syrup 250 mg/mL; injection 250 mg/mL.

Notes: Administer for 8 hours or until bleeding is controlled. Contraindicated in disseminated intravascular coagulation. Not for upper urinary tract bleeding.

AMINOPHYLLINE

Indications: Asthma and bronchospasm; neonatal apnea of prematurity.

Actions: Relaxes smooth muscle of bronchi and pulmonary blood vessels.

Dosage: Acute bronchospasm: Load 6 mg/kg IV, then 0.4–1.2 mg/kg/h IV continuous infusion.
Apnea of prematurity: Load 5 mg/kg, then 5 mg/kg/day IV or PO divided q12h.

Supplied: Tablets 100 mg, 200 mg; solution 105 mg/5 mL; injection 25 mg/mL.

Notes: Individualize dosage. Signs of toxicity include nausea and vomiting, irritability, tachycardia, ventricular arrhythmias, and seizures. Follow serum levels carefully (asthma 10–20 mcg/mL; apnea 6–13 mcg/mL). Aminophylline is about 85% theophylline.

AMIODARONE (CORDARONE, PACERONE)

Indications: Recurrent ventricular fibrillation or hemodynamically unstable ventricular tachycardia and supraventricular arrhythmias; PALS algorithm for pulseless ventricular tachycardia or ventricular fibrillation.

Actions: Class III antiarrhythmic.

Dosage: Ventricular arrhythmias: Intravenous or intraosseous (PALS): 5 mg/kg rapid bolus; *Continuous infusion:* 5–15 mcg/kg/min IV; *Oral:* 10–15 mg/kg/day in 1–2 divided doses for 4–14 days or until arrhythmia is controlled or adverse effects occur; dose should then be reduced to 5 mg/kg/day for several weeks.

Supplied: Tablet 200 mg; injection 50 mg/mL.

Notes: Average half-life is 53 days. Potentially toxic effects include pulmonary fibrosis, liver failure, and ocular opacities, as well as exacerbation of arrhythmias. Routine use with drugs that prolong QT interval is not recommended.

AMITRIPTYLINE (ELAVIL)

Indications: Depression; peripheral neuropathy; chronic pain; tension and migraine headaches.

Actions: Tricyclic antidepressant; inhibits reuptake of serotonin and norepinephrine by presynaptic neuronal membrane.

Dosage: Chronic pain: Initial 0.1 mg/kg per dose PO at bedtime; may increase to 0.5–2 mg/kg at bedtime.

   Depression: Children 9–12 years: Initial 1 mg/kg/day in 3 divided doses up to 5 mg/kg/day; *Adolescents:* Initial 25–50 mg/day, may increase up to 100 mg/day, max 200 mg/day.
   Migraine prophylaxis: 0.25–1.5 mg/kg/day PO at bedtime.

Supplied: Tablets 10 mg, 25 mg, 50 mg, 75 mg, 100 mg, 150 mg; injection 10 mg/mL.

Notes: Strong anticholinergic side effects. May cause urine retention and sedation. Overdose can cause arrhythmias and seizures and may be fatal.

AMLODIPINE (NORVASC)

Indications: Treatment of hypertension and angina.

Actions: Calcium channel blocking agent; produces relaxation of coronary vascular smooth muscle.

Dosage: 0.05 mg/kg PO once daily, max 0.5 mg/kg/day.

Supplied: Tablets 2.5 mg, 5 mg, 10 mg.

Notes: May be taken without regard to meals.

AMMONIUM ALUMINUM SULFATE (ALUM)

Indications: Hemorrhagic cystitis when bladder irrigation fails.

Actions: Astringent.

Dosage: 1–2% solution used with constant bladder irrigation with NS.

Supplied: Powder for reconstitution.

Notes: Can be used safely without anesthesia and in presence of vesi-coureteral reflux. Encephalopathy has been reported. Obtain aluminum levels, especially in patients with renal insufficiency. Alum solution often precipitates and occludes catheters.

AMOXICILLIN (AMOXIL, POLYMOX, OTHERS)

Indications: Infections resulting from susceptible gram-positive bacteria (streptococci) and gram-negative bacteria (*Haemophilus influenzae, E coli, Proteus mirabilis*).

Actions: Beta-lactam antibiotic; inhibits cell wall synthesis.

Dosage: 25–50 mg/kg/day PO divided q12h.
  Acute otitis media from resistant Streptococcus pneumoniae: 80–90 mg/kg/day PO divided q12h.

Supplied: Capsules 250 mg, 500 mg; chewable tablets 125 mg, 200 mg, 250 mg, 400 mg; suspension 125 mg/5 mL, 200 mg/5 mL, 250 mg/5 mL, 400 mg/5 mL; tablets 500 mg, 875 mg.

Notes: Cross-hypersensitivity with penicillin. May cause diarrhea. Skin rash is common. Many hospital strains of *E coli* are resistant.

AMOXICILLIN AND CLAVULANIC ACID (AUGMENTIN, AUGMENTIN ES-600, AUGMENTIN XR)

Indications: Infections caused by beta-lactamase–producing strains of *Haemophilus influenzae, Staphylococcus aureus,* and *E coli*.

Actions: Combination of beta-lactam antibiotic and beta-lactamase inhibitor.

Dosage: 20–45 mg/kg/day PO divided q8–12h.
  Multidrug-resistant pneumococcal otitis media: 80–90 mg/kg/day PO divided q12h (use 7:1 twice daily formulation).
  Bacterial sinusitis or community-acquired pneumonia: Children > 16 years and adults: Extended-release tablet: 2000 mg PO q12h for 10 days.

Supplied: Expressed as mg amoxicillin/mg clavulanic acid: Tablets 250/125, 500/125, **875/125, XR 1000/62.5;** chewable tablets 125/31.25, **200/28.5,** 250/62.5, **400/57;** suspension per 5 mL 125/31.25, 250/62.5, **200/28.5, 400/57, ES-600 600/42.9 (twice daily formulations).**

Notes: Do not substitute two 250-mg tablets for one 500-mg tablet or over-dose of clavulanic acid will occur. May cause diarrhea and GI intolerance.

AMPHOTERICIN B (FUNGIZONE)

Indications: Severe, systemic fungal infections; oral and cutaneous candidiasis.

Actions: Binds to ergosterol in fungal membrane, altering membrane permeability.

Dosage: Intravenous: Test dose of 0.1 mg/kg (max dose 1 mg) IV over 20–60 minutes, then 0.25–1.5 mg/kg/24 h IV over 2–6 hours; doses may be administered on an every-other-day basis at 1–1.5 mg/kg per dose.
   Intrathecal, intraventricular, or intracisternal: 25–100 mcg q48–72h, increase to 500 mcg as tolerated.
   Bladder irrigation: 5–15 mg amphotericin/100 mL sterile water irrigation solution at 100–300 mL/day, irrigate 3–4 times daily for 2–5 days.
   Topical: Apply 2–4 times daily for 1–4 weeks depending on infection.

Supplied: Powder for injection 50 mg per vial; cream 3%, lotion 3%.

Notes: Total dose varies with indication. Monitor renal function; hypokalemia and hypomagnesemia may occur from renal wasting. Pretreatment with acetaminophen and diphenhydramine helps minimize adverse effects associated with IV infusion.

AMPHOTERICIN B LIPID COMPLEX (ABELCET)

Indications: Invasive fungal infection in patients refractory or intolerant to conventional amphotericin B.

Actions: Binds to sterols in cell membrane, resulting in changes in membrane permeability.

Dosage: 2.5–5 mg/kg/day IV administered as single daily dose; infuse at rate of 2.5 mg/kg/h.

Supplied: Injection 5 mg/mL.

Notes: Do not use an in-line filter less than 5 microns. *Do not* mix in electrolyte-containing solutions. If infusion exceeds 2 hours, mix bag due to settling.

AMPHOTERICIN B LIPOSOMAL (AMBISOME)

Indications: Invasive fungal infection in patients refractory or intolerant to conventional amphotericin B.

Actions: Binds to sterols in cell membrane, resulting in changes in membrane permeability.

Dosage: 3–5 mg/kg IV once daily, infused over 60–120 minutes.

Supplied: Powder for injection 50 mg.

Notes: Do not use an in-line filter less than 1 micron; doses up to 6 mg/kg/day have been used for *Aspergillus.*

AMPICILLIN (PRINCIPEN, OTHERS)

Indications: Infections caused by susceptible gram-negative (*Shigella, Salmonella, E coli, Haemophilus influenzae,* and *Proteus mirabilis*) and gram-positive (streptococci) bacteria.

Actions: Beta-lactam antibiotic; inhibits cell wall synthesis.

Dosage: Intramuscular or intravenous: 100–400 mg/kg/day divided q6h; *Oral:* 50–100 mg/kg/day divided q6h.

Supplied: Capsules 250 mg, 500 mg; suspension 125 mg/5 mL, 250 mg/5 mL; powder for injection 125 mg, 250 mg, 500 mg, 1 g, 2 g, 10 g per vial.

Notes: Cross-hypersensitivity with penicillin. Can cause diarrhea and skin rash. Neonates may require less-frequent dosing (q8h or q12h), depending on postnatal age and weight.

AMPICILLIN AND SULBACTAM (UNASYN)

Indications: Infections caused by beta-lactamase–producing strains of *Staphylococcus aureus, Enterococcus, Haemophilus influenzae, Proteus mirabilis,* and *Bacteroides* spp.

Actions: Combination of beta-lactam antibiotic and beta-lactamase inhibitor.

Dosage: Infants ≥ *1 month:* 100–400 mg/kg/day (based on ampicillin) IV or IM divided q6h, max 8 g/day; *Adults:* 1–2 g ampicillin IV or IM q6–8h, max 12 g/day.

Supplied: Powder for injection 1.5-g vial (1 g ampicillin plus 0.5 g sulbactam); 3-g vial (2 g ampicillin plus 1 g sulbactam).

Notes: Adjust dose in patients with renal failure. Observe for hypersensitivity reactions. Use higher end of dosage range for patients with meningitis.

ANTIHEMOPHILIC FACTOR (FACTOR VIII) (AHF) (MONOCLATE)

Indications: Classical hemophilia A.

Actions: Provides factor VIII needed to convert prothrombin to thrombin.

Dosage: 1 antihemophilic factor (AHF) unit/kg increases factor VIII concentration in body by ~2%. Units required = (body weight in kg) × (desired factor VIII increase as % normal) × (0.5).

- *Minor hemorrhage:* 10–20 units/kg.
- *Moderate hemorrhage:* 15–30 units/kg.
- *Severe or life threatening hemorrhage:* 30–50 units/kg.
- *Minor surgery:* 15–40 units/kg.
- *Major surgery:* 40–50 units/kg.

Patient's percentage of normal level of factor VIII concentration must be ascertained prior to dosing for these calculations.

Supplied: Check each vial for number of units contained within vial.

Notes: May repeat doses q12–24h until bleeding or healing resolves. AHF is not effective in controlling bleeding in patients with von Willebrand disease.

ANTITHYMOCYTE GLOBULIN (ATG) (ATGAM)

Indications: Management of allograft rejection in transplant patients; treatment of aplastic anemia; prevention of graft-versus-host disease following bone marrow transplantation.

Actions: Reduces number of circulating, thymus-dependent lymphocytes.

Dosage: Test dose: 0.1 mL of 1:1000 dilution of ATG in NS intradermally.
Aplastic anemia: 10–20 mg/kg/day IV for 8–14 days, or 40 mg/kg/day once daily over 4 hours for 4 days, then 10–30 mg/kg/day every other day for 7 doses.
Rejection treatment: 10–15 mg/kg/day IV for 14 days, then give every other day for 7 doses.

Supplied: Injection 50 mg/mL.

Notes: Positive skin test: > 10-mm diameter wheal or erythema. *Do not* administer to patient with prior history of severe systemic reaction to any other equine gamma globulin preparation. Discontinue treatment if severe, unremitting thrombocytopenia or leukopenia occurs.

ARTIFICIAL TEARS (TEARS NATURALE, OTHERS)*

Indications: Dry eyes.

Actions: Ocular lubricant.

Dosage: 1–2 drops 3–4 times daily.

Supplied: OTC solution.

Ascorbic Acid (see Vitamins, p. 745)*
Asparaginase

Indications: Acute lymphocytic leukemia; lymphoma.

Actions: Antineoplastic agent that inhibits protein synthesis by deaminating the essential amino acid asparagine.

Dosage: *Intramuscular:* 6000–10,000 units/m^2 per dose 3 times per week for 3 weeks; *Intravenous:* 1000 units/kg/day for 10 days (combination therapy) or 200 units/kg/day for 28 days (if combination therapy inappropriate).

Supplied: Injection 10,000 units per vial.

Notes: Perform intradermal sensitivity testing with 2 units asparaginase before initial dose and ≥ 7 days between doses.

ASPIRIN (BAYER, ST. JOSEPH, OTHERS)*

Indications: Mild to moderate pain, fever, inflammation; adjunctive treatment of Kawasaki disease; management of rheumatoid arthritis; prevention of emboli; prevention of myocardial infarction.

Actions: Prostaglandin inhibitor.

Dosage: *Analgesic or antipyretic:* 10–15 mg/kg per dose PO or PR q4–6h, max 4 g/day.
　Anti-inflammatory: 60–100 mg/kg/day PO in divided doses.
　Antiplatelet effects: 3–10 mg/kg/day PO once daily.
　Kawasaki disease: 80–100 mg/kg/day PO divided q6h until fever resolves, then lower to 3–5 mg/kg/day PO once daily; continue lower dose for 6–8 weeks or until ESR and platelet count are normal; in patients with cardiovascular abnormalities continue low dose indefinitely.

Supplied: Tablets 325 mg, 500 mg; chewable tablets 81 mg; enteric-coated tablets 81 mg, 325 mg, 500 mg, 650 mg, 975 mg; sustained-release tablets 800 mg; suppositories 200 mg, 300 mg, 600 mg.

Notes: GI upset and erosion are common adverse reactions. Discontinue use 1 week prior to surgery to avoid postoperative bleeding complications. Monitor serum salicylate concentration with chronic use.

ATENOLOL (TENORMIN)

Indications: Hypertension; angina; postmyocardial infarction.

Actions: β_1-Selective blocker.

Dosage: Initial 0.8–1 mg/kg per dose PO daily; range 0.8–1.5 mg/kg/day, max 2 mg/kg/day or 100 mg/day.

Supplied: Tablets 25 mg, 50 mg, 100 mg.

Notes: Adjust dose in patients with renal impairment. Abrupt withdrawal should be avoided.

ATOVAQUONE (MEPRON)

Indications: Treatment and prevention of mild to moderate *Pneumocystis carinii* pneumonia.

Actions: Inhibits nucleic acid and ATP synthesis.

Dosage: Treatment: Children: 40 mg/kg/day PO divided twice daily; *Adolescents and adults:* 750 mg PO twice daily for 21 days.
   Prevention: Infants 1–3 months and children > 24 months: 30 mg/kg/day PO once daily; *Infants and children 4–24 months:* 45 mg/kg/day PO once daily; *Adolescents:* 1500 mg PO once daily, max 1500 mg/day.

Supplied: Suspension 750 mg/5 mL.

Notes: Should be taken with food or high-fat meal.

ATRACURIUM (TRACRIUM)

Indications: Adjunct to anesthesia to facilitate endotracheal intubation.

Actions: Nondepolarizing neuromuscular blocker.

Dosage: 0.3–0.5 mg/kg IV bolus, then 0.08–0.1 mg/kg q20–45min prn; *Continuous IV infusion:* 0.4–1.2 mg/kg/h or 6–20 mcg/kg/min.

Supplied: Injection 10 mg/mL.

Notes: Patient must be intubated and on controlled ventilation. Use adequate amounts of sedation and analgesia. Undergoes rapid nonenzymatic degradation (Hofmann elimination) making dosage adjustment in renal or hepatic impairment unnecessary.

ATROPINE

Indications: Preanesthetic; symptomatic bradycardia and asystole.

Actions: Antimuscarinic agent; blocks acetylcholine at parasympathetic sites.

Dosage: Bradycardia: 0.02 mg/kg IV, IO, or ET q5min up to 1 mg in children or 2 mg in adolescents total; minimum dose 0.1 mg.

Preanesthetic: 0.01–0.02 mg/kg per dose PO, IM, IV, or SQ 30–60 minutes preoperatively, then q4–6h prn; max dose 0.4 mg, minimum dose 0.1 mg.

Bronchospasm: 0.03–0.05 mg/kg per dose via inhalation 3–4 times daily; max dose 2.5 mg.

Supplied: Tablet 0.4 mg; injection 0.1 mg/mL, 0.4 mg/mL, 0.5 mg/mL, 1 mg/mL.

Notes: Can cause blurred vision, urinary retention, and dried mucous membranes.

AZATHIOPRINE (IMURAN)

Indications: Adjunct for prevention of rejection following organ transplantation; rheumatoid arthritis; systemic lupus erythematosus.

Actions: Immunosuppressive agent; antagonizes purine metabolism.

Dosage: Transplantation: 2–5 mg/kg per dose IV or PO daily.
    Lupus nephritis: 2–3 mg/kg per dose PO once daily.
    Rheumatoid arthritis: 1 mg/kg per dose PO once daily for 6–8 weeks; increase by 0.5 mg/kg every 4 weeks until response or up to 2.5 mg/kg/day.

Supplied: Tablet 50 mg; powder for injection 100 mg.

Notes: Do not administer vaccines to patient taking azathioprine. Reduce dose to 25–33% of usual dose in patients receiving allopurinol. Reduce dose in patients with renal impairment.

AZITHROMYCIN (ZITHROMAX)

Indications: Treatment of community-acquired pneumonia, pharyngitis, otitis media, skin and skin structure infections, urethritis, cervicitis; treatment and prevention of *Mycobacterium avium*–complex (MAC) infections in HIV-infected persons.

Actions: Macrolide antibiotic; inhibits protein synthesis.

Dosage: Oral:
- *Respiratory tract:* 10 mg/kg PO on day 1, followed by 5 mg/kg PO daily on days 2–5.
- *Otitis media:* 30 mg/kg PO as single dose, or 10 mg/kg PO daily for 3 days, or 10 mg/kg PO on day 1, followed by 5 mg/kg PO daily on days 2–5.
- *Pharyngitis and tonsillitis:* 12 mg/kg/day PO daily for 5 days.

- *Nongonococcal urethritis:* 10 mg/kg or 1 g PO as single dose.
- *Gonococcal urethritis:* 2 g PO as single dose.
- *Primary prevention of MAC:* 5 mg/kg/day PO once daily or 20 mg/kg PO once weekly alone or in combination with rifabutin.
- *Treatment and secondary prevention of MAC:* 5 mg/kg/day PO once daily in combination with ethambutol with or without rifabutin.

Intravenous: Adolescents > 16 years and adults: 500 mg for at least 2 days, followed by 500 mg PO for total of 7–10 days.

Supplied: Tablets 250 mg, 500 mg; suspension 1 g single-dose packet, 100 mg/5 mL, 200 mg/5 mL; injection 500 mg.

Notes: Suspension should be taken on an empty stomach; tablets may be taken with or without food.

AZTREONAM (AZACTAM)

Indications: Infections caused by aerobic gram-negative bacteria, including *Pseudomonas aeruginosa.*

Actions: Monobactam antibiotic; inhibits cell wall synthesis.

Dosage: 90–120 mg/kg/day IV or IM divided q6–8h.
   Cystic fibrosis: 50 mg/kg per dose IV or IM q6–8h; max 800 mg/day.

Supplied: Injection 500 mg, 1 g, 2 g.

Notes: Not effective against gram-positive or anaerobic bacteria. May be given to penicillin-allergic patients. Adjust dose in patients with renal impairment.

BACITRACIN (BACIGUENT)

Indications: Treatment or prevention of superficial skin or eye infections.

Actions: Inhibits cell wall synthesis.

Dosage: Topical: Apply sparingly 1–5 times daily.
   Ophthalmic: Instill 1/4–1/2-inch ribbon directly into conjunctival sac q3–4h until improvement occurs then reduce frequency to 1–3 times daily.
   Irrigation: 50–100 units/mL in NS, LR, or sterile water for irrigation 1–5 times daily.

Supplied: Ointment (ophthalmic and topical*) 500 units/g; powder for injection 50,000 units.

Notes: Systemic and irrigation forms of bacitracin are not generally used due to potential toxicity.

BACITRACIN AND POLYMYXIN B (POLYSPORIN)

Indications: Treatment of eye infections; prevention and treatment of minor cuts, scrapes, and burns.

Actions: Inhibits cell wall synthesis (bacitracin) and alters permeability of bacterial cytoplasmic membrane (polymyxin B).

Dosage: Ophthalmic: Instill 1/4–1/2-inch ribbon directly into conjunctival sac q3–4h.
   Topical: Apply sparingly 1–3 times daily.

Supplied: Bacitracin 500 units/polymyxin B sulfate 10,000 units/g ointment (topical* and ophthalmic) and powder.

Notes: Do not use topical ointment in eyes.

BACITRACIN, NEOMYCIN, AND POLYMYXIN B (NEOSPORIN, TRIPLE ANTIBIOTIC)

Indications: Treatment of eye infections; prevention and treatment of minor cuts, scrapes, and burns.

Actions: Inhibits cell wall synthesis (bacitracin), alters permeability of bacterial cytoplasmic membrane (polymyxin B), and inhibits bacterial protein synthesis (neomycin).

Dosage: Ophthalmic: Instill 1/4–1/2-inch ribbon directly into conjunctival sac q3–4h for 7–10 days.
   Topical: Apply sparingly 1–3 times daily.

Supplied: Bacitracin 400 units/neomycin 3.5 mg/polymyxin B 5000 units/g topical ointment*; ophthalmic ointment same as above except 10,000 units/g polymyxin B.

Notes: Do not use topical ointment in eyes.

BACLOFEN (LIORESAL, OTHERS)

Indications: Management of spasticity; trigeminal neuralgia.

Actions: Centrally acting skeletal muscle relaxant; inhibits transmission of both monosynaptic and polysynaptic reflexes at the spinal cord.

Dosage: Children 2–7 years: Initial 10–15 mg/day PO divided q8h; increase every 3 days to maximum effect; max 40 mg/day. *Children ≥ 8 years:* Titrate as above to max of 60–80 mg/day.

Intrathecal: Single dose ranges between 25 and 100 mcg per dose or between 4 and 33 mcg/h continuous intrathecal infusion through implantable pump.

Supplied: Tablets 10 mg, 20 mg; intrathecal injection 0.05 mg/mL, 0.5 mg/mL, 2 mg/mL.

Notes: Use with caution in patients with epilepsy and neuropsychiatric disturbances; withdrawal may occur with abrupt discontinuation.

BASILIXIMAB (SIMULECT)

Indications: Prevention of acute organ transplant rejections.

Actions: Interleukin-2 receptor antagonist.

Dosage: 20 mg IV 2 hours prior to transplantation, then 20 mg IV for 4 days post-transplantation.

Supplied: Injection 20 mg.

Notes: Murine/human monoclonal antibody.

BECLOMETHASONE (BECONASE, BECONASE AQ, VANCENASE NASAL INHALER, VANCENASE AQ NASAL SPRAY)

Indications: Allergic rhinitis refractory to conventional therapy with anti-histamines and decongestants.

Actions: Inhaled corticosteroid.

Dosage: Intranasal inhaler: Children 6–12 years: 1 inhalation/nostril 3 times daily; *Children ≥ 12 years:* 2 inhalations/nostril twice daily.
   Aqueous inhalation, nasal spray: Children 6–12 years: 1 spray/nostril twice daily; *Children ≥ 12 years:* 1–2 inhalations/nostril twice daily.

Supplied: Nasal metered-dose inhaler 42 mcg per dose; nasal spray 42 mcg per dose, 84 mcg per dose.

Notes: Clear nasal passages before administration.

BECLOMETHASONE (BECLOVENT INHALER, VANCERIL INHALER)

Indications: Chronic asthma.

Actions: Inhaled corticosteroid.

Dosage: Oral inhalation: Children 6–12 years: 2–4 inhalations twice daily, max 10 inhalations per day; *Children ≥ 12 years:* 4 inhalations twice daily, max 20 inhalations per day; patients with severe asthma 12–16 inhalations per day divided 3–4 times daily; adjust dose downward according to response.

Supplied: Oral metered-dose inhaler 42 mcg per inhalation.

Notes: Not effective for acute asthmatic attacks. May cause oral candidiasis; instruct patients to rinse mouth after use.

BELLADONNA AND OPIUM SUPPOSITORIES (B & O SUPPRETTES) [C]

Indications: Bladder spasms; moderate to severe pain.

Actions: Antispasmodic.

Dosage: 1 suppository PR q6h prn.
- 15A = 30 mg powdered opium; 16.2 mg belladonna extract.
- 16A = 60 mg powdered opium; 16.2 mg belladonna extract.

Supplied: Suppositories 15A, 16A.

Notes: Anticholinergic side effects. Caution patients about sedation, urinary retention, and constipation.

BENZOCAINE AND ANTIPYRINE (AURALGAN)

Indications: Analgesia in severe otitis media; facilitate ear wax removal.

Actions: Anesthetic and local decongestant.

Dosage: Analgesia: Fill ear canal and insert moist cotton plug; repeat 1–2 hours prn until pain is relieved.
   Ear wax removal: 3–4 drops each ear 3–4 times daily for 2–3 days.

Supplied: Solution benzocaine 1.4% and antipyrine 5.4%, 10 mL and 15 mL.

Notes: Do not use in patients with perforated eardrum.

BENZTROPINE (COGENTIN)

Indications: Parkinsonism; drug-induced extrapyramidal effects; acute dystonic reactions.

Actions: Partially blocks striatal cholinergic receptors.

Dosage: Drug-induced extrapyramidal reaction: Children > 3 years: 0.02–0.05 mg/kg per dose PO, IM, or IV 1–2 times daily; *Adults:* 1–4 mg per dose 1–2 times daily.

Acute dystonia: Adults: 1–2 mg IV or IM single dose.
Parkinsonism: Adults: Initial 0.5 mg/day PO in 1–2 divided doses, increase in 0.5-mg increments every 5–6 days to effect up to 6 mg/day.

Supplied: Tablets 0.5 mg, 1 mg, 2 mg; injection 1 mg/mL.

Notes: Anticholinergic side effects. Reserve use in children < 3 years for life-threatening emergencies.

BERACTANT (SURVANTA)

Indications: Prevention and treatment of acute respiratory distress syndrome in premature neonates.

Actions: Surfactant replacement.

Dosage: Prophylactic treatment: 4 mL/kg as soon after birth as possible, may give up to 4 doses q6h during first 48 hours of life; need for additional doses determined by evidence of continued respiratory distress.
Rescue treatment: 4 mL/kg as soon as diagnosis is made, may repeat q6h up to 4 doses.

Supplied: Suspension for inhalation 25 mg/mL.

Notes: Suction infant prior to administration. Administer through 5-Fr end-hole catheter inserted into endotracheal tube in four 1 mL/kg aliquots. Each aliquot should be given with infant in different position.

BETAMETHASONE (CELESTONE, CELESTONE SOLUSPAN)

Indications: Anti-inflammatory, steroid-replacement, or immunosuppressant agent.

Actions: Adrenal corticosteroid.

Dosage: Intramuscular: Children: 0.0175–0.125 mg/kg/day divided q6–12h or 0.5–7.5 mg base/m^2/day divided q6–12h; *Adolescents and adults:* 0.6–9 mg/day divided q12–24h.
Oral: Children: 0.0175–0.25 mg/kg/day divided q6–8h or 0.5–7.5 mg/day divided q6–8h; *Adolescents and adults:* 2.4–4.8 mg/day in 2–4 doses; range 0.6–7.2 mg/day.

Supplied: Injectable solution 3 mg base/mL; injectable suspension (Soluspan) 6 mg/mL; syrup 0.6 mg base/5 mL; tablet 0.6 mg base.

Notes: Use lowest dose listed as initial dose and titrate to response.

BETHANECHOL (URECHOLINE)

Indications: Nonobstructive urinary retention due to neurogenic bladder; gastroesophageal reflux disease (GERD).

Actions: Stimulates cholinergic receptors in smooth muscle of bladder and GI tract.

Dosage: Urinary retention: 0.6 mg/kg/day PO divided 3–4 times daily.
  GERD: 0.1–0.2 mg/kg per dose before each meal to max of 4 times daily.

Supplied: Tablets 5 mg, 10 mg, 25 mg, 50 mg.

Notes: Contraindicated in bladder outlet obstruction, asthma, and coronary artery disease.

BISACODYL (DULCOLAX)*

Indications: Constipation; preoperative bowel preparation.

Actions: Stimulates peristalsis.

Dosage: 5–10 mg PO or PR daily prn.

Supplied: Enteric-coated tablet 5 mg; suppository 10 mg; enema 10 mg/30 mL.

Notes: Do not use with an acute abdomen or bowel obstruction. Instruct patient *not* to chew tablets. *Do not* administer within 1 hour of giving antacids or milk.

BISMUTH SUBSALICYLATE (PEPTO-BISMOL, KAOPECTATE)*

Indications: Indigestion; nausea; diarrhea; in combination for treatment of *Helicobacter pylori* infection.

Actions: Antisecretory and anti-inflammatory effects.

Dosage: Nonspecific diarrhea: 100 mg/kg/day PO divided into 5 doses for 5 days, max 4.19 g/day.
  Chronic infantile diarrhea: Infants and children 2–24 months: 2.5 mL PO q4h; *Children 2–4 years:* 5 mL PO q4h; *Children > 4 years:* 10 mL PO q4h.
  H pylori: Children ≤ 10 years: 15 mL of 262 mg/15 mL solution PO 4 times daily for 6 weeks; *Children > 10 years and adults:* 30 mL of 262 mg/15 mL solution or two 262-mg tablets PO 4 times daily for 6 weeks.

Supplied: Chewable tablet 262 mg; liquid 262 mg/15 mL, extra strength 524 mg/15 mL.

Notes: May turn tongue and stools black. Avoid use in patients with renal failure. *Do not* use in children with viral illness due to risk of Reye syndrome. Use with caution if patient is taking aspirin.

BLEOMYCIN

Indications: Hodgkin lymphoma; non-Hodgkin lymphoma; renal cell carcinoma; soft tissue sarcoma; sclerosing agent for malignant effusions.

Actions: Antineoplastic antibiotic inhibits DNA synthesis.

Dosage: Refer to individual protocols. Range 10–20 units/m^2 per dose IV, IM, or SQ.
   Test dose for lymphoma patients: 1–2 units for first 2 doses, monitor vital signs q15min; wait 1 hour before giving remainder of dose.
   Pleural effusion: Adults: 15–60 units (not to exceed 1 unit/kg) diluted in 50–100 mL NS intracavitary via thoracostomy tube.

Supplied: Injection 15 units, 30 units.

Notes: 1 unit = 1 mg. Reduce dose in patients with renal impairment.

BRETYLIUM

Indications: Ventricular tachycardia or fibrillation.

Actions: Class III antiarrhythmic.

Dosage: Intramuscular: 2–5 mg/kg as single dose; *Intravenous:* 5 mg/kg per dose, may repeat q10–20min up to 30 mg/kg total dose.

Supplied: Injection 50 mg/mL.

Notes: Bretylium has been removed from the 2000 Adult ACLS and PALS Guidelines due to limited supply, high incidence of adverse effects, and availability of safer agents. Effectiveness in children has not been demonstrated. Reduce dose in patients with renal impairment.

BRIMONIDINE (SEE TABLE VIII–6, P. 754)
BROMPHENIRAMINE AND PSEUDOEPHEDRINE (BROMFED, BROMFED PD, DIMETAPP, RONDEC)*

Indications: Nasal congestion; rhinorrhea; sneezing; itchy, watery eyes.

Actions: Antihistamine/decongestant combination.

Dosage: Dose according to pseudoephedrine component. *Infants and children < 2 years:* 4 mg/kg/day PO divided q6h; *Children 2–5 years:* 15 mg PO q6h, max 60 mg/day; *Children 6–12 years:* 30 mg PO q6h or 60 mg extended-release capsule PO q12h, max 120 mg/day; *Children > 12 years and adults:* 30–60 mg PO q6h or 120 mg extended-release capsule q12h, max 240 mg/day.

Supplied: Extended-release capsule (Bromfed) brompheniramine 12 mg and pseudoephedrine 120 mg, (Bromfed PD) brompheniramine 6 mg and pseudoephedrine 60 mg; elixir (Dimetapp) brompheniramine 1 mg and pseudoephedrine 15 mg/5 mL; syrup (Rondec) brompheniramine 4 mg and pseudoephedrine 45 mg/5 mL.

Notes: Use with caution in patients with hypertension or asthma.

BUDESONIDE (ENTOCORT EC, RHINOCORT, RHINOCORT AQUA, PULMICORT RESPULES OR TURBUHALER)

Indications: Management of allergic and nonallergic rhinitis; management of asthma; treatment of mild to moderate active Crohn disease.

Actions: Adrenal corticosteroid.

Dosage: Intranasal: Children ≥ 6 years and adults: 2 sprays in each nostril twice daily or 4 sprays per nostril once daily.
Intranasal, aqueous: Children ≥ 6 years and adults: 32 mcg spray/nostril once daily; max < 12 years: 128 mcg/day, max > 12 years: 256 mcg/day.
Oral inhaled: Children ≥ 6 years and adults: 200–400 mcg twice daily.
Nebulization: Children 1–8 years: 0.25 mg twice daily or 0.5 mg once daily, max 1 mg/day.
Oral for Crohn disease: Children 9–18 years: 0.45 mg/kg/day once daily, max 9 mg/day.

Supplied: Powder for oral inhalation (Pulmicort Turbuhaler) 200 mcg per inhalation; suspension for metered-dose nasal inhalation (Rhinocort) 50 mcg per inhalation; nasal aqueous spray (Rhinocort Aqua) 32 mcg per spray; suspension for nebulization (Pulmicort Respules) 0.25 mg/2 mL or 0.5 mg/2 mL; capsule (Entocort EC) 3 mg.

Notes: Not indicated for acute bronchospasm. May cause oral candidiasis. Instruct patients to rinse mouth after use. When switching from oral prednisolone to oral budesonide, taper prednisolone at same time budesonide is started.

BUMETANIDE (BUMEX)

Indications: Management of edema from congestive heart failure, hepatic or renal disease.

Actions: Loop diuretic; inhibits reabsorption of sodium and chloride in ascending loop of Henle and distal renal tubule.

Dosage: 0.015–0.1 mg/kg per dose PO, IV, or IM q6–24h, max 10 mg/day.

Supplied: Tablets 0.5 mg, 1 mg, 2 mg; injection 0.25 mg/mL.

Notes: Monitor fluid and electrolyte status during treatment. Injection contains 1% benzyl alcohol. Reduce dose in patients with hepatic impairment. Potency of 1 mg bumetanide is approximately equal to 40 mg furosemide.

BUPIVACAINE (MARCAINE)

Indications: Peripheral nerve block.

Actions: Local anesthetic.

Dosage: Dose is dependent on procedure, vascularity of tissues, depth of anesthesia, and degree of muscle relaxation required.
   Continuous epidural infusion: Loading dose 2–2.5 mg/kg, followed by 0.4–0.5 mg/kg/h.

Supplied: Injection 0.25%, 0.5%, 0.75% with and without preservatives.

Notes: Solutions containing preservatives should not be used for epidural or caudal blocks.

BUSULFAN (MYLERAN)

Indications: Chronic myelogenous leukemia; prior to bone marrow transplantation for refractory leukemias, lymphomas, and pediatric solid tumors.

Actions: Antineoplastic alkylating agent.

Dosage: Refer to individual protocols.

Supplied: Injection 6 mg/mL; tablet 2 mg.

Notes: Dose based on ideal body weight. Prophylactic anticonvulsant therapy should be initiated prior to high-dose therapy. High doses may cause hepatic veno-occlusive disease. Discontinue if leukocyte count falls to $< 20,000/mm^3$.

CAFFEINE (CAFCIT)

Indications: Treatment of apnea of prematurity; diuretic; treatment of spinal puncture headache.

Actions: Phosphodiesterase inhibitor; CNS stimulant that increases medullary respiratory center sensitivity to carbon dioxide, stimulates central inspiratory drive, and improves diaphragmatic contractility.

Dosage: Apnea of prematurity: Loading dose 10–20 mg/kg IV or PO as **caffeine citrate** (5–10 mg/kg as caffeine base), maintenance dose 5 mg/kg/day as **caffeine citrate** (2.5 mg/kg/day as caffeine base) PO or IV once daily starting 24 hours after load.

Stimulant and diuretic: Adults: 500 mg **caffeine sodium benzoate** IV or IM as single dose.

Treatment of spinal puncture headache: Adults: 500 mg **caffeine sodium benzoate** IV as single dose, may repeat in 4 hours if no relief.

Supplied: Injection, as **caffeine sodium benzoate** 125 mg/mL, as **caffeine citrate** 20 mg/mL (10 mg/mL caffeine base); oral solution, as **caffeine citrate** 20 mg/mL (10 mg/mL caffeine base).

Notes: Caffeine is a significant metabolite of theophylline in the newborn. Caffeine citrate and caffeine sodium benzoate are *not* interchangeable. Therapeutic levels are 8–20 mcg/mL for apnea of prematurity.

CALCITONIN (MIACALCIN)

Indications: Paget disease of bone; hypercalcemia; osteogenesis imperfecta; postmenopausal osteoporosis.

Actions: Polypeptide hormone.

Dosage: Dose not established in children.

Adults:

- *Paget disease:* Initial dose 100 units/day IM or SQ, maintenance dose 50 units/day or 50–100 units every 1–3 days; *Intranasal:* 200–400 units (1–2 sprays)/day.
- *Osteogenesis imperfecta:* 2 units/kg IM or SQ 3 times per week.
- *Hypercalcemia:* 4 units/kg IM or SQ q12h; increase to 8 units/kg q12h, max q6h.
- *Osteoporosis:* 100 units/day IM or SQ; *Intranasal:* 200 units (1 spray)/day.

Supplied: Spray, nasal 200 units per activation; injection salmon, 200 units/mL (2 mL).

Notes: Alternate spray in each nostril daily. Maintain adequate vitamin D and calcium intake for osteoporosis.

CALCITRIOL (ROCALTROL)

Indications: Hyperparathyroidism; pseudohypoparathyroidism; metabolic bone disease; hypocalcemia associated with dialysis.

Actions: 1,25-Dihydroxycholecalciferol, a vitamin D analogue.

Dosage: Hypocalcemia:

- *In hemodialysis patients: Children:* 0.01–0.05 mcg/kg IV 3 times per week or 0.25–2 mcg/day PO; *Adults:* 0.5 mcg 3 times per week IV, increase as needed or 0.25–1 mcg/day PO.
- *In nonhemodialysis patients: Children < 3 years:* 0.01–0.015 mcg/kg PO once daily; *Children ≥ 3 years and adults:* 0.25 mcg/day PO, max 0.5 mcg/day.
- *In premature infants:* 1 mcg PO once daily for 5 days.

Hypocalcemic tetany in premature infants: 0.05 mcg/kg IV once daily for 5–12 days.

Hypoparathyroidism and pseudohypoparathyroidism: Infants < 1 year: 0.04–0.08 mcg/kg PO once daily; *Children 1–5 years:* 0.25–0.75 mcg PO once daily; *Children > 6 years and adults:* 0.5–2.0 mcg PO once daily.

Vitamin D–dependent rickets: Children and adults: 1 mcg PO once daily.

Vitamin D–resistant rickets: Children and adults: Initial dose 0.015–0.02 mcg/kg PO once daily, maintenance dose 0.03–0.06 mcg/kg once daily, max dose 2 mcg/day.

Supplied: Injection 1 mcg/mL, 2 mcg/mL; capsules 0.25 mcg, 0.5 mcg; solution 1 mcg/mL.

Notes: Monitor dosing to keep calcium levels within 9–10 mg/dL. Maintain adequate calcium intake. Both 0.25 and 0.5 mcg liquid-filled capsules contain 0.17 mL.

CALCIUM CARBONATE (TUMS)*

Indications: Hyperacidity associated with peptic ulcer disease.

Actions: Neutralizes gastric acid.

Dosage: 500 mg to 1 g calcium carbonate PO prn.

Supplied: Chewable tablets 500 mg, 650 mg, 750 mg, 1000 mg; suspension 1250 mg/5 mL.

Notes: Calcium carbonate contains 20 mEq elemental calcium per gram.

CALCIUM SALTS

Indications: Electromechanical dissociation secondary to hypocalcemia or calcium channel blocker toxicity; life-threatening hypocalcemia; symptomatic hypocalcemia; hypocalcemic tetany.

Actions: Dietary supplement; increased myocardial contractility, binding phosphate.

Dosage: Hypocalcemia: Oral:

- As **calcium gluconate:** *Neonates:* 500–1500 mg/kg/day in 4–6 divided doses; *Infants and children:* 500–725 mg/kg/day in 3–4 divided doses; *Adults:* 10–20 g/day in 3–4 divided doses.
- As **calcium glubionate:** *Neonates:* 1200 mg/kg/day in 4–6 divided doses; *Infants and children:* 600–2000 mg/kg/day in 4 divided doses, max 9 g/day; *Adults:* 6–18 g/day in divided doses.

Intravenous:

- As **calcium chloride:** *Neonates, infants, children:* 10–20 mg/kg per dose, repeat q4–6h prn; *Adults:* 500 mg to 1 g per dose q6h.
- As **calcium gluconate:** *Neonates:* 200–800 mg/kg/day as continuous infusion or divided q6h; *Children:* 200–500 mg/kg/day as continuous infusion or divided q6h; *Adults:* 2–15 g/day as continuous infusion or in divided doses.

Cardiac arrest or calcium channel blocker toxicity: Intravenous or intraosseous:

- As **calcium chloride:** *Neonates, infants, children:* 20 mg/kg per dose, may repeat in 10 minutes; *Adults:* 2–4 mg/kg, may repeat in 10 minutes.
- As **calcium gluconate:** *Neonates, infants, children:* 60–100 mg/kg per dose, max 3 g per dose; *Adults:* 500–800 mg per dose, max 3 g per dose.

Tetany: Intravenous:

- As **calcium chloride:** *Neonates, infants, children:* 10 mg/kg over 5–10 minutes, may repeat in 6 hours or follow with max infusion of 200 mg/kg/day; *Adults:* 1 g over 10–30 minutes, may repeat in 6 hours.
- As **calcium gluconate:** *Neonates:* 100–200 mg/kg per dose, may follow with 500 mg/kg/day in divided doses or as continuous infusion; *Infants and children:* 100–200 mg/kg per dose over 5–10 minutes, may repeat after 6 hours or follow with infusion of 500 mg/kg/day; *Adults:* 1–3 g until therapeutic response occurs.

Hyperphosphatemia in end-stage renal disease: Oral:

- As **calcium acetate:** *Adults:* 1334–2668 mg PO with meals.
- As **calcium carbonate:** *Children and adults:* 1 g PO with each meal, range 4–7 g/day.

Supplied: **Calcium acetate** gelcaps, tablets 667 mg (169 mg elemental calcium). **Calcium carbonate** chewable tablets 500, 650, 750, 1000 mg; tablets 650, 1250, 1500 mg; suspension 1250 mg/5 mL. **Calcium chloride** injection 10% (100 mg/mL). **Calcium glubionate** syrup 1.8 g/5 mL. **Calcium gluconate** injection 10% (100 mg/mL).

Notes: Elemental calcium (mg/mEq) content per 1 g calcium salts: acetate 250/12.7; carbonate 400/20; chloride 270/13.5; glubionate 64/3.2; gluconate 90/4.5.

CALFACTANT (INFASURF)

Indications: Prevention and treatment of acute respiratory distress syndrome in premature neonates.

Actions: Surfactant replacement.

Dosage: Intratracheal: 3 mL/kg q12h up to total of 3 doses; repeat doses have been given as early as 6 hours after previous doses for total of 4 doses (if still intubated and requiring at least 30% inspired oxygen to maintain $PaO_2 \leq 80$ torr).

Supplied: Suspension, intratracheal 35 mg/mL.

Notes: Suction infant prior to administration. Administer dose in two 1.5 mL/kg aliquots into endotracheal tube. Each aliquot should be given with infant in different position.

CAPTOPRIL (CAPOTEN)

Indications: Management of hypertension; congestive heart failure.

Actions: ACE inhibitor.

Dosage: Infants: 0.1–0.3 mg/kg per dose PO, titrate dose upward to max of 6 mg/kg/day in 2–4 divided doses; *Children:* 0.3–0.5 mg/kg per dose PO, titrate same as infants; *Adolescents and adults:* 12.5–25 mg per dose PO q8–12h, titrate upward by 25 mg per dose to max of 450 mg/day.

Supplied: Tablets 12.5 mg, 25 mg, 50 mg, 100 mg.

Notes: Reduce dose in patients with renal impairment. Use ¹/₂ dose in patients who are sodium or volume depleted, or both. Administer on empty stomach.

CARBAMAZEPINE (TEGRETOL)

Indications: Epilepsy; trigeminal neuralgia.

Actions: Anticonvulsant.

Dosage: Children < 6 years: 10–20 mg/kg/day PO divided 2–3 times daily, increase weekly until response, max 35 mg/kg/day; *Children 6–12 years:* 100 mg PO twice daily, increase by 100 mg/day, usual 400–800 mg/day, max 1 g/day; *Children > 12 years and adults:* Initial dose 200 mg PO twice daily, increase by 200 mg/day, usual 800–1200 mg/day in divided doses, max 1.6–2.4 g/day.

Supplied: Extended-release capsule (Carbatrol) 200, 300 mg; tablet 200 mg; chewable tablet 100 mg; extended-release tablets 100 mg, 200 mg, 400 mg; suspension 100 mg/5 mL.

Notes: Can cause severe hematologic side effects; monitor CBC. Therapeutic serum levels are 4–12 mcg/mL. Generic products are not interchangeable. Reduce dose in patients with renal impairment.

CARBOPLATIN (PARAPLATIN)

Indications: Pediatric brain tumor, neuroblastoma, bony and soft tissue sarcomas, and germ cells tumors; high-dose therapy with stem cell and bone marrow transplantation.

Actions: Antineoplastic alkylating agent.

Dosage: Refer to individual protocols.

Supplied: Powder for injection 50 mg, 150 mg, 450 mg.

Notes: Toxicity includes myelosuppression, nausea, vomiting, diarrhea, nephrotoxicity, hematuria, neurotoxicity, and hepatic enzyme elevations. Some investigators calculate pediatric doses using modified Calvert formula.

CARNITINE (CARNITOR)

Indications: Carnitine deficiency.

Actions: Endogenous substance required in energy metabolism; facilitates long-chain fatty acid entry into mitochondria.

Dosage: *Oral:* 50–100 mg/kg/day divided 2–3 times daily, max 3 g/day; *Intravenous:* 50 mg/kg/day divided q4–6h, max 300 mg/kg/day.
 Supplement to parenteral nutrition in neonates: 10–20 mg/kg/day.

Supplied: Capsule 250 mg; injection 200 mg/mL; liquid 100 mg/mL; tablets 330 mg, 500 mg.

Notes: Use with caution in patients with seizure disorders. Toxic metabolites may accumulate in renally impaired patients.
Cefaclor (Ceclor) (see Table VIII–4, p. 752)
Cefadroxil (Duricef, Ultracef) (see Table VIII–3, p. 751)
Cefazolin (Ancef, Kefzol) (see Table VIII–3, p. 751)
Cefdinir (Omnicef) (see Table VIII–5, p. 753)
Cefepime (Maxipime) (see Table VIII–5, p. 753)
Cefixime (Suprax) (see Table VIII–5, p. 753)
Cefotaxime (Claforan) (see Table VIII–5, p. 753)
Cefoxitin (Mefoxin) (see Table VIII–4, p. 752)
Cefpodoxime (Vantin) (see Table VIII–5, p. 753)
Cefprozil (Cefzil) (see Table VIII–4, p. 752)
Ceftazidime (Fortaz, Ceptaz, Tazidime, Tazicef) (see Table VIII–5, p. 753)

Ceftriaxone (Rocephin) (see Table VIII–5, p. 753)
Cefuroxime (Ceftin, Zinacef) (see Table VIII–4, p. 752)
Cephalexin (Keflex, Keftab) (see Table VIII–3, p. 752)
Cetirizine (Zyrtec)

Indications: Allergic rhinitis; chronic urticaria.

Actions: Nonsedating antihistamine.

Dosage: Infants 6–12 months: 2.5 mg PO once daily; *Children 1–5 years:* 2.5 mg PO 1–2 times daily; *Children > 6 years and adults:* 5–10 mg/day as single dose or divided twice daily.

Supplied: Tablets 5 mg, 10 mg; syrup 5 mg/5 mL.
Charcoal, Activated (Actidose, Liqui-Char)

Indications: Emergency treatment in poisoning by most drugs and chemicals.

Actions: Adsorbent detoxicant.

Dosage: Acute intoxication: Children 1–12 years: 1–2 g/kg as single dose or q2–6h.
  GI dialysis in adults: 25–50 g q4–6h.

Supplied: Tablets 250 mg; liquid 25 g, 50 g.

Notes: Liquid dosage forms are in a water or sorbitol base. Use of repeated charcoal with sorbitol is *not* recommended. Protect airway in lethargic or comatose patients.

CHLORAL HYDRATE (SOMNOTE)[C]

Indications: Short-term (< 2 weeks) sedative and hypnotic, often used prior to procedures.

Actions: CNS depressant.

Dosage: Infants and children: 25–50 mg/kg/day PO or PR divided q6–8h, max 500 mg per dose.
  Prior to EEG: 25–50 mg/kg per dose PO or PR 30–60 minutes prior to EEG; may repeat in 30 minutes to max of 100 mg/kg.
  Sedation, nonpainful procedure: 50–75 mg/kg per dose PO or PR 30–60 minutes prior to procedure; may repeat in 30 minutes to max of 120 mg/kg.

Supplied: Capsule 500 mg; suppositories 325 mg, 650 mg; syrup 500 mg/5 mL.

Notes: Avoid use in patients with hepatic or renal impairment. Syrup contains benzyl alcohol.

CHLORAMBUCIL (LEUKERAN)

Indications: Chronic lymphocytic leukemia (CLL); Hodgkin and non-Hodgkin lymphoma; nephrotic syndrome unresponsive to conventional therapy.

Actions: Antineoplastic alkylating agent (nitrogen mustard).

Dosage: Refer to individual protocols for chemotherapy.
  Nephrotic syndrome: 0.1–0.2 mg/kg/day once daily for 5–12 weeks with low-dose prednisone.

Supplied: Tablet 2 mg.

Notes: Use with caution in patients with seizure disorder and bone marrow suppression. Onset of myelosuppression 7 days, nadir 14–21 days.

CHLORAMPHENICOL (CHLOROMYCETIN)

Indications: Serious infections caused by gram-positive and gram-negative aerobic and anaerobic bacteria; can be used to treat *Enterococcus* resistant to ampicillin and vancomycin.

Actions: Interferes with protein synthesis.

Dosage: 50–100 mg/kg/day IV divided 4 times daily.

Supplied: Powder for injection 1 g.

Notes: Aplastic anemia has been associated with use of this drug; monitor hematology lab results closely. Reduce dosage in patients with renal or hepatic impairment, or both.

CHLOROTHIAZIDE (DIURIL)

Indications: Hypertension; edema; congestive heart failure.

Actions: Thiazide diuretic.

Dosage: 20–40 mg/kg/day PO or 2–8 mg/kg/day IV in 1–2 divided doses.

Supplied: Tablets 250 mg, 500 mg; suspension 250 mg/5 mL; injection 500 mg per vial.

Notes: Contraindicated in anuria.

CHLORPHENIRAMINE (CHLOR-TRIMETON, OTHERS)*

Indications: Allergic rhinitis and other allergic symptoms, including urticaria.

Actions: Antihistamine.

Dosage: Children 2–5 years: 1 mg PO 4–6h; *Children 6–11 years:* 2 mg PO q4–6h or timed release 8 mg PO q12h, max 12 mg/day; *Children ≥ 12 years and adults:* 4 mg PO q4–6h or timed release 8–12 mg, max 24 mg/day.

Supplied: Tablet 4 mg; sustained-release tablets 8 mg, 12 mg; syrup 2 mg/5 mL.

Notes: Anticholinergic side effects and sedation are common.

CHOLESTYRAMINE (QUESTRAN)

Indications: Adjunct in management of primary hypercholesterolemia; pruritus associated with elevated bile acids; diarrhea associated with excess fecal bile acids.

Actions: Binds bile acids in intestine to form insoluble complexes.

Dosage: 240 mg/kg/day PO divided 3 times daily, range 1–4 g/day.

Supplied: 4 g of cholestyramine resin/9 g of powder; *With aspartame:* 4 g of resin/5 g of powder.

Notes: Mix 4 g cholestyramine in 2–6 oz noncarbonated beverage or applesauce; other medications should be taken 1–2 hours before or 6 hours after cholestyramine.

CIPROFLOXACIN (CIPRO)

Indications: Broad-spectrum activity against various gram-positive and gram-negative aerobic bacteria, including *Pseudomonas aeruginosa;* therapy or postexposure prophylaxis for anthrax.

Actions: Quinolone antibiotic; inhibits DNA gyrase.

Dosage: 20–30 mg/kg/day IV or PO divided twice daily, max 1.5 g/day PO or 800 mg/day IV.
  Cystic fibrosis: 40 mg/kg/day PO divided twice daily or 30 mg/kg/day IV divided q8–12h, max 2 g/day PO or 1.2 g/day IV.

Supplied: Tablets 100 mg, 250 mg, 500 mg, 750 mg; suspension 5 g/100 mL, 10 g/100 mL; injection 200 mg, 400 mg.

Notes: Has little activity against streptococci. Drug interactions occur with theophylline, caffeine, sucralfate, warfarin, didanosine, and antacids. Should be taken on empty stomach. Adjust dose in patients with renal impairment.

CIPROFLOXACIN, OPHTHALMIC (CILOXAN) (SEE TABLE VIII–6, P. 754)
CIPROFLOXACIN, OTIC (CIPRO HC OTIC)

Indications: Otitis externa.

Actions: Quinolone antibiotic; inhibits DNA gyrase.

Dosage: 3 drops in affected ear(s) twice daily for 7 days.

Supplied: Suspension ciprofloxacin 0.2% and hydrocortisone 1%.
Cisatracurium (Nimbex)

Indications: Adjunct to anesthesia to facilitate endotracheal intubation.

Actions: Nondepolarizing neuromuscular blocker.

Dosage: Initial 0.1 mg/kg IV, followed by 0.03 mg/kg prn; *Continuous infusion:* 1–4 mcg/kg/min IV or 6–20 mcg/kg/min.

Supplied: Injection 2 mg/mL, 10 mg/mL.

Notes: Patient must be intubated and on controlled ventilation. Intermediate onset; not recommended for rapid sequence intubation. Undergoes rapid nonenzymatic degradation (Hofmann elimination), making dosage adjustment in patients with renal or hepatic impairment unnecessary.

CISPLATIN (PLATINOL-AQ)

Indications: Treatment of Hodgkin and non-Hodgkin lymphoma; head or neck cancer; cervical, testicular, ovarian, and breast cancer; lung cancer; brain tumors; neuroblastoma; osteosarcoma.

Actions: Antineoplastic alkylating agent.

Dosage: Refer to individual protocols. Verify doses > 120 mg/m^2 per course to prevent overdose.

Supplied: Injection 1 mg/mL.

Notes: Adjust dose in patients with renal impairment. Maintain adequate hydration and urine output to prevent nephrotoxicity. Toxicities include allergic reactions, high-frequency hearing loss, peripheral "stocking-glove" type neuropathy, cardiotoxicity, hypomagnesemia, mild myelosuppression, and hepatotoxicity.

CITRATE AND CITRIC ACID (BICITRA)

Indications: Metabolic acidosis.

Actions: Alkalinizing agent.

Dosage: 2–3 mEq/kg/day PO divided 3–4 times daily or 5–15 mL after meals and at bedtime.

Supplied: Oral solution 1 mEq/mL sodium and 1 mEq/mL bicarbonate.

Notes: Dilute in water or juice. Contraindicated in patients with severe renal impairment or sodium-restricted diets.

CLARITHROMYCIN (BIAXIN)

Indications: Upper and lower respiratory tract infections; acute otitis media; skin and skin structure infections; *Helicobacter pylori* infections caused by susceptible strains of *Staphylococcus aureus, Streptococcus pyogenes, S pneumoniae, Haemophilus influenzae, Moraxella catarrhalis, Mycoplasma pneumoniae, Chlamydia trachomatis,* and *Legionella* spp; prevention and treatment of *Mycobacterium avium*–complex (MAC) infections in HIV-infected individuals; prophylaxis of bacterial endocarditis in penicillin-allergic patients.

Actions: Macrolide antibiotic; inhibits protein synthesis.

Dosage: Infants and children: 15 mg/kg/day PO twice daily; *Bacterial endocarditis prophylaxis:* 15 mg/kg PO 1 hour before procedure; *MAC prophylaxis:* 15 mg/kg/day PO twice daily, max 1 g/day.
  Adolescents and adults: 250–500 mg PO twice daily or 1000 mg (2 × 500 mg extended-release tablets) PO daily; *Bacterial endocarditis prophylaxis:* 500 mg PO 1 hour before procedure; *MAC prophylaxis:* 500 mg PO twice daily; *H pylori:* 250 mg PO twice daily up to 500 mg PO 3 times daily.

Supplied: Tablets 250 mg, 500 mg; suspension 125 mg/5 mL, 250 mg/5 mL; extended-release tablet 500 mg.

Notes: Increases theophylline and carbamazepine levels. Avoid concurrent use with cisapride. Causes metallic taste. Reduce dose in patients with renal impairment.

CLINDAMYCIN (CLEOCIN, CLEOCIN-T)

Indications: Susceptible strains of streptococci, pneumococci, staphylococci, and gram-positive and gram-negative anaerobes (no activity against gram-negative aerobes); bacterial vaginosis; topical therapy for severe acne and vaginal infections.

Actions: Bacteriostatic; interferes with protein synthesis.

Dosage: Oral: 10–30 mg/kg/day PO divided 3–4 times daily, max 1.8 g/day.
Intravenous: 25–40 mg/kg/day IV divided q6–8h, max 4.8 g/day.
Vaginal: 1 applicatorful at bedtime for 7 days.
Topical: Apply 1% gel, lotion, or solution twice daily.

Supplied: Capsules 75 mg, 150 mg, 300 mg; suspension 75 mg/5 mL; injection 300 mg/2 mL; vaginal cream 2%; topical gel, lotion, or solution 1%.

Notes: Beware of diarrhea that may represent pseudomembranous colitis caused by *Clostridium difficile.*

CLONAZEPAM (KLONOPIN) [C]

Indications: Lennox-Gastaut syndrome; akinetic and myoclonic seizures; absence seizures.

Actions: Benzodiazepine anticonvulsant.

Dosage: Infants and children < 10 years (< 30 kg): Initial dose 0.01–0.03 mg/kg/day (max initial dose 0.05 mg/kg/day) PO divided 2–3 times daily, increase by no more than 0.5 mg every 3 days prn up to 0.2 mg/day; *Children ≥ 10 years (> 30 kg):* 0.5 mg PO 3 times daily, increase by 0.5–1 mg every 3 days prn up to 20 mg/day.

Supplied: Tablets 0.5 mg, 1 mg, 2 mg.

Notes: CNS side effects, including sedation.

CLONIDINE (CATAPRES)

Indications: Hypertension; alternative treatment of attention-deficit/hyperactivity disorder (ADHD); adjunct in treatment of neuropathic pain; epidural form used in combination with opiates for analgesia in cancer patients; opioid, alcohol, and tobacco withdrawal in adults.

Actions: Centrally acting α_2-adrenergic stimulant.

Dosage: Hypertension: Children: 5–10 mcg/kg/day PO divided q8–12h, increase gradually prn to 5–25 mcg/kg/day divided q6h, max 0.9 mg/day;

Adults: 0.1 mg PO twice daily adjusted daily by 0.1–0.2-mg increments, max 2.4 mg/day.

ADHD: Children: 0.05 mg/day PO, increase every 3–7 days by 0.05 mg/day to 3–5 mcg/kg/day divided 3–4 times daily, max 0.5 mg/day.

Epidural: Children: 0.5 mcg/kg/h continuous infusion, increase up to 2 mcg/kg/h prn; *Adults:* 30–40 mcg/h.

Transdermal: Children may switch to transdermal from an equivalent, stable PO dose; *Adults:* 0.1 mg/day patch every 7 days, titrate to response.

Supplied: Tablets 0.1 mg, 0.2 mg, 0.3 mg; transdermal patch TTS-1, TTS-2, TTS-3 deliver 0.1, 0.2, 0.3 mg/day respectively; epidural injection 100 mcg/mL, 500 mcg/mL.

Notes: Dry mouth, drowsiness, and sedation occur frequently. Adjust dose in patients with renal impairment. Rebound hypertension can occur with abrupt cessation. Hypotensive action may not begin until 2–3 days after transdermal application. Apply patch at bedtime to hairless area (arm; chest).

CLORAZEPATE (TRANXENE) [C]

Indications: Acute anxiety disorders; adjunctive therapy for partial seizures.

Actions: Benzodiazepine; antianxiety agent.

Dosage: Initial dose 0.3 mg/kg/day PO 2–3 times daily up to 0.5–3 mg/kg/day.

Supplied: Tablets 3.75 mg, 7.5 mg, 15 mg; extended-release tablets 11.25 mg, 22.5 mg.

Notes: Monitor patients with renal or hepatic impairment. Has CNS depressant effects.

CLOTRIMAZOLE (LOTRIMIN, MYCELEX)*

Indications: Candidiasis and tinea infections; troches may be effective for prophylaxis against oropharyngeal candidiasis in immunosuppressed patients.

Actions: Antifungal agent; alters cell wall permeability.

Dosage: *Oral:* 1 troche dissolved slowly in mouth 5 times per day for 14 days.

Vaginal:

- *Cream:* 1 applicatorful at bedtime for 7–14 days.
- *Tablets:* 100 mg vaginally at bedtime for 7 days; or 200 mg (2 tablets) vaginally at bedtime for 3 days; or 500-mg tablet vaginally at bedtime one time.

Topical: Apply twice daily for 10–14 days.

Supplied: Cream 1%; solution 1%; lotion 1%; troche 10 mg; vaginal tablets 100 mg, 500 mg; vaginal cream 1%.

Notes: Dissolve troche in mouth over 15–30 minutes; troches should not be used for treatment of systemic fungal infections.

COCAINE [C]

Indications: Topical anesthetic for mucous membranes.

Actions: Narcotic analgesic; local vasoconstrictor.

Dosage: Apply lowest amount of topical solution that provides relief; max 1 mg/kg.

Supplied: Topical solution 4%, 10%; powder 5 g, 125 g.

Notes: *Do not* use on extensive areas of broken skin. Solutions > 4% are not recommended due to increased risk of systemic toxicities.

CODEINE [C]

Indications: Mild to moderate pain; symptomatic relief of cough.

Actions: Narcotic analgesic; depresses cough reflex.

Dosage: *Analgesic:* 0.5–1 mg/kg per dose PO, IM, SQ divided q4–6h prn, max 60 mg per dose.
   Antitussive: Children ≥ 2 years: 1–1.5 mg/kg/day PO divided q4–6 hours prn; max 30–60 mg/day.

Supplied: Tablets 15 mg, 30 mg, 60 mg; solution 15 mg/5 mL; injection 15 mg/mL, 30 mg/mL.

Notes: Most often used in combination with acetaminophen for pain or with agents such as guaifenesin as an antitussive; 120 mg IM is equivalent to 10 mg morphine IM.

COLFOSCERIL (EXOSURF)

Indications: Prevention and treatment of acute respiratory distress syndrome in premature neonates.

Actions: Surfactant replacement.

Dosage: Prophylactic treatment: 5 mL/kg as soon after birth as possible, may give 1–2 more doses q12h to infants who remain on ventilators.

Rescue treatment: 5 mL/kg as soon as diagnosis is made, may repeat in 12 hours for 1 more dose.

Supplied: Powder for intratracheal suspension 108 mg.

Notes: Suction infant prior to administration. Administer via sideport on special endotracheal tube adapter without interrupting mechanical ventilation. Administer dose in two 2.5 mL/kg aliquots. Each aliquot should be given with infant in different position.

CORTICOTROPIN (H.P. ACTHAR GEL)

Indications: Infantile spasms.

Actions: Stimulates adrenal cortex to secrete adrenal steroids, androgenic substances, and small amount of aldosterone.

Dosage: Infantile spasms: Various regimens have been used. *Low dose/short term:* 5–40 units IM daily for 1–6 weeks; or *High dose/long term:* 40–160 units IM daily for 3–12 months.

Supplied: Injection, repository 80 units/mL.

Notes: Do not give IV; *do not* abruptly discontinue.

CROMOLYN SODIUM (INTAL, NASALCROM, OPTICROM)

Indications: Adjunct to prophylaxis of asthma; prevention of exercise-induced asthma; allergic rhinitis; ophthalmic allergic manifestations; systemic treatment of inflammatory bowel disease.

Actions: Antiasthmatic; mast cell stabilizer.

Dosage: Nebulization: Children > 2 years and adults: 20 mg inhaled 4 times daily.

Metered-dose inhaler (MDI): Children ≤ 12 years: 1–2 puffs 3–4 times daily; *Children > 12 years and adults:* 2–4 puffs 3–4 times daily.

Inflammatory bowel disease: Children > 2 years: 100 mg PO 4 times daily, may double dose if needed up to 40 mg/kg/day; *Children > 12 years and adults:* 200 mg PO 4 times daily, may double dose if needed up to 400 mg 4 times daily.

Nasal instillation: Children > 2 years and adults: Spray once in each nostril 2–6 times daily.

Ophthalmic: Children > 4 years and adults: 1–2 drops in each eye 4–6 times daily.

Prevention of allergen- or exercise-induced bronchospasm: Children > 2 years and adults: 20 mg nebulization or 2 puffs from MDI 10–15 minutes prior exposure or exercise.

Supplied: Oral concentrate 100 mg/5 mL; solution for nebulization 10 mg/mL; MDI 800 mcg/inhalation; nasal spray 40 mg/mL; ophthalmic solution 4%.

Notes: Has no benefit in acute situations. May require 2–4 weeks for maximal effect in patients with perennial allergic disorders.

CYANOCOBALAMIN (VITAMIN B₁₂) (SEE VITAMINS, P. 745)
CYCLOPENTOLATE OPHTHALMIC (AK-PENTOLATE, CYCLOGYL)

Indications: Mydriasis and cycloplegia.

Actions: Prevents ocular muscles from responding to cholinergic stimulation.

Dosage: Neonates and infants: 1 drop in eye q5–10min, up to 3 doses, 40–50 minutes before procedure of cyclopentolate 0.2% and phenylephrine 1% combination (recommended in this age group due to lower cyclopentolate concentration); *Children:* 1 drop of 0.5% or 1% solution in eye, may repeat if necessary in 5 minutes, approximately 40–50 minutes before procedure; *Adults:* 1 drop of 1% solution followed by another drop in 5 minutes, approximately 40–50 minutes before procedure.

Supplied: Ophthalmic solution 0.5%, 1%, 2%.

Notes: Pilocarpine ophthalmic drops applied after the exam may reduce recovery time to 3–6 hours.

CYCLOPHOSPHAMIDE (CYTOXAN, NEOSAR)

Indications: Hodgkin disease; malignant lymphomas; multiple myeloma; leukemias; sarcomas; mycosis fungoides; neuroblastoma; ovarian and breast cancer; conditioning regimen for bone marrow transplantation; nephrotic syndrome; lupus erythematosus; severe rheumatoid arthritis and vasculitis.

Actions: Antineoplastic alkylating agent (nitrogen mustard).

Dosage: Refer to individual protocols.

Supplied: Tablets 25 mg, 50 mg; Powder for injection 100 mg, 200 mg, 500 mg, 1 g, 2 g.

Notes: Toxicity includes myelosuppression (leukopenia and thrombocytopenia), hemorrhagic cystitis, SIADH, alopecia, anorexia, nausea, and vomiting. Second malignancies (bladder cancer and leukemias) have been reported. Continuous bladder irrigation and mesna uroprotection are used in high-dose regimens to prevent hemorrhagic cystitis. Reduce dose if creatinine clearance ≤ 10 mL/min.

CYCLOSPORINE (SANDIMMUNE, NEORAL)

Indications: Prophylaxis of organ rejection in kidney, liver, heart, and bone marrow transplantation in conjunction with adrenal corticosteroids; treatment of nephrotic syndrome in patients with focal glomerulosclerosis; severe psoriasis; severe rheumatoid arthritis; severe autoimmune disease; prevention of graft-versus-host disease in bone marrow transplant patients.

Actions: Immunosuppressant; reversible inhibition of immunocompetent lymphocytes.

Dosage: Transplantation: Oral: 14–18 mg/kg per dose beginning 4–12 hours prior to transplantation followed postoperatively by 5–15 mg/kg/day divided q12–24h; after 2 weeks, taper dose to 3–10 mg/kg/day. *Intravenous:* If patient is unable to take drug orally, give 1/3 of oral dose IV.
   Rheumatoid arthritis and psoriasis: 2.5 mg/kg/day PO divided q12h, may increase by 0.5–0.75 mg/kg/day if insufficient response is seen after 4–8 weeks of treatment to max of 4 mg/kg/day.
   Focal glomerulosclerosis: 3 mg/kg/day PO divided q12h.
   Autoimmune diseases: 1–3 mg/kg/day PO divided q12h.

Supplied: Capsules 25 mg, 100 mg; oral solution 100 mg/mL; injection 50 mg/mL.

Notes: May elevate BUN and creatinine, which may be confused with renal transplant rejection. Should be administered in glass containers. Has many drug interactions. Neoral and Sandimmune are not interchangeable. Therapeutic levels depend on organ transplanted and time after transplantation; range 100–400 ng/mL.

CYPROHEPTADINE (PERIACTIN)

Indications: Allergic reactions, including urticaria; appetite stimulant for anorexia nervosa.

Actions: Phenothiazine antihistamine.

Dosage: Allergic conditions: 0.25 mg/kg/day PO divided q8–12h; max 0.5 mg/kg/day.
   Appetite stimulation: Adolescents > 13 years: 2 mg PO 4 times daily, may increase gradually over 3 weeks up to 8 mg PO 4 times daily.

Supplied: Tablet 4 mg; syrup 2 mg/5 mL.

Notes: Anticholinergic side effects and drowsiness are common.

CYTARABINE (CYTOSAR-U, ARA-C)

Indications: Leukemias; Hodgkin lymphoma; non-Hodgkin lymphoma.

Actions: Antineoplastic antimetabolite agent.

Dosage: Refer to individual protocols.

Supplied: Powder for injection 100 mg, 500 mg, 1 g, 2 g.

Notes: Toxicity includes myelosuppression, nausea, vomiting, and diarrhea, stomatitis, flulike syndrome, rash of palms and soles of feet, and hepatic dysfunction. High-dose toxicities include conjunctivitis, cerebellar dysfunction, and noncardiogenic pulmonary edema.

CYTOMEGALOVIRUS IMMUNE GLOBULIN [CMV-IVIG] (CYTOGAM)

Indications: Prophylaxis against cytomegalovirus (CMV) disease associated with transplantation.

Actions: Provides exogenous IgG antibodies to CMV.

Dosage: Administer for 16 weeks post-transplantation; see product information for dosing schedule.

Supplied: Injection 50 mg/mL.
Daclizumab (Zenapax)

Indications: Prevention of acute organ rejection.

Actions: Interleukin-2 receptor antagonists.

Dosage: 1 mg/kg IV per dose; first dose prior to transplantation followed by 4 doses 14 days apart post-transplantation.

Supplied: Injection 5 mg/mL.
Dactinomycin (Cosmegen)

Indications: Wilms tumor; rhabdomyosarcoma; neuroblastoma; retinoblastoma; Ewing sarcoma; testicular tumors; uterine sarcomas.

Actions: Antineoplastic antibiotic.

Dosage: Refer to individual protocols.

Supplied: Injection 0.5 mg.

Notes: Toxicity includes myelosuppression, nausea, vomiting, alopecia, acneiform skin changes and hyperpigmentation, radiation recall phenomenon, phlebitis, and tissue damage with extravascular extravasation and hepatic dysfunction.

DANTROLENE (DANTRIUM)

Indications: Clinical spasticity resulting from upper motor neuron disorders such as spinal cord injuries, strokes, cerebral palsy, or multiple sclerosis; malignant hyperthermic crisis.

Actions: Skeletal muscle relaxant.

Dosage: Spasticity: Initial dose 0.5 mg/kg per dose PO twice daily, increase frequency to 3–4 times daily at 4–7 day intervals, then increase dose by 0.5 mg/kg to max of 3 mg/kg per dose 2–4 times daily up to 400 mg/day.

Malignant hyperthermia:
- *Preoperative prophylaxis:* 4–8 mg/kg/day PO divided 4 times daily 1–2 days prior to surgery, with last dose 3–4 hours prior to surgery or 2.5 mg/kg IV 1 1/4 hours prior to surgery.
- *Treatment:* Continuous rapid IV push beginning at 1 mg/kg until symptoms subside or 10 mg/kg is reached.
- *Post-crisis follow-up:* 4–8 mg/kg/day PO in 3–4 divided doses for 1–3 days to prevent recurrence.

Supplied: Capsules 25 mg, 50 mg, 100 mg; powder for injection 20 mg per vial.

Notes: Monitor ALT and AST closely.

DAPSONE

Indications: Treatment and prevention of *Pneumocystis carinii* pneumonia (PCP); toxoplasmosis prophylaxis; leprosy.

Actions: Sulfone antimicrobial competitive antagonist of PABA and inhibits folic acid synthesis.

Dosage: Toxoplasmosis prophylaxis: 2 mg/kg PO daily, max 25 mg per dose.
    PCP Prophylaxis: 2 mg/kg PO daily, max 100 mg per dose, or 4 mg/kg PO once weekly, max 200 mg per dose.

Leprosy: 1–2 mg/kg PO daily, max 100 mg per dose.

Supplied: Tablets 25 mg, 100 mg.

Notes: Absorption is enhanced by an acidic environment.

DAUNORUBICIN (CERUBIDINE, DAUNOMYCIN)

Indications: Leukemias (ALL, AML).

Actions: Antineoplastic anthracycline antibiotic.

Dosage: Refer to individual protocols.

Supplied: Solution for injection 5 mg/mL; powder for injection 20 mg.

Notes: Toxicity includes myelosuppression, mucositis, nausea, vomiting, alopecia, radiation recall phenomenon, hepatotoxicity (hyperbilirubinemia), tissue necrosis with extravascular extravasation, and total cumulative dose-related irreversible cardiotoxicity. Reduce dose in patients with hepatic or renal impairment.

DESMOPRESSIN (DDAVP, STIMATE)

Indications: Diabetes insipidus; bleeding due to hemophilia A; type I von Willebrand disease; primary nocturnal enuresis.

Actions: Synthetic analogue of vasopressin, a naturally occurring human antidiuretic hormone; increases factor VIII.

Dosage: Diabetes insipidus:
- *Intranasal:* 5 mcg/day in 1–2 divided doses, titrate to response (range 5–30 mcg/day).
- *Oral:* Initial 0.05 mg PO twice daily, titrate to response (range 0.1–0.8 mg/day).
- *Parenteral:* 2–4 mcg/day IV or SQ in 2 divided doses or 1/10th of intranasal dose.

Hemophilia A:
- *Intranasal: Children ≤ 50 kg:* 150 mcg (1 spray); *Children > 50 kg:* 300 mcg (1 spray in each nostril). If preoperative, give intranasal dose 2 hours prior to procedure.
- *Parenteral:* 0.3 mcg/kg IV 30 minutes prior to procedure, may repeat dose if needed.

Nocturnal enuresis: Children ≥ 6 years:
- *Intranasal:* 10 mcg each nostril at bedtime, range 10–40 mcg.
- *Oral:* 0.2–0.6 mg PO before bedtime.

Supplied: Tablets 0.1 mg, 0.2 mg; injection 4 mcg/mL; nasal solution 100 mcg/mL with rhinal tube; nasal spray 100 mcg/mL (10 mcg/spray), 1.5 mg/mL (150 mcg/spray).

Notes: Adjust fluid intake to avoid water intoxication and hyponatremia.

DEXAMETHASONE (DECADRON)

Indications: Chronic inflammation; airway edema prior to extubation; chemotherapy-induced emesis; bacterial meningitis; cerebral edema; facilitates ventilator weaning in neonates with bronchopulmonary dysplasia (BPD).

Actions: Anti-inflammatory corticosteroid.

Dosage: Neonatal BPD: 0.5–0.6 mg/kg/day PO or IV q12h for 3–7 days, taper over 1–6 weeks.
   Airway edema or extubation: 0.5–2 mg/kg/day PO or IV q6h, begin 24 hours prior to extubation and continue for 4–6 doses after extubation.
   Antiemetic: Initial 10 mg/m^2 per dose IV, max dose 20 mg, then 5 mg/m^2 per dose IV q6h.
   Anti-inflammatory: 0.08–0.3 mg/kg/day or 2.5–10 mg/m^2/day PO, IM, or IV.
   Bacterial meningitis: 0.6 mg/kg/day IV divided q6h for 16 doses, start at time of first dose of antibiotic.
   Cerebral edema: 1–2 mg/kg load PO, IM, or IV followed by 1–1.5 mg/kg/day divided q4–6h, max 16 mg/day.

Supplied: Tablets 0.25 mg, 0.5 mg, 0.75 mg, 1 mg, 1.5 mg, 2 mg, 4 mg, 6 mg; elixir 0.5 mg/5 mL; injection 4 mg/mL, 10 mg/mL.

Notes: Elixir contains benzoic acid (use with caution in neonates). *Do not* discontinue abruptly.

DEXAMETHASONE OPHTHALMIC (AK-DEX OPHTHALMIC, DECADRON OPHTHALMIC, OTHERS) (SEE TABLE VIII–6, P. 754)

DEXTROAMPHETAMINE (DEXEDRINE)

Indications: Attention-deficit/hyperactivity (ADHD) disorder; narcolepsy; exogenous obesity.

Actions: CNS stimulant, amphetamine.

Dosage: ADHD: Children 3–5 years: Initial dose 2.5 mg/day PO q AM, increase by 2.5 mg/day every 7 days until response obtained, max 40 mg/day given in 1–3 divided doses. *Children ≥ 6 years:* 5 mg once or twice daily, increase by 5 mg/day every 7 days until response obtained, max 40 mg/day given in 1–3 divided doses.

Narcolepsy: Children 6–12 years: Initial dose 5 mg/day, increase by 5 mg/ day every 7 days until response obtained, max 60 mg/day; *Children > 12 years and adults:* Initial dose 10 mg/day, increase by 10 mg/day every 7 days until response obtained, max 60 mg/day.

Exogenous obesity: Children > 12 years: 5–30 mg in divided doses 30–60 minutes before meals.

Supplied: Sustained-release capsule 5 mg, 10 mg, 15 mg; tablet 5 mg, 10 mg.

Notes: May be habit-forming; avoid abrupt discontinuation. Periodic "drug holidays" are recommended for ADHD patients.

DEXTROAMPHETAMINE AND AMPHETAMINE (ADDERALL, ADDERALL XR)

Indications: Attention-deficit/hyperactivity disorder; narcolepsy.

Actions: CNS stimulant; amphetamine.

Dosage: ADHD: Children 3–5 years: Initial dose 2.5 mg/day PO q AM, increase by 2.5 mg/day every 7 days until response obtained, max 40 mg/day given in 1–3 divided doses; *Children ≥ 6 years:* 5 mg once or twice daily, increase by 5 mg/day every 7 days until response obtained, max 40 mg/day given in 1–3 divided doses.

Narcolepsy: Children 6–12 years: Initial dose 5 mg/day, increase by 5 mg/day every 7 days until response obtained, max 60 mg/day given in 1–3 divided doses; *Children > 12 years and adults:* Initial 10 mg/day, increase by 10 mg/day every 7 days until response obtained, max 60 mg/day given in 1–3 divided doses.

Supplied: Extended-release capsules 5 mg, 10 mg, 15 mg, 20 mg, 25 mg, 30 mg; tablets 5 mg, 7.5 mg, 10 mg, 12.5 mg, 15 mg, 20 mg, 30 mg.

Notes: May be habit-forming; avoid abrupt discontinuation. Periodic "drug holidays" are recommended for ADHD patients.

DEXTROMETHORPHAN (BENYLIN, DELSYM)

Indications: Control of nonproductive cough.

Actions: Depresses cough center in medulla.

Dosage: Oral:
- *Infants 1–3 months:* 0.5–1 mg q6–8h.
- *Infants 3–6 months:* 1–2 mg q6–8h.
- *Infants 7–12 months:* 2–4 mg q6–8h.
- *Children ≥ 2–6 years:* 2.5–7.5 mg q4–8h, extended-release formulation: 15 mg twice daily, max 30 mg/day.

- *Children 7–12 years:* 5–10 mg q4h or 15 mg q6–8h, extended-release formulation: 30 mg twice daily, max 60 mg/day.
- *Children > 12 years and adults:* 10–30 mg q4–8h, extended-release formulation: 60 mg twice daily, max 120 mg/day.

Supplied: Capsule 30 mg; lozenge 5 mg; syrup 7.5 mg/5 mL, 15 mg/5 mL, 7.5 mg/mL, 20 mg/15 mL, 5 mg/mL, 15 mg per 5 mL, 15 mg/15 mL; sustained-action liquid 30 mg/5 mL.

Notes: May be found in combination products with guaifenesin.

Diazepam (Valium, Others) [C]

Indications: Anxiety; alcohol withdrawal; muscle spasm; status epilepticus; panic disorders; amnesia; preoperative sedation.

Actions: Benzodiazepine.

Dosage: Status epilepticus: Children 1 month to 5 years: 0.1–0.3 mg/kg per dose IV q15–30min to max total dose of 5 mg, may repeat in 2–4 hours prn; *Children ≥ 5 years:* Same dose except max total dose of 10 mg.
  Anticonvulsant: Rectal gel: Children 2–5 years: 0.5 mg/kg PR; *Children 6–11 years:* 0.3 mg/kg PR; *Children ≥ 12 years:* 0.2 mg/kg, may repeat PR doses q4–12h prn.
  Anxiety or muscle spasm: 0.12–0.8 mg/kg/day PO divided 3–4 times daily or 0.04–0.3 mg/kg per dose IM or IV q2–4h prn, max 0.6 mg/kg within 8-hour period.
  Preoperative: 0.2–0.3 mg/kg, max 10 mg per dose, PO 45–60 minutes before procedure.

Supplied: Tablets 2 mg, 5 mg, 10 mg; solution 1 mg/mL, concentrated solution 5 mg/mL; injection 5 mg/mL; gel for rectal delivery 5 mg/mL.

Notes: Do not exceed 5 mg/min IV, as respiratory arrest can occur. Absorption of IM dose may be erratic. *Do not* use rectal gel > 5 times per month.

DIAZOXIDE (HYPERSTAT, PROGLYCEM)

Indications: Emergency lowering of BP (IV); management of hypoglycemia caused by hyperinsulinism (PO).

Actions: Direct smooth muscle relaxation of peripheral arterioles; inhibits pancreatic insulin release.

Dosage: Hypertension: 1–3 mg/kg IV, max 150 mg per dose, may repeat in 5–15 minutes until BP reduced, give q4–24h.
  Hyperinsulinemic hypoglycemia: Newborns and infants: 8–15 mg/kg/day PO divided q8–12h; *Children and adults:* 3–8 mg/kg/day PO divided q8–12h.

Supplied: Injection 15 mg/mL; oral suspension 50 mg/mL.

Notes: Sodium retention and hyperglycemia frequently occur. Possible thiazide diuretic cross-hypersensitivity. Use for > 10 days is *not* recommended.

DICLOXACILLIN (DYCILL)

Indications: Skin and soft tissue infections; pneumonia and follow-up therapy of osteomyelitis caused by susceptible penicillinase-producing staphylococci.

Actions: Inhibits bacterial wall synthesis.

Dosage: Children < 40 kg: 25–50 mg/kg/day PO q6h, doses of 50–100 mg/kg/day in divided doses q6h have been used for osteomyelitis, max 2 g/day; *Children ≥ 40 kg and adults:* 125–500 mg PO q6h, max 2 g/day.

Supplied: Capsules 250 mg, 500 mg.

Notes: Administer on an empty stomach.
Dicyclomine (Bentyl)

Indications: Treatment of functional irritable bowel syndromes.

Actions: Smooth muscle relaxant.

Dosage: Infants > 6 months: 5 mg PO 3–4 times daily; *Children:* 10 mg PO 3–4 times daily; *Adults:* 20 mg PO or IM 4 times daily, titrate to max dose of 160 mg/day.

Supplied: Capsule 10 mg; tablet 20 mg; syrup 10 mg/5 mL; injection 10 mg/mL.

Notes: Anticholinergic side effects may limit dose.
Didanosine [ddl] (Videx)

Indications: HIV infection in patients who are zidovudine intolerant.

Actions: Nucleoside antiretroviral agent.

Dosage: Neonates < 90 days: 50 mg/m^2 per dose PO q12h.
  Children < 13 years: 180–300 mg/m^2/day PO divided q12h.
  Children ≥ 13 years and adults:
  - *< 60 kg:* 250 mg PO daily or 125 mg PO twice daily; *Buffered powder for oral solution:* 167 mg PO q12h; *Delayed-release capsule:* 250 mg PO daily.

- ≥ 60 kg: 200 mg PO q12h or 400 mg PO daily; *Buffered powder for oral solution:* 250 mg PO q12h; *Delayed-release capsule:* 400 mg PO daily.

Supplied: Delayed-release capsules 125 mg, 200 mg, 250 mg, 400 mg; chewable tablets 25 mg, 50 mg, 100 mg, 150 mg, 200 mg; powder packets 100 mg, 167 mg, 250 mg; powder for solution 10 mg/mL.

Notes: Reconstitute powder with water; *do not* mix powder with fruit juice or other acidic beverages. Side effects include pancreatitis, peripheral neuropathy, diarrhea, and headache. Give 2 tablets for each administration. Adjust dose in patients with renal impairment.

DIGOXIN (LANOXIN, LANOXICAPS)

Indications: Congestive heart failure; atrial fibrillation and flutter; paroxysmal atrial tachycardia.

Actions: Positive inotrope; increases refractory period of AV node.

Dosage: Total digitalizing dose (TDD):

- *Preterm neonates:* 20–30 mcg/kg PO or 15–25 mcg/kg IV or IM.
- *Full-term neonates:* 25–35 mcg/kg PO or 20–30 mcg/kg IV or IM.
- *Infants and children 1 month to 2 years:* 35–60 mcg/kg PO or 30–50 mcg/kg IV or IM.
- *Children 2–5 years:* 30–40 mcg/kg PO or 25–35 mcg/kg IV or IM.
- *Children 5–10 years:* 20–35 mcg/kg PO or 15–30 mcg/kg IV or IM.
- *Children > 10 years:* 10–15 mcg/kg PO or 8–12 mcg/kg IV or IM.
- *Adults:* 0.75–1.5 mg PO or 0.5–1 mg IV or IM.

Give $\frac{1}{2}$ of TDD in initial dose, then give $\frac{1}{4}$ of TDD in each of 2 subsequent doses at 6- to 12-hour intervals. Obtain ECG 6 hours after each dose to assess potential toxicity.

Daily maintenance dose:

- *Preterm neonates:* 5–7.5 mcg/kg PO or 4–6 mcg/kg IV or IM.
- *Full-term neonates:* 6–10 mcg/kg PO or 5–8 mcg/kg IV or IM.
- *Infants and children 1 month to 2 years:* 10–15 mcg/kg PO or 7.5–12 mcg/kg IV or IM.
- *Children 2–5 years:* 7.5–10 mcg/kg PO or 6–9 mcg/kg IV or IM.
- *Children 5–10 years:* 5–10 mcg/kg PO or 4–8 mcg/kg IV or IM.
- *Children > 10 years:* 2.5–5 mcg/kg PO or 2–3 mcg/kg IV or IM.
- *Adults:* 0.125–0.5 mg PO or 0.1–0.4 mg IV or IM.

Give maintenance dose q12h in infants and children < 10 years age, and daily to older children and adults.

Supplied: Capsules 0.05 mg, 0.1 mg, 0.2 mg; tablets 0.125 mg, 0.25 mg, 0.5 mg; elixir 0.05 mg/mL; injection 0.1 mg/mL, 0.25 mg/mL.

Notes: Can cause heart block. Low potassium can potentiate toxicity. Reduce dose in patients with renal failure. Symptoms of toxicity include nausea, vomiting, headache, fatigue, visual disturbances (yellow-green halos around lights), cardiac arrhythmias. IM injection can be painful, has erratic absorption, and should not be used. Therapeutic levels are 0.5–2 ng/mL.

DIGOXIN IMMUNE FAB (DIGIBIND)

Indications: Digoxin intoxication; hyperkalemia in the setting of digoxin toxicity.

Actions: Binds free (unbound) digoxin, which is then removed through renal excretion.

Dosage: Determine total body load (TBL) of digoxin, as follows:

- TBL of digoxin (mg) = serum digoxin concentration (ng/mL) $\times$ 5.6 $\times$ body weight (kg)/1000.
- Intravenous dose of Digibind (mg) = TBL $\times$ 76.
- Intravenous dose of Digibind (number of vials) = TBL/0.5.

Supplied: Injection 38 mg.

Notes: Each 38 mg vial Digibind will bind approximately 0.5 mg digoxin.

DILTIAZEM (CARDIZEM, DILACOR, TIAZAC)

Indications: Treatment of angina pectoris; prevention of reinfarction, hypertension, atrial fibrillation or flutter, and paroxysmal supraventricular tachycardia.

Actions: Calcium channel blocking agent.

Dosage: *Children:* 1.5–2 mg/kg/day PO divided 3–4 times daily or 1–2 times daily if extended-release formulation used, max 6 mg/kg/day up to 360 mg/day.
Adolescents and adults: Oral: Initial dose 30 mg PO 4 times daily, titrate to 180–360 mg/day divided 3–4 times daily prn; *Sustained-release:* 60–120 mg PO twice daily, titrate to effect, max 360 mg/day; *Extended-release (CD or XR):* 120–360 mg once daily, max 480 mg/day; *Intravenous:* 0.25 mg/kg IV bolus over 2 minutes, may repeat dose in 15 minutes at 0.35 mg/kg, may begin continuous infusion of 5–15 mg/h.

Supplied: Tablets 30 mg, 60 mg, 90 mg, 120 mg; long-acting tablets 120 mg, 180 mg, 240 mg, 300 mg, 360 mg, 420 mg; sustained-release capsules 60 mg, 90 mg, 120 mg; CD or XR capsules 120 mg, 180 mg, 240 mg, 300 mg, 360 mg, 420 mg; injection 5 mg/mL.

Notes: Contraindicated in sick sinus syndrome, AV block, and hypotension. Cardizem CD, Dilacor XR, and Tiazac are *not* interchangeable.

DIMENHYDRINATE (DRAMAMINE, OTHER)*

Indications: Prevention and treatment of nausea, vomiting, dizziness, or vertigo of motion sickness.

Actions: Antiemetic; antihistamine.

Dosage: 50–100 mg PO q4–6h to max of 400 mg/day; 50 mg IM or IV prn.

Supplied: Tablet 50 mg; chewable tablet 50 mg; liquid 12.5 mg/4 mL, 12.5 mg/5 mL, 15.62 mg/5 mL; injection 50 mg/mL.

Notes: Anticholinergic side effects.

DIPHENHYDRAMINE (BENADRYL, OTHERS)

Indications: Allergic reactions; motion sickness; potentiate narcotics; sedation; cough suppression; treatment of extrapyramidal reactions.

Actions: Antihistamine; antiemetic.

Dosage: 5 mg/kg/day PO, IV, or IM divided q6–8h.

Supplied: Tablets and capsules 25 mg*, 50 mg; chewable tablet 12.5 mg*; elixir/syrup 12.5 mg/5 mL*; injection 10 mg/mL, 50 mg/mL.

Notes: Anticholinergic side effects, including dry mouth and urinary retention; causes sedation. Increase dosing interval in patients with moderate to severe renal failure.

DIPHENOXYLATE AND ATROPINE (LOMOTIL) [C]

Indications: Diarrhea.

Actions: A constipating meperidine congener, reduces GI motility.

Dosage: *Children > 2 years:* 0.3–0.4 mg/kg/day PO divided 4 times daily, max 20 mg/day.

Supplied: Tablet 2.5 mg diphenoxylate/0.025 mg atropine; liquid 2.5 mg diphenoxylate/0.025 mg atropine per 5 mL.

Notes: Atropine-type side effects (headache, drowsiness). Reduce dose once symptoms are controlled.

Diphtheria, Tetanus Toxoid, Acellular Pertussis Vaccine (see Appendix D, p. 759)
   Diphtheria and Tetanus Toxoid (see Appendix D, p. 759)
   Dobutamine (Dobutrex)

Indications: Short-term use in patients with cardiac decompensation secondary to depressed contractility.

Actions: Positive inotropic agent.

Dosage: Continuous IV infusion of 2.5–15 mcg/kg/min; rarely 40 mcg/kg/min may be required; titrate according to response.

Supplied: Injection 12.5 mg/mL.

Notes: Monitor ECG for increase in heart rate, BP, and increased ectopic activity. Monitor pulmonary wedge pressure and cardiac output if possible.

DOCUSATE (DOS, COLACE, OTHERS)*

Indications: Constipation-prone patient; adjunct to painful anorectal conditions (hemorrhoids).

Actions: Softens stools.

Dosage: 5 mg/kg/day PO in 1–4 divided doses.

Supplied: *Docusate calcium:* Capsule 240 mg; *Docusate sodium:* Capsules 50 mg, 100 mg, 250 mg; syrup 50 mg/15 mL, 60 mg/15 mL; liquid 150 mg/15 mL; tablet 100 mg.

Notes: No significant side effects; no laxative action.

DOPAMINE (INTROPIN)

Indications: Short-term use in patients with cardiac decompensation secondary to decreased contractility; increases organ perfusion.

Actions: Positive inotropic agent with dose-related response.
- *Low dose:* 1–5 mcg/kg/min increases renal blood flow and urine output.
- *Intermediate dose:* 5–15 mcg/kg/min increases renal blood flow, heart rate, cardiac contractility, cardiac output, and BP.
- *High dose:* > 15 mcg/kg/min produces peripheral and renal vasoconstriction, increased BP.

Dosage: 5 mcg/kg/min by continuous infusion, titrated by increments of 5 mcg/kg/min to max of 50 mcg/kg/min based on effect.

Supplied: Injection 40 mg/mL, 80 mg/mL, 160 mg/mL.

Notes: Dosage > 10 mcg/kg/min may decrease renal perfusion. Monitor urinary output. Monitor ECG for increases in heart rate, BP, and ectopic activity. Monitor pulmonary capillary wedge pressure and cardiac output if possible.

DORNASE ALFA (PULMOZYME)

Indications: To reduce frequency of respiratory infections in patients with cystic fibrosis.

Actions: Enzyme selectively cleaves DNA.

Dosage: Children > 5 years and adults: 2.5 mg inhaled once daily.

Supplied: Solution for inhalation 1 mg/mL.

Notes: To be used with recommended nebulizer.

DOXORUBICIN (ADRIAMYCIN)

Indications: Ovarian, breast, and bladder tumors; various lymphomas and leukemias (ALL, AML); soft tissue sarcomas; neuroblastoma; osteosarcoma.

Actions: Antineoplastic anthracycline antibiotic.

Dosage: Refer to individual protocols.

Supplied: Solution for injection 2 mg/mL; powder for injection 10 mg, 20 mg, 50 mg.

Notes: Toxicity includes myelosuppression, mucositis, nausea, vomiting, diarrhea, mucositis, radiation recall phenomenon, and tissue necrosis with extravascular extravasation. Cardiomyopathy is rare but dose related. Reduce dose in patients with hepatic impairment.

DOXYCYCLINE (VIBRAMYCIN)

Indications: Broad-spectrum antibiotic, including activity against *Rickettsiae, Chlamydia,* and *Mycoplasma pneumoniae.*

Actions: Tetracycline; interferes with protein synthesis.

Dosage: Children ≥ 8 years: 2–4 mg/kg/day PO or IV divided q12–24h, max 200 mg/day.

Supplied: Tablets 50 mg, 100 mg; capsules 50 mg, 100 mg; syrup 50 mg/ 5 mL; suspension 25 mg/5 mL; injection 100 mg.

Notes: Useful for chronic bronchitis. Tetracycline of choice for patients with renal impairment. May discolor teeth in children < 8 years; may cause photosensitivity.

DROPERIDOL (INAPSINE)

Indications: Nausea and vomiting; premedication for anesthesia.

Actions: Tranquilizer, sedative, antiemetic.

Dosage: Postoperative nausea and vomiting: Children 2–12 years:
- *Prophylaxis:* 0.015–0.06 mg/kg per dose IV or IM once, max 0.1 mg/kg.
- *Treatment:* 0.01–0.03 mg/kg per dose IV, max 0.1 mg/kg.

Nausea: Adults: 2.5–5 mg IV or IM q3–4h prn or as premedication 30–60 minutes preoperatively.

Supplied: Injection 2.5 mg/mL.

Notes: Administer additional doses with caution, only if benefits outweigh risks. May cause drowsiness, moderate hypotension, occasionally tachycardia, and possible QT prolongation.

DROTRECOGIN ALFA (XIGRIS)

Indications: Sepsis associated with acute organ dysfunction.

Actions: Human recombinant activated protein C; has profibrinolytic, antithrombic, and anti-inflammatory activities.

Dosage: 24 mcg/kg/h IV infusion for 96 hours.

Supplied: Powder for injection 5 mg, 20 mg.

Notes: Infusion should start within 24 hours of onset of at least 3 signs of systemic inflammation and evidence of at least one organ system dysfunction. Monitor for bleeding.

EDROPHONIUM (ENLON, REVERSOL)

Indications: Diagnosis of myasthenia gravis; acute myasthenic crisis; reversal of nondepolarizing neuromuscular blockers.

Actions: Anticholinesterase.

Dosage: Diagnosis of myasthenia gravis: Infants: 0.5–1 mg IM or SQ or 0.1 mg IV followed by 0.4 mg (if no response); *Children ≤ 34 kg:* 1 mg IV, if no response within 45 seconds may repeat dose in 1-mg increments every 30–45 seconds to total of 5 mg; *Children > 34 kg:* 2 mg IV, if no response repeat as above to total of 10 mg.

Reversal of neuromuscular blockade: Adults: 10 mg IV over 30–45 seconds, may repeat q5–10 min up to 40-mg total dose.

Supplied: Injection 10 mg/mL.

Notes: Can cause severe cholinergic effects; keep atropine available.

ENALAPRIL AND ENALAPRILAT (VASOTEC, VASOTEC IV)

Indications: Hypertension; congestive heart failure; asymptomatic left ventricular dysfunction; proteinuria in steroid-resistant nephrotic syndrome.

Actions: ACE inhibitor.

Dosage: Neonates: 0.1 mg/kg/day PO daily or 5–10 mcg/kg per dose IV q8–24h; *Infants and children:* same PO dose as neonates given in 1–2 divided doses, may increase prn over 2 weeks to max of 0.5 mg/kg/day; IV dose same as neonates; *Adolescents and adults:* 2.5–5 mg/day PO then increase prn to 10–40 mg/day in 1–2 divided doses or 0.625–1.25 mg per dose IV q6h.
  Asymptomatic left ventricular dysfunction: 2.5 mg PO twice daily, increase as tolerated up to 20 mg/day.

Supplied: Injection, enalaprilat 1.25 mg/1 mL; tablets, enalapril 2.5 mg, 5 mg, 10 mg, 20 mg.

Notes: Adjust dose in patients with renal impairment. Use with caution in patients with renal artery stenosis. Injection contains benzyl alcohol.

ENOXAPARIN (LOVENOX)

Indications: Prevention of deep venous thrombosis (DVT); treatment of DVT and pulmonary embolus (PE); unstable angina and non–Q-wave myocardial infarction.

Actions: Low-molecular-weight heparin.

Dosage: DVT prevention: Infants ≤ 2 months: 0.75 mg/kg SQ q12h; *Infants > 2 months, children, and adolescents ≤ 18 years:* 0.5 mg/kg q12h; *Adults:* 30 mg SQ twice daily or 40 mg SQ q24h.
  DVT and PE treatment: Infants ≤ 2 months: 1.5 mg/kg SQ q12h; *Infants > 2 months, children, and adolescents ≤ 18 years:* 1 mg/kg SQ q12h; *Adults:* 1 mg/kg SQ q12h or 1.5 mg/kg SQ q24h.

Supplied: Injection 10 mg/0.1 mL (30-mg, 40-mg, 60-mg, 80-mg, 100-mg syringes).

Notes: Does not significantly affect bleeding time, platelet function, PT, or APTT.

EPINEPHRINE (ADRENALIN, SUS-PHRINE, OTHERS)

Indications: Bronchospasm; cardiac arrest; anaphylactic reactions; upper airway obstruction; croup.

Actions: β-Adrenergic agonist with some α-agonist effects.

Dosage: Asystole, pulseless arrest, or bradycardia: 0.01 mg/kg (0.1 mL/kg) of **1:10,000** solution IV or IO q3–5min prn, max dose 1 mg or 10 mL; *Intratracheal:* 0.1 mg/kg (0.1 mL/kg) of **1:1000** solution, doses as high as 0.2 mg/kg may be effective.
  Anaphylaxis: 0.01 mg/kg (0.01 mL/kg) of **1:1000** solution SQ not to exceed 0.5 mg or 0.005 mL/kg/dose of **1:200** suspension SQ, not to exceed 0.15 mL q8–12h; *EpiPen and EpiPen Jr: Children < 30 kg:* 0.15 mg IM; *Children ≥ 30 kg:* 0.3 mg IM.
  Nebulization: 0.25–0.5 mL of 2.25% **racemic epinephrine** solution diluted in 3 mL saline.
  Continuous IV infusion: 0.1–1 mcg/kg/min titrate to effect.

Supplied: EpiPen 0.3 mg/0.3 mL [1:1000]; EpiPen Jr 0.15 mg/0.3 mL [1:2000]; Injection 1 mg/mL [1:1000], 0.1 mg/mL [1:10,000]; suspension for injection [1:200]; aerosol for oral inhalation 0.2 mg per inhalation; solution for oral inhalation 2.25%.

Notes: Sus-Phrine offers sustained action. Dilute intratracheal doses with 3–5 mL saline and follow with several positive pressure ventilations. Tissue irritant.

EPOETIN ALFA [ERYTHROPOIETIN, EPO] (EPOGEN, PROCRIT)

Indications: Treatment of anemia associated with chronic renal failure, anemia of prematurity, zidovudine treatment in HIV-infected patients, and patients receiving cancer chemotherapy; reduction in transfusions associated with surgery.

Actions: Recombinant erythropoietin induces erythropoiesis.

Dosage: Neonatal anemia of prematurity: 25–100 units/kg per dose SQ 3 times per week or 100 units/kg per dose 5 times per week or 200 units/kg per dose every other day for 10 doses.
  Anemia in cancer patients: 150 units/kg per dose SQ 3 times per week, max 1200 units/kg/wk.
  Anemia in chronic renal failure: 50–150 units/kg per dose SQ 3 times per week.
  Zidovudine-treated HIV-infected patients: 100 units/kg per dose SQ 3 times per week for 8 weeks.
  Surgery: Adults: 300 units/kg/day for 10 days prior to surgery.

Supplied: Injection 2000 units/mL, 3000 units/mL, 4000 units/mL, 10,000 units/mL, 20,000 units/mL.

Notes: Onset of action is several days, max effect 2–6 weeks. Target Hct range 30–33%; reduce dose when target range is reached or Hct increases > 4 points in a 2-week period; increase dose when Hct does not increase by 5–6 points after 8 weeks; stop therapy when Hct > 40%. May cause hypertension, headache, tachycardia, and nausea and vomiting.

ERGOCALCIFEROL (CALCIFEROL, DRISDOL) (SEE VITAMINS, P. 745)
ERYTHROMYCIN (E-MYCIN, ILOSONE, ERYTHROCIN, PCE, OTHERS)

Indications: Infections caused by group A streptococci, α-hemolytic streptococci, and *Neisseria gonorrhoeae* infections in penicillin-allergic patients, *Streptococcus pneumoniae, Mycobacterium pneumoniae, Legionella,* and *Chlamydia;* Lyme disease; diphtheria; pertussis; chancroid; *Campylobacter gastroenteritis;* used in conjunction with neomycin for preoperative bowel decontamination; used to improve gastric emptying time and intestinal motility.

Actions: Bacteriostatic; interferes with protein synthesis.

Dosage: Infants and children:
- *Base and ethylsuccinate:* 30–50 mg/kg/day PO divided q6–8h, max 2 g/day (base) or 3.2 g/day (ethylsuccinate).
- *Estolate and stearate:* 30–50 mg/day PO divided q6h, max 2 g/day.
- *Lactobionate:* 15–50 mg/kg/day IV divided q6h, max 4 g/day.
- *Pertussis:* 40–50 mg/kg/day PO divided q6h for 2 weeks (estolate salt recommended).
- *Prokinetic agent:* 3 mg/kg IV over 60 minutes followed by 20 mg/kg/day PO divided 3–4 times daily before meals and bedtime.
- *Prophylaxis of neonatal gonococcal ophthalmia:* 0.5–1 cm ointment instilled in each conjunctival sac once.
- *Preoperative bowel preparation:* 20 mg/kg base PO at 1, 2, and 11 PM on day before surgery.

Adults: 250–500 mg PO 4 times daily or 500 mg to 1 g IV 4 times daily.

Supplied: Powder for injection as lactobionate salt: 500 mg, 1 g; *Base:* Tablets 250 mg, 333 mg (PCE), 500 mg; capsule 250 mg; *Estolate:* Tablet 500 mg; capsule 250 mg; suspension 125 mg/5 mL, 250 mg/5 mL; *Stearate:* Tablets 250 mg, 500 mg; *Ethylsuccinate:* Chewable tablet 200 mg; tablet 400 mg; suspension 200 mg/5 mL, 400 mg/5 mL; ophthalmic ointment 5 mg/g.

Notes: Some frequent mild GI disturbances. Estolate salt is associated with cholestatic jaundice. Erythromycin base is not well absorbed from GI tract; some forms, such as PCE, are better tolerated with respect to GI irritation.

ESMOLOL (BREVIBLOC)

Indications: Supraventricular tachycardia (SVT); noncompensatory sinus tachycardia.

Actions: β-Adrenergic blocking agent; class II antiarrhythmic.

Dosage: SVT: Children: 100–500 mcg/kg IV over 1 minute followed by continuous infusion of 200 mcg/kg/min, titrate infusion upward by 50–100 mcg/kg/min q5–10 min until > 10% reduction in heart rate or mean BP occurs; *Adults:* Initiate treatment with 500 mcg/kg load over 1 minute, then 50 mcg/kg/min for 4 minutes. If inadequate response, repeat loading dose and follow with maintenance infusion of 100 mcg/kg/min for 4 minutes; continue titration process by repeating loading dose followed by incremental increases in maintenance dose of 50 mcg/kg/min for 4 minutes until desired heart rate is reached or a decrease in BP occurs.

Supplied: Injection 10 mg/mL, 250 mg/mL.

Notes: Monitor closely for hypotension; decreasing or discontinuing infusion will reverse hypotension in about 1 minute.

ETANERCEPT (ENBREL)

Indications: Polyarticular-course juvenile rheumatoid arthritis in patients who have had inadequate response to other therapies; to delay structural damage in patients with moderately to severely active rheumatoid arthritis.

Actions: Binds tumor necrosis factor (TNF), thus blocking its interaction at TNF receptors.

Dosage: Children and adolescents 4–17 years: 0.4 mg/kg per dose SQ twice weekly given 72–96 hours apart; *Adults:* 25 mg given SQ twice weekly given 72–96 hours apart.

Supplied: Dose tray: Contains 25-mg single-use vial of etanercept and 1 syringe of sterile bacteriostatic water for injection.

Notes: Serious infections and sepsis have been reported. Avoid use in patients with active infections or with underlying conditions that predispose them to infection.

ETHACRYNIC ACID (EDECRIN)

Indications: Edema, congestive heart failure, and ascites; need for rapid diuresis.

Actions: Loop diuretic; inhibits reabsorption of sodium and chlorine in ascending loop of Henle and distal renal tubule.

Dosage: Children: 1 mg/kg per dose PO once daily, increase every 2–3 days to max of 3 mg/kg/day or 1 mg/kg per dose IV, repeat doses not recommended but may be given q8–12h; *Adults:* 50–200 mg PO once daily or 50 mg IV prn.

Supplied: Tablets 25 mg, 50 mg; powder for injection 50 mg.

Notes: Contraindicated in anuria. Severe side effects have been reported.

ETHAMBUTOL (MYAMBUTOL)

Indications: Pulmonary tuberculosis and other mycobacterial infections.

Actions: Inhibits cellular metabolism.

Dosage: 15–25 mg/kg PO daily or 50 mg/kg per dose PO twice weekly, max 2.5 g per dose.

Supplied: Tablets 100 mg, 400 mg.

Notes: May cause vision changes and GI upset. Reduce dose in patients with renal impairment.

ETHOSUXIMIDE (ZARONTIN)

Indications: Management of seizures.

Actions: Anticonvulsant; increases seizure threshold.

Dosage: Children < 6 years: Initial 15 mg/kg/day PO divided twice daily, max 250 mg per dose, increase every 4–7 days prn up to 40 mg/kg/day, max 1.5 g/day; *Children ≥ 6 years and adults:* Initial dose 500 mg PO divided twice daily; increase by 250 mg/day every 4–7 days as needed, max 1.5 g/day.

Supplied: Capsule 250 mg; syrup 250 mg/5 mL.

Notes: Blood dyscrasias as well as CNS and GI side effects may occur. Use with caution in patients with renal or hepatic impairment.

ETOPOSIDE (TOPOSAR, VEPESID)

Indications: Testicular and lung carcinoma; malignant lymphoma; Hodgkin disease; leukemias; neuroblastoma; Ewing sarcoma; rhabdomyosarcoma; osteosarcoma; Wilms tumor; brain tumors.

Actions: Antineoplastic mitotic inhibitor.

Dosage: Refer to individual protocols.

Supplied: Capsule 50 mg; injection 20 mg/mL.

Notes: Toxicities include myelosuppression, nausea and vomiting, and alopecia. Hypotension may occur if infused too rapidly. Anaphylaxis or lesser hypersensitivity reactions (wheezing) rarely occurs. Potential for secondary leukemias. Reduce dose in patients with renal impairment.

FAMOTIDINE (PEPCID)

Indications: Short-term treatment of active duodenal ulcer and benign gastric ulcer; maintenance therapy for duodenal ulcer, hypersecretory conditions, gastroesophageal reflux disease (GERD), and heartburn.

Actions: H_2-antagonist; inhibits gastric acid secretion.

Dosage: Ulcer: Children < 16 years: 0.5 mg/kg/day PO or IV divided twice daily, max 40 mg/day; *Adults:* 20–40 mg PO at bedtime or 20 mg IV q12h.
  GERD: Children < 16 years: 1 mg/kg/day PO or IV divided twice daily, max 80 mg/day; *Adults:* 20 mg PO twice daily for 6 weeks.
  Hypersecretory conditions: Adults: 20–160 mg PO q6h.
  Heartburn: Adults: 10 mg PO prn.

Supplied: Gel capsule 10 mg*; tablets 10 mg*, 20 mg*, 40 mg; chewable tablet 10 mg*; suspension 40 mg/5 mL; injection 10 mg/2 mL.

Notes: Decrease dose in patients with renal insufficiency.

FELBAMATE (FELBATOL)

Indications: Partial and generalized seizures; Lennox-Gastaut syndrome; not a first-line agent, reserved for patients who do not respond to alternative agents.

Actions: Anticonvulsant.

Dosage: Children 2–14 years: Initial 15 mg/kg/day PO divided 3–4 times daily, increase dose by 15 mg/kg/day at weekly intervals, max 45 mg/kg/day or 3.6 g/day (whichever is less); *Children > 14 years and adults:* Initial 1200 mg/day PO divided 3–4 times daily, increase daily dose by 1200 mg at weekly intervals to max of 3.6 g/day.

Supplied: Tablets 400 mg, 600 mg; suspension 600 mg/5 mL.

Notes: Causes hepatic failure and aplastic anemia. Benefit should outweigh risk. Monitor patients closely. Obtain written informed consent prior to starting therapy.

FENTANYL (SUBLIMAZE, DURAGESIC) [C]

Indications: Short-acting analgesic used in conjunction with anesthesia; management of chronic pain (transdermal system).

Actions: Narcotic.

Dosage: Sedation and analgesia: 1–2 mcg/kg per dose IV or IM, may repeat q30–60min.
   Continuous IV infusion: Bolus 1–2 mcg/kg followed by 1–5 mcg/kg/h infusion.
   Transdermal patch: Children > 12 years: Initial 25 mcg/h system every 3 days, dose may be increased after 72 hours.

Supplied: Injection 0.05 mg/mL; transdermal patches 25, 50, 75, and 100 mcg/h.

Notes: Causes significant sedation; 0.1 mg of fentanyl is equivalent to 10 mg of morphine IM. Apply patch to upper torso every 72 hours. Dose is calculated from narcotic requirements for previous 24 hours.

FERROUS SULFATE* (SEE MINERALS, P. 740)
FILGRASTIM [G-CSF] (NEUPOGEN)

Indications: To decrease incidence of infection in febrile neutropenic patients; treatment of chronic neutropenia.

Actions: Recombinant granulocyte colony-stimulating factor.

Dosage: 5–10 mcg/kg/day SQ or IV as single daily dose.

Supplied: Injection 300 mcg/mL.

Notes: May cause bone pain. Discontinue therapy when ANC > 10,000/mm^3.

FLUCONAZOLE (DIFLUCAN)

Indications: Oropharyngeal and esophageal candidiasis; cryptococcal meningitis; *Candida* infections of lungs, peritoneum, and urinary tract; prevention of candidiasis in bone marrow transplant patients receiving chemotherapy or radiation; *Candida* vaginitis.

Actions: Antifungal; inhibits fungal cytochrome P-450 sterol demethylation.

Dosage: Children: 6–12 mg/kg/day PO or IV once daily, max 600 mg/day; *Adults:* Usual 100–400 mg PO or IV once daily, max 800 mg/day.
   Vaginitis: 150 mg PO as single dose.

Supplied: Tablets 50 mg, 100 mg, 150 mg, 200 mg; suspension 10 mg/mL, 40 mg/mL; injection 2 mg/mL.

Notes: Adjust dose in patients with renal insufficiency. Oral dosing produces same blood levels as intravenous; therefore, oral route should be used whenever possible.

FLUCYTOSINE (ANCOBON)

Indications: Serious infections caused by susceptible strains of *Candida* or *Cryptococcus.*

Actions: Antifungal.

Dosage: 50–150 mg/kg/day PO divided q6h.

Supplied: Capsules 250 mg, 500 mg.

Notes: May cause nausea, vomiting, diarrhea, and photosensitivity. Adjust dose in patients with renal impairment. Instruct patient to take capsules a few at a time over 15 minutes.

FLUDROCORTISONE ACETATE (FLORINEF)

Indications: Partial treatment of adrenocortical insufficiency; treatment of salt-losing forms of congenital adrenogenital syndrome.

Actions: Mineralocorticoid replacement.

Dosage: Infants and children: 0.05–0.1 mg PO once daily; *Adults:* 0.05–0.2 mg PO once daily.
   Congenital adrenal hyperplasia (salt losers): 0.05–0.3 mg PO once daily.

Supplied: Tablet 0.1 mg.

Notes: For adrenal insufficiency, must be used in conjunction with a glucocorticoid supplement. Dosage changes are based on plasma renin activity.

FLUMAZENIL (ROMAZICON)

Indications: For complete or partial reversal of sedative effects of benzodiazepines.

Actions: Benzodiazepine receptor antagonist.

Dosage: Children: 0.01 mg/kg IV over 15 seconds, max dose 0.2 mg, may repeat after 45 seconds, then every minute until max total dose of 0.05 mg/kg or 1 mg, whichever is lower; *Adults:* 0.2 mg IV over 15 seconds;

dose may be repeated if desired level of consciousness is not obtained, to max dose of 1 mg.

Supplied: Injection 0.1 mg/mL.

Notes: Does not reverse narcotics.

FLUNISOLIDE (AEROBID, NASALIDE)

Indications: Chronic treatment of asthma; seasonal or perennial allergic rhinitis.

Actions: Topical steroid.

Dosage: Metered-dose inhaler: Children > 6 years: 2 inhalations twice daily, max 8 inhalations per day.

Nasal: Children 6–14 years: 1 spray in each nostril 3 times daily or 2 sprays in each nostril twice daily, max 4 sprays to each nostril per day; *Adults:* 2 sprays in each nostril twice daily, max 8 sprays to each nostril per day.

Supplied: Metered-dose aerosol 250 mcg per actuation; nasal solution 25 mcg per spray.

Notes: May cause oral candidiasis; instruct patients to rinse mouth after use. Not for acute asthma attack. Dose should be titrated to lowest effective dose.

FLUORIDE (SEE MINERALS, P. 740)
FLUOROMETHOLONE (FML, FLAREX) (SEE TABLE VIII–6, p. 754)
FLUOROURACIL (ADRUCIL, CARAC, EFUDEX, FLUOROPLEX)

Indications: Stomach, colon, rectal, breast, and pancreatic cancer; topically for multiple actinic keratoses and superficial basal cell carcinomas.

Actions: Antineoplastic antimetabolite agent.

Dosage: Refer to individual protocols.

Supplied: Injection 50 mg/mL; topical cream 0.5%, 1%, 5%; topical solution 1%, 2%.

Notes: If intractable vomiting, diarrhea, or hemorrhage occurs discontinue immediately. Adjust dose in patients with renal or hepatic impairment.

FLUOXETINE (PROZAC, SARAFEM)

Indications: Depression; obsessive-compulsive disorders; bulimia; premenstrual dysphoric disorder (PMDD).

Actions: SSRI.

Dosage: Children 5–18 years: 5–10 mg/day, titrate to 20 mg/day prn.

Depression: Adults: Initial 20 mg PO once daily; titrate to max of 80 mg/24 h; doses of > 20 mg/day should be divided.
  Bulimia: 60 mg once daily in AM.
  PMDD: 20 mg once daily.

Supplied: Capsules 10 mg, 20 mg; tablet 10 mg; solution 20 mg/5 mL.

Notes: May cause nausea, nervousness, and weight loss. Adjust dose in patients with hepatic failure. Can cause insomnia or hypersomnia and sexual dysfunction.

FLUTICASONE NASAL (FLONASE)

Indications: Seasonal allergic rhinitis.

Actions: Topical steroid.

Dosage: Children ≥ 4 years and adults: 1–2 sprays (50–100 mcg) in each nostril once daily.

Supplied: Nasal spray 50 mcg per actuation.

FLUTICASONE ORAL (FLOVENT, FLOVENT ROTADISK)

Indications: Chronic treatment of asthma.

Actions: Topical steroid.

Dosage: Oral inhalation, divided twice daily: Children: Low dose 88–176 mcg/day; Medium dose 176–440 mcg/day; High dose > 440 mcg/day; *Adults:* Low dose 88–264 mcg/day; Medium dose 264–660 mcg/day; High dose > 660 mcg/day.
  Inhalation powder: Children 4–11 years: 50–100 mcg twice daily; *Adolescents and adults:* 100–500 mcg twice daily.

Supplied: Metered dose inhaler: 44 mcg, 110 mcg, or 220 mcg per activation; *Rotadisk dry powder:* 50 mcg, 100 mcg, and 250 mcg per activation.

Notes: May cause oral candidiasis; instruct patients to rinse mouth after use. Counsel patients carefully on use of delivery system.

FOLIC ACID (SEE VITAMINS, P. 739)
FOSCARNET (FOSCAVIR)

Indications: Cytomegalovirus (CMV) infection; acyclovir-resistant herpes simplex virus (HSV) infections.

Actions: Inhibits viral DNA polymerase and reverse transcriptase.

Dosage: Children and adults:
- *CMV retinitis: Induction:* 60 mg/kg IV q8h for 14–21 days; *Maintenance:* 90–120 mg/kg IV once daily.
- *Acyclovir-resistant HSV infection:* 40 mg/kg q8h or 40–60 mg/kg q12h for 3 weeks or until lesions heal.

Supplied: Injection 24 mg/mL.

Notes: Dosage must be adjusted for renal function; nephrotoxic. Monitor ionized calcium closely. Administer through a central line.

FOSPHENYTOIN (CEREBYX)

Indications: Status epilepticus.

Actions: Inhibits seizure spread in motor cortex.

Dosage: Limited data in children; some centers use phenytoin dosing guidelines. *Children 5–18 years:* Load 10–20 mg phenytoin equivalents (PE)/kg IV; *Adults:* Load 15–20 mg PE/kg IV.

Maintenance: 4–6 mg PE/kg/day IV or IM in 1–2 divided doses.

Supplied: Injection 50 mg PE/mL.

Notes: Dosed as phenytoin equivalents (PE). Requires 15 minutes to convert prodrug fosphenytoin to phenytoin. Administer at < 150 mg PE/min to prevent hypotension. Adjust dose in patients with renal or hepatic impairment.

FUROSEMIDE (LASIX)

Indications: Congestive heart failure; edema; hypertension.

Actions: Loop diuretic; inhibits sodium and chloride reabsorption in ascending loop of Henle and distal renal tubule.

Dosage: Children: 1–6 mg/kg/day PO divided q6–12h or 1–2 mg/kg per dose IV or IM q12–24h; *Adults:* 20–80 mg PO, IV, or IM 1–2 times daily.; *Continuous IV infusion:* 0.05–0.1 mg/kg/h, titrate to effect.

Supplied: Tablets 20 mg, 40 mg, 80 mg; solution 10 mg/mL, 40 mg/5 mL; injection 10 mg/mL.

Notes: Monitor for hypokalemia. Use with caution in patients with hepatic disease. High doses of IV form may cause ototoxicity.

GABAPENTIN (NEURONTIN)

Indications: Adjunctive therapy in treatment of partial seizures; adjunct in treatment of neuropathic pain.

Actions: Anticonvulsant.

Dosage: Anticonvulsant: Children 3–12 years: Initial 10–15 mg/kg/day PO divided 3 times daily, titrate every 3 days to 35–50 mg/kg/day; *Adolescents and adults:* 900–1800 mg/day PO in 3 divided doses.
  Neuropathic pain: Children: 5 mg/kg per dose PO at bedtime on day 1, increase to twice daily day 2, increase to 3 times daily on day 3, titrate to effect 8–35 mg/kg/day; *Adults:* 100 mg PO 3 times daily, titrate at weekly intervals by 300 mg/day, max 1.8 g/day.

Supplied: Capsules 100 mg, 300 mg, 400 mg.

Notes: Not necessary to monitor serum gabapentin levels. Adjust dose in patients with renal impairment.

GANCICLOVIR (CYTOVENE, VITRASERT)

Indications: Treatment and prevention of cytomegalovirus (CMV) retinitis; prevention of CMV disease in transplant recipients.

Actions: Inhibits viral DNA synthesis.

Dosage: Congenital CMV infection: 15 mg/kg/day IV divided q12h.
  CMV retinitis: Infants > 3 months and adults: 5 mg/kg IV q12h for 14–21 days, then maintenance of 5 mg/kg IV once daily for 7 days/wk or 6 mg/kg IV once daily for 5 days/wk.
  Oral, following IV induction: Children: 30 mg/kg per dose PO three times daily; *Adults:* 1000 mg PO three times daily.
  Prevention of CMV in transplant recipients: 5 mg/kg IV q12h for 7–14 days, followed by 5 mg/kg IV once daily for 7 days/wk or 6 mg/kg IV once daily for 5 days/wk for 100 days.
  Ocular implant: Children > 9 years: One implant every 6–9 months plus age-appropriate oral dose.

Supplied: Capsules 250 mg, 500 mg; injection 500 mg; ocular implant 4.5 mg.

Notes: Not a cure for CMV. Granulocytopenia and thrombocytopenia are the major toxicities. Injection should be handled with cytotoxic precautions. Administer capsules with food. Implant confers no systemic benefit. Adjust dose in patients with renal impairment.

GENTAMICIN (GARAMYCIN)

Indications: Serious infections caused by susceptible strains of *Pseudomonas, Proteus, E coli, Klebsiella, Enterobacter,* and *Serratia;* initial treatment of gram-negative sepsis.

Actions: Bactericidal; inhibits protein synthesis.

Dosage: Infants and children < 5 years: 2.5 mg/kg per dose IM or IV q8h; *Children ≥ 5 years:* 2–2.5 mg/kg per dose IM or IV q8h or 5–7.5 mg/kg per dose once daily; *Adults:* 1–2 mg/kg per dose IM or IV q8h or 4–6.6 mg/kg per dose once daily.
   Cystic fibrosis: 2.5–3.3 mg/kg per dose IV or IM q6–8h.
   Intraventricular and intrathecal: Infants > 3 months and children: 1–2 mg/day; *Adults:* 4–8 mg/day.

Supplied: Injection 10 mg/mL, 40 mg/mL; intrathecal preservative free 2 mg/mL.

Notes: Nephrotoxic and ototoxic. Decrease dose in patients with renal insufficiency. Monitor creatinine clearance and serum concentration for dosage adjustments.

GENTAMICIN, OPHTHALMIC (GARAMYCIN, GENOPTIC, GENTACIDIN, GENTAK, OTHERS) (SEE TABLE VIII–6, P. 754)
GENTAMICIN, TOPICAL (GARAMYCIN, G-MYTICIN)

Indications: Skin infections caused by susceptible organisms.

Actions: Bactericidal; inhibits protein synthesis.

Dosage: Apply 3–4 times daily.

Supplied: Cream 0.1%, ointment 0.1%.

GENTAMICIN AND PREDNISOLONE, OPHTHALMIC (PRED-G OPHTHALMIC)
(SEE TABLE VIII–6, P. 754)

GLUCAGON

Indications: Management of hypoglycemia; cardiac stimulant in β-blocker overdose.

Actions: Accelerates liver gluconeogenesis.

Dosage: Hypoglycemia: Neonates, infants, and children ≤ 20 kg: 0.5 mg IM, IV, or SQ; *Children > 20 kg and adults:* 1 mg IM, IV, or SQ; repeat after 20 minutes prn.

    β-Blocker overdose: 3–10 mg IV; repeat in 10 minutes prn; may be given as continuous infusion.

Supplied: Injection 1 mg (1 unit).

Notes: Administration of glucose IV is necessary. Ineffective in states of starvation, adrenal insufficiency, or chronic hypoglycemia.

GLYCERIN SUPPOSITORY*

Indications: Constipation.

Actions: Osmotic dehydrating agent; draws fluid into colon, stimulating evacuation.

Dosage: Children < 6 years: 1 infant suppository PR prn; *Children ≥ 6 years and adults:* 1 adult suppository PR prn.

Supplied: Suppositories adult, infant.

GLYCOPYRROLATE (ROBINUL)

Indications: Inhibition of salivation and excessive secretions of respiratory tract; reversal of muscarinic effects of cholinergic agents during reversal of neuromuscular blockade.

Actions: Inhibits muscarinic action of acetylcholine at postganglionic parasympathetic neuroeffector sites in smooth muscle, secretory glands, and CNS.

Dosage: Control of secretions: Children: 40–100 mcg/kg per dose PO 3–4 times daily or 4–10 mcg/kg per dose IM or IV q3–4h.

    Preoperative: Children < 2 years: 4.4–8.8 mcg/kg IM 30–60 minutes before procedure; *Children ≥ 2 years:* 4.4 mcg/kg IM 30–60 minutes before procedure.
    Reversal of muscarinic effects of cholinergic agents: Children and adults: 0.2 mg IV for each 1 mg of neostigmine or 5 mg of pyridostigmine administered.

Supplied: Injection 0.2 mg/mL, tablet 1 mg, 2 mg.

Notes: Infants and patients with Down syndrome, spastic paralysis, or brain damage may be hypersensitive to antimuscarinic effects. PO dose is 10 times IV dose.

GRANISETRON (KYTRIL)

Indications: Prevention and treatment of nausea and vomiting.

Actions: Serotonin receptor antagonist.

Dosage: Children ≥ 2 years: 10 mcg/kg IV 15–60 minutes prior to initiation of chemotherapy; *Adults:* 10 mcg/kg or 1 mg IV, or 2 mg PO once daily, or 1 mg PO twice daily.

Supplied: Tablet 1 mg; injection 1 mg/mL.

Notes: Use with caution in patients with liver disease.

GRISEOFULVIN (GRIS-PEG, FULVICIN P/G, GRIFULVIN V)

Indications: Tinea infections of skin, hair, and nails.

Actions: Inhibits fungal cell mitosis.

Dosage: Microsize: Children: 10–20 mcg/kg/day PO in 1 or 2 divided doses; *Adults:* 500–1000 mg/day PO in 1 or 2 divided doses.

Ultramicrosize: Children: 5–10 mg/kg/day PO in 1 or 2 divided doses; *Adults:* 330–375 mg/day PO in 1 or 2 divided doses.

Supplied: Tablets, microsize 250 mg, 500 mg; tablet, ultramicrosize 125 mg, 250 mg, 330 mg; suspension, microsize 125 mg/5 mL.

Notes: Administer with fatty meal to increase absorption. Causes photosensitivity.

GUAIFENESIN (ROBITUSSIN, OTHERS)*

Indications: Symptomatic relief of dry, nonproductive cough.

Actions: Expectorant.

Dosage: Children < 2 years: 12 mg/kg/day PO in 6 divided doses; *Children 2–5 years:* 50–100 mg PO q4h, max 600 mg/day; *Children 6–11 years:* 100–200 mg PO q4h, max 1.2 g/day; *Children ≥ 12 years and adults:* 200–400 mg PO q4h, max 2.4 g/day.

Supplied: Tablets 100 mg, 200 mg, 1200 mg; sustained-release tablets 600 mg, 1200 mg; capsules 200 mg; sustained-release capsule 300 mg; liquid 100 mg/5 mL.

GUAIFENESIN AND CODEINE (ROBITUSSIN AC, BRONTEX, OTHERS) [C]*

Indications: Symptomatic relief of dry, nonproductive cough.

Actions: Antitussive with expectorant.

Dosage: Children 2–6 years: 1–1.5 mg/kg codeine per day PO divided into 4 doses, max 30 mg/day; *Children 6–12 years:* 5 mL PO q4h, max 30 mL/day; *Adults:* 5–10 mL or 1 tablet PO q4–6h, max 120 mg or 6 tablets per day.

Supplied: Tablet guaifenesin 300 mg/10 mg codeine; liquid guaifenesin 75 mg/codeine 2.5 mg/5 mL, guaifenesin 100 mg/codeine 10 mg/5 mL.
Guaifenesin and Dextromethorphan (Many OTC Brands)*

Indications: Cough due to upper respiratory irritation.

Actions: Antitussive with expectorant.

Dosage: Dose expressed as dextromethorphan: Children: 1–2 mg/kg/day PO divided q6–8h; *Adults:* 60–120 mg/day PO divided q6–8h or 30–60 mg extended-release product PO q12h, max 120 mg/day.

Supplied: Guaifenesin/dextromethorphan dose: 100 mg/5 mg per 5 mL; 100 mg/15 mg per 5 mL; 200 mg/20 mg per 5 mL.

Haemophilus influenzae Type b Conjugate Vaccine (ProHIBiT, Comvax, Others) (see Appendix D, p. 759)
Haloperidol (Haldol)

Indications: Psychotic disorders; agitation; Tourette syndrome.

Actions: Antipsychotic, neuroleptic.

Dosage: Children 3–12 years: 0.01–0.15 mg/kg/day PO divided 2–4 times daily; *Children 6–12 years:* 1–3 mg per dose IM (as lactate) q4–8h prn, max 0.15 mg/kg/day; *Adults:* 0.5–5 mg PO 2–4 times daily, max 100 mg/day or 2–5 mg IM (as lactate) q4–8h prn or 10–15 times PO dose IM (as decanoate) given at 3–4-week intervals.

Supplied: Tablets 0.5 mg, 1 mg, 2 mg, 5 mg, 10 mg, 20 mg; concentrate liquid 2 mg/mL; lactate injection 5 mg/mL; decanoate injection 50 mg/mL, 100 mg/mL.

Notes: Can cause extrapyramidal symptoms and hypotension.

HEPARIN

Indications: Treatment and prevention of thromboembolic disorders.

Actions: Acts with antithrombin III to inactivate thrombin and inhibit thromboplastin formation.

Dosage: Line flushing: Infants < 10 kg: 10 units/mL; *Infants ≥ 10 kg, children, and adults:* 100 units/mL; volume is similar to or slightly greater than catheter size.
   TPN: 0.5–1 unit/mL.
   Arterial lines: 0.5–2 units/mL.
   Prophylaxis for cardiac catheterization: 100–150 units/kg via an artery.
Treatment of thrombosis: Neonates and infants < 1 year: Load 75 units/kg IV over 10 minutes then 28 units/kg/h IV infusion (adjust to maintain APTT of 60–85 seconds); *Children ≥ 1 year:* Load same as above, then 20 units/kg/h IV infusion, adjust to same APTT.

Supplied: Injection 10 units/mL, 100 units/mL, 1000 units/mL, 2000 units/mL, 2500 units/mL, 5000 units/mL, 7500 units/mL, 10,000 units/mL, 20,000 units/mL.

Notes: Follow APTT, Hgb, Hct, platelets, and signs of bleeding. Heparin has little effect on PT. Obtain APTT 4 hours postload and 4 hours after every rate change. Can cause thrombocytopenia.

HEPATITIS A VACCINE (HAVRIX, VAQTA) (SEE APPENDIX D, P. 759)
HEPATITIS B IMMUNE GLOBULIN (HYPERHEP, H-BIG) (SEE APPENDIX D, P. 759)
HEPATITIS B VACCINE (ENGERIX-B, RECOMBIVAX HB) (SEE APPENDIX D, P. 759)
HETASTARCH (HESPAN)

Indications: Plasma volume expansion as adjunct in treatment of shock.

Actions: Synthetic colloid with actions similar to those of albumin.

Dosage: Volume expansion: Children: 10 mL/kg per dose IV infusion, not to exceed 20 mL/kg; *Adults:* 500–1000 mL (*do not* exceed 1500 mL per dose) IV at a rate not to exceed 20 mL/kg/h.

Supplied: Injection 6 g/100 mL.

Notes: Hetastarch is not a substitute for blood or plasma. Contraindicated in patients with severe bleeding disorders, severe congestive heart failure, or renal failure with oliguria or anuria.

HYDRALAZINE (APRESOLINE, OTHERS)

Indications: Moderate to severe hypertension.

Actions: Peripheral vasodilator.

Dosage: Infants and children: Initial 0.75–1 mg/kg/day PO divided 2–4 times daily, max 25 mg per dose; increase over 3–4 weeks to max of 5 mg/kg/day in infants and 7.5 mg/kg/day in children, max of 200 mg/day; or 0.1–0.2 mg/kg per dose IV or IM q4–6h prn up to 1.7–3.5 mg/kg/day, max 20 mg per dose; *Adults:* Initial 10 mg PO 4 times daily, then increase by 10–25 mg per dose every 2–5 days to max of 300 mg/day or 10–20 mg IV q4–6h prn.

Supplied: Tablets 10 mg, 25 mg, 50 mg, 100 mg; injection 20 mg/mL.

Notes: Use with caution in patients with hepatic impairment and coronary artery disease. Compensatory sinus tachycardia can be eliminated with addition of a β-blocker. Chronically high doses can cause lupus-like syndrome. Adjust dose in patients with renal impairment.

HYDROCHLOROTHIAZIDE (HYDRODIURIL)

Indications: Edema; hypertension; congestive heart failure.

Actions: Thiazide diuretic; inhibits sodium reabsorption in distal tubule.

Dosage: Neonates and infants < 6 months: 2–4 mg/kg/day PO divided twice daily, max 37.5 mg/day; *Infants ≥ 6 months and children:* 2 mg/kg/day PO divided twice daily, max 200 mg/day; *Adults:* 12.5–100 mg PO once daily in single or divided doses.

Supplied: Tablets 25 mg, 50 mg, 100 mg; capsule 12.5 mg; oral solution: 50 mg/5 mL.

Notes: Hypokalemia is frequent; hyperglycemia, hyperuricemia, hyperlipidemia, and hyponatremia are common side effects.

HYDROCODONE AND ACETAMINOPHEN (LORTAB, VICODIN, OTHERS) [C]

Indications: Moderate to severe pain; hydrocodone has antitussive properties.

Actions: Narcotic analgesic with nonnarcotic analgesic.

Dosage: Antitussive (dose based on hydrocodone): Children < 2 years: 0.6 mg/kg/day PO divided 3–4 times daily, max 1.25 mg per dose; *Children 2–12 years:* Same dose, but max 5 mg per dose. *Children > 12 years:* Same dose, but max 10 mg per dose.
   Analgesic: Children < 50 kg: 0.2 mg/kg PO q3–4h prn; *Adults:* 1–2 capsules or tablets PO q4–6h prn.

Supplied: Many different combinations; specify hydrocodone/acetaminophen dose: capsules 5/500; tablets 2.5/500, 5/325, 5/400, 5/500, 7.5/400, 10/400, 7.5/500, 7.5/650, 7.5/750, 10/325, 10/500, 10/650; elixir and solution (fruit punch flavored) 2.5 mg hydrocodone/167 mg acetaminophen per 5 mL.

HYDROCORTISONE (CORTEF, SOLU-CORTEF)

Indications: Adrenocortical insufficiency; inflammation.

Actions: Adrenal corticosteroid.

Dosage: Acute adrenal insufficiency: Infants and young children: 1–2 mg/kg IV bolus followed by 25–150 mg/day divided q6–8h; *Older children:* Same load followed by 150–250 mg/day divided q6–8h; *Adults:* 100 mg IV bolus followed by 100 mg IV q8h, when stable change to 50 mg PO q8h for 6 doses, then taper to 30–50 mg/day in divided doses.
   Anti-inflammatory and immunosuppressive: Infants and children: 2.5–10 mg/kg/day PO divided q6–8h or 1–5 mg/kg/day IM or IV divided q12–24h; *Adolescents and adults:* 15–240 mg PO, IM, or IV q12h.
   Congenital adrenal hyperplasia: Infants: 2.5–5 mg PO 3 times daily; *Children:* 5–10 mg PO 3 times daily.
   Physiologic replacement: Children: 0.5–0.75 mg/kg/day PO divided q8h or 0.25–0.35 mg/kg/day IM once daily.
   Shock: Sodium succinate: Children: 50 mg/kg IV repeat in 4 hours and/or q24h prn; *Adolescents and adults:* 500 mg–2 g IV q2–6h.
   Status asthmaticus: Children: Optional load 4–8 mg/kg IV, max 250 mg, then 2 mg/kg per dose q6h; *Adults:* 100–500 mg IV q6h.
   Topical: Children and adults: Apply 3–4 times daily.

Supplied: Tablets 5 mg, 10 mg, 20 mg; solution for injection 50 mg/mL; powder for injection 100 mg, 250 mg, 500 mg, 1 g; suspension 10 mg/5 mL; topical cream/ointment 0.1% (butyrate), 0.2% (valerate), 0.5% (base/acetate)*, 1% (base/acetate)*, 2.5% (base); topical spray/gel 1%; lotion 0.5%, 1%, 2.5%.

Notes: Various salt forms can lead to confusion in prescribing; use appropriate salt/dosage form for proper indication. Tablets may result in more reliable serum concentrations than suspension. After long-term therapy *do not* abruptly withdraw.

HYDROCORTISONE, RECTAL (ANUSOL-HC SUPPOSITORY, CORTIFOAM RECTAL, PROCTOCORT, OTHERS)

Indications: Adjunct to painful anorectal conditions; radiation proctitis; management of ulcerative colitis.

Actions: Anti-inflammatory steroid.

Dosage: Ulcerative colitis: Adolescents and adults: 10–100 mg PR 1–2 times daily for 2–3 weeks.

Supplied: Hydrocortisone acetate rectal aerosol 90 mg per applicator*; suppository 25 mg, 30 mg*; hydrocortisone base rectal cream 1% and 2.5%*; rectal solution 100 mg/60 mL.

Notes: Patient should lie on left side during administration and for 30 minutes after; retain enema for at least 1 hour, preferably all night.

HYDROMORPHONE (DILAUDID) [C]

Indications: Moderate to severe pain; antitussive at low doses.

Actions: Narcotic analgesic.

Dosage: Antitussive: Children 6–12 years: 0.5 mg PO q3–4h prn; *Children > 12 years and adults:* 1 mg PO q3–4h prn.
   Analgesia: Young children: 0.03–0.08 mg/kg per dose PO q4–6h prn, max 5 mg per dose; or 0.015 mg/kg per dose IV q4–6h prn; *Older children and adults:* 1–4 mg PO, IM, IV, or SQ q4–6h prn; 3 mg PR q6–8h prn.

Supplied: Tablets 2 mg, 4 mg, 8 mg; liquid 1 mg/mL; injection 1 mg/mL, 2 mg/mL, 4 mg/mL, 10 mg/mL; suppositories: 3 mg.

Notes: 1.5 mg IM is equivalent to 10 mg of morphine IM. Side effects include sedation, dizziness, and GI upset.

HYDROXYUREA (HYDREA, DROXIA)

Indications: Chronic myelocytic leukemia, melanoma, and ovarian carcinoma; adjunct in management of sickle cell crisis; combination therapy for treatment of HIV infection.

Actions: Interferes with DNA synthesis; in patients with sickle cell disease increases production of fetal hemoglobin.

Dosage: Antineoplastic: Refer to individual protocols.
   Sickle cell anemia: Children and adults: Initial 15 mg/kg/day PO once daily, increase in 5 mg/kg/day increments every 12 weeks to max dose of 35 mg/kg/day.

Supplied: Tablet 1000 mg; capsules 200 mg, 300 mg, 400 mg, 500 mg.

Notes: Adjust dose in patients with renal impairment. Causes myelosuppression (leukopenia and thrombocytopenia); may cause elevated hepatic enzymes, rash, hyperuricemia, or seizures.

HYDROXYZINE (ATARAX, VISTARIL)

Indications: Anxiety; sedation; itching; emesis.

Actions: Antihistamine; antianxiety agent.

Dosage: Children: 2 mg/kg/day PO q6–8h or 0.5–1 mg/kg per dose IM q4–6h prn.
   Adults: Anxiety or sedation: 25–100 mg PO or IM 4 times daily or prn, max 600 mg/day; *Itching:* 25–50 mg PO or IM 3–4 times daily; *Antiemetic:* 25–100 mg IM q4–6h prn.

Supplied: Tablets 10 mg, 25 mg, 50 mg, 100 mg; capsules 25 mg, 50 mg, 100 mg; syrup 10 mg/5 mL; suspension 25 mg/5 mL; injection 25, 50 mg/mL.

Notes: Useful in potentiating effects of narcotics. Not for IV use. Drowsiness and anticholinergic effects are common.

HYOSCYAMINE (LEVSIN, OTHERS)

Indications: Spasm associated with GI and bladder disorders.

Actions: Anticholinergic; antispasmodic.

Dosage: Infants < 2 years: 3–11 drops (depending on weight) PO q4h prn; *Children 2–12 years:* 0.0625–0.125 mg PO q4h prn, max dose 0.75 mg/day; *Adults:* 0.125–0.25 mg PO before meals and at bedtime; sustained-release 0.0375 mg PO q12h; max dose 1.5 mg/day; or 0.25–0.5 mg IV, IM, or SQ q4h for 1–4 doses.

Supplied: Capsule/tablet, sustained-release 0.375 mg; injection 0.5 mg/mL; tablets 0.15 mg, 0.125 mg; elixir 0.125 mg/5 mL; drops 0.125 mg/mL, 0.125 mg/5 mL.

Notes: May cause dry mouth, drowsiness, dizziness, or blurred vision.

HYOSCYAMINE, ATROPINE, SCOPOLAMINE, AND PHENOBARBITAL (DONNATAL, OTHERS)

Indications: Irritable bowel; spastic colitis; peptic ulcer; spastic bladder.

Actions: Anticholinergic.

Dosage: Children: 0.1 mL/kg per dose PO q4h, max 5 mL per dose; *Adults:* Tablets: 0.125–0.25 mg (1–2 tablets) 3–4 times per day; sustained-release capsule: 1 capsule q12h; elixir: 5–10 mL q8h.

Supplied: Hyoscyamine/atropine/scopolamine/phenobarbital capsules, tablets 0.1037 mg/0.0194 mg/0.0065 mg/16.2 mg; elixir same per 5 mL.

Notes: Do not crush or chew extended-release tablets. May cause dry mouth, drowsiness, dizziness, or blurred vision.

IBUPROFEN (MOTRIN, RUFEN, ADVIL, OTHERS)

Indications: Inflammatory diseases and rheumatoid disorders; mild to moderate pain; fever; dysmenorrhea; gout.

Actions: NSAID.

Dosage: Infants and children: Analgesic and antipyretic: 5–10 mg/kg per dose PO q6–8h, max 40 mg/kg/day; *Juvenile rheumatoid arthritis:* 30–50 mg/kg/day PO divided 4 times daily, max 2.4 g/day.

Adolescents and adults: Anti-inflammatory: 400–800 mg per dose PO 3–4 times daily, max dose 3.2 g/day; *Analgesic and antipyretic:* 200–400 mg per dose PO q4–6h, max dose 1.2 g/day.

Supplied: Tablets 200 mg*, 400 mg, 600 mg, 800 mg; chewable tablets 50 mg*, 100 mg*; capsule 200 mg*; caplets 100 mg*, 200 mg*; suspension 100 mg/5 mL*; infant drops 40 mg/mL*.

Notes: Give with food. Tablets contain phenylalanine. Use with caution if patient has a history of GI bleeding.

IDARUBICIN (IDAMYCIN)

Indications: Acute myelocytic leukemia, chronic myelogenous leukemia, and acute lymphocytic leukemia.

Actions: Antineoplastic anthracycline agent; inhibits DNA topoisomerases I and II.

Dosage: Refer to individual protocols.

Supplied: Powder for injection 20 mg; solution for injection 1 mg/mL.

Notes: Toxicity includes myelosuppression, cardiotoxicity, nausea and vomiting, mucositis, alopecia, and irritation at sites of IV administration. Adjust dose in patients with renal or hepatic dysfunction.

IFOSFAMIDE (IFEX)

Indications: Lung cancer; Hodgkin and non-Hodgkin lymphoma; acute and chronic lymphocytic leukemia; ovarian, breast, and testicular cancers and sarcomas.

Actions: Antineoplastic alkylating agent.

Dosage: Refer to individual protocols.

Supplied: Powder for injection 1 g, 3 g.

Notes: Toxicity includes mild to moderate leukopenia, hemorrhagic cystitis, nephrotoxicity, alopecia, nausea and vomiting, lethargy, confusion, and hepatic enzyme elevations. Adjust dose in patients with renal impairment.

IMIPENEM AND CILASTATIN (PRIMAXIN)

Indications: Serious infections caused by wide variety of susceptible bacteria; inactive against *Staphylococcus aureus,* group A and B streptococci, and others.

Actions: Bactericidal; interferes with cell wall synthesis.

Dosage: *Infants* $\geq$ *3 months and children:* 60–100 mg/kg/day (imipenem) IV divided q6h; *Adults:* 250–500 mg IV q6h.

Supplied: Injection (imipenem/cilastatin) 250 mg/250 mg, 500 mg/500 mg.

Notes: Seizures may occur if drug accumulates. Adjust dosage for renal insufficiency to avoid drug accumulation if calculated creatinine clearance is < 70 mL/min.

IMIPRAMINE (TOFRANIL)

Indications: Depression; panic attacks; enuresis; chronic pain.

Actions: Tricyclic antidepressant; increases synaptic concentration of serotonin and/or norepinephrine in CNS.

Dosage: *Children: Depression:* 1.5 mg/kg/day PO in 1–4 divided doses, increase dose gradually by 1 mg/kg every 3–4 days to max of 5 mg/kg/day; *Enuresis: Children* $\geq$ *6 years:* 10–25 mg PO at bedtime, may increase by 25 mg/day if inadequate response within 1 week, max dose 2.5 mg/kg/day.
    Adolescents: 25–50 mg/day PO in single or divided doses, can increase over several weeks to 200 mg/day.
    Adults: 25 mg PO 3–4 times daily, increase dose gradually, may be given as a single bedtime dose, max 300 mg/day.

Supplied: Tablets 10 mg, 25 mg, 50 mg; capsules 75 mg, 100 mg, 125 mg, 150 mg.

Notes: Do not use with MAO inhibitors; provides less sedation than amitriptyline.

IMMUNE GLOBULIN, INTRAVENOUS (GAMIMUNE N, SANDOGLOBULIN, GAMMAR IV)

Indications: IgG antibody deficiency disease states; Kawasaki disease; pediatric HIV infection; idiopathic thrombocytopenic purpura (ITP); bone marrow transplantation (BMT).

Actions: IgG supplementation.

Dosage: Immunodeficiency: 300–400 mg/kg IV monthly at rate of 0.01–0.04 mL/kg/min to maintain IgG concentration of 500 mg/dL.
 Kawasaki disease: 2 g/kg IV as single dose over 10–12 hours, may repeat dose if signs and symptoms persist.
 Pediatric HIV infection: 400 mg/kg per dose IV every 4 weeks.
 ITP: 400–1000 mg/kg per dose IV once daily for 2–5 days; repeat dose every 3–6 weeks based on clinical response and platelet count.
 BMT: 400–500 mg/kg/wk IV for 3 months and then every month.

Supplied: Injection 5%, 10%.

Notes: Adverse effects are associated mostly with rate of infusion.

INAMRINONE (INOCOR)

Indications: Short-term management of low cardiac output states and pulmonary hypertension.

Actions: Positive inotrope with vasodilator activity.

Dosage: Initial dose as IV bolus of 0.75 mg/kg over 2–3 minutes, followed by maintenance dose of 5–10 mcg/kg/min; not to exceed 10 mg/kg/day.

Supplied: Injection 5 mg/mL.

Notes: Incompatible with dextrose-containing solutions. Monitor for fluid and electrolyte changes and renal function during therapy.

INDINAVIR (CRIXIVAN)

Indications: Antiretroviral therapy for HIV infection.

Actions: Protease inhibitor; inhibits maturation of immature noninfectious virions to mature infectious virus.

Dosage: *Children:* 500 mg/m^2 per dose PO q8h, max 800 mg per dose; *Adolescents and adults:* 800 mg PO q8h.

Supplied: Capsules 100 mg, 200 mg, 333 mg, 400 mg.

Notes: Use in combination with other antiretroviral agents. Should be taken on an empty stomach. May cause nephrolithiasis. Advise patient to drink six 8-oz glasses of water per day. Numerous drug interactions. Adjust dose in patients with hepatic impairment.

INDOMETHACIN (INDOCIN)

Indications: Inflammatory diseases and rheumatoid disorders; moderate pain; gout; IV form for patent ductus arteriosus (PDA) closure in neonates.

Actions: NSAID.

Dosage: *Neonates:* *PDA closure:* Initial 0.2 mg/kg IV followed by 2 doses of 0.1–0.25 mg/kg given 12 hours apart, depending on postnatal age.
Children ≥ 2 years: *Anti-inflammatory:* 1–2 mg/kg/day PO 2–4 times daily, max dose 150–200 mg/day.
Adults: 25–50 mg per dose PO 2–3 times daily, max dose 200 mg/day.

Supplied: Capsules 25 mg, 50 mg; sustained-release capsule 75 mg; powder for injection 1 mg; suspension 25 mg/5 mL.

Notes: Administer with food. Sustained-release capsules should be swallowed whole. Use with caution in patients with a history of GI bleeding.

INFLIXIMAB (REMICADE)

Indications: Moderate to severe Crohn disease; rheumatoid arthritis (in combination with methotrexate).

Actions: IgG1κ neutralizes biologic activity of tumor necrosis factor-α.

Dosage: *Crohn disease:* 5 mg/kg IV infusion, may follow with subsequent doses given at 2 and 6 weeks after initial infusion.
Rheumatoid arthritis: 3 mg/kg IV infusion at 0, 2, and 6 weeks, followed by every 8 weeks.

Supplied: Injection 100 mg.

Notes: May cause hypersensitivity reaction; made up of human constant and murine variable regions. Patients are predisposed to infection. Active tuberculosis may develop soon after initiating therapy with infliximab. Screening for latent tuberculosis before initiation of therapy is recommended. *Influenza Vaccine (Fluzone, Fluogen, FluShield, Fluvirin) (see Appendix D, p. 759)*
Insulin (see Table VIII–1, p. 750)

Indications: Type 1 and type 2 diabetes mellitus that cannot be controlled by diet or oral hypoglycemic agents; adjunct in management of acute life-threatening hyperkalemia.

Actions: Insulin supplementation.

Dosage: Children and adults: 0.5–1 unit/kg/day SQ, IV, or IM (only regular insulin can be given IV) in divided doses; *Adolescents:* 0.8–1.2 units/kg/day.

Diabetic ketoacidosis: 0.1 unit/kg IV load followed by 0.05–0.2 unit/kg/h continuous infusion.

Supplied: See Table VIII–1, p. 744.

Notes: The highly purified insulins provide an increase in free insulin. Monitor patients closely for several weeks when changing doses. Adjust dose in patients with renal impairment.

IPECAC SYRUP*

Indications: To induce vomiting in treatment of drug overdose and certain cases of poisoning.

Actions: Irritation of GI mucosa; stimulation of chemoreceptor trigger zone.

Dosage: Infants 6–12 months: 5–10 mL PO, followed by 120–240 mL water, if no emesis occurs within 20 minutes, may repeat 1 time; *Adolescents and adults:* 15–30 mL PO, followed by 200–300 mL of water, if no emesis occurs in 20 minutes, may repeat 1 time.

Supplied: Syrup 70 mg/mL.

Notes: Do not use for ingestion of petroleum distillates or strong acid, base, or other corrosive or caustic agents. Not for use in comatose or unconscious patients. Use with caution in patients with CNS depressant overdose. Routine use in emergency department has been abandoned unless patient presents within 60 minutes of ingestion.

IPRATROPIUM (ATROVENT)

Indications: Bronchospasm associated with chronic obstructive pulmonary disease, bronchitis, and emphysema; rhinorrhea.

Actions: Synthetic anticholinergic agent similar to atropine.

Dosage: Nebulization: Children < 12 years: 250 mcg q20 min for 3 doses for acute asthma exacerbation then q2–4h; *Children > 12 years and* *adults:* 500 mcg q30min for 3 doses for acute asthma exacerbation then q2–4h prn.

   Metered-dose inhaler: 4–8 puffs prn for acute exacerbations, then 1–2 puffs 3 times daily, max 6 puffs per day.

   Nasal: 2 sprays in each nostril 2–4 times daily.

Supplied: Metered-dose inhaler 18 mcg per dose; solution for nebulization 0.02%; nasal spray 0.03%, 0.06%.

Notes: Not for initial treatment of acute episodes of bronchospasm.

IRON DEXTRAN (DEXFERRUM, INFED) (SEE MINERALS, P. 740)
IRON SUCROSE (VENOFER) (SEE MINERALS, P. 740)
ISONIAZID (INH)

Indications: Treatment and prophylaxis of *Mycobacterium* infections.

Actions: Bactericidal; interferes with mycolic acid synthesis, thus disrupting bacterial cell wall.

Dosage: *Active tuberculosis (TB): Infants and children:* 10–15 mg/kg/day PO or IM in 1–2 divided doses, max dose 300 mg/day; *Adults:* 5 mg/kg/24 h PO or IM once daily, max 300 mg/day.

   Prophylaxis: Infants and children: 10 mg/kg/day PO once daily; *Adults:* 300 mg PO once daily for 6–12 months.

Supplied: Tablets 100 mg, 300 mg; syrup 50 mg/5 mL; injection 100 mg/mL.

Notes: Can cause severe hepatitis. Given with other antituberculous drugs for active TB; consult MMWR for latest recommendations on treatment and prophylaxis of TB. Prophylaxis is usually with INH alone, and treatment for active TB includes INH plus two or three other antituberculous drugs pending drug sensitivity results. IM route is rarely used. To prevent peripheral neuropathy, can give pyridoxine 50–100 mg/day. Adjust dose in patients with hepatic impairment.

ISOPROTERENOL (ISUPREL, MEDIHALER-ISO)

Indications: Shock; cardiac arrest; AV nodal block.

Actions: β_1- and β_2-Receptor stimulant.

Dosage: *Shock: Infants and children:* 0.05–0.2 mcg/kg/min IV infusion; *Adults:* 2–20 mcg/min titrate to effect.

Supplied: Injection 0.02 mg/mL, 0.2 mg/mL.

Notes: Contraindications include tachycardia. Pulse > 130 beats/min may induce ventricular arrhythmias.

ISOTRETINOIN (13-CIS RETINOIC ACID) (ACCUTANE)

Indications: Severe acne unresponsive to conventional therapy.

Actions: Retinoic acid derivative.

Dosage: 0.5–2 mg/kg/day PO divided twice daily.

Supplied: Capsules 10 mg, 20 mg, 40 mg.

Notes: Contraindicated in pregnancy and lactation. Isolated reports of depression, psychosis, and suicidal thoughts. Adjust dose in patients with hepatic impairment.

ITRACONAZOLE (SPORANOX)

Indications: Systemic fungal infections caused by *Aspergillus, Blastomyces,* and *Histoplasma.*

Actions: Inhibits synthesis of ergosterol.

Dosage: Children: 3–10 mg/kg/day PO once daily; *Adults:* 200 mg PO or IV 1–2 times daily.

Supplied: Capsule 100 mg; solution 10 mg/mL; injection 10 mg/mL.

Notes: Administer with meals or cola. Should not be used concurrently with H_2-antagonist, omeprazole, antacids; numerous other drug interactions (a potent CYP3A4 inhibitor). Advise patient to avoid grapefruit juice. Watch for signs and symptoms of congestive heart failure with IV use. Not recommended for use when creatinine clearance < 30 mL/min.

KAOLIN AND PECTIN (KAODENE, KAO-SPEN, KAPECTOLIN)*

Indications: Diarrhea.

Actions: Adsorbent demulcent.

Dosage: Children 3–6 years: 15–30 mL PO prn after each bowel movement (BM); *Children 6–12 years:* 30–60 mL PO prn after each BM; *Adults:* 60–120 mL PO after each BM or q3–4h prn.

Supplied: Multiple OTC forms.

Notes: Also available with opium (Parepectolin).

KETAMINE (KETALAR)

Indications: Anesthesia; short surgical procedures; dressing changes.

Actions: Dissociative anesthetic.

Dosage: Children: 6–10 mg/kg PO mixed in cola or other beverage 30 minutes prior to procedure, or 3–7 mg/kg IM, or 0.5–2 mg/kg IV, or 5–20 mcg/kg/min continuous IV infusion; *Adults:* 3–8 mg/kg IM or 1–4.5 mg/kg IV.

Supplied: Injection 10 mg/mL, 50 mg/mL, 100 mg/mL.

Notes: Supplemental doses may be given at $^1/_3$—$^1/_2$ of initial dose. May impair mental alertness for up to 24 hours postdose.

KETOCONAZOLE (NIZORAL)

Indications: Systemic fungal infections (candidiasis, chronic mucocutaneous candidiasis, blastomycosis, coccidioidomycosis, histoplasmosis, and paracoccidioidomycosis); topical cream for localized fungal infections due to dermatophytes and yeast.

Actions: Inhibits fungal cell wall synthesis.

Dosage: Infants and children: 3.3–6.6 mg/kg/day PO once daily; *Adults:* 200–400 mg PO once daily.
   Shampoo: Twice weekly at least 3 days apart for 4 weeks.
   Topical: Apply to affected area 1–2 times daily.

Supplied: Tablet 200 mg; topical cream 2%; shampoo 1%.

Notes: Systemic use is associated with hepatotoxicity; monitor liver function tests. Avoid concurrent use with any agent that increases gastric pH (preventing absorption of ketoconazole). Avoid concurrent use with cisapride. Ketoconazole may enhance activity of oral anticoagulants; may react with alcohol to produce a disulfiram-like reaction; and has numerous other drug interactions.

KETOROLAC (TORADOL)

Indications: Moderate to severe pain.

Actions: NSAID.

Dosage: Children 2–16 years: 0.5 mg/kg per dose IV or IM q6h; *Adults:* 30–60 mg IM or IV as single dose or 30 mg IV or IM q6h, max 120 mg/day or 20 mg PO, then 10 mg PO q4–6h, max 40 mg/day.

Supplied: Tablet 10 mg; injection 15 mg/mL, 30 mg/mL.

Notes: Do not exceed adult doses in children. Adjust dose in patients with renal impairment. *Do not* exceed 5 days total use.

LABETALOL (TRANDATE, NORMODYNE)

Indications: Hypertension and hypertensive emergencies.

Actions: α- and β-Adrenergic blocking agent.

Dosage: Children: Hypertension: 3–4 mg/kg/day PO divided twice daily, up to 40 mg/kg/day or 0.2–0.5 mg/kg per dose IV, max 20 mg per dose; *Hypertensive emergency:* 0.4–1 mg/kg/h IV continuous infusion, max 3 mg/kg/h.
   Adults: Hypertension: Initial dose 100 mg PO twice daily; then 200–400 mg PO twice daily; *Hypertensive emergency:* 20–80 mg IV bolus, then 2 mg/min IV infusion, titrated to effect.

Supplied: Tablets 100 mg, 200 mg, 300 mg; injection 5 mg/mL.

Notes: May cause dry mouth. *Do not* abruptly discontinue. May mask signs of diabetes mellitus.

LACTIC ACID AND AMMONIUM HYDROXIDE [AMMONIUM LACTATE] (LAC-HYDRIN)*

Indications: Severe xerosis and ichthyosis.

Actions: Emollient moisturizer.

Dosage: Apply twice daily.

Supplied: Lactic acid 12% with ammonium hydroxide.

LACTOBACILLUS ACIDOPHILUS AND LACTOBACILLUS BULGARICUS (LACTINEX GRANULES)*

Indications: Control of diarrhea, especially after antibiotic therapy.

Actions: Replaces normal intestinal flora.

Dosage: 1 packet, 2 capsules, or 4 tablets with meals or liquids 3–4 times daily.

Supplied: Tablet; capsule; enteric-coated capsule; powder in packets.
Lactulose (Chronulac, Cephulac)

Indications: Hepatic encephalopathy; laxative.

Actions: Acidifies colon, allowing ammonia to diffuse into colon.

Dosage: Acute hepatic encephalopathy: Infants: 2.5–10 mL/day PO divided 3–4 times daily; *Children:* 40–90 mL/day PO divided 3–4 times daily; *Adults:* 30–45 mL PO q1h until soft stools are observed, then 3–4 times daily.
   Constipation: Children: 7.5 mL/day PO after breakfast; *Adults:* 15–30 mL/day PO; adjust dosage every 1–2 days to produce 2–3 soft stools daily.
   Rectal: 200 g diluted with 700 mL of water instilled into rectum.

Supplied: Syrup 10 g/15 mL.

Notes: Adjust doses to produce 2–3 soft stools per day. Can cause severe diarrhea and life-threatening hypernatremia with an excessive number of stools per day.

LAMIVUDINE (EPIVIR, EPIVIR-HBV)

Indications: Treatment of HIV infection when therapy is warranted based on clinical or immunologic evidence of disease progression, or both; chronic hepatitis B.

Actions: Inhibits HIV reverse transcriptase, resulting in viral DNA chain termination.

Dosage: HIV: Neonates: 2 mg/kg PO twice daily; *Infants and children:* 4 mg/kg PO twice daily, max 150 mg per dose; *Adolescents and adults:* 150 mg PO twice daily or 300 mg PO daily.
   Hepatitis B: 100 mg once daily.

Supplied: Tablets 100 mg, 150 mg; solution 5 mg/mL, 10 mg/mL.

Notes: Used in combination with zidovudine. Adjust dose in patients with renal dysfunction.

LAMOTRIGINE (LAMICTAL)

Indications: Partial seizures.

Actions: Phenyltriazine antiepileptic.

Dosage: Dose depends on patient's concomitant antiepileptic drug (AED) including valproic acid (VPA) and enzyme-inducing agents (phenytoin, phenobarbital, primidone, carbamazepine).

Patients on AED regimens with VPA:

- *Children 2–12 years:* 0.15 mg/kg/day PO divided 1–2 times daily for 2 weeks, then 0.3 mg/kg/day for 2 weeks, then titrate to effect every 1–2 weeks to maintenance of 1–5 mg/kg/day, max 200 mg/day.

- *Children > 12 years and adults:* 25 mg PO every other day for 2 weeks, then 25 mg daily for 2 weeks, then titrate to effect every 1–2 weeks to maintenance of 100–400 mg/day.

Patients on enzyme-inducing AED without VPA:

- *Children 2–12 years:* 0.6 mg/kg/day PO divided twice daily for 2 weeks, then 1.2 mg/kg/day for 2 weeks, then titrate to effect every 1–2 weeks to maintenance of 5–15 mg/kg/day, max 400 mg/day.
- *Children > 12 years and adults:* 50 mg PO daily for 2 weeks, then 50 mg twice daily for 2 weeks, then titrate to effect every 1–2 weeks to maintenance of 300–500 mg/day.

Monotherapy: Children > 16 years and adults: 50 mg PO once daily, followed by 50 mg twice daily for 2 weeks, then maintenance of 500 mg/day in two divided doses.

Supplied: Tablets 25 mg, 100 mg, 150 mg, 200 mg; chewable tablets 2 mg, 5 mg, 25 mg.

Notes: Only whole tablets should be used for dosing; round dose down to the nearest whole tab. May cause photosensitivity and rash severe enough to warrant drug discontinuance. Value of therapeutic monitoring has not been established. Interacts with other antiepileptics. Reduce dose in patients with hepatic impairment.

LANSOPRAZOLE (PREVACID)

Indications: Gastroesophageal reflux disease; duodenal ulcer; erosive esophagitis; hypersecretory conditions (Zollinger-Ellison syndrome); *Helicobacter pylori*–associated gastritis.

Actions: Proton pump inhibitor.

Dosage: Children 3 months to 12 years: 0.5–1.6 mg/kg PO daily; *Children > 12 years and adults:* 15–60 mg PO daily.

Supplied: Delayed-release capsules 15 mg, 30 mg; granules for suspension 15 mg, 30 mg.

Notes: Adjust dose in patients with severe hepatic impairment. Patients with hypersecretory conditions may need higher twice daily dosing. *Do not* crush or chew granules.

LEVETIRACETAM (KEPPRA)

Indications: Partial-onset seizures.

Actions: Unknown.

Dosage: 500 mg PO twice daily, may be increased to max of 3000 mg/day.

Supplied: Tablets 250 mg, 500 mg, 750 mg.

Notes: May cause dizziness and somnolence; may impair coordination. Requires renal dosage adjustment.

LEVOFLOXACIN (LEVAQUIN)

Indications: Lower respiratory tract infections; sinusitis; UTIs.

Actions: Quinolone antibiotic; inhibits DNA gyrase.

Dosage: Children: 5–10 mg/kg/day PO or IV once daily, max 500 mg per dose; *Adults:* 250–500 mg PO or IV once daily, max dose 1 g/day.

Supplied: Tablets 250 mg, 500 mg, 750 mg; injection 5 mg/mL, 25 mg/mL.

Notes: Reliable activity against *Streptococcus pneumoniae.* Drug interactions with cation-containing products. Requires renal dosage adjustment.

LEVOTHYROXINE (SYNTHROID)

Indications: Hypothyroidism.

Actions: Supplementation of L-thyroxine.

Dosage: Oral:
- *Infants ≤ 6 months:* 8–10 mcg/kg or 25–50 mcg/day.
- *Infants 6–12 months:* 6–8 mcg/kg or 50–75 mcg/day.
- *Children 1–5 years:* 5–6 mcg/kg or 75–100 mcg/day.
- *Children 6–12 years:* 4–5 mcg/kg or 100–150 mcg/day.
- *Children and adolescents > 12 years:* 2–3 mcg/kg or > 150 mcg/day.
- *Adults:* Initial dose 25–50 mcg/day; increase by 25–50 mcg/day every month; usual dose 100–200 mcg/day.

Supplied: Tablets 25 mcg, 50 mcg, 75 mcg, 88 mcg, 100 mcg, 112 mcg, 125 mcg, 137 mcg, 150 mcg, 175 mcg, 200 mcg, 300 mcg; injection 200 mcg, 500 mcg.

Notes: Titrate dosage based on clinical response and thyroid function tests. Intravenous or intramuscular dose is 50–75% of oral dose.

LIDOCAINE (ANESTACON TOPICAL, XYLOCAINE, OTHERS)

Indications: Local anesthetic; treatment of cardiac arrhythmias.

Actions: Anesthetic; class IB antiarrhythmic.

Dosage: Antiarrhythmic: Endotracheal: 5 mg/kg; follow with 0.5 mg/kg in 10 minutes if effective.

Intravenous: Load 1 mg/kg per dose bolus over 2–3 minutes; repeat in 5–10 minutes up to 200–300 mg/h; continuous infusion of 20–50 mcg/kg/min or 1–4 mg/min.

Topical: Apply to affected area prn, *do not* repeat within 2 hours, max 3 mg/kg per dose.

Local injection anesthetic: Dose varies with procedure, max 4.5 mg/kg.

Supplied: Injection (local) 0.5%, 1%, 1.5%, 2%, 4 %, 10%, 20%; injection IV 1% (10 mg/mL), 2% (20 mg/mL); admixture 4%, 10%, 20%; IV infusion 0.2%, 0.4%; cream 2%; gel 2%, 2.5%; ointment 2.5%, 5%; liquid 2.5%; solution 2%, 4%; viscous 2%.

Notes: Dilute endotracheal doses to 1–2 mL with NS. Epinephrine may be added for local anesthesia to prolong effect and help decrease bleeding. *Do not* use lidocaine with epinephrine on digits, ears, or nose because vasoconstriction may cause necrosis. For IV forms, dosage reduction is required with liver disease or congestive heart failure. Dizziness, paresthesias, and convulsions are associated with toxicity.

LIDOCAINE AND PRILOCAINE (EMLA)

Indications: Topical anesthetic; adjunct to phlebotomy or invasive dermal procedures.

Actions: Topical anesthetic.

Dosage: Cream and anesthetic disc (1 g/10 cm²): Apply thick layer of cream 2–2.5 g to intact skin and cover with occlusive dressing (Tegaderm) for at least 1 hour.

Anesthetic disc: 1 g per 10 cm² for at least 1 hour.

Supplied: Cream 2.5% lidocaine/2.5% prilocaine; anesthetic disc (1 g).

Notes: Not for use on mucous membranes or eyes. Use with caution in patients at risk of methemoglobinemia. Longer contact time gives greater effect.

LINDANE (KWELL)

Indications: Eradication of head lice, crab lice, and scabies.

Actions: Ectoparasiticide and ovicide.

Dosage: Lotion: Apply thin layer after bathing and leave in place for 8–12 hours, pour on laundry.

Shampoo: Apply 15–30 mL and lather with warm water for 4 minutes; comb out nits.

Supplied: Lotion 1%; shampoo 1%.

Notes: Caution patient about overuse. Drug may be absorbed into blood. *Do not* repeat sooner than 7 days if necessary. *Do not* apply lotion immediately after hot bath.

LINEZOLID (ZYVOX)

Indications: Infections caused by gram-positive bacteria, including vancomycin-resistant and methicillin-resistant strains.

Actions: Inhibits bacterial protein synthesis.

Dosage: *Children:* 10 mg/kg per dose IV or PO q12h; *Adults:* 400–600 mg IV or PO q12h.

Supplied: Injection 2 mg/mL; tablets 400 mg, 600 mg; suspension 100 mg/ 5 mL.

Notes: Reversible inhibitor of MAO; avoid foods that contain tyramine. Avoid cough and cold products containing pseudoephedrine. Myelosuppression may occur; monitor CBC weekly.

LITHIUM CARBONATE (ESKALITH, OTHERS)

Indications: Manic episodes of manic-depressive illness; maintenance therapy in recurrent disease.

Actions: Effects shift toward intraneuronal metabolism of catecholamines.

Dosage: *Children:* 15–60 mg/kg/day PO divided 3–4 times daily; *Adults:* 600 mg PO 3 times daily or 900 mg sustained-release tablets twice daily. *Maintenance:* 300 mg PO 3–4 times daily.

Supplied: Capsules 150 mg, 300 mg, 600 mg; tablet 300 mg; sustained-release tablets 300 mg, 450 mg; syrup 300 mg/5 mL.

Notes: Dosage must be titrated; therapeutic levels 0.6–1.2 mEq/L. Common side effects are polyuria and tremor. Adjust dose in patients with renal impairment. Sodium retention or diuretic use may potentiate toxicity.

LOPERAMIDE (IMODIUM)*

Indications: Diarrhea.

Actions: Slows intestinal motility.

Dosage: *Children:* Initial 1–2 mg PO, then 0.1 mg/kg per dose prn after each loose stool, but not to exceed initial dosage; *Adults:* Initial 4 mg PO; then 2 mg after each loose stool, up to 16 mg/day.

Supplied: Capsule 2 mg; tablet 2 mg; liquid 1 mg/5 mL.

Notes: Do not use in acute diarrhea caused by *Salmonella, Shigella,* or *Clostridium difficile.*

LORATADINE (CLARITIN)*

Indications: Allergic rhinitis.

Actions: Nonsedating antihistamine.

Dosage: Children 2–5 years: 5 mg PO daily; *Children ≥ 6 years and adults:* 10 mg PO daily.

Supplied: Tablet 10 mg; syrup 1 mg/mL.

Notes: Should be taken on an empty stomach.

LORAZEPAM (ATIVAN, OTHERS) [C]

Indications: Anxiety; preoperative sedation; control of status epilepticus; antiemetic.

Actions: Benzodiazepine; antianxiety agent.

Dosage: Anxiety: Children: 0.05 mg/kg per dose PO and IV q4–8h, max 2 mg per dose; *Adults:* 1–10 mg/day PO in 2–3 divided doses.
    Preoperative sedation: Children and adults: 0.02–0.05 mg/kg IV, IM, or PO, max dose 2–4 mg.
    Insomnia: Adults: 2–4 mg PO at bedtime.
    Status epilepticus: Infants and children: 0.1 mg/kg slow IV over 2–5 minutes, max 4 mg per dose, may repeat dose at 0.05 mg/kg in 10–15 minutes if needed; *Adults:* 4 mg per dose IV may be repeated at 10- to 15-minute intervals; usual total dose 8 mg.
    Antiemetic: Children: 0.04–0.08 mg/kg per dose IV q6h prn, max 4 mg per dose; *Adults:* 0.5–2 mg IV or PO q4–6h prn.

Supplied: Tablets 0.5 mg, 1 mg, 2 mg; solution, oral concentrate 2 mg/mL; injection 2 mg/mL, 4 mg/mL.

Notes: Do not administer intravenously faster than 2 mg/min or 0.05 mg/kg/min. Effects of drug may not be apparent for as long as 10 minutes when given intravenously. Avoid abrupt discontinuance.

MAGNESIUM HYDROXIDE (MILK OF MAGNESIA)*

Indications: Constipation.

Actions: Saline laxative.

Dosage: Children < 2 years: 0.5 mL/kg per dose PO; *Children 2–5 years:* 5–15 mL or 311–622 mg (1–2 tablets) PO once or in divided doses; *Children ≥ 6 years:* 15–30 mL or 933–1244 mg (3–4 tablets) PO prn; *Adults:* 30–60 mL or 1866–2488 mg (6–8 tablets) PO prn.

Supplied: Tablet 311 mg; liquid 400 mg/5 mL, 800 mg/5 mL.

Notes: *Do not* use in patients with renal insufficiency or intestinal obstruction.

MAGNESIUM OXIDE (MAG-OX 400, OTHERS)

Indications: Replacement for low plasma levels.

Actions: Magnesium supplementation.

Dosage: Children: 10–20 mg/kg elemental magnesium per dose PO 4 times daily; *Adults:* 400–800 mg magnesium oxide per day divided 1–4 times daily.

Supplied: Capsule 140 mg (84 mg elemental mag); tablet 400 mg (242 elemental mag).

Notes: May cause diarrhea. *Do not* use in patients with renal insufficiency or intestinal obstruction.

MAGNESIUM SULFATE

Indications: Replacement for low plasma levels; refractory hypokalemia and hypocalcemia.

Actions: Magnesium supplement.

Dosage: Children: 25–50 mg/kg per dose IV or IM q4–6h for 3–4 doses, max 2 g per dose; *Adults:* 1–2 g IM or IV; repeat dosing based on response and continued hypomagnesemia.

Supplied: Injection 10 mg/mL, 20 mg/mL, 40 mg/mL, 80 mg/mL, 125 mg/mL, 500 mg/mL.

Notes: Reduce dose in patients with low urine output or renal insufficiency.

MANNITOL

Indications: Cerebral edema; oliguria; anuria; myoglobinuria.

Actions: Osmotic diuretic.

Dosage: Children and adults: Initial 0.5–1 g/kg per dose IV over 3–5 minutes then 0.25–0.5 g/kg IV q4–6h.

Cerebral edema: 0.25 g/kg per dose IV push, repeated at 5-minute intervals prn; increase incrementally to 1 g/kg per dose prn for increased intracranial pressure.

Supplied: Injection 5%, 10%, 15%, 20%, 25%.

Notes: Use with caution in patients with congestive heart failure or volume overload.

MEDROXYPROGESTERONE (PROVERA, DEPO PROVERA)

Indications: Secondary amenorrhea and abnormal uterine bleeding caused by hormonal imbalance; contraception.

Actions: Progestin supplement.

Dosage: *Secondary amenorrhea:* 5–10 mg PO daily for 5–10 days.
Abnormal uterine bleeding: 5–10 mg PO daily for 5–10 days beginning on 16th or 21st day of menstrual cycle.
Contraception: 150 mg IM every 3 months.

Supplied: Tablets 2.5 mg, 5 mg, 10 mg; Depo-injection 150 mg/mL, 400 mg/mL.

Notes: Contraindicated in patients with histories of past thromboembolic disorders or hepatic disease. If used for contraception, obtain pregnancy test if last injection was more than 3 months ago.

MEGESTROL ACETATE (MEGACE)

Indications: Breast and endometrial cancers; appetite stimulant in patients with cancer and HIV-related cachexia.

Actions: Hormone; progesterone analogue.

Dosage: *Cancer:* 40–320 mg/day PO in divided doses.
Appetite regulation: 800 mg PO daily.

Supplied: Tablets 20 mg, 40 mg; solution 40 mg/mL.

Notes: May induce deep venous thrombosis. *Do not* abruptly discontinue therapy.

MELPHALAN (ALKERAN, L-PAM)

Indications: Multiple myeloma; breast cancer; testicular cancer; ovarian cancer; melanoma; allogenic and autologous bone marrow transplantation (BMT) in high doses.

Actions: Antineoplastic alkylating agent.

Dosage: Refer to individual protocols.

Supplied: Tablet 2 mg; powder for injection 50 mg.

Notes: Toxicity includes myelosuppression (leukopenia and thrombocytopenia), secondary leukemia, alopecia, dermatitis, stomatitis, and pulmonary fibrosis; very rare hypersensitivity reactions.

MEPERIDINE (DEMEROL) [C]

Indications: Moderate to severe pain.

Actions: Narcotic analgesic.

Dosage: *Children:* 1–1.5 mg/kg per dose IV, IM, SQ, or PO q3–4h prn, max 100 mg per dose; *Adults:* 50–150 mg IV, IM, SQ, or PO q3–4h prn; *Continuous infusion:* 0.5–1 mg/kg IV load then 0.3 mg/kg/h, may titrate to 0.7 mg/kg/h.

Supplied: Tablets 50 mg, 100 mg; syrup 50 mg/mL; injection 10 mg/mL, 25 mg/mL, 50 mg/mL, 75 mg/mL, 100 mg/mL.

Notes: Meperidine 75 mg IM = 10 mg of morphine IM. Beware of respiratory depression. Reduces seizure threshold. Normeperidine (active metabolite) may accumulate in patients with renal failure; reduce dose with renal impairment.

MERCAPTOPURINE (6-MP) (PURINETHOL)

Indications: Acute leukemias; second-line treatment of chronic myelogenous leukemia and non-Hodgkin lymphoma; immunosuppressant therapy for autoimmune diseases (Crohn disease).

Actions: Antineoplastic antimetabolite; mimics hypoxanthine.

Dosage: Refer to individual protocols.

Supplied: Tablet 50 mg.

Notes: Toxicity includes mild hematologic toxicity; GI toxicity is uncommon, except mucositis, stomatitis, and diarrhea. Rash, fever, eosinophilia, jaundice, and hepatitis have been reported. Concurrent allopurinol therapy requires a 67–75% dose reduction of 6-MP because of interference with metabolism by xanthine oxidase.

MEROPENEM (MERREM)

Indications: Serious infections caused by a wide variety of bacteria, including intra-abdominal and polymicrobic; bacterial meningitis.

Actions: Carbapenem; inhibition of cell wall synthesis.

Dosage: Children > 3 months: 60 mg/kg/day IV divided q8h; *Meningitis:* 120 mg/kg/day IV divided q8h.
    Adults: 1 g IV q8h.

Supplied: Injection 500 mg, 1 g.

Notes: Adjust dose in patients with impaired renal function. Has less seizure potential than imipenem.

MESALAMINE (ROWASA, ASACOL, PENTASA)

Indications: Mild to moderate distal ulcerative colitis; proctosigmoiditis; proctitis.

Actions: Unknown; may topically inhibit prostaglandins.

Dosage: Capsule: Children: 50 mg/kg/day PO divided q6–12h; *Adults:* 1 g PO 4 times daily for up to 8 weeks.
    Tablet: Children: 50 mg/kg/day PO divided q8–12h; *Adults:* 800 mg PO 3 times daily for up to 6 months.
    Retention enema: Adults: 60 mL PR at bedtime, retained overnight or insert 1 suppository twice daily.

Supplied: Delayed-release enteric-coated tablet 400 mg; controlled-release capsule 250 mg; suppository 500 mg; rectal suspension 4 g/60 mL.

Notes: May discolor urine yellow-brown; may cause pancreatitis.

MESNA (MESNEX)

Indications: Reduction of incidence of ifosfamide- and cyclophosphamide-induced hemorrhagic cystitis.

Actions: Binds to urotoxic metabolites of ifosfamide and cyclophosphamide in bladder.

Dosage: 20% (w/w) of ifosfamide dose or cyclophosphamide dose IV at 15 minutes prior to and 4 and 8 hours after chemotherapy; *Continuous infusion:* 60–100% of ifosfamide or cyclophosphamide dose; *Oral:* 40% (w/w) of antineoplastic agent q4h for 3 doses or 20 mg/kg per dose q4h for 3 doses.

Supplied: Tablet 400 mg; injection 100 mg/mL.

Metformin (Glucophage)

Indications: Type 2 diabetes mellitus.

Actions: Decreases hepatic glucose production; decreases intestinal absorption of glucose; improves insulin sensitivity.

Dosage: Children > 10 years and adults: Initial dose of 500 mg PO twice daily; dose may be increased to max daily dose of 2500 mg. *Extended-release:* 500–2000 mg PO q PM.

Supplied: Tablets 500 mg, 850 mg, 1000 mg; extended-release tablet 500 mg.

Notes: Administer with morning and evening meals. May cause lactic acidosis. *Do not use metformin* if serum creatinine is > 1.3 in females or > 1.4 in males. Withhold prior to and following IV contrast studies. Contraindicated in hypoxemic conditions, including acute congestive heart failure and sepsis.

METHADONE (DOLOPHINE) [C]

Indications: Severe pain; detoxification and maintenance of narcotic addiction.

Actions: Narcotic analgesic.

Dosage: Children: 0.1 mg/kg per dose IV, IM, SQ, or PO q4h for 2–3 doses, then q6–12h prn, max 10 mg per dose; *Adults:* 5–10 mg IM q3–8h or 5–15 mg PO q8h; titrate as needed.

Supplied: Tablets 5 mg, 10 mg, 40 mg; oral solution 5 mg/5 mL, 10 mg/5 mL; oral concentrate 10 mg/mL; injection 10 mg/mL.

Notes: Equianalgesic with parenteral morphine. Has long half-life. Increase dose slowly to avoid respiratory depression. Dose must be individualized when used for iatrogenic narcotic dependency.

METHOTREXATE (FOLEX, RHEUMATREX)

Indications: Acute lymphoblastic and myelogenous leukemias; leukemic meningitis; trophoblastic tumors (chorioepithelioma, choriocarcinoma, chorioadenoma destruens, hydatidiform mole); breast cancer; Burkitt lymphoma; mycosis fungoides; osteosarcoma; head and neck cancers; Hodgkin and non-Hodgkin lymphoma; lung cancer; psoriasis; rheumatoid arthritis.

Actions: Inhibits dihydrofolate reductase–mediated generation of tetrahydrofolate.

Dosage: Cancer: Refer to specific protocol.

Rheumatoid arthritis: 5–15 mg/m^2/wk PO, IM, or SQ as single dose each week or give in 3 divided doses 12 hours apart each week.

Supplied: Tablets 2.5 mg, 5 mg, 7.5 mg, 10 mg; injection 25 mg/mL; preservative-free injection 25 mg/mL; powder for injection 20 mg, 1 g.

Notes: Toxicity includes myelosuppression, nausea and vomiting, anorexia, mucositis, diarrhea, hepatotoxicity (transient and reversible; may progress to atrophy, necrosis, fibrosis, cirrhosis), rashes, dizziness, malaise, blurred vision, renal failure, pneumonitis, and, rarely, pulmonary fibrosis. Chemical arachnoiditis and headache may occur with intrathecal delivery. High-dose therapy requires leucovorin rescue to prevent severe hematologic and mucosal toxicity. Monitor blood counts and methotrexate levels carefully. Adjust dose in patients with renal failure.

METHYLPHENIDATE (RITALIN, CONCERTA)

Indications: Attention-deficit/hyperactivity disorder.

Actions: CNS stimulant; blocks reuptake mechanism of dopaminergic neurons.

Dosage: Immediate release: Children > 6 years: Initial 2.5–5 mg per dose PO before breakfast and lunch, increase by 5–10 mg/day at weekly intervals, max 60 mg/day.

Concerta: Children > 6 years: Initial 18 mg PO daily, may increase by 18 mg/day at weekly intervals, max 54 mg/day.

Supplied: Immediate-release tablets 5 mg, 10 mg, 20 mg; extended-release capsules 20 mg, 30 mg, 40 mg; sustained-release tablet 20 mg; extended-release tablets 10 mg, 18 mg, 20 mg, 27 mg, 36 mg, 54 mg.

Notes: Sustained-release and extended-release tablets may be given in place of immediate-release tablets once daily dose is titrated; some patients may require a 4 PM dose.

METHYLPREDNISOLONE (SOLU-MEDROL)

Indications: Anti-inflammatory or immunosuppressant agent.

Actions: Adrenal corticosteroid.

Dosage: Children:

- *Anti-inflammatory or immunosuppressive:* 0.5–1.7 mg/kg/day PO, IM, or IV divided q6–12h.
- *Pulse therapy:* 15–30 mg/kg per dose IV over ≥ 30 minutes once daily for 3 days.

- *Status asthmaticus:* Initial 2 mg/kg per dose then 0.5–1 mg/kg per dose IV q6h.
- *Lupus nephritis:* 30 mg/kg IV over ≥ 30 minutes every other day for 6 doses.
- *Acute spinal cord injury:* 30 mg/kg IV over 15 minutes then follow in 45 minutes with a continuous infusion of 5.4 mg/kg/h IV for 23 hours.

Adults: 2–60 mg/day PO in 1–4 divided doses or 40–250 mg IV q4–6h.

Supplied: Tablets 2 mg, 4 mg, 8 mg, 16 mg, 32 mg; injection as sodium succinate 40 mg, 125 mg, 500 mg, 1 g, 2 g; suspension for injection as acetate (Depo-Medrol) 20 mg/mL, 40 mg/mL, 80 mg/mL.

Notes: Only the sodium succinate injection may be given IV.

METOCLOPRAMIDE (REGLAN)

Indications: Gastroesophageal reflux disease (GERD); Cancer chemotherapy-induced nausea and vomiting.

Actions: Stimulates motility of upper GI tract and blocks dopamine in chemoreceptor trigger zone.

Dosage: *GERD: Children:* 0.4–0.8 mg/kg/day PO, IM, or IV in 4 divided doses; *Adults:* 10–15 mg PO 30 minutes before meals and bedtime.
  Postoperative nausea and vomiting: Children: 0.1–0.2 mg/kg per dose IV, repeat q6–8h prn; *Children > 14 years and adults:* 10 mg IV, repeat 6–8h prn.
  Chemotherapy-induced emesis: Children and adults: 1–2 mg/kg per dose IV 30 minutes prior to antineoplastic agent, then q2h for 2 doses, then q3h for 3 doses.

Supplied: Tablets 5 mg, 10 mg; syrup 5 mg/5 mL; solution 10 mg/mL; injection 5 mg/mL.

Notes: Dystonic reactions are common with high doses; can be pretreated with IV diphenhydramine. Metoclopramide can also be used to facilitate small bowel intubation and radiologic evaluation of upper GI tract.

METOLAZONE (ZAROXOLYN)

Indications: Mild to moderate essential hypertension; edema of renal disease or cardiac failure.

Actions: Thiazide-like diuretic; inhibits reabsorption of sodium in distal tubules.

Dosage: *Children:* 0.2–0.4 mg/kg/day PO divided q12–24h.
  Adults: Hypertension: 2.5–5 mg PO daily; *Edema:* 5–20 mg PO daily.

Supplied: Tablets 0.5 mg, 2.5 mg, 5 mg, 10 mg.

Notes: Monitor fluid and electrolyte status during treatment.

METRONIDAZOLE (FLAGYL, METROGEL)

Indications: Amebiasis; trichomoniasis; *Clostridium difficile; Helicobacter pylori;* anaerobic infections; bacterial vaginosis.

Actions: Interferes with DNA synthesis.

Dosage: Anaerobic infections: Children: 30 mg/kg/day IV or PO divided q6h; *Adults:* 500 mg IV q6–8h.
    Amebiasis: Children: 35–50 mg/kg/day PO divided q8h; *Adults:* 750 mg PO daily for 5–10 days.
    Parasitic infections: Children: 15–30 mg/kg/day PO divided q8h; *Adults:* 250 mg PO 3 times daily for 7 days or 2 g PO single dose.
    C difficile: Children: 30 mg/kg/day PO divided q6h; *Adults:* 500 mg PO q8h for 7–10 days.
    Bacterial vaginosis: 1 applicatorful intravaginally twice daily or 500 mg PO twice daily for 7 days.
    Topical: Apply twice daily.

Supplied: Tablets 250 mg, 500 mg; extended-release tablet 750 mg; capsule 375 mg; topical lotion and gel 0.75%; vaginal gel 0.75% (5 g per applicator; 37.5 mg in 70-g tube).

Notes: Reduce dose in patients with hepatic failure. Has no activity against aerobic bacteria; use in combination in serious mixed infections. May cause a disulfiram-like reaction; avoid concurrent use of alcohol.

MICONAZOLE (MONISTAT, OTHERS)*

Indications: Topical treatment of vulvovaginal candidiasis and superficial fungal infections.

Actions: Fungicidal; alters permeability of fungal cell membrane.

Dosage: Dermatologic use: Apply to affected area twice daily for 2–4 weeks.
    Intravaginal: Insert 1 applicatorful or suppository at bedtime for 7 days.

Supplied: Topical cream 2%; lotion 2%; powder 2%; spray 2%; vaginal suppository 100 mg, 200 mg; vaginal cream 2%, 4%.
Midazolam (Versed) [C]

Indications: Sedation; anxiolysis; amnesia prior to procedures or before induction of general anesthesia; status epilepticus.

Actions: Short-acting benzodiazepine.

Dosage: Infants and children:

- *Status epilepticus:* 0.15 mg/kg IV load followed by continuous infusion of 1 mcg/kg/min; titrate dose upward q5min until seizures controlled.
- *Sedation preprocedure or prior to induction of anesthesia:* 0.25–0.5 mg/kg PO, max 20 mg per dose.
- *Conscious sedation:* 0.05–0.1 mg/kg IM or IV, max 6 mg per dose.
- *Intranasal:* 0.2 mg/kg may repeat in 5–15 min.

Adults: 1–5 mg IV or IM, titrate to effect.

Supplied: Injection 1 mg/mL, 5 mg/mL; syrup 2 mg/mL.

Notes: Monitor patient for respiratory depression. May produce hypotension in conscious sedation.

MILRINONE (PRIMACOR)

Indications: Congestive heart failure.

Actions: Positive inotrope and vasodilator, with little chronotropic activity.

Dosage: Loading dose of 50 mcg/kg IV over 15 minutes, followed by continuous infusion of 0.375–0.75 mcg/kg/min.

Supplied: Injection 1 mg/mL, premixed in D_5W 200 mcg/mL.

Notes: Carefully monitor fluid and electrolyte status. Adjust dose in patients with renal impairment.

MINERAL OIL (FLEET MINERAL OIL, KONDREMUL)*

Indications: Constipation.

Actions: Emollient laxative.

Dosage: *Children:* 5–15 mL PO daily or 30–60 mL PR as single dose; *Adults:* 5–45 mL PO prn or 60–150 mL/day PR as single dose.

Supplied: Oral, topical, or rectal liquid or oral emulsion 55% (Kondremul).

Notes: Should not be used longer than 1 week.

MINOXIDIL (LONITEN, ROGAINE)

Indications: Severe hypertension; treatment of male- and female-pattern baldness.

Actions: Peripheral vasodilator; stimulates vertex hair growth.

Dosage: Oral: Children: Initial 0.1–0.2 mg/kg per dose once daily, max 5 mg/day, increase gradually every 3 days to usual dose of 0.25–1 mg/kg/day divided 1–2 times daily; *Adults:* 2.5–10 mg 2–4 times daily.
   Topical (Alopecia): Adults: Apply twice daily to affected area.

Supplied: Tablets 2.5 mg, 10 mg; topical solution (Rogaine) 2%*.

Notes: Pericardial and pleural effusions and volume overload may occur with oral use; hypertrichosis after chronic use.

MONTELUKAST (SINGULAIR)

Indications: Prophylaxis and treatment of chronic asthma.

Actions: Leukotriene receptor antagonist.

Dosage: Children 2–5 years: 4 mg/day PO; *Children 6–14 years:* 5 mg/day PO; *Adults:* 10 mg PO daily taken in evening.

Supplied: Tablet 10 mg; chewable tablets 4 mg, 5 mg.

Notes: Not for acute asthma attacks.

MORPHINE SULFATE (ROXANOL, DURAMORPH, MS CONTIN) [C]

Indications: Severe pain.

Actions: Narcotic analgesic.

Dosage: Oral: Infants and children: 0.2–0.5 mg/kg per dose q4–6h prn; *Adults:* 10–30 mg q4h prn; sustained-release tablets 30–60 mg q8–12h.
   Intravenous or intramuscular: Infants and children: 0.1–0.2 mg/kg per dose q2–4h prn; *Adults:* 2–15 mg q2–6h.

Supplied: Tablets or capsules 15 mg, 30 mg; sustained-release tablets 15 mg, 30 mg, 60 mg, 100 mg; extended-release tablets 15 mg, 30 mg 60 mg, 100 mg, 200 mg; oral solution 10 mg/5 ml, 20 mg/5 mL, 20 mg/mL; 100 mg/5 ml; suppositories 5, 10, 20, 30 mg; injection 2 mg/mL, 4 mg/mL, 5 mg/mL, 8 mg/mL, 10 mg/mL, 15 mg/mL, 25 mg/mL; preservative-free injection 0.5 mg/mL, 1 mg/mL.

Notes: Morphine has many narcotic side effects; may require scheduled dosing to relieve severe chronic pain. Duramorph and MS Contin are commonly used sustained-release forms.

MUPIROCIN (BACTROBAN)

Indications: Impetigo; eradication of methicillin-resistant *Staphylococcus aureus* (MRSA) nasal carrier state.

Actions: Inhibits bacterial protein synthesis.

Dosage: *Topical:* Apply small amount to affected area.
  Nasal: Apply twice daily in nostrils.

Supplied: Ointment 2%; cream 2%.

Notes: *Do not* use concurrently with other nasal products.

MUROMONAB-CD3 (ORTHOCLONE OKT3)

Indications: Acute rejection following organ transplantation.

Actions: Blocks T-cell function.

Dosage: *Children < 30 kg:* 2.5 mg IV daily for 10–14 days; *Children > 12 years, ≥ 30 kg, and adults:* 5 mg IV daily for 10–14 days.

Supplied: Injection 5 mg/5 mL.

Notes: Muromonab is a murine antibody; may cause significant fever and chills after first dose. Premedicate with methylprednisolone. Requires close patient monitoring for anaphylaxis or pulmonary edema.

MYCOPHENOLATE MOFETIL (CELLCEPT)

Indications: Prevention of organ rejection following transplantation.

Actions: Inhibits immunologically mediated inflammatory responses.

Dosage: *Children:* 600 mg/m^2 per dose PO twice daily, max 2 g/day; *Adults:* 1 g PO or IV twice daily.

Supplied: Capsule 250 mg; tablet 500 mg; oral suspension 200 mg/mL; injection 500 mg.

Notes: Switch from IV to PO as soon as tolerated. Used in conjunction with corticosteroids and cyclosporine.

NAFCILLIN (NAFCIL, UNIPEN, NALLPEN)

Indications: Osteomyelitis, septicemia, endocarditis and CNS infections due to susceptible strains of penicillinase-producing *Staphylococcus*.

Actions: Antistaphylococcal penicillin antibiotic.

Dosage: *Children: Mild to moderate infections:* 50–100 mg/kg/day IV divided q6h; *Severe infections:* 100–200 mg/kg/day IV divided q4–6h, max 12 g/day.
  Adults: 500 mg to 2 g IV q4–6h.

Supplied: Powder for injection 1 g, 2 g, 10 g; premixed in D_5W 100 mg/mL.

Notes: Adjust dose in patients with hepatic or renal impairment.

NALBUPHINE (NUBAIN)

Indications: Moderate to severe pain; preoperative and obstetric analgesia.

Actions: Narcotic agonist-antagonist; inhibits ascending pain pathways.

Dosage: Children: 0.1–0.15 mg/kg IV q3–6h prn, max 20 mg per dose; *Adults:* 10–20 mg IM or IV q4–6h prn, max 160 mg/day.

Supplied: Injection 10 mg/mL, 20 mg/mL.

Notes: Causes CNS depression and drowsiness. Use with caution in patients receiving opiate drugs.

NALOXONE (NARCAN)

Indications: Reversal of narcotic effect.

Actions: Competitive narcotic antagonist.

Dosage: Opiate intoxication: Neonates and children ≤ 5 years: 0.1 mg/kg, repeat q2–3min prn; *Children > 5 years:* 2 mg per dose, repeat q2–3min prn; *Adults:* 0.4–2 mg IV, IM, or SQ q5min; max total dose 10 mg; *Continuous IV infusion:* 2.5–160 mcg/kg/h.

Supplied: Injection 0.4 mg/mL, 1 mg/mL.

Notes: May precipitate acute withdrawal in addicts. If no response after 10 mg, suspect a nonnarcotic cause.

NAPROXEN (ALEVE, NAPROSYN, ANAPROX)

Indications: Inflammatory diseases and rheumatoid disorders; mild to moderate pain; fever; dysmenorrhea; gout.

Actions: NSAID.

Dosage: Children > 2 years: Analgesia: 5–7 mg/kg per dose PO q8h; *Anti-inflammatory:* 10–15 mg/kg/day PO divided twice daily, max 1 g/day.
  Adolescents and adults: Analgesia: Initial 500 mg, then 250 mg PO q6–8h, max dose 1.25 g/day; *Anti-inflammatory:* 500–1000 mg per dose PO twice daily.

Supplied: Tablets 220 mg, 250 mg, 375, 500 mg; gelcap 220 mg; caplet 220 mg; suspension 125 mg/5 mL.

Notes: Give with food. Use with caution if patient has history of GI bleeding.

NEDOCROMIL (TILADE)

Indications: Mild to moderate asthma.

Actions: Anti-inflammatory agent.

Dosage: Children > 6 years and adults: 2 inhalations 4 times daily.

Supplied: Metered-dose inhaler, 1.75 mg per actuation.

NELFINAVIR (VIRACEPT)

Indications: HIV infection.

Actions: Protease inhibitor; results in formation of immature, noninfectious virion.

Dosage: Children: 20–30 mg/kg per dose PO 3 times daily; *Adolescents and adults:* 750 mg PO 3 times daily or 1250 mg PO twice daily.

Supplied: Tablet 250 mg; oral powder.

Notes: Food is necessary to increase absorption. Interacts with St. John's wort.

NEOSPORIN (SEE BACITRACIN, NEOMYCIN, AND POLYMYXIN B)*
NEOMYCIN AND POLYMYXIN B BLADDER IRRIGANT

Indications: Continuous irrigant for prophylaxis against bacteriuria and gram-negative bacteremia associated with indwelling catheter use.

Actions: Bactericidal antibiotic.

Dosage: Children and adults: 1 mL irrigant added to 1 L of 0.9% NaCl; continuous irrigation of bladder with 1–2 L of solution per 24 hours.

Supplied: Solution, urogenital irrigant neomycin 40 mg/polymyxin B 200,000 units/mL.

Notes: Potential for bacterial or fungal superinfection. Slight possibility of neomycin-induced ototoxicity or nephrotoxicity.

NEOMYCIN (BACITRACIN), POLYMYXIN B, AND HYDROCORTISONE (CORTISPORIN)*

Indications: Inflammatory condition for which a corticosteroid is indicated and where bacterial infection exists.

Actions: Inhibits cell wall synthesis (bacitracin), alters permeability of bacterial cytoplasmic membrane (polymyxin B), inhibits bacterial protein synthesis (neomycin), decreases inflammation (hydrocortisone).

Dosage: Otic: 3 drops into affected ear 3–4 times daily.
    Topical: Apply sparingly 2–4 times daily.
    Ophthalmic: Instill $^{1}/_{2}$-inch ribbon to inside of lower lid q3–4h until improvement occurs, then reduce frequency to 1–3 times daily.

Supplied: Topical cream and ointment; otic suspension and solution; ophthalmic ointment and solution. Bacitracin 400 units, neomycin sulfate 5 mg, polymyxin 10,000 units, and hydrocortisone 10 mg per gram or per milliliter.

Notes: Otic suspension is preferred otic preparation; otic solution is used only for superficial infections of auditory canal (eg, swimmer's ear).

NEOMYCIN, POLYMYXIN B, AND PREDNISOLONE (POLY-PRED OPHTHALMIC) (SEE TABLE VIII–6, P. 754)
NEOMYCIN SULFATE

Indications: Hepatic coma; preoperative bowel preparation.

Actions: Aminoglycoside; suppresses GI bacterial flora.

Dosage: Children: Oral: 50–100 mg/kg/day in divided doses q6–8h; *Preoperative bowel cleansing:* 90 mg/kg/day divided q4h for 2 days; *Hepatic coma:* 2.5–7 g/m²/day divided q4–6h for 5–6 days, max 12 g/day.
    Adults: 3–12 g/24 h PO divided 3–4 times daily.

Supplied: Tablet 500 mg; oral solution 125 mg/5 mL.

Notes: Part of the Condon bowel prep.

NIACIN (VITAMIN B₃)* (SEE VITAMINS, P. 745)
NIFEDIPINE (PROCARDIA, PROCARDIA XL, ADALAT, ADALAT CC)

Indications: Vasospastic or chronic stable angina and hypertension.

Actions: Calcium channel blocking agent.

Dosage: Children: Hypertensive emergencies: 0.25–0.5 mg/kg per dose, max 10 mg per dose; *Hypertrophic cardiomyopathy:* 0.6–0.9 mg/kg/day PO divided 3 times daily; *Hypertension:* 0.25–0.5 mg/kg/day PO once daily using extended-release tablet, titrate to effect, max 3 mg/kg/day.
    Adults: Sustained-release tablets: 30–90 mg once daily.

Supplied: Capsules 10 mg, 20 mg; sustained-release tablets 30 mg, 60 mg, 90 mg.

Notes: Headaches are common side effect of initial treatment; lower-extremity edema is also common. Reflex tachycardia may occur with regular-release dosage forms. Adalat CC and Procardia XL are not interchangeable dosage forms. Capsules are not recommended for acute reduction of BP.

NITROFURANTOIN (MACRODANTIN, FURADANTIN, MACROBID)

Indications: Prevention and treatment of UTIs.

Actions: Bacteriostatic; interferes with carbohydrate metabolism.

Dosage: Children: 5–7 mg/kg/day PO divided q6h, max 400 mg/day.
  Adults: Prophylaxis of UTI: 50–100 mg PO once daily; *Treatment:* 50–100 mg PO 4 times daily.

Supplied: Capsules 25 mg, 50 mg, 100 mg; capsules, macrocrystals 50 mg, 100 mg; sustained-release capsule 100 mg; suspension 25 mg/5 mL.

Notes: GI side effects are common; drug should be taken with food, milk, or antacid. Macrocrystals (Macrodantin) cause less nausea than other forms of drug. Avoid use if creatinine clearance < 50 mL/min.

NITROGLYCERIN (NITROSTAT, NITROLINGUAL, NITRO-BID OINTMENT, NITRO-BID IV, NITRODISC, TRANSDERM-NITRO, OTHERS)

Indications: Angina pectoris, acute and prophylactic therapy; congestive heart failure; BP control.

Actions: Relaxation of vascular smooth muscle.

Dosage: Children: Initial 0.25–0.5 mcg/kg/min continuous IV infusion, titrate by 0.5–1 mcg/kg/min q3–5min prn, max dose 5 mcg/kg/min.
  Adults:
- *Sublingual:* 1 tablet q5min prn for 3 doses.
- *Translingual:* 1–2 metered doses sprayed onto oral mucosa q3–5min, max 3 doses.
- *Oral:* 2.5–9 mg 3 times daily.
- *Intravenous:* 5–20 mcg/min, titrated to effect.
- *Topical:* Apply 1–2 inches of ointment to chest wall q6h, then wipe off at night.
- *Transdermal:* 0.1–0.6 mg/h patch daily.

Supplied: Sublingual tablets 0.3 mg, 0.4 mg, 0.6 mg; translingual spray 0.4 mg per dose; sustained-release capsules 2.5 mg, 6.5 mg, 9 mg;

sustained-release tablets 2.6 mg, 6.5 mg, 9 mg; injection 5 mg/mL; ointment 2%; transdermal patches 2.5 mg/24 h, 5 mg/24 h, 7.5 mg/24 h, 10 mg/24 h, 15 mg/24 h; buccal controlled release 2 mg, 3 mg.

Notes: Tolerance to nitrates will develop with chronic use after 1–2 weeks; this can be avoided by providing a nitrate-free period each day. Shorter-acting nitrates should be used on a 3 times daily basis, and long-acting patches and ointment should be removed before bedtime to prevent development of tolerance.

NITROPRUSSIDE (NIPRIDE, NITROPRESS)

Indications: Pulmonary edema.

Actions: Reduces systemic vascular resistance.

Dosage: Children and adults: 0.3–10 mcg/kg/min IV infusion, titrated to desired effect; usual dose 3 mcg/kg/min.

Supplied: Injection 25 mg/mL, powder for injection 50 mg.

Notes: Thiocyanate (metabolite) is excreted by kidney; thiocyanate toxicity occurs at plasma levels of 5–10 mg/dL; more likely to occur when used for > 2–3 days.

NOREPINEPHRINE (LEVOPHED)

Indications: Acute hypotensive states.

Actions: Peripheral vasoconstrictor acting on both arterial and venous beds.

Dosage: Children: 0.05–2 mcg/kg/min IV infusion; *Adults:* 8–12 mcg/min IV, titrated to desired effect.

Supplied: Injection 1 mg/mL.

Notes: Correct blood volume depletion as much as possible prior to initiation of vasopressor therapy. Drug may interact with tricyclic antidepressants to produce severe profound hypertension. Infuse into large vein to avoid extravasation; phentolamine 5–10 mg/10 mL NS may be injected locally as antidote to extravasation.

NORTRIPTYLINE (AVENTYL, PAMELOR)

Indications: Endogenous depression; nocturnal enuresis.

Actions: Tricyclic antidepressant; increases synaptic concentrations of serotonin or norepinephrine, or both, in CNS.

Dosage: *Nocturnal enuresis:* *Children 20–25 kg:* 10 mg/day 30 min prior to bedtime; *Children 25–35 kg:* 10–20 mg/day 30 min prior to bedtime; *Children 35–54 kg:* 25–35 mg/day 30 minutes before bedtime.
Depression: *Children 6–12 years:* 10–20 mg/day PO in 3–4 divided doses; *Adults:* 25 mg PO 3–4 times daily, max 150 mg/day.

Supplied: Capsules 10 mg, 25 mg, 50 mg, 75 mg; solution 10 mg/5 mL.

Notes: Many anticholinergic side effects, including blurred vision, urinary retention, and dry mouth. Max effect is seen after 2 weeks of therapy. Adjust dose in patients with hepatic impairment.

NYSTATIN (MYCOSTATIN, NILSTAT, OTHERS)

Indications: Mucocutaneous *Candida* infections (thrush, vaginitis).

Actions: Alters membrane permeability.

Dosage: *Oral:* *Neonates and infants:* 100,000–200,000 units swab to each side of mouth 4 times daily; *Children and adults:* 400,000–600,000 units PO swish and swallow 4 times daily.
Intravaginal: 1 tablet per vagina at bedtime for 2 weeks.
Topical: Apply 2–3 times daily to affected area.

Supplied: Oral suspension 100,000 units/mL; oral tablet 500,000 units; lozenge 200,000 units; vaginal tablet 100,000 units; topical cream and ointment 100,000 units/g.

Notes: Not absorbed orally; therefore, not effective for systemic infections.

OCTREOTIDE (SANDOSTATIN)

Indications: Suppression or inhibition of severe diarrhea associated with carcinoid and neuroendocrine tumors of intestinal tract; treatment of bleeding esophageal varices.

Actions: Long-acting peptide that mimics the natural hormone somatostatin.

Dosage: *Diarrhea:* *Children:* 1–10 mcg/kg IV or SQ q12h or 1 mcg/kg/h IV continuous infusion; *Adults:* 50 mcg SQ 1–2 times daily or 50–100 mcg IV q8h, increase by 100 mcg per dose q48h, max 500 mcg q8h.
Bleeding: *Children:* 1 mcg/kg IV bolus, then 1 mcg/kg/h continuous infusion; *Adults:* 25–50 mcg IV bolus, then 25–50 mcg/h for 48 hours.

Supplied: Injection 0.05 mg/mL, 0.1 mg/mL, 0.2 mg/mL, 0.5 mg/mL, 1 mg/mL.

Notes: May cause nausea, vomiting, and abdominal discomfort.

OMEPRAZOLE (PRILOSEC)

Indications: Gastroesophageal reflux disease; duodenal ulcer; erosive esophagitis; hypersecretory conditions (Zollinger-Ellison syndrome); *Helicobacter pylori*–associated gastritis.

Actions: Proton pump inhibitor.

Dosage: Children: 1 mg/kg/day PO once or twice daily; *Adults:* 20–60 mg PO daily.

Supplied: Delayed-release capsule 10 mg*, 20 mg*, 40 mg.

Notes: Administration via NG tube should be in acidic juice. *Do not* crush or chew granules.

ONDANSETRON (ZOFRAN)

Indications: Prevention of nausea and vomiting associated with cancer chemotherapy; prevention of postoperative nausea and vomiting.

Actions: Serotonin receptor antagonist.

Dosage: Chemotherapy: Children and adults: 0.15 mg/kg per dose IV prior to chemotherapy; then repeated 4 and 8 hours after first dose; or 4–8 mg PO 3 times daily; administer first dose 30 minutes prior to chemotherapy.
  Postoperative: Children < 40 kg: 0.1 mg/kg IV; *Adults:* 4 mg IV immediately before induction of anesthesia or postoperatively.

Supplied: Tablets 4 mg, 8 mg; injection 2 mg/mL.

Notes: May cause diarrhea and headache. Should be administered on a schedule, not prn.

OSELTAMIVIR (TAMIFLU)

Indications: Influenza A and B.

Actions: Inhibition of viral neuraminidase.

Dosage: Children ≤ 15 kg: 2 mg/kg per dose PO twice daily for 5 days, max 30 mg per dose; *Children 15–23 kg:* 45 mg per dose PO twice daily for 5 days; *23–40 kg:* 60 mg per dose PO twice daily for 5 days; *Children > 12 years and adults:* 75 mg PO twice daily for 5 days.

Supplied: Capsule 75 mg; oral suspension 12 mg/mL.

Notes: Initiate within 36 hours of symptom onset. Reduce dose in patients with renal impairment.

OXACILLIN (BACTOCILL)

Indications: Osteomyelitis, septicemia, endocarditis, and CNS infections due to susceptible strains of penicillinase-producing *Staphylococcus*.

Actions: Antistaphylococcal penicillin antibiotic.

Dosage: Children: Mild to moderate infections: 100–150 mg/kg/day IV divided q6h; *Severe infections:* 150–200 mg/kg/day IV divided q4–6h, max 12 g/day.
  Adults: 250 mg to 2 g IV q4–6h.

Supplied: Injection 1 g, 2 g, 10 g.

Notes: Reduce dose in patients with renal impairment.

OXCARBAZEPINE (TRILEPTAL)

Indications: Partial seizures.

Actions: Produce blockage of voltage-sensitive sodium channels, resulting in stabilization of hyperexcited neural membranes.

Dosage: Children 4–16 years: Initial 8–10 mg/kg/day PO divided twice daily, max 600 mg/day, increase slowly over 2 weeks to weight-dependent maintenance dose:

- *20–29 kg:* 900 mg/day.
- *29.1–39 kg:* 1200 mg/day.
- *> 39 kg:* 1800 mg/day.

  Adults: 300 mg twice daily; increase dose weekly to usual dose of 1200–2400 mg/day.

Supplied: Tablets 150 mg, 300 mg, 600 mg, suspension 300 mg/5 mL.

Notes: May cause clinically significant hyponatremia. Has possible cross-sensitivity to carbamazepine. Adjust dose in patients with renal impairment.

OXYBUTYNIN (DITROPAN, DITROPAN XL)

Indications: Symptomatic relief of urgency, nocturia, and incontinence associated with neurogenic or reflex neurogenic bladder.

Actions: Direct antispasmodic effect on smooth muscle; increases bladder capacity.

Dosage: Children 1–5 years: 0.2 mg/kg per dose PO divided 2–4 times daily; *Children > 5 years and adults:* 5 mg PO 2–4 times daily; *Extended-release:* 5 mg PO daily; can titrate up to 30 mg PO daily.

Supplied: Tablet 5 mg; extended-release tablets 5 mg, 10 mg, 15 mg; syrup 5 mg/5 mL.

Notes: Anticholinergic side effects.

OXYCODONE (DIHYDROHYDROXYCODEINONE) (OXYCONTIN, OXYIR, ROXICODONE) [C]

Indications: Moderate to severe pain; normally used in combination with nonnarcotic analgesics.

Actions: Narcotic analgesic.

Dosage: Immediate-release products: Children: 0.05–0.15 mg/kg per dose PO q4–6h prn; *Adults:* 5 mg PO q6h prn.
    Controlled-release product: Adolescents > 18 years and adults: Initial 10 mg PO q12h, adjust dose every 1–2 days by 25–50%.
    Breakthrough pain: Use immediate-release form prn for breakthrough; dose should be 1/4–1/3 of controlled-release dose.

Supplied: Immediate-release capsule 5 mg; immediate-release tablet 5 mg, 15 mg, 30 mg; controlled-release tablet 10 mg, 20 mg, 40 mg, 80 mg, 160 mg; solution 5 mg/5 mL, 20 mg/mL.

Notes: Usually prescribed in combination with acetaminophen or aspirin. Useful for chronic cancer pain. In some parts of the United States, OxyContin is highly sought after as a drug of abuse. Tablets can be crushed and snorted or injected.

OXYCODONE AND ACETAMINOPHEN (PERCOCET, TYLOX) [C]

Indications: Moderate to severe pain.

Actions: Narcotic analgesic.

Dosage: Children (based on oxycodone component): 0.05–0.15 mg/kg per dose PO q4–6h prn, max 5 mg per dose; *Adults:* 1–2 tablets or capsules PO q4–6h prn.

Supplied: Percocet tablet: oxycodone/acetaminophen 2.5 mg/325 mg, 5 mg/325 mg, 7.5 mg/325 mg, 10 mg/650 mg; Tylox capsule: 5 mg/500 mg; solution 5 mg oxycodone/325 mg acetaminophen/5 mL.

Notes: Acetaminophen max dose of 4 g/day.

PALIVIZUMAB (SYNAGIS)

Indications: Prevention of serious lower respiratory infection caused by respiratory syncytial virus (RSV).

Actions: Humanized monoclonal antibody with inhibitory activity against RSV.

Dosage: 15 mg/kg IM once monthly during RSV season.

Supplied: Injection 50 mg, 100 mg.

Notes: May cause anaphylaxis or allergic reactions.

PANCRELIPASE (PANCREASE, COTAZYM, CREON, ULTRASE)

Indications: Patients deficient in exocrine pancreatic secretions (cystic fibrosis, chronic pancreatitis, other pancreatic insufficiency); steatorrhea of malabsorption syndrome.

Actions: Pancreatic enzyme supplementation.

Dosage: Infants: 2000–4000 lipase units per 120 mL formula; *Children < 4 years:* 1000 lipase units/kg per meal, $\frac{1}{2}$ dose with each snack, max 2500 lipase units/kg; *Children ≥ 4 years and adults:* 400–500 lipase units/kg per meal, $\frac{1}{2}$ dose with snacks.

Supplied: Capsules, tablets, and powder with various lipase, amylase, and protease content.

Notes: Instruct patient to avoid antacids. *Do not* crush or chew enteric-coated products. May cause nausea, abdominal cramps, or diarrhea; dosage is dependent on patient's digestive requirements.

PANCURONIUM (PAVULON)

Indications: Aids in management of patients on mechanical ventilation.

Actions: Nondepolarizing neuromuscular blocker.

Dosage: Children: 0.15 mg/kg IV q30–60min prn or continuous infusion of 0.03–0.1 mg/kg/h (0.5–1.7 mcg/kg/min); *Adults:* 0.15 mg/kg IV q2–4h prn or continuous infusion of 0.02–0.04 mg/kg/h (0.4–0.6 mcg/kg/min).

Supplied: Injection 1 mg/mL, 2 mg/mL.

Notes: Patient must be intubated and on controlled ventilation. Use adequate amount of sedation or analgesia. Adjust dose in patients with renal or hepatic impairment.

PANTOPRAZOLE (PROTONIX)

Indications: Gastroesophageal reflux disease; duodenal ulcer; erosive esophagitis; hypersecretory conditions (Zollinger-Ellison syndrome); *Helicobacter pylori*–associated gastritis.

Actions: Proton pump inhibitor.

Dosage: Children: 0.5–1 mg/kg/day PO once daily; *Adults:* 40–80 mg PO daily.

Supplied: Injection 40 mg; enteric-coated tablets 20 mg, 40 mg.

Notes: May cause dry mouth. *Do not* crush or chew tablets.

PAREGORIC [C]

Indications: Diarrhea; pain; neonatal opiate withdrawal syndrome.

Actions: Narcotic.

Dosage: Children: 0.25–0.5 mL/kg PO 1–4 times daily; *Adults:* 5–10 mL PO 1–4 times daily prn.

Notes: Contains opium. Drug is for short-term use only.

PAROXETINE (PAXIL)

Indications: Depression; obsessive-compulsive disorder; panic disorder; social anxiety disorder.

Actions: Serotonin reuptake inhibitor.

Dosage: Adolescents and adults: 10–60 mg PO as single daily dose.

Supplied: Tablets 10 mg, 20 mg, 30 mg, 40 mg; suspension 10 mg/5 mL.

Notes: Administer in the morning; may cause insomnia or hypersomnia. Adjust dose in patients with severe hepatic or renal impairment.

PENICILLIN G, AQUEOUS (POTASSIUM OR SODIUM) (PFIZERPEN)

Indications: Most gram-positive infections (except penicillin-resistant staphylococci), including streptococci, *Neisseria meningitidis,* syphilis, clostridia, and some coliforms.

Actions: Bactericidal; inhibits cell wall synthesis.

Dosage: Infants and children: 100,000–400,000 units/kg/day IV or IM q4–6h, max 24 million units/day; *Adults:* 400,000–800,000 units PO 4 times daily; IV doses vary depending on indications; range 1.2–24 million units/day in divided doses q4h.

Supplied: Powder for injection 5 million units, 20 million units.

Notes: Beware of hypersensitivity reactions. Adjust dose in patients with renal impairment.

PENICILLIN G BENZATHINE (BICILLIN L-A)

Indications: Useful as single-dose treatment regimen for streptococcal pharyngitis, rheumatic fever and glomerulonephritis prophylaxis, and syphilis.

Actions: Bactericidal; inhibits cell wall synthesis.

Dosage: Infants and children: 25,000–50,000 units/kg IM single dose, max 1.2 million units per dose; *Adults:* 1.2–2.4 million units deep IM injection every 2–4 weeks.

Supplied: Suspension for injection 600,000 units/mL.

Notes: Has sustained action with detectable levels up to 4 weeks. Considered drug of choice for treatment of noncongenital syphilis. Not for IV injection.

PENICILLIN G PROCAINE (WYCILLIN)

Indications: Moderately severe infections caused by penicillin G–sensitive organisms that respond to low, persistent serum levels.

Actions: Bactericidal; inhibits cell wall synthesis.

Dosage: Infants and children: 25,000–50,000 units/kg/day IM in divided doses q12–24h, max 4.8 million units/day; *Adults:* 0.6–4.8 million units/day IM in divided doses q12–24h.

Supplied: Injection 600,000 units/mL.

Notes: Long-acting parenteral penicillin; provides measurable blood levels up to 15 hours. Give at least 30 minutes prior to administration of penicillin to prolong action. Not for IV injection.

PENICILLIN V POTASSIUM (PEN-VEE K, VEETIDS)

Indications: Most gram-positive infections, including streptococci, *Neisseria meningitidis,* syphilis, clostridia, and some coliforms.

Actions: Bactericidal; inhibits cell wall synthesis.

Dosage: Children: 25–50 mg/kg/day PO in divided doses q6–8h, max 3 g/day; *Adults:* 250–500 mg PO q6h.

Supplied: Tablets 250 mg, 500 mg; suspension 125 mg/5 mL, 250 mg/5 mL.

Notes: A well-tolerated oral penicillin; 250 mg = 400,000 units of penicillin.

PENTAMIDINE (PENTAM 300, NEBUPENT)

Indications: Treatment and prevention of *Pneumocystis carinii* pneumonia.

Actions: Inhibits DNA, RNA, phospholipid, and protein synthesis.

Dosage: Treatment: Children and adults: 4 mg/kg/day IV daily for 14–21 days.
Prevention: 4 mg/kg per dose IV or IM every 2–4 weeks.
Inhalation: Children > 5 years and adults: 300 mg every 4 weeks administered via Respirgard II nebulizer.

Supplied: Injection 300 mg per vial; aerosol 300 mg.

Notes: Monitor patient for severe hypotension following IV administration. Drug is associated with pancreatic islet cell necrosis leading to hypoglycemia and hyperglycemia. Monitor hematology lab results for leukopenia and thrombocytopenia. IV route requires dosage adjustment in patients with renal impairment.

PENTOBARBITAL (NEMBUTAL, OTHERS) [C]

Indications: Insomnia; convulsions; induced coma following severe head injury.

Actions: Barbiturate.

Dosage: Preoperative sedation: Children: 2–6 mg/kg IM, max 100 mg per dose or 1–3 mg/kg IV to max of 100 mg until asleep; *Adults:* 150–200 mg IM.
Hypnotic: Children: 2–6 mg/kg IM, max 100 mg per dose; *Adults:* 100–200 mg IV or IM at bedtime prn.
Induced coma: Loading dose 10–15 mg/kg IV given slowly over 1–2 hours, then maintenance 1–3 mg/kg/h IV continuous infusion to keep serum level between 20 and 50 mg/mL.

Supplied: Injection 50 mg/mL.

Notes: May cause respiratory depression. May produce profound hypotension when used aggressively intravenously for cerebral edema. Tolerance to sedative-hypnotic effect is acquired within 1–2 weeks. Reduce dose in patients with severe hepatic impairment.

PERMETHRIN (NIX, ELIMITE)*

Indications: Eradication of lice and scabies.

Actions: Pediculicide.

Dosage: Saturate hair and scalp; allow to remain in hair for 10 minutes before rinsing out.

Supplied: Topical liquid 1%; cream 5%, shampoo 0.33%.

PHENAZOPYRIDINE (PYRIDIUM, OTHERS)*

Indications: Symptomatic relief of discomfort from lower urinary tract irritation.

Actions: Local anesthetic on urinary tract mucosa.

Dosage: Children: 12 mg/kg/day PO divided 3 times daily for 2 days; *Adults:* 100–200 mg PO 3 times daily for 2–3 days.

Supplied: Tablets 100 mg, 200 mg.

Notes: Side effects include GI disturbances. Drug causes red-orange discoloration to body secretions, may stain clothing, contacts, etc. Adjust dose in patients with renal impairment. Use in conjunction with an antibacterial agent for UTI.

PHENOBARBITAL [C]

Indications: Seizure disorders; insomnia; anxiety.

Actions: Barbiturate.

Dosage: Sedative-hypnotic: Children: 2 mg/kg PO 3 times daily or 3–5 mg/kg IM, IV or SQ at bedtime; *Adults:* 30–120 mg PO or IM daily prn.
  Hyperbilirubinemia: 3–12 mg/kg/day PO divided 2–3 times daily.
  Anticonvulsant:
  • *Loading dose: Neonates, infants, children, adults:* 15–20 mg/kg in single or divided dose.
  • *Maintenance dose in 1–2 divided doses: Neonates:* 3–5 mg/kg/day PO or IV once daily; *Infants:* 5–6 mg/kg/day PO or IV; *Children 1–5 years:* 6–8 mg/kg/day; *Children 5–12 years:* 4–6 mg/kg/day; *Adults:* 1–3 mg/kg/24 h PO or IV.

Supplied: Tablets 15 mg, 30 mg, 32 mg, 60 mg, 65 mg, 100 mg; elixir 20 mg/ 5 mL; injection 60 mg/mL, 130 mg/mL.

Notes: Give maintenance dose 12 hours after loading dose. Tolerance develops to sedation. Long half-life allows single daily dosing. Follow levels as needed; therapeutic range 15–40 mcg/mL.

PHENYLEPHRINE (NEO-SYNEPHRINE)

Indications: Vascular failure in shock, hypersensitivity, or drug-induced hypotension; nasal congestion; mydriatic.

Actions: α-Adrenergic agonist.

Dosage: Mild to moderate hypotension: 2–5 mg IM or SQ elevates BP for 2 hours; 0.1–0.5 mg IV elevates BP for 15 minutes.
Severe hypotension or shock: Children: 5–20 mcg/kg per dose IV q10–15min prn or 0.1–0.5 mcg/kg/min continuous IV infusion; *Adults:* 0.1–0.5 mg per dose q10–15min prn or continuous IV infusion at 100–180 mcg/min; once stabilized, lower to maintenance rate of 40–60 mcg/min.
Nasal congestion: Infants > 6 months: 1–2 drops of 0.16% q3h; *Children 1–6 years:* 2–3 drops of 0.125% q4h prn; *Children 6–12 years:* 2–3 drops of 0.25% q4h prn; *Children > 12 years and adults:* 2–3 drops or 1–2 sprays of 0.25–0.5% solution q4h into each nostril prn.
Ophthalmologic: Infants < 1 year: 1 drop of 2.5% 15–30 minutes before exam; *Children and adults:* 1 drop of 2.5% or 10% solution, may repeat in 10–60 minutes as needed.

Supplied: Injection 10 mg/mL; nasal solution* 0.125%, 0.16%, 0.25%, 0.5%, 1%; ophthalmic solution* 0.12%, 2.5%, 10%.

Notes: Promptly restore blood volume if loss has occurred. Use with extreme caution in patients with hyperthyroidism, bradycardia, partial heart block, myocardial disease, or severe arteriosclerosis. Use large veins for infusion to avoid extravasation; phentolamine 10 mg in 10–15 mL of NS may be injected locally as antidote for extravasation. Activity of drug is potentiated by oxytocin, MAO inhibitors, and tricyclic antidepressants.

PHENYTOIN (DILANTIN)

Indications: Seizure disorders.

Actions: Inhibits seizure spread in motor cortex.

Dosage: Neonates: Load 15–20 mg/kg IV in single or divided dose followed by maintenance dose of 5–8 mg/kg/day divided q8–12h.
Infants, children, and adults: Load 15–20 mg/kg IV at max infusion rate of 25 mg/min in single or divided dose followed by age-dependent maintenance dose:

- *0.5–3 years:* 8-10 mg/kg/day.
- *4–6 years:* 7.5–9 mg/kg/day.

- *7–9 years:* 7–8 mg/kg/day.
- *10–16 years:* 6–7 mg/kg/day.
- *Adolescents > 15 years and adults:* 300 mg/day or 4–6 mg/kg/day in 2–3 divided doses; Oral dosing same as IV.

Supplied: Capsules 30 mg, 100 mg; chewable tablet 50 mg; oral suspension 125 mg/5 mL; injection 50 mg/mL.

Notes: Be alert for cardiac depressant side effects, especially with IV administration; follow levels as needed. Nystagmus and ataxia are early signs of toxicity. Gum hyperplasia occurs with long-term use. Avoid use of oral suspension if possible because of erratic absorption. Some patients may require q8h dosing.

PHOSPHATE SUPPLEMENTS

Indications: Treatment and prevention of hypophosphatemia; short-term treatment of constipation; urinary acidifier for reduction in formation of calcium stones.

Actions: Participates in bone deposition and calcium metabolism; acts as buffer in acid-base equilibrium; acts as laxative by exerting osmotic effect in small intestine.

Dosage: Hypophosphatemia: Children: 0.08–0.36 mmol/kg IV over 6 hours; *Adults:* 0.16–0.64 mmol/kg IV over 6–12 hours; *Maintenance: Children:* 0.5–1.5 mmol/kg/day IV or 2–3 mmol/kg/day PO in divided doses; *Adults:* 50—70 mmol/day IV or 50–150 mmol/day PO in divided dose.
    Laxative: Children < 4 years: 250 mg (8 mmol) PO 4 times daily; *Children ≥ 4 years and adults:* 250–500 mg (8–16 mmol) PO 4 times daily; *Oral solution: Children 5–9 years:* 5 mL PO 1 time; *Children 10–12 years:* 10 mL PO 1 time; *Children > 12 years and adults:* 20–30 mL PO 1 time.
    Enema: Children 2–11 years: One 2.25-oz pediatric enema 1 time; *Children > 12 years and adults:* One 4.5-oz adult enema 1 time.
    Urinary acidification: Adults: 2 tablets PO 4 times daily.

Supplied: Tablet phosphorous 114 mg (3.7 mmol), 125.6 mg (4 mmol), 250 mg (8 mmol); enema pediatric (66 mL) or adult (133 mL); injection as potassium or sodium phosphate 3 mmol phosphate per mL; powder phosphorous 250 mg (8 mmol) per packet; oral solution phosphate 4 mmol and sodium 4.82 mEq per mL.

Notes: Give with food to reduce risk of diarrhea. Dilute each packet in 75 mL of water. Maintain adequate fluid intake. Max rate of IV infusion is 0.06 mmol/kg/h.

PHYSOSTIGMINE (ANTILIRIUM, ISOPTO ESERINE)

Indications: Antidote for tricyclic antidepressant, atropine, and scopolamine overdose.

Actions: Reversible cholinesterase inhibitor.

Dosage: Reversal of toxic anticholinergic effects: Children: 0.01–0.03 mg/kg per dose IV, may repeat after 15–20 min to max total dose of 2 mg; *Adults:* 2 mg IV, IM, or SQ q20min until response occurs.
   Preanesthetic reversal: Children and adults: Twice the dose, on a weight basis, of the anticholinergic drug (atropine, scopolamine).

Supplied: Injection 1 mg/mL.

Notes: Rapid IV administration is associated with convulsions. Max rate of infusion is 0.5–1 mg/min. Has cholinergic side effects; may cause asystole.

PHYTONADIONE (VITAMIN K) (AQUAMEPHYTON, OTHERS)

Indications: Coagulation disorders caused by faulty formation of factors II, VII, IX, and X; hemorrhagic disease of newborn; oral anticoagulant overdose.

Actions: Supplementation; needed for production of factors II, VII, IX, and X.

Dosage: Hemorrhagic disease of newborn: Prophylaxis: 0.5–1 mg SQ or IM within 1 hour of birth; *Treatment:* 1–2 mg/day SQ or IM.
   Oral anticoagulant overdose: Infants and children: 0.5–5 mg SQ or IV; Adults: 2.5–10 mg PO or IV.
   Vitamin K deficiency: Infants and children: 2.5–5 mg PO daily or 1–2 mg SQ, IM, or IV; *Adults:* 2.5–25 mg PO daily or 10 mg SQ, IM, or IV.

Supplied: Tablet 5 mg; injection 2 mg/mL, 10 mg/mL.

Notes: With parenteral treatment, first change in prothrombin is usually seen in 12–24 hours. SQ route is preferred. Anaphylaxis can result from IV dosage; drug should therefore be administered slowly if IV route is used.

PILOCARPINE (ISOPTO CARPINE, PILOCAR, PILOPINE HS GEL) (SEE TABLE VIII–6, P. 748) PIPERACILLIN (PIPRACIL)

Indications: Serious infections caused by susceptible strains of gram-positive, gram-negative (including *Pseudomonas aeruginosa*), and anaerobic bacilli.

Actions: Inhibits bacterial cell wall synthesis by binding to penicillin-binding proteins.

Dosage: Infants and children: 200–300 mg/kg/day IV divided q4–6h, max 24 g/day; *Adults:* 2–4 g IV q4–8h, max 24 g/day.

Supplied: Powder for reconstitution 2 g, 3 g, 4 g.

Notes: Reduce dose in patients with renal dysfunction. Use with caution in patients allergic to cephalosporins.

PIPERACILLIN AND TAZOBACTAM (ZOSYN)

Indications: Sepsis; gynecologic, intra-abdominal, skin and skin structure, and lower respiratory infections; and UTIs caused by piperacillin-resistant, β-lactamase–producing strains that are piperacillin-tazobactam susceptible.

Actions: Inhibits bacterial cell wall synthesis by binding to penicillin-binding proteins; tazobactam prevents degradation of piperacillin by binding to β-lactamases.

Dosage: Infants and children: 240–400 mg/kg/day of piperacillin IV divided q6–8h, max 18 g/day; *Adults:* 3.375 g (3 g piperacillin/0.375 g tazobactam) IV q6h, max 18 g/day.

Supplied: Injection 2.25 g, 3.375 g, 4.5 g.

Notes: Reduce dose in patients with renal dysfunction. Use with caution in patients who are allergic to cephalosporins. 8:1 ratio of piperacillin to tazobactam.

PNEUMOCOCCAL CONJUGATE VACCINE, 7 VALENT (PREVNAR) (SEE APPENDIX D, P. 759)
PNEUMOCOCCAL VACCINE, POLYVALENT (PNEUMOVAX-23) (SEE APPENDIX D, P. 759)
POLIOVIRUS VACCINE, INACTIVATED (SEE APPENDIX D, P. 759)
POLYETHYLENE GLYCOL [PEG]-ELECTROLYTE SOLUTION (GOLYTELY, MIRALAX)

Indications: Bowel cleansing prior to examination or surgery.

Actions: Osmotic cathartic.

Dosage: Bowel cleansing: Children: 25–40 mL/kg/h PO or NG until rectal effluent is clear; *Adults:* 240 mL PO q10min until 4 L consumed or rectal effluent is clear.
　Constipation (MiraLax): 17 g PO daily.

Supplied: Powder for reconstitution in 4 L container; MiraLax 17 g/tbsp.

Notes: No solid foods 2 hours prior to administration. First bowel movement should occur in approximately 1 hour. Solution may cause some cramping or nausea.

POLYMYXIN B AND HYDROCORTISONE (OTOBIOTIC OTIC)

Indications: Superficial bacterial infections of external ear canal.

Actions: Antibiotic anti-inflammatory combination.

DOSAGE: 4 drops in ear(s) 3–4 times daily.

Supplied: Solution: Polymyxin B 10,000 units/hydrocortisone 0.5%/mL.

Notes: Useful in neomycin allergy.

POTASSIUM CITRATE AND CITRIC ACID (POLYCITRA-K)

Indications: Alkalinization of urine; prevention of urinary stones (uric acid, calcium stones if hypocitraturic).

Actions: Urinary alkalinizer.

Dosage: Infants and children: 2–3 mEq/kg/day PO divided 3–4 times daily; *Adults:* 10–20 mEq PO 3 times daily with meals, max 100 mEq/day.

Supplied: Solution 2 mEq/mL potassium and 2 mEq/mL bicarbonate.

POTASSIUM IODIDE (LUGOL'S SOLUTION, SSKI)

Indications: Thyroid crisis; reduction of vascularity before thyroid surgery; blocking thyroid uptake of radioactive isotopes of iodine; thinning of bronchial secretions; sporotrichosis.

Actions: Iodine supplement.

Dosage: Preoperative thyroidectomy: Children and adults: 50–250 mg (1–5 drops SSKI; or 2–6 drops Lugol's solution) PO 3 times daily for 10 days prior to surgery.
   Thyroid crisis: Infants < 1 year: 150–250 mg (3–5 drops SSKI) PO 3 times daily; *Children and adults:* 300–500 mg (6–10 drops SSKI) PO 3 times daily.
   Expectorant: Children: 60–250 mg PO 4 times daily; *Adults:* 300–650 mg PO 3–4 times daily.
   Sporotrichosis: Children and adults: 250–500 mg PO 3 times daily.

Supplied: Tablets 60 mg, 130 mg; solution SSKI 1 g/mL; Lugol's solution, strong iodine: potassium iodide 100 mg and iodine 50 mg per mL; syrup 325 mg/5 mL.

Notes: 10 drops SSKI = 500 mg potassium iodide.

POTASSIUM SUPPLEMENTS (KAON, KAOCHLOR, K-LOR, SLOW-K, MICRO-K, KLORVESS, OTHERS)

Indications: Prevention or treatment of hypokalemia (often related to diuretic use).

Actions: Supplementation of potassium.

Dosage: Treatment of hypokalemia:
- *Oral: Infants and children:* 2–5 mEq/kg/day in divided doses; *Adults:* 40–100 mEq/day in divided doses.
- *IV intermittent infusion: Infants and children:* 0.5–1 mEq/kg per dose IV over 30–60 minutes; *Adults:* 10–20 mEq IV over 2–3 hours, max 40 mEq per dose.

Supplied: As potassium chloride: Sustained-release tablets 8 mEq, 10 mEq, 20 mEq; sustained-release capsules 8 mEq, 10 mEq; liquid 10 mEq/15 mL, 20 mEq/15 mL, 30 mEq/mL, 40 mEq/15 mL; powder packets 20 mEq, 25 mEq; effervescent tablets as potassium bicarbonate 25 mEq.

Notes: Must dilute prior to use. Maximum concentration via peripheral line is 80 mEq/mL; via central line, 200 mEq/mL. Maximum infusion rate is 1 mEq/kg/h. Oral supplements can cause GI irritation. Powder and liquids must be mixed with water or juice. Use with caution in patients with renal insufficiency, and along with NSAIDs, potassium-sparing diuretics, and ACE inhibitors. Chloride salt is recommended in patients with coexisting alkalosis; for coexisting acidosis use acetate, bicarbonate, citrate, or gluconate salt.

PRAMOXINE (ANUSOL OINTMENT, PROCTOFOAM-NS, OTHERS)*

Indications: Pain and itching from external and internal hemorrhoids and anorectal surgery; topical for burns and dermatosis.

Actions: Topical anesthetic.

Dosage: Apply cream, ointment, gel, or spray freely to anal area q3–4h.

Supplied: Foam (Proctofoam NS) 1%; cream 1%; ointment 1%; lotion 1%; gel 1%; pads 1%; spray 1%.

PRAMOXINE AND HYDROCORTISONE (ENZONE, PROCTOFOAM-HC)

Indications: Pain and itching from hemorrhoids.

Actions: Topical anesthetic.

Dosage: Apply freely to anal area 3–4 times daily.

Supplied: Cream: Pramoxine hydrochloride 1% hydrocortisone acetate 0.5/1%; *Foam:* Pramoxine 1% hydrocortisone 1%; *Lotion:* Pramoxine 1% hydrocortisone 0.25/1/2.5%; pramoxine 2.5% and hydrocortisone 1%.
Prazosin (Minipress)

Indications: Hypertension; congestive heart failure.

Actions: Peripherally acting α-adrenergic blocker.

Dosage: Children: Initial 5 mcg/kg per dose, increase gradually up to 25 mcg/kg per dose PO q6h, max dose 15 mg/day; *Adults:* 1 mg PO 3 times daily, may increase to total daily dose of up to 20 mg/day.

Supplied: Capsules 1 mg, 2 mg, 5 mg.

Notes: May cause orthostatic hypotension; therefore, patient should take first dose at bedtime. Tolerance develops to this effect. Tachyphylaxis may result.

PREDNISOLONE (PEDIAPRED, PRELONE, ORAPRED)

Indications: Endocrine disorders; rheumatic disorders; collagen diseases; dermatologic diseases; allergic states; ophthalmic diseases; respiratory diseases; hematologic disorders; neoplastic diseases; edematous states; GI diseases.

Actions: Anti-inflammatory.

Dosage: Children: 0.1–2 mg/kg/day PO in divided doses; *Adults:* 5–60 mg/day PO.

Supplied: Tablet 5 mg; syrup 5 mg/5 mL, 15 mg/5 mL.

Notes: Administer after meals or with food to decrease GI upset.

PREDNISOLONE (AK-PRED, PRED FORTE) (SEE TABLE VIII-6, p. 754) PREDNISONE (DELTASONE)

Indications: Management of adrenocortical insufficiency, used for anti-inflammatory or immunosuppressant effects.

Actions: Anti-inflammatory.

Dosage: Anti-inflammatory or immunosuppressive: Children: 0.1–2 mg/kg/day PO in divided doses; *Adults:* 5–60 mg/day PO.

Supplied: Tablets 1 mg, 2.5 mg, 5 mg, 10 mg, 20 mg, 50 mg; oral solution 1 mg/1 mL, 5 mg/mL.

Notes: Dose depends on condition being treated and patient response. Administer after meals or with food to decrease GI upset.

PRIMIDONE (MYSOLINE)

Indications: General tonic-clonic, complex partial, and simple partial seizures.

Actions: Decreases neuron excitability; raises seizure threshold.

Dosage: Children < 8 years: Initial 50–125 mg/day PO at bedtime; increase by 50–125 mg/day increments every 3–7 days; usual dose 10–25 mg/kg/day divided 3–4 times daily.
  Children ≥ 8 years and adults: Initial 125–250 mg/day PO at bedtime; increase by 125–250 mg/day every 3–7 days; usual dose 750–1500 mg/day divided 3–4 times daily, max 2 g/day.

Supplied: Tablets 50 mg, 250 mg.

Notes: Metabolized in liver to phenobarbital. Monitor both primidone and phenobarbital concentrations. Therapeutic level is 5–12 mcg/mL.

PROCAINAMIDE (PRONESTYL, PROCAN)

Indications: Supraventricular and ventricular arrhythmias.

Actions: Class 1a antiarrhythmic.

Dosage: Children: 15–50 mg/kg/day PO in divided doses q3–6h, max 4 g/day; *Adults: Immediate release:* 250–500 mg PO q3–6h; *Sustained-release:* 500 mg to 1 g PO q6h.
  Intravenous loading dose: Children: 3–6 mg/kg per dose over 5 minutes, max 100 mg per dose, followed by continuous IV infusion of 20–80 mcg/kg/min; *Adults:* 50–100 mg IV load followed by infusion of 1–6 mg/min.

Supplied: Tablets 250 mg, 375 mg, 500 mg; capsules 250 mg, 500 mg; sustained-release tablets 500 mg, 750 mg, 1000 mg; injection 100 mg/mL, 500 mg/mL.

Notes: Titrate to patient's response. Can cause hypotension and lupus-like syndrome. Adjust dose in patients with renal or hepatic impairment.

PROCHLORPERAZINE (COMPAZINE)

Indications: Nausea and vomiting; agitation; psychotic disorders.

Actions: Phenothiazine; blocks postsynaptic mesolimbic dopaminergic receptors in brain.

Dosage: Antiemetic: Children > 10 kg: 0.4 mg/kg/day PO or PR divided 3–4 times daily; *Adults:* 5–10 mg PO 3–4 times daily; or 25 mg PR twice daily; or 5–10 mg deep IM q4–6h, max 40 mg/day.
Antipsychotic: Children 2–12 years: 2.5 mg PO or PR 2–3 times daily, increase to max dose prn of 20 mg for 2–5 years or 25 mg for 6–12 years; *Adults:* 10–20 mg IM in acute situations; or 5–10 mg PO 3–4 times daily for maintenance.

Supplied: Tablets 5 mg, 10 mg; sustained-release capsules 10 mg, 15 mg; syrup 5 mg/5 mL; suppositories: 2.5 mg, 5 mg, 25 mg; injection 5 mg/mL.

Notes: Much larger dose may be required for antipsychotic effect. Extrapyramidal side effects are common. Treat acute extrapyramidal reactions with diphenhydramine. Not recommended for IV use.

PROMETHAZINE (PHENERGAN)

Indications: Management of nausea and vomiting and motion sickness; symptomatic treatment of various allergic conditions; sedative.

Actions: Phenothiazine; blocks postsynaptic mesolimbic dopaminergic receptors in brain.

Dosage: Antihistamine: Children: 0.1 mg/kg per dose (max 12.5 mg per dose) PO q6h during the day and 0.5 mg/kg per dose (max 25 mg per dose) at bedtime prn; *Adults:* 6.25–12.5 mg PO 3 times daily and 25 mg at bedtime.
Antiemetic: Children: 0.25 mg to 1 mg/kg PO, PR, IM, or IV (max 25 mg per dose) 4–6 times daily prn; *Adults:* 12.5–25 mg PO, PR, or IM q4h prn.
Motion sickness: Children: 0.5 mg/kg (max 25 mg per dose) PO or PR 30 minutes to 1 hour prior to departure, then q12h prn; *Adults:* 25 mg PO twice daily with first dose 30 minutes to 1 hour prior to departure, then q8–12h prn.
Sedation: Children: 0.5–1 mg/kg per dose PO, PR, IM, IV (max 50 mg per dose) q6h prn; *Adults:* 25–50 mg PO, PR, IM, or IV q4–6h prn.

Supplied: Tablets 25 mg, 50 mg; syrup 6.25 mg/5 mL; suppositories 25 mg, 50 mg; injection 25 mg/mL, 50 mg/mL.

Notes: High incidence of drowsiness.

PROPOFOL (DIPRIVAN)

Indications: Induction or maintenance of anesthesia; continuous sedation in intubated patients.

Actions: Sedative hypnotic; mechanism unknown.

Dosage: Children: Anesthesia: 2.5–3.5 mg/kg induction, then 125–300 mcg/kg/min continuous infusion; *ICU sedation:* 1 mg/kg IV bolus followed by 50–150 mcg/kg/min IV continuous infusion.
  Adults: Anesthesia: 2–2.5 mg/kg induction, then 0.1–0.2 mg/kg/min continuous infusion; *ICU sedation:* 5–50 mcg/kg/min continuous infusion.

Supplied: Injection 10 mg/mL.

Notes: 1 mL of propofol contains 0.1 g of fat. Drug may increase serum triglycerides when administered for extended periods. May discolor urine green.

PROPRANOLOL (INDERAL)

Indications: Hypertension; tetralogy of Fallot cyanotic spells; migraine headache prophylaxis; arrhythmias; thyrotoxicosis.

Actions: Competitively blocks β-adrenergic receptors, β_1, β_2. Decreases conversion of T_4 to T_3.

Dosage: Arrhythmia: Children: Initial 0.5–1 mg/kg/day PO divided q6–8h, then titrate every 3–5 days to 2–4 mg/kg/day, max 16 mg/kg/day; or 0.01–0.1 mg/kg slow IV over 10 minutes, max dose 1 mg (infants) or 3 mg (children); *Adults:* 10–80 mg PO 3–4 times daily; or 1 mg IV slowly; repeat q5min up to 5 mg.
  Hypertension: Children: Initial 0.5–1 mg/kg/day PO divided q6–12h, then titrate every 3–5 days to 1–5 mg/kg/day, max 8 mg/kg/day; *Adults:* 40 mg PO twice daily; or 60–80 mg sustained release once daily; increase weekly to max of 640 mg/day.
  Migraine headache prophylaxis: Children: 0.6–1.5 mg/kg/day PO q8h, max 4 mg/kg/day; *Adults:* 80 mg/day PO divided 3–4 times daily; increase weekly to max of 160–240 mg/day divided 3–4 times daily; wean off if no response in 6 weeks.
  Thyrotoxicosis: Neonates: 2 mg/kg/day PO divided q6–12h; *Adolescents and adults:* 1–3 mg IV single dose; 10–40 mg PO q6h.
  Tetralogy spells: Infants and children: 1–2 mg/kg per dose PO q6h, may increase by 1 mg/kg/day q24h to max of 5 mg/kg/day; or 0.15–0.25 mg/kg per dose slow IV, may repeat in 15 minutes.

Supplied: Tablets 10 mg, 20 mg, 40 mg, 60 mg, 80 mg; sustained-release capsules 60 mg, 80 mg, 120 mg, 160 mg; oral solution 4 mg/mL, 8 mg/mL, 80 mg/mL; injection 1 mg/mL.

Notes: Adjust dose in patients with renal impairment.

PROPYLTHIOURACIL

Indications: Hyperthyroidism; thyrotoxic crisis.

Actions: Inhibits synthesis of thyroid hormones.

Dosage: Children: 5–7 mg/kg/day PO divided q8h; *Adults:* Initial 300–450 mg/day PO divided q8h; maintenance 100–150 mg/day divided q8–12h.

Supplied: Tablet 50 mg.

Notes: Give with food. Enhances anticoagulant activity; may cause bleeding.

PROTAMINE SULFATE

Indications: Reversal of heparin effect.

Actions: Neutralizes heparin by forming stable complex.

Dosage: Based on amount of heparin reversal desired; given slow IV; 1 mg will reverse approximately 100 units of heparin given in preceding 3–4 hours, to max dose of 50 mg.

Supplied: Injection 10 mg/mL.

Notes: Follow coagulation studies. Drug may have anticoagulant effect if given without heparin.

PSEUDOEPHEDRINE (SUDAFED, NOVAFED, AFRINOL, OTHERS)*

Indications: Decongestant.

Actions: Stimulates α-adrenergic receptors, resulting in vasoconstriction.

Dosage: Children < 2 years: 4 mg/kg/day PO divided q6h; *Children 2–5 years:* 15 mg PO q6h, max 60 mg/day; *Children 6–12 years:* 30 mg PO q6h, max 120 mg/day; *Children > 12 years and adults:* 30–60 mg PO q6–8h, max 240 mg/day; sustained-release capsules 120 mg PO q12h.

Supplied: Tablets 30 mg, 60 mg; chewable tablet 15 mg; capsule 30 mg; sustained-release tablets 120 mg, 240 mg; oral drops 7.5 mg/0.8 mL; liquid 15 mg/5 mL, 30 mg/5 mL.

Notes: Contraindicated in patients with poorly controlled hypertension or coronary artery disease and in patients taking MAO inhibitors. Pseudoephedrine is an ingredient in many cough and cold preparations.

PSYLLIUM (METAMUCIL, SERUTAN)*

Indications: Constipation; diverticular disease of colon.

Actions: Bulk laxative.

Dosage: Children 6–11 years: 1/2–1 rounded teaspoonful in 4 oz liquid PO 1–3 times per day; *Adults:* 1–2 teaspoonfuls or 1–2 packets or 1–2 wafers PO 1–4 times daily or 5 capsules PO 3 times daily.

Supplied: Capsule 0.52 g; granules 4 g/tsp, 2.5 g/tsp; powder 3.5 g per packet; wafers 3.4 g per dose.

Notes: Do not use if bowel obstruction is suspected. Effervescent form (Effer-Syllium) usually contains potassium and should be used with caution in patients with renal failure. Psyllium 3.4 g = 1 tsp = 1 packet = 1 wafer.

PYRAZINAMIDE

Indications: Active tuberculosis.

Actions: Bacteriostatic; mechanism unknown.

Dosage: Infants, children, and adolescents: 20–40 mg/kg/day PO divided q12–24h for first 2 months of active treatment, max 2 g/day; *Adults:* 15–30 mg/kg/24 h PO daily, max 3 g/day.

Supplied: Tablet 500 mg.

Notes: May cause hepatotoxicity. Use in combination with other antituberculosis drugs; consult *MMWR* for latest recommendations on treatment of tuberculosis. Dosage regimen differs for directly observed therapy. Adjust dose in patients with renal or hepatic impairment.

PYRIDOXINE (VITAMIN B6) (SEE VITAMINS, P. 745)
QUINUPRISTIN AND DALFOPRISTIN (SYNERCID)

Indications: Infections caused by vancomycin-resistant *Enterococcus faecium* (VREF); complicated skin and skin structure infections caused by *Staphylococcus aureus* and *Streptococcus pyogenes*.

Actions: A streptogramin antimicrobial agent; acts on bacterial ribosome to inhibit protein synthesis.

Dosage: Children and adults: 7.5 mg/kg IV over 60 minutes q8–12h.

Supplied: 500 mg (150 mg quinupristin and 350 mg dalfopristin) per 10-mL vial.

Notes: Significantly inhibits CYP3A4 isoenzymes. Use with caution when coadministered with drugs metabolized by this isoenzyme (eg, cyclosporine). May cause venous irritation, elevation in bilirubin, and arthralgias or myalgias. Administer through central line if possible; not compatible with saline or heparin; therefore, flush IV lines with dextrose. Adjust dose in patients with hepatic impairment.

RANITIDINE (ZANTAC)

Indications: Duodenal ulcer; active benign ulcers; hypersecretory conditions; gastroesophageal reflux disease (GERD).

Actions: H_2-receptor antagonist.

Dosage: Children > 1 month to 16 years:

- *Gastric or duodenal ulcer:* 2–4 mg/kg/day PO divided twice daily, max 300 mg/day or 2–4 mg/kg/day IV divided q6–8h, max 200 mg/day.
- *GERD or erosive esophagitis:* 4–10 mg/kg/day PO divided twice daily, max 300–600 mg/day or 2–4 mg/kg/day IV divided q6–8h, max 200 mg/day.
- *Continuous IV infusion:* 1 mg/kg per dose 1 time, followed by 0.08–0.17 mg/kg/h or 2–4 mg/kg/day.

Children > 16 years and adults:

- *Ulcer:* 150 mg PO twice daily, 300 mg PO at bedtime, or 50 mg IV q6–8h; or 400 mg/day IV via continuous infusion, followed by maintenance of 150 mg PO at bedtime.
- *Hypersecretion:* 150 mg PO twice daily, max 600 mg/day.
- *GERD:* 300 mg PO twice daily, maintenance 300 mg PO at bedtime.

Supplied: Tablets 75 mg*, 150 mg, 300 mg; syrup 15 mg/mL; injection 1 mg/mL, 25 mg/mL.

Notes: Reduce dose in patients with renal failure. Note that oral and parenteral doses are different.

RESPIRATORY SYNCYTIAL VIRUS IMMUNE GLOBULIN (RESPIGAM)

Indications: Prevention of serious lower respiratory infection caused by respiratory syncytial virus (RSV).

Actions: Immune globulin.

Dosage: 750 mg/kg IV infusion once monthly during RSV season (Nov–April). *Rate of infusion:* 1.5 mL/kg/h for 15 minutes, then 3 mL/kg/h for 15 minutes, then 6 mL/kg/h.

Supplied: Injection 50 mg/mL.

Notes: Adverse reactions are rate related; anaphylactic medications should be available. Live virus vaccines should be deferred until 9 months after last dose.

RIBAVIRIN (VIRAZOLE)

Indications: Respiratory syncytial virus; influenza A and B; hepatitis C; adenovirus.

Actions: Inhibits DNA and RNA virus replication.

Dosage: Aerosolization: 6 g diluted in 300 mL sterile water or NS for 12–18 h/day for 3–7 days.
   Hepatitis C: 600 mg PO twice daily in combination with interferon alfa-2b.

Supplied: Powder for aerosol 6 g; capsule 200 mg.

Notes: Aerosolized by a SPAG generator; may accumulate on soft contact lenses. Monitor Hct and Hgb frequently.

RIFAMPIN (RIFADIN)

Indications: Tuberculosis (treatment and prophylaxis); prophylaxis for exposure to *Meningococcus* and *Haemophilus influenzae;* treatment of *Staphylococcus aureus* nasal carriers.

Actions: Inhibits DNA-dependent RNA polymerase activity.

Dosage: Meningococcal prophylaxis: Children: 20 mg/kg/day PO divided q12h for 2 days; *Adults:* 600 mg PO q12h for 2 days.
   H influenzae prophylaxis: Children: 20 mg/kg/day PO daily for 4 days; *Adults:* 600 mg PO daily for 4 days.
   S aureus nasal carrier dose: Children: 15 mg/kg/day PO divided q12h for 5–10 days; *Adults:* 600 mg PO daily for 5–10 days.
   Tuberculosis: Infants and children: 10–20 mg/kg/day PO or IV divided q12–24h or given twice weekly; *Adults:* 10 mg/kg PO or IV once daily or twice weekly, max 600 mg/day.

Supplied: Capsules 150 mg, 300 mg; injection 600 mg.

Notes: Multiple drug interactions; causes orange-red discoloration of bodily secretions, including tears. Never used as a single agent to treat active tuberculosis infections.

RIMANTADINE (FLUMADINE)

Indications: Prophylaxis and treatment of influenza A infection.

Actions: Prevents penetration of virus into cell.

Dosage: Prophylaxis: Children: 5 mg/kg PO daily, max 150 mg per dose; *Adults: Prophylaxis and treatment:* 100 mg PO twice daily.

Supplied: Tablet 100 mg; syrup 50 mg/5 mL.

Notes: Give prophylaxis at least 10 days after exposure.

RITONAVIR (NORVIR)

Indications: Treatment of HIV infection when therapy is warranted.

Actions: Protease inhibitor; inhibits maturation of immature noninfectious virions to mature infectious virus.

Dosage: Children: Initial 250 mg/m^2 per dose PO twice daily then titrate up to 400 mg/m^2 per dose PO twice daily, max 600 mg per dose; *Adults:* 600 mg PO twice daily; or 400 mg PO twice daily in combination with saquinavir.

Supplied: Capsule 100 mg; solution 80 mg/mL.

Notes: Titrate dose over 1 week to avoid GI complications; should be taken with food. Has many drug interactions; may cause perioral and peripheral paresthesias. Store in refrigerator.

ROCURONIUM (ZEMURON)

Indications: Skeletal muscle relaxation during rapid-sequence intubation, surgery, or mechanical ventilation.

Actions: Nondepolarizing neuromuscular blockade.

Dosage: Rapid sequence intubation: Children and adults: 0.6–1.2 mg/kg IV; *Continuous infusion:* 4–16 mcg/kg/min IV.

Supplied: Injection 10 mg/mL.

Notes: Reduce dose in patients with hepatic impairment.

SALMETEROL (SEREVENT, SEREVENT DISKUS)

Indications: Asthma; exercise-induced bronchospasm.

Actions: Sympathomimetic bronchodilator.

Dosage: Metered-dose inhaler: 2 inhalations twice daily; *Diskus:* 1 inhalation twice daily.

Supplied: Metered-dose inhaler 25 mcg per spray; inhalation powder 50 mcg per inhalation.

Notes: Not for relief of acute attacks.

SERTRALINE (ZOLOFT)

Indications: Depression.

Actions: Inhibits neuronal uptake of serotonin.

Dosage: 50–200 mg PO daily.

Supplied: Tablets 25 mg, 50 mg, 100 mg.

Notes: Can activate manic and hypomanic state; has caused weight loss in clinical trials. Use with caution in patients with hepatic impairment. Can cause insomnia or hypersomnia and sexual dysfunction.

SILVER NITRATE (DEY-DROP)

Indications: Removal of granulation tissue and warts; cauterization of wounds.

Actions: Caustic antiseptic and astringent.

Dosage: Apply to moist surface 2–3 times per week for several weeks or until desired effect.

Supplied: Topical: Impregnated applicator sticks, 10% ointment, 10%, 25%, 50% solution.

Notes: May stain tissue black; usually resolves.

SILVER SULFADIAZINE (SILVADENE)

Indications: Prevention of sepsis in second- and third-degree burns.

Actions: Bactericidal.

Dosage: Aseptically cover affected area with 1/16-inch coating twice daily.

Supplied: Cream 1%.

Notes: Can have systemic absorption with extensive application.

SIMETHICONE (MYLICON)*

Indications: Symptomatic treatment of flatulence.

Actions: Defoaming action.

Dosage: 40–125 mg PO after meals and at bedtime prn.

Supplied: Tablets 40 mg, 80 mg, 125 mg; capsule 125 mg; drops 40 mg/ 0.6 mL.

SIROLIMUS (RAPAMUNE)

Indications: Prophylaxis of organ rejection.

Actions: Inhibits T-lymphocyte activation.

Dosage: 2 mg/day PO.

Supplied: Solution 1 mg/mL.

Notes: Instruct patient to dilute drug in water or orange juice and not to drink grapefruit juice while taking drug. Drug should be taken 4 hours after cyclosporine. Adjust dose in patients with hepatic impairment.

SODIUM BICARBONATE

Indications: Alkalinization of urine; renal tubular acidosis (RTA); treatment of metabolic acidosis; hyperkalemia.

Dosage: Emergency cardiac care: Initiate adequate ventilation, 1 mEq/kg per dose IV; can repeat 0.5 mEq/kg in 10 minutes 1 time or based on acid-base status.
Metabolic acidosis: 2–5 mEq/kg IV over 8 hours and prn based on acid-base status.
Alkalinize urine: 4 g (48 mEq) PO, then 1–2 g q4h; adjust dose based on urine pH.
Chronic renal failure: 1–3 mEq/kg/day.
Distal RTA: 1 mEq/kg/day PO.

Supplied: Injection 0.5 mEq/mL, 1 mEq/mL; tablets 325 mg, 650 mg.

Notes: 1 g neutralizes 12 mEq of acid. Supplied as IV infusion, powder, and tablets 300 mg = 3.6 mEq; 325 mg = 3.8 mEq; 520 mg = 6.3 mEq; 600 mg = 7.3 mEq; 650 mg = 7.6 mEq. Avoid use of multiple ampules; can cause hyperosmolar state.

SODIUM CHLORIDE

Indications: Restoration of sodium ion in hyponatremia.

Actions: Functions in fluid and electrolyte balance, osmotic pressure control, and water distribution.

Dosage: Maintenance requirements: Infants and children: 2–4 mEq/kg/day PO or IV, max dose 100–150 mg/day; *Adults:* 154 mEq/day.

To correct acute hyponatremia:

$$\text{mEq sodium} = [\text{Desired sodium (mEq/L)} - \text{Actual sodium (mEq/L)}] \times 0.6 \times \text{wt (kg)}$$

Supplied: Injection 0.45%, 0.9%, 3%; tablet 1 g (17 mEq).

Notes: Hypertonic solutions (> 0.9%) should only be used for treatment of symptomatic hyponatremia. Normal saline (0.9%) = 154 mEq/L; 3% NaCl = 513 mEq/L. Acutely correct serum sodium in 5 mEq/L per dose increments; more gradual correction can occur for asymptomatic patients.

SODIUM POLYSTYRENE SULFONATE (KAYEXALATE)

Indications: Hyperkalemia.

Actions: Sodium and potassium ion exchange resin.

Dosage: 15–60 g PO; or 30–60 g PR q6h based on serum potassium.

Supplied: Powder; suspension 15 g/60 mL sorbitol.

Notes: Can cause hypernatremia. Should be given with an agent such as sorbitol to promote movement through the bowel.

SPIRONOLACTONE (ALDACTONE)

Indications: Hyperaldosteronism; essential hypertension; edematous states (congestive heart failure, cirrhosis, nephrotic syndrome).

Actions: Aldosterone antagonist; potassium-sparing diuretic.

Dosage: *Children:* 1.5–3.3 mg/kg/day PO divided q6–24h; *Adults:* 25–400 mg PO once daily.

Supplied: Tablets 25 mg, 50 mg, 100 mg.

Notes: Can cause hyperkalemia and gynecomastia. Reduce dose in patients with renal impairment.

SUCCINYLCHOLINE (ANECTINE, QUELICIN, SUCOSTRIN)

Indications: Adjunct to general anesthesia to facilitate endotracheal intubation and to induce skeletal muscle relaxation during surgery or mechanically supported ventilation.

Actions: Depolarizing neuromuscular blocking agent.

Dosage: *Children:* 1–2 mg/kg IV followed by 0.3–0.6 mg/kg q5–10min prn or 2.5–4 mg/kg IM, max 150 mg per dose; *Adults:* 0.6 mg/kg IV or IM followed by 0.04–0.07 mg/kg prn to maintain muscle relaxation.

Supplied: Injection 20 mg/mL, 50 mg/mL, 100 mg/mL.

Notes: May precipitate malignant hyperthermia. Respiratory depression or prolonged apnea may occur. Has many drug interactions potentiating its activity; monitor patient for cardiovascular effects. Decrease dosage in patients with severe liver disease.

SUCRALFATE (CARAFATE)

Indications: Duodenal and gastric ulcers.

Actions: Forms ulcer-adherent complex that protects it against acid, pepsin, and bile acid.

Dosage: Children: 40–80 mg/kg/day PO divided q6h; *Adults:* 1 g PO 4 times daily, 1 hour prior to meals and at bedtime.

Supplied: Tablets 1 g; suspension 1 g/10 mL.

Notes: Treatment should be continued for 4–8 weeks unless healing is demonstrated by x-ray or endoscopy. Constipation is most frequent side effect. Aluminum salt is minimally absorbed, but may accumulate in patients with renal failure.

SULFACETAMIDE (BLEPH-10, CETAMIDE, SODIUM SULAMYD) (SEE TABLE VIII–6, P. 754)
SULFACETAMIDE AND PREDNISOLONE (BLEPHAMIDE, OTHERS) (SEE TABLE VIII–6, P. 754)
SULFASALAZINE (AZULFIDINE)

Indications: Ulcerative colitis; Crohn disease; juvenile rheumatoid arthritis.

Actions: Anti-inflammatory 5-aminosalicylic acid derivative.

Dosage: Ulcerative colitis: Children > 2 years: Mild exacerbation: 40–50 mg/kg/day PO divided q6h; *Moderate-severe exacerbation:* 50–75 mg/kg/day PO divided q6h, max 6 g/day; *Maintenance:* 30–50 mg/kg/day PO divided q8h, max 2 g/day.
Juvenile rheumatoid arthritis: Initial 10 mg/kg/day, increase weekly by 10 mg/kg/day to 30–50 mg/kg/day divided twice daily, max 2 g/day.
Adults: Initial dose 1 g 3–4 times daily; increase to max of 6 g/day in 3–4 divided doses; maintenance 500 mg PO 4 times daily.

Supplied: Tablet 500 mg; enteric-coated tablets 500 mg.

Notes: Can cause severe GI upset; discolors urine orange-yellow.

TACROLIMUS (FK 506) (PROGRAF, PROTOPIC)

Indications: Prophylaxis of organ rejection; topical for atopic dermatitis.

Actions: Macrolide immunosuppressant.

Dosage: Children and adults: Intravenous: 0.03–0.15 mg/kg/day as continuous infusion.
  Oral: 0.15–0.4 mg/kg/day divided into 2 doses.
  Topical: Apply to affected area twice daily.

Supplied: Capsules 0.5 mg, 1 mg, 5 mg; injection 5 mg/mL; ointment 0.03%, 0.1%.

Notes: Children may require higher doses on a milligram-per-kilogram basis than adults. May cause neurotoxicity and nephrotoxicity; use lower doses in patients with renal impairment. May need to reduce dose in patients with hepatic impairment. Monitor serum drug levels; range 5–20 ng/mL.

TERBUTALINE (BRETHINE)

Indications: Reversible bronchospasm (asthma, chronic obstructive pulmonary disease).

Actions: β_2-Adrenergic agonist bronchodilator.

Dosage: Bronchodilator: Oral: Children < 12 years: 0.05 mg/kg per dose PO q8h, increase gradually up to 0.15 mg/kg per dose, max 5 mg/day; *Adults:* 2.5–5 mg PO 4 times daily, max 15 mg per dose.
  Subcutaneous: Children: 0.005–0.01 mg/kg per dose SQ q15–20min for 3 doses, may repeat q2–6h prn, max 0.4 mg per dose; *Adults:* 0.25 mg SQ; may repeat in 20 minutes for 3 doses, max total dose 7.5 mg.
  Nebulization: Children and adults: 0.01–0.03 mL/kg, max 2.5 mL q4–6h.
  Continuous IV infusion: 2–10 mcg/kg load followed by 0.08–0.4 mcg/kg/min, titrate to response, max 10 mcg/kg/min.

Supplied: Tablets 2.5 mg, 5 mg; injection 1 mg/mL.

Notes: Use with caution in patients with diabetes, hypertension, or hyperthyroidism. High doses may precipitate β_1-adrenergic effects.

TETANUS IMMUNE GLOBULIN (SEE APPENDIX L, P. 771)
TETANUS TOXOID (SEE APPENDIX L, P. 771)
TETRACYCLINE (ACHROMYCIN V, SUMYCIN)

Indications: Broad-spectrum antibiotic treatment against *Staphylococcus, Streptococcus, Chlamydia, Rickettsia,* and *Mycoplasma.*

Actions: Bacteriostatic; inhibits protein synthesis.

Dosage: Children > 8 years: 25–50 mg/kg/day PO divided q6h, max 3 g/day; *Adolescents and adults:* 250–500 mg PO 2–4 times daily.

Supplied: Capsules 250 mg, 500 mg; tablets 250 mg, 500 mg; oral suspension 125 mg/5 mL.

Notes: Do not use in pregnancy. *Do not* use in patients with impaired renal function. *Do not* use with antacids or milk products.

THEOPHYLLINE (THEOLAIR, THEO-DUR, UNIPHYL, OTHERS)

Indications: Asthma; bronchospasm; apnea of prematurity.

Actions: Relaxes smooth muscle of bronchi and pulmonary blood vessels; stimulates CNS respiratory drive; increases diaphragmatic contraction.

Dosage: Apnea of prematurity: 4 mg/kg per dose PO load.
    Bronchospasm: Infants and children: 5 mg/kg PO load, followed by maintenance dose dependent on age, range 10–24 mg/kg/day divided q6–8h; *Adults:* 900 mg PO divided q6h; sustained-release products may be divided q8–12h.

Supplied: Elixir 80 mg/15 mL; extended-release capsules 100 mg, 200 mg, 300 mg, 400 mg; immediate-release tablets, 125 mg, 250 mg, 300 mg; sustained-release tablets 100 mg, 200 mg, 300 mg, 400 mg, 450 mg, 500 mg, 600 mg.

Notes: Use $\frac{1}{2}$ loading dose if patient is currently taking theophylline. Therapeutic range, asthma 10–20 mcg/mL, apnea of prematurity 6–14 mcg/mL. Has many drug interactions; side effects include nausea, vomiting, tachycardia, and seizures.

THIAMINE (VITAMIN B1) (SEE VITAMINS, P. 745)
THIOGUANINE

Indications: Acute and chronic myelogenous leukemia; acute lymphocytic leukemia.

Actions: Antineoplastic purine antimetabolite.

Dosage: Refer to individual protocols.

Supplied: Tablet 40 mg.

Notes: Toxicity includes myelosuppression (leukopenia, thrombocytopenia), nausea, vomiting, anorexia, stomatitis, diarrhea, and rare hepatotoxicity. Adjust dose in patients with renal or hepatic impairment.

THIOTEPA (THIOPLEX)

Indications: Hodgkin and non-Hodgkin lymphomas; leukemia; breast, ovarian, and bladder cancer; preparative for allogeneic and autologous bone marrow transplantation.

Actions: Antineoplastic alkylating agent.

Dosage: Refer to individual protocols.

Supplied: Powder for injection 15 mg.

Notes: Toxicity includes myelosuppression, nausea, vomiting, dizziness, headache, allergy, and paresthesias.

TIAGABINE (GABITRIL)

Indications: Adjunctive therapy in treatment of partial seizures.

Actions: Inhibition of GABA.

Dosage: Children 12–18 years: Initial 4 mg PO once daily for 1 week, then 4 mg PO twice daily for 1 week, then increase weekly by 4–8 mg/day until clinical response is achieved, max dose 32 mg/day; *Adults:* Initial 4 mg PO once daily for 1 week, may keep increasing by 4–8 mg/day weekly until clinical response is achieved, max dose 56 mg/day; 3 times daily dosing is preferred frequency for maintenance doses.

Supplied: Tablets 2 mg, 4 mg, 12 mg, 16 mg.

Notes: Use gradual withdrawal; lower doses or slower titration may be required in patients not receiving enzyme-inducing anticonvulsants.

TICARCILLIN (TICAR)

Indications: Serious gram-negative infections caused by *Pseudomonas, Proteus, E coli,* and *Enterobacter.*

Actions: Antipseudomonal penicillin antibiotic.

Dosage: Infants and children: 200–400 mg/kg/day IV divided q4–6h, max 24 g/day; *Adults:* 1–4 g IV q4–6h, max 24 g/day.

Supplied: Powder for injection 3 g.

Notes: Adjust dose in patients with renal impairment.

TICARCILLIN AND POTASSIUM CLAVULANATE (TIMENTIN)

Indications: Serious gram-negative infections caused by *Pseudomonas, Proteus, E coli,* and *Enterobacter.*

Actions: Antipseudomonal penicillin and beta-lactamase combination antibiotic.

Dosage: Infants and children: 200–300 mg/kg/day of ticarcillin IV divided q4–6h, max 18–24 g/day; *Adults:* 3.1 g (3 g ticarcillin plus 0.1 g clavulanate) IV q4–6h, max 18–24 g/day.

Supplied: Powder for injection 3 g ticarcillin/0.1 g clavulanate.

Notes: Sodium content of 1 g = 4.75 mEq; potassium content of 1 g = 0.15 mEq. Adjust dose in patients with renal impairment.

TOBRAMYCIN (NEBCIN)

Indications: Serious gram-negative infections, especially *Pseudomonas.*

Actions: Aminoglycoside; inhibits protein synthesis.

Dosage: Infants and children < 5 years: 2.5 mg/kg per dose IV or IM q8h; *Children ≥ 5 years:* 2–2.5 mg/kg per dose IV or IM q8h.
   Cystic fibrosis: Children: 2.5–3.3 mg/kg per dose IV or IM q6–8h; *Adults:* 3–6 mg/kg/day IV or IM divided q8–24h.
   Inhalation: Children: 40–80 mg aerosolized 2–3 times daily; *Adults:* 60–80 mg aerosolized 3 times daily.
   High-dose inhalation: Children ≥ 6 years and adults: 300 mg q12h.

Supplied: Injection 10 mg/mL, 40 mg/mL; solution for nebulization 60 mg/mL.

Notes: Drug is nephrotoxic and ototoxic. Decrease dose in patients with renal insufficiency. Monitor creatinine clearance and serum concentrations for dosage adjustments.

TOBRAMYCIN OPHTHALMIC (AK TOB, TOBREX) (SEE TABLE VIII–6, P. 754)
TOBRAMYCIN AND DEXAMETHASONE OPHTHALMIC (TOBRADEX) (SEE TABLE VIII–6, P. 754)
TOLMETIN (TOLECTIN)

Indications: Inflammatory and rheumatoid disorders, including juvenile rheumatoid arthritis.

Actions: NSAID.

Dosage: Anti-inflammatory: Children > 2 years: Initial 20 mg/kg/day PO in 3–4 divided doses, then 15–30 mg/kg/day, max 1800 mg/day; *Analgesic:* 5–7 mg/kg per dose PO q6–8h.
    Adults: 400 mg PO 3 times daily, max 2 g/day.

Supplied: Capsule 400 mg, tablet 600 mg.

Notes: Give with food. Use with caution in patients with GI disease or renal dysfunction.

TOLNAFTATE (TINACTIN)*

Indications: Tinea pedis; tinea cruris; tinea corporis; tinea manuum; tinea versicolor.

Actions: Topical antifungal.

Dosage: Apply to area 2–3 times daily for 2–4 weeks.

Supplied: 1% gel*, 1% powder*, 1% cream*, 1% solution*.

TOPIRAMATE (TOPAMAX)

Indications: Partial-onset seizures.

Actions: Anticonvulsant.

Dosage: 8-week titration schedule: Children 2–16 years: 1–3 mg/kg/day PO nightly for 1 week, increase at 1–2-week intervals by 1–3 mg/kg/day in 1–2 divided doses, titrate to response, usual maintenance 5–9 mg/kg/day in 2 divided doses; *Adults:* 25–50 mg PO daily for 1 week, increase by 25–50 mg/day at weekly intervals, titrate to response, usual maintenance 200 mg PO twice daily, max 1600 mg/day.

Supplied: Tablets 25 mg, 100 mg, 200 mg; capsule sprinkles 15 mg, 25 mg.

Notes: May precipitate kidney stones; adjust dose in patients with renal impairment. Acute myopia associated with secondary angle-closure glaucoma has been reported; discontinue to reverse symptoms.

TRAZODONE (DESYREL)

Indications: Depression.

Actions: Antidepressant; inhibits reuptake of serotonin and norepinephrine.

Dosage: Children 6–18 years: Initial 1.5–2 mg/kg/day PO in divided doses, increase gradually every 3–4 days prn, max 6 mg/kg/day divided 3 times daily; *Adolescents and adults:* 50–150 mg PO 1–3 times daily; max 600 mg/day.

Supplied: Tablets 50 mg, 100 mg, 150 mg, 300 mg.

Notes: May take 2–6 weeks for symptomatic improvement. Anticholinergic side effects.

TRETINOIN, TOPICAL [RETINOIC ACID] (RETIN-A, AVITA)

Indications: Acne vulgaris; sun-damaged skin; some skin cancers.

Actions: Exfoliant retinoic acid derivative.

Dosage: Apply daily at bedtime; if irritation develops, decrease frequency.

Supplied: Cream 0.025%; 0.05%; 0.1%; Gel 0.01%, 0.025%, 0.04%, 0.1%; liquid 0.05%.

Notes: Begin with weaker concentration and increase as tolerated. Instruct patients to avoid sunlight.

TRIAMCINOLONE (AZMACORT, NASACORT)

Indications: Chronic treatment of asthma.

Actions: Topical steroid.

Dosage: *Intranasal: Children 6–12 years:* 2 sprays each nostril once daily, titrate to response; *Children > 12 years and adults:* 2 sprays each nostril once daily, may increase to 4 sprays each nostril in 4–7 days, maintenance dose may be given in 1–4 divided doses.
   Oral inhalation: Children 6–12 years: 4–12 inhalations per day divided 3–4 times daily; *Children > 12 years and adults:* 4–16 inhalations per day divided 3–4 times daily.

Supplied: Metered-dose inhaler 100 mcg per spray; nasal spray 55 mcg per inhalation.

Notes: Use lowest effective dose. May cause oral candidiasis; instruct patients to rinse mouth after use. Not for acute asthma.

TRIMETHOPRIM (PRIMSOL, PROLOPRIM)

Indications: Acute otitis media and UTIs caused by susceptible gram-positive and gram-negative organisms; often used for suppression of UTIs.

Actions: Inhibits dihydrofolate reductase.

Dosage: *Acute otitis media:* 10 mg/kg/d PO divided q12h for 10 days.
   UTI: 4–6 mg/kg/d PO divided q12h for 10 days;
   Adults: 200 mg/d divided qd–bid.

Supplied: Tablets 100 mg, 200 mg; oral solution: 50 mg/5 mL.

Notes: Reduce dose in patients with renal failure.

TRIMETHOPRIM-SULFAMETHOXAZOLE (CO-TRIMOXAZOLE, BACTRIM, SEPTRA)

Indications: UTI; otitis media; sinusitis; bronchitis; *Shigella; Pneumocystis carinii.*

Actions: Dual effect of sulfamethoxazole (SMX)-inhibiting synthesis of dihydrofolic acid and trimethoprim (TMP)-inhibiting dihydrofolate reductase to cause impaired protein synthesis.

Dosage: Mild to moderate infections: 6–12 mg TMP/kg/day PO or IV divided q12h.
    Serious infections and Pneumocystis: 15–20 mg TMP/kg/day PO or IV divided q6–8h.
    Pneumocystis prophylaxis: 150 mg TMP/m^2/day PO divided q12h 3 days/wk.
    UTI prophylaxis: 2 mg TMP/kg per dose PO daily or 5 mg TMP/kg per dose twice weekly.
    Adults: 1 double-strength (DS) tablet PO twice daily or 5–20 mg TMP/kg/day IV in 3–4 divided doses.

Supplied: Single-strength tablet 80 mg TMP/400 mg SMX; double-strength tablet 160 mg TMP/800 mg SMX; oral suspension 40 mg TMP/200 mg SMX per 5 mL; injection 80 mg TMP/400 mg SMX per 5 mL.

Notes: Synergistic combination. Reduce dose in patients with renal failure. Maintain adequate hydration.

TRIPROLIDINE AND PSEUDOEPHEDRINE (ACTIFED)*

Indications: Temporary relief of nasal congestion, runny nose, sneezing, and itchiness due to common cold, hay fever, or allergies.

Actions: Antihistamine and decongestant combination.

Dosage: Children: (Dose according to pseudoephedrine component) 4 mg/kg/day PO divided 3–4 times daily; *Children > 12 years and adults:* 10 mL or 1 tablet PO 3–4 times daily.

Supplied: Tablet 2.5 mg triprolidine/60 mg pseudoephedrine; syrup 1.25 mg triprolidine/30 mg pseudoephedrine per 5 mL.

Notes: Contraindicated in patients with severe hypertension. Not for use in infants < 4 months.

UROKINASE (ABBOKINASE)

Indications: Pulmonary embolism; deep venous thrombosis; to restore patency to IV catheters.

Actions: Converts plasminogen to plasmin that causes clot lysis.

Dosage: Systemic effect: 4400 units/kg IV over 10 minutes, followed by 4400–6000 units/kg/h for 6–12 hours; longer infusions (12–72 hours) may be necessary.
Restore catheter patency: Inject 5000 units into catheter and gently aspirate.

Supplied: Powder for injection 5000 units, 250,000 units.

Notes: Do not use systemically within 10 days of surgery, delivery, or organ biopsy.

URSODIOL (ACTIGALL, URSO)

Indications: Dissolution and prevention of gallstones; to facilitate bile excretion in biliary atresia; TPN-induced cholestasis; to improve fatty acid metabolism in cystic fibrosis.

Actions: Decreases cholesterol content of bile and bile stones.

Dosage: Biliary atresia: Infants: 10–15 mg/kg/day PO daily.
Cystic fibrosis: 30 mg/kg/day PO divided twice daily.
TPN-induced cholestasis: 30 mg/kg/day PO divided 3 times daily.
Gallstones: Dissolution: Adults: 8–10 mg/kg/day PO divided 2–3 times daily, then 250 mg/day at bedtime for 6 months to 1 year; *Prevention:* 300 mg PO twice daily.

Supplied: Capsule 300 mg, tablet 250 mg.

Notes: 30–50% of patients have stone recurrence after dissolution. Effect of drug is decreased in combination with aluminum-containing antacids and cholestyramine.

VALPROIC ACID AND DIVALPROEX (DEPAKENE, DEPAKOTE)

Indications: Epilepsy; prophylaxis of migraines.

Actions: Anticonvulsant; increases availability of gamma-aminobutyric acid (GABA).

Dosage: Seizures: Children and adults:
- *Oral:* Initial 10–15 mg/kg/day in 1–3 divided doses, then increase weekly by 5–10 mg/kg/day to 30–60 mg/kg/day maintenance.
- *Parenteral:* Total IV dose is equal to total PO dose divided q6h.

- *Rectal:* Dilute syrup 1:1 with water as retention enema, loading dose is 17–20 mg/kg, followed by maintenance of 10–15 mg/kg per dose q8h.

Migraines: Adults: 250 mg PO twice daily, increased to 1000 mg/day.

Extended-release tablets (Depakote ER): 500 mg PO daily for 7 days, then may increase up to 1000 mg/day if needed.

Supplied: *Valproic acid:* capsules 250 mg; syrup 250 mg/5 mL. *Divalproex:* enteric-coated tablets 125 mg, 250 mg, 500 mg; extended-release tablet (Depakote ER) 500 mg; sprinkle capsule 125 mg; injection 100 mg/mL.

Notes: Monitor liver function and serum levels (range 50–100 mcg/mL). Concurrent use of phenobarbital and phenytoin may alter serum levels of these agents. Reduce dose in patients with hepatic impairment. Hemodialysis reduces levels by 20%. Use of Depakote ER is not recommended in children.

VANCOMYCIN (VANCOCIN, VANCOLED)

Indications: Serious infections caused by methicillin-resistant staphylococci and ampicillin-resistant enterococcal infections and in enterococcal endocarditis in combination with aminoglycosides in penicillin-allergic patients; oral treatment of *Clostridium difficile* pseudomembranous colitis.

Actions: Inhibits cell wall synthesis.

Dosage: *Infants > 1 month and children:* 40 mg/kg/day IV divided q6–8h. *Staphylococcal CNS infection:* 60 mg/kg/day IV divided q6h, max 1 g per dose; *Adults:* 1 g IV q12h, max 4 g/day.

C difficile colitis: Children: 40 mg/kg/day PO divided q6h for 7–10 days; *Adults:* 125–500 mg PO q6h.

Intrathecal and intraventricular: Neonates: 5–10 mg/day; *Children:* 5–20 mg/day; *Adults:* 20 mg/day.

Supplied: Capsules 125 mg, 250 mg; powder for oral solution 250 mg/5 mL; powder for injection 500 mg, 1 g, 10 g per vial.

Notes: Drug is ototoxic and nephrotoxic. Not absorbed orally; oral dose provides local effect in gut only. IV dose must be given slowly over 1 hour to prevent "red-man syndrome." Adjust dose in patients with renal failure. Peak 25–40 mcg/mL; trough 5–10 mcg/mL.

VARICELLA VACCINE (VARIVAX) (SEE APPENDIX D, P. 759)
VASOPRESSIN (ANTIDIURETIC HORMONE) (PITRESSIN)

Indications: Diabetes insipidus; postoperative abdominal distention; severe GI bleeding.

Actions: Posterior pituitary hormone; potent GI vasoconstrictor.

Dosage: Diabetes insipidus: Children and adults: 2.5–10 units SQ or IM 3–4 times daily or 0.0005 unit/kg/h IV continuous infusion, double dose q30min prn to max of 0.01 units/kg/h.

GI hemorrhage: Children: 0.002–0.005 units/kg/min IV continuous infusion, titrate prn to max of 0.01 units/kg/min; *Adults:* 0.2–0.4 units/min, max 0.9 unit/min.

Supplied: Injection 20 units/mL.

Notes: Continue dose for 12 hours once bleeding stops, then taper off over 24–48 hours. Use with caution in patients with any vascular disease.

VECURONIUM (NORCURON)

Indications: Skeletal muscle relaxation during surgery or mechanical ventilation.

Actions: Nondepolarizing neuromuscular blocker.

Dosage: Children and adults: 0.1 mg/kg IV, repeat q1h prn, or 1.5–2.5 mcg/kg/min IV continuous infusion.

Supplied: Powder for injection 10 mg.

Notes: Drugs leading to potentiation of effect include aminoglycosides, diuretics, and succinylcholine. Has fewer cardiac effects than pancuronium. Reduce in patients with hepatic dysfunction. Concomitant analgesia or sedation is required.

VERAPAMIL (CALAN, ISOPTIN)

Indications: Angina; essential hypertension; arrhythmias (paroxysmal supraventricular tachycardia [PSVT], atrial fibrillation, atrial flutter).

Actions: Calcium channel blocker.

Dosage: Arrhythmias (SVT): Children 1–16 years: 0.1–0.3 mg/kg per dose IV, max 5 mg per dose, may repeat in 30 minutes if inadequate response, or 4–8 mg/kg/day PO divided 3 times daily; *Adults:* 5–10 mg IV over 2 minutes followed by 10 mg in 15–30 minutes if tolerated but not responding to initial dose.

Hypertension: Adults: 80–180 mg PO 3 times daily; or sustained-release tablet 120–240 mg PO once daily to 240 mg twice daily.

Supplied: Tablets 40 mg, 80 mg, 120 mg; sustained-release tablets 120 mg, 180 mg, 240 mg; sustained-release capsules 120 mg, 180 mg, 240 mg, 360 mg; injection 5 mg/2 mL.

Notes: Reduce dose in patients with renal or hepatic failure. Constipation is a common side effect. Instruct patients to avoid grapefruit juice.

VITAMIN B$_1$ (SEE VITAMINS, P. 745)
VITAMIN B$_6$ (SEE VITAMINS, P. 745)
VITAMIN B$_{12}$ (SEE VITAMINS, P. 745)
VITAMIN K (SEE VITAMINS, P. 745)
WARFARIN (COUMADIN)

Indications: Prophylaxis and treatment of pulmonary embolism and venous thrombosis; prevention and treatment of arterial thromboembolism in patients with prosthetic heart valves or atrial fibrillation; other postoperative indications.

Actions: Inhibits vitamin K–dependent synthesis of clotting factors in the following order: VII, IX, X, II.

Dosage: Individualize dose to keep international normalized ratio (INR) 2–3 for most indications. *Infants and children:* Day 1 0.2 mg/kg, max dose 10 mg; Days 2–4 dose dependent on patient's INR.
   For mechanical heart valves: Desired INR is 2.5–3.5.
   ACCP guidelines: Recommend initiation with 5 mg, unless rapid attainment of therapeutic INR is necessary, then use 7.5–10 mg. If bleeding risk is present, reduce dosing. *Maintenance:* 2–10 mg PO, IV, or IM once daily; follow daily INR during initial phase to guide dosage change, then every 1–4 weeks when INR is stable.

Supplied: Tablets 1 mg, 2 mg, 2.5 mg, 3 mg, 4 mg, 5 mg, 6 mg, 7.5 mg, 10 mg; injection 5 mg.

Notes: INR is now preferred test rather than PT. Check INR periodically in patients receiving maintenance dose. Beware of bleeding caused by over-anticoagulation (PT > 3 × control or INR > 5.0–6.0). To rapidly correct over-coumadinization, use vitamin K or fresh-frozen plasma, or both. Drug is highly teratogenic; *do not* use in pregnancy. Caution patients who take warfarin with other medications, especially aspirin. **Common warfarin drug interactions: Potentiated by:** Acetaminophen, alcohol (with liver disease), amiodarone, cimetidine, ciprofloxacin, co-trimoxazole, erythromycin, fluconazole, isoniazid, itraconazole, metronidazole, omeprazole, phenytoin, propranolol, quinidine, tetracycline. **Inhibited by:** Barbiturates, carbamazepine, chlordiazepoxide, cholestyramine, dicloxacillin, nafcillin, rifampin, sucralfate, food high in vitamin K. Avoid IM injection of drugs.

ZAFIRLUKAST (ACCOLATE)

Indications: Prophylaxis and chronic treatment of asthma.

Actions: Selective and competitive inhibitor of leukotriene D4 and E4.

Dosage: Children 7–11 years: 10 mg PO twice daily; *Children ≥ 12 years and adults:* 20 mg PO twice daily.

Supplied: Tablets 10 mg, 20 mg.

Notes: Not for acute exacerbations of asthma. Contraindicated in breast-feeding. Increases anticoagulant effect of warfarin.

ZALCITABINE (HIVID)

Indications: HIV infection, in combination with other agents.

Actions: Nucleotide reverse transcriptase inhibitor.

Dosage: Infants and children < 13 years: 0.01 mg/kg PO 3 times daily; *Adolescents and adults:* 0.75 mg PO 3 times daily.

Supplied: Tablets 0.375 mg, 0.75 mg.

Notes: Adjust dose in patients with renal impairment. Administer on empty stomach. *Do not* administer with antacids. Use with extreme caution in patients with preexisting peripheral neuropathy. Discontinue use in patients with clinical or laboratory signs of pancreatitis or hepatotoxicity.

ZIDOVUDINE (RETROVIR)

Indications: HIV infection, in combination with other agents.

Actions: Nucleotide reverse transcriptase inhibitor.

Dosage: Neonates: 2 mg/kg per dose PO q6h or 1.5 mg/kg per dose IV q6h; *Children:* 160 mg/m^2 per dose PO q8h or 120 mg/m^2 per dose IV q6h; *Children > 12 years and adults:* 600 mg/day PO in 2–3 divided doses or 1–2 mg/kg per dose IV q4h.
   HIV postexposure prophylaxis: 600 mg/day PO in 2–3 divided doses in combination with lamivudine and indinavir.

Supplied: Capsule 100 mg; tablet 300 mg; syrup 50 mg/5 mL; injection 10 mg/mL.

Notes: Reduce dose by 30% in children with Hgb < 8 g/dL. Adjust dose in patients with renal impairment. Administer dose in upright position to minimize esophageal ulceration.

ZIDOVUDINE AND LAMIVUDINE (COMBIVIR)

Indications: HIV infection.

Actions: Combination inhibitors of reverse transcriptase.

Dosage: Adolescents and adults: 1 tablet twice daily.

Supplied: Capsules zidovudine 300 mg/lamivudine 150 mg.

Notes: Alternative used to reduce number of capsules required for combination therapy with these two agents.

ZONISAMIDE (ZONEGRAN)

Indications: Partial seizures; infantile spasms.

Actions: Anticonvulsant.

Dosage: Infants and children: Initial 1–4 mg/kg/day PO divided twice daily, titrate dose upward if needed every 2 weeks to max dose of 12 mg/kg/day; *Adolescents > 16 years and adults:* Initial 100 mg once daily; may be increased to 400 mg/day.

Supplied: Capsule 100 mg.

Notes: Contraindicated if patient is hypersensitive to sulfonamides. Use with caution in patients with hepatic or renal dysfunction. *Do not* use if creatinine clearance < 50 mL/min. *Do not* crush, chew, or break capsule.

3. MINERALS: INDICATIONS/EFFECTS, RDA/DOSAGE, SIGNS/SYMPTOMS OF DEFICIENCY AND TOXICITY, AND NOTES

CALCIUM

Indications/Effects: Strengthens bones and teeth; used as adjunct with osteoporosis medications to promote bone rebuilding; may decrease BP; aids premenstrual symptoms (pain, cramping, mood swings).

RDA/Dosage: (Expressed as elemental calcium) *Infants < 6 months:* 400 mg/day; *Infants 6–12 months:* 600 mg/day; *Children 1–10 years:* 800 mg/day; *Children and adolescents 11–24 years:* 1200 mg/day; *Adults > 24 years:* 800 mg/day.

S/Sx of Deficiency: Osteoporosis (over time) leading to increased risk of fractures and breaks.

S/Sx of Toxicity: > 2500 mg/day: Constipation, anorexia, dry mouth, nausea, polyuria, renal calculi.

Notes: Avoid calcium sources from dolomite, oyster shell, and bone meal as they may contain heavy metal contamination (lead, arsenic). Caffeine and cigarette smoking may reduce calcium absorption. Hyperthyroidism, diabetes mellitus, use of corticosteroids, and use of loop diuretics all either reduce calcium absorption or increase excretion. Calcium supplementation should be strongly considered in these cases. Vitamin D plus calcium combination decreases fracture rate and increases absorption.

CHROMIUM

Indications/Effects: Required for normal glucose metabolism (trace element).

RDA/Dosage: Infants: 0.2 mcg/kg; *Children ≥ 3 months and ≤ 5 years:* 0.14–0.2 mcg/kg (max 5 mcg/kg); *Children > 5 years and adults:* 10–15 mcg.

S/Sx of Deficiency: Rare; may cause development of adult diabetes mellitus and atherosclerosis, peripheral neuropathy.

S/Sx of Toxicity: Irritation of GI tract (nausea, vomiting, ulcers), renal damage, eczema or dermatitis from occupational exposure.

Notes: Balanced diet fulfills RDA.

COPPER

Indications/Effects: Bone formation; hematopoiesis; enzyme component.

RDA/Dosage: Infants: 20 mcg/kg; *Children ≥ 3 months and ≤ 5 years:* 20 mcg/kg (max 300 mcg); *Children > 5 years and adults:* 0.3–0.5 mg.

S/Sx of Deficiency: Anemia in malnourished children.

S/Sx of Toxicity: Self-limiting nausea, vomiting, diarrhea (usually caused by occupational exposure).

Notes: Balanced diet fulfills RDA.

FLUORIDE

Indications/Effects: Prevention of dental caries; promotes remineralization of decalcified enamel; inhibits the cariogenic microbial process in dental plaque; increases tooth resistance to acid dissolution.

RDA/Dosage: Recommended daily intake is adjusted based on fluoride content of drinking water.

< 0.3 parts per million (ppm):

- Birth to 6 months: 0 mg.
- 6 months to 3 years: 0.25 mg.
- 3–6 years: 0.5 mg.
- 6–16 years: 1 mg.

0.3–0.6 ppm:

- Birth to 3 years: 0 mg.
- 3–6 years: 0.25 mg.
- 6–16 years: 0.5 mg.

0.6 ppm: All ages: 0 mg.

S/Sx of Deficiency: Tooth decay; rarely osteoporosis.

S/Sx of Toxicity: Nausea, vomiting, dysplegia, electrolyte imbalances, muscle weakness or spasms, headaches, behavioral changes, cardiac arrhythmias including arrest.

Notes: Do not administer with milk.

IRON

Indications/Effects: Energy transfer and carrying oxygen; prevention of microcytic anemia.

RDA/Dosage: (Expressed as elemental iron) *Infants < 5 months:* 5 mg; *Infants 5 months to children 10 years:* 10 mg; *Male children and adolescents 11–18 years:* 12 mg; *Male adolescents and adults > 18 years:* 10 mg; *Female children, adolescents, and adults 11–50 years:* 15 mg; *Female adults > 50 years:* 10 mg.

S/Sx of Deficiency: Microcytic, hypochromic anemia; fatigue, breathlessness, pallor, dizziness, headache.

S/Sx of Toxicity: > 75 mg/day: Nausea, diarrhea, abdominal pain, anorexia.

Notes: Iron may decrease absorption of other minerals when given concomitantly, has numerous drug interactions, and should not be given at the same time as other prescribed medications (eg, antacids, tetracycline). Concern exists regarding risk of hemochromatosis when supplementing iron in males. Iron is the most common cause of pediatric poisonings in the home. It is available in numerous salt forms with differing elemental iron content:

- Iron Salt Elemental Iron
- Fumarate 33%
- Gluconate 12%
- Sulfate 20–30%

FERROUS SULFATE

Indications/Effects: Iron deficiency anemia and iron supplementation; dietary supplementation.

RDA/Dosage: Premature neonates: 2–4 mg elemental iron/kg/day PO divided q12–24h, max 15 mg/day.

Infants and children:

- *Severe iron deficiency anemia:* 4–6 mg elemental iron/kg/day PO divided 3 times a day.
- *Mild to moderate iron deficiency anemia:* 3 mg elemental iron/kg/day PO 1–2 times a day.
- *Prophylaxis:* 1–2 mg elemental iron/kg/day PO daily, max 15 mg/day.

Notes: May turn stools and urine dark; can cause GI upset and constipation. Vitamin C taken with ferrous sulfate will increase absorption of iron, especially in patients with atrophic gastritis.

IRON DEXTRAN (DEXFERRUM, INFED)

Indications/Effects: Iron deficiency when oral supplementation is not possible; parenteral iron supplementation.

RDA/Dosage: Test dose: Infants: 12.5 mg (0.25 mL) IM or IV; *Children, adolescents, and adults:* 25 mg (0.5 mL) IM or IV 1 hour prior to starting iron dextran therapy.
Total replacement dose for iron deficiency anemia:

$$\text{Iron dextran (mL)} = 0.0476 \times \text{LBW (kg)} \times [\text{Hbn} - \text{Hbo}] + 1\ \text{mL/5 kg LBW (up to max of 14 mL).}$$

In which LBW = lean body weight; Hbn = desired Hgb (g/dL) = 12 if < 15 kg or 14.8 if > 15 kg; and Hbo = measured Hgb (g/dL).
Intramuscular: Maximum daily dose: Infants < 5 kg: 25 mg; *Children 5–10 kg:* 50 mg; *Children > 10 kg and adults:* 100 mg.

Notes: Test dose must be administered because anaphylaxis is common. Iron dextran may be given deep IM using the z-track technique, although IV administration is preferred.

IRON SUCROSE (VENOFER)

Indications/Effects: Iron deficiency anemia in patients undergoing chronic hemodialysis who are receiving supplemental erythropoietin therapy; iron replacement.

RDA/Dosage: Expressed as elemental iron: Adults: 5 mL (100 mg) IV 1–3 times per week during dialysis, given no faster than 1 mL (20 mg) per minute, for total dose of 1000 mg (10 doses).

Notes: Most patients require cumulative doses of 1000 mg; anaphylaxis and significant hypotension may follow administration. Test doses of 50 mg may be administered but not required by product labeling.

MAGNESIUM

Indications/Effects: Strengthens bones and teeth; reduces neurologic irritability in patients at risk for seizures (ie, eclampsia); may reduce pre-menstrual symptoms (headache, fluid retention, mood changes); maintains normal sinus rhythm.

RDA/Dosage: (Expressed as elemental magnesium) *Infants < 6 months:* 40 mg; *Infants 6–12 months:* 60 mg; *Children 1–3 years:* 80 mg; *Children 4–8 years:* 130 mg; *Male children and adolescents 9–13 years:* 240 mg; *Male adolescents 14–18 years:* 410 mg; *Male adolescents and adults ≥19 years:* 400; *Female children and adolescents 9–13 years:* 240 mg; *Female adolescents 14–18 years:* 360 mg; *Female adolescents and adults ≥19 years:* 310 mg.

S/Sx of Deficiency: Weakness, confusion, tingling, muscle contractions, cramps.

S/Sx of Toxicity: (> 350 mg/day): Diarrhea, nausea, drowsiness, lethargy, sweating, slurred speech.
Selenium

Indications/Effects: Decreases risk of heart disease (antioxidant); essential for normal function of immune system and thyroid gland.

RDA/Dosage: *Infants:* 2–3 mcg/kg; *Children ≥ 3 months and ≤ 5 years:* 2–3 mcg/kg (max 30 mcg); *Children > 5 years and adults:* 20–60 mcg.

S/Sx of Deficiency: Rare, due to TPN or GI malabsorptive diseases; can cause cardiomyopathy.

S/Sx of Toxicity: *> 400 mg/day:* "Selenosis": GI upset, hair loss, white-blotchy nails, mild nerve damage.

Notes: Balanced diet meets RDA requirements (dietary source: plant foods).

ZINC

Indications/Effects: Supplementation strengthens immune system if patient is zinc deficient; may prevent macular degeneration; may improve cognition; supports normal growth and development during pregnancy, childhood, and adolescence.

Dosage: Zinc deficiency: Oral: Infants and children: 0.5–1 elemental zinc/kg/day divided 1–3 times a day, *Adults:* 25–50 mg elemental zinc per dose 3 times a day.

Supplemental to parenteral nutrition solutions, as elemental zinc: Premature infants: 400 mcg/kg/day; *Term infants < 3 months:* 300 mcg/kg/day; *Infants ≥ 3 months and children ≤ 5 years:* 100 mcg/kg/day, max 5 mg/day; *Children > 5 years and adolescents:* 2.5–5 mg/day.

S/Sx of Deficiency: Impaired night vision, immune function, taste; also poor appetite, poor growth, delayed wound healing, anemia, hyperpigmentation, hepatosplenomegaly.

S/Sx of Toxicity: Altered iron function, reduced immune function, lowered HDL levels, GI intolerance, anemia, copper deficiency.

Notes: High calcium intake (> 1400 mg/day) reduces zinc absorption, requiring increased zinc intake of 18 mg/day.

4. VITAMINS: INDICATIONS/EFFECTS, RDA/DOSAGE, SIGNS/SYMPTOMS OF DEFICIENCY AND TOXICITY, AND NOTES

VITAMIN A

Indications/Effects: *General:* Healthy skin and vision; resistance to infection; bone and sperm development. *Pregnancy:* Maintains healthy fetus and prevents neural tube defects; may decrease maternal transmission of AIDS to fetus.

RDA/Dosage: *Oral: Infants < 1 year:* 375 mcg retinol equivalent (RE) (1250 units vitamin A); *Children 1–3 years:* 400 mcg RE (1330 units); *Children 4–6 years:* 500 mcg RE (1670 units); *Children 7–10 years:* 700 mcg RE (2330 units); *Children and adolescents > 10 years: Male:* 1000 mcg (2670 units); *Female:* 800 mcg (3330 units).

S/Sx of Deficiency: Rare; anemia, night blindness, diarrhea, renal calculi, tooth decay, flaking skin.

S/Sx of Toxicity: *> 3000 mcg/day:* Fatigue, night sweats, GI upset, headache, dry skin, alopecia, pruritus, hepatotoxicity; in pregnancy can result in birth defects (head, heart, brain, spinal column).

Notes: Patients who smoke or drink > 2 drinks/day should avoid vitamin A supplementation; 0.3 mcg retinol =1 unit Vitamin A.

CYANOCOBALAMIN (VITAMIN B$_{12}$)

Indications/Effects: Pernicious anemia and other vitamin B$_{12}$ deficiency states; dietary supplement of vitamin B$_{12}$.

RDA/Dosage: Oral: Children: 0.3–2 mcg; *Adults:* 2 mcg.
   Pernicious anemia: Neonates and infants: 1000 mcg/day IM or SQ for 2 weeks, then 50 mcg per month maintenance; *Children:* 30–50 mcg/day IM or SQ for 2 or more weeks to total dose of 1000 mcg, then 100 mcg per month maintenance; *Adults:* 100 mcg IM or SQ daily for 7 days, then 100 mcg IM twice a week for 1 month, then 100 mcg IM weekly for 1 month, then 1000 mcg IM monthly.

S/Sx of Deficiency: Macrocytic anemia, mental status changes, neuropathy (in elderly).

Notes: Oral absorption highly erratic, altered by many drugs and not recommended; for use with hyperalimentation.

FOLATE (FOLIC ACID, PTEROYLGLUTAMIC ACID)

Indications/Effects: Prevention of stroke, heart disease (via decreased homocysteine levels), dementia, cancer (antioxidant effect); prevention of neural tube defects in pregnancy; treatment of megaloblastic anemia.

RDA/Dosage: Oral: Premature neonates: 50 mcg; *Neonates ≤ 6 months:* 25–25 mcg; *Infants and children 6 months to 3 years:* 50 mcg; *Children 4–6 years:* 75 mcg; *Children 7–10 years:* 100 mcg; *Children and adolescents 11–14 years:* 150 mcg; *Adolescents ≥15 years and adults:* 200 mcg; *Pregnancy:* 400 mcg.
   Folate deficiency: Infants: 15 mcg/kg per dose PO, IM, IV, or SQ daily or 50 mcg/day; *Children 1–10 years:* Initial 1 mg PO daily, maintenance 0.1–0.4 mg/day; *Children ≥ 11 years and adults:* 1 mg/day initial, maintenance 0.5 mg/day.

S/Sx of Deficiency: Megaloblastic and macrocytic anemia, glossitis; risk of deficiency increased in patients receiving methotrexate.

S/Sx of Toxicity: Few (irritability, nausea), but doses of > 1000 mcg/day can mask vitamin B$_{12}$ deficiency.

Notes: Enhances metabolism of phenytoin. Recommended for all women of childbearing years; will decrease fetal neural tube defects by 50%.

NIACIN (VITAMIN B$_3$)

Indications/Effects: Adjunctive therapy in patients with significant hyperlipidemia who do not respond adequately to diet and weight loss; inhibits lipolysis; decreases esterification of triglycerides; increases lipoprotein lipase activity.

RDA/Dosage: Infants ≤ 6 months: 5 mg; *Infants 6 months to 1 year:* 6 mg; *Children 1–3 years:* 9 mg; *Children 4–6 years:* 12 mg; *Children 7–10 years:* 13 mg; *Male children and adolescents 11–14 years:* 17 mg; *Male adolescents 15–18 years:* 20 mg; *Male adolescents ≥ 19 years and adults:* 19 mg; *Female children ≥ 11 years, adolescents, and adults:* 15 mg.

S/Sx of Deficiency: Pellagra (dermatitis, diarrhea, dementia).

S/Sx of Toxicity: Flushing, pruritus, hyperglycemia, liver damage (rare).

Notes: May cause upper body and facial flushing and warmth following dose. May cause hepatitis, exacerbate peptic ulcer disease and gout, and worsen glucose control in patients with diabetes mellitus.

RIBOFLAVIN (VITAMIN B_2)

Indications/Effects: Prevention of riboflavin deficiency and treatment of ariboflavinosis; microcytic anemia associated with glutathione reductase deficiency.

RDA/Dosage: Children 1–3 years: 0.5 mg; *Children 4–8 years:* 0.6 mg; *Children 9–13 years:* 0.9 mg; *Adolescents 14–18 years: Male:* 1.3 mg; *Female:* 1 mg; *Adolescents ≥ 19 years and adults: Male:* 1.3 mg; *Female:* 1 mg.

S/Sx of Deficiency: Microcytic anemia.

S/Sx of Toxicity: Discoloration of urine (bright yellow) with large doses.

THIAMINE (VITAMIN B_1)

Indications/Effects: Carbohydrate metabolism; myocardial function.

RDA/Dosage: Children 1–3 years: 0.5 mg; *Children 4–8 years:* 0.6 mg; *Children 9–13 years:* 0.9 mg; *Adolescents 14–18 years: Male:* 1.2 mg; *Female:* 1 mg; *Adolescents ≥ 19 years and adults: Male:* 1.2 mg; *Female:* 1.1 mg.
   Thiamine deficiency: Children: 10–25 mg per dose IM or IV daily (if critically ill) or 10–50 mg per dose PO daily for 2 weeks, then 5–10 mg per dose PO daily for 1 month; *Adults:* 5–30 mg per dose IM or IV 3 times a day (if critically ill), then 5–30 mg/day PO 1–3 times a day for 1 month.
   Wernicke encephalopathy: 100 mg IV in single dose, then 100 mg IV or IM daily for 2 weeks.

S/Sx of Deficiency: Most likely to occur in chronic alcoholics and/or those with poor nutritional intake (eg, cachectic elderly in nursing home); peripheral neuropathy, nystagmus, confusion, ataxia, high-output heart failure. Early stages of deficiency known as Wernicke encephalopathy, which is reversible, may progress to Korsakoff psychosis, which is not.

S/Sx of Toxicity: Unknown.

Notes: IV thiamine administration is associated with anaphylactic reaction; must be given slowly IV.

VITAMIN B$_6$ (PYRIDOXINE)

Indications/Effects: Reduces severity and risk of depression, premenstrual syndrome, hypertension, carpal tunnel syndrome, and morning sickness; may help reduce cardiovascular disease through effects on homocysteine levels.

RDA/Dosage: Oral: Children 1–3 years: 0.5 mg; *Children 4–8 years:* 0.6 mg; *Children 9–13 years:* 1 mg; *Adolescents 14–19 years: Male:* 1.3 mg; *Female:* 1.2 mg; *Adults 20–50 years:* 1.3 mg; *Adults > 50 years: Male:* 1.7 mg; *Female:* 1.5 mg.
   Drug-induced neuritis: Children: 10–50 mg/day PO for treatment and 1–2 mg/kg/day for prophylaxis; *Adults:* 100–200 mg/day or 25–100 mg/day prophylaxis.

S/Sx of Deficiency: Microcytic anemia, glossitis, cheilosis, irritability, muscle fasciculations, dermatitis, neuritis, seizures, renal calculi.

S/Sx of Toxicity: > 2 g/day: Ataxia, distal paresthesias, muscle weakness, nerve damage.

Notes: May reduce effect of levodopa in patients with Parkinson disease; avoid use in these patients. Often prescribed concomitantly with isoniazid, cycloserine, or penicillamine to prevent CNS adverse effects (pyridoxine dose 10–50 mg/day).

VITAMIN C (ASCORBIC ACID)

Indications/Effects: Antioxidant; promotes healthy gums; assists in collagen formation; improves iron absorption; may improve wound healing; may shorten duration of viral upper respiratory infection.

RDA/Dosage: Oral, intramuscular, intravenous, or subcutaneous: Children 1–3 years: 15 mg; *Children 4–8 years:* 25 mg; *Children 9–13 years:* 45 mg; *Children 14–18 years: Male:* 75 mg; *Female:* 65 mg; *Adolescents ≥ 19 years and adults: Male:* 90 mg; *Female:* 75 mg.

S/Sx of Deficiency: Anemia, hemorrhage, muscle weakness, gum disease (scurvy), delayed wound healing, skin changes (including perifollicular hyperkeratotic papules, hemorrhage, purpura).

S/Sx of Toxicity: > 2000 mg/day: Abdominal cramps, nausea, diarrhea, nosebleeds; may increase risk of renal calculi and exacerbate hemochromatosis; interferes with absorption of vitamin B_{12}.

VITAMIN D_2 (ERGOCALCIFEROL)

Indications/Effects: Assists in calcium and phosphorus absorption; may reduce risks of colon and breast cancer.

RDA/Dosage: Neonates, children, and adults: 200 IU/day.

S/Sx of Deficiency: Osteomalacia, increased risk of fractures (especially in postmenopausal women), muscle spasms.

S/Sx of Toxicity: > 1000 IU/day: Nausea, headache, fatigue, heart irregularities, anorexia, metallic taste, increased calcium levels with subsequent renal disease.

Notes: Requires UV light to convert to active forms (sufficient amount of sun exposure: 5–15 minutes, 2–3 times per week); 1.25 mg ergocalciferol provides 50,000 IU vitamin D activity.

VITAMIN E (D-ALPHA TOCOPHEROL)

Indications/Effects: Cardioprotective (decreases LDL oxidation, anticoagulant); immunostimulant; protects against cataracts; slows progression of Alzheimer disease; reduces premenstrual symptoms.

RDA/Dosage: Oral: Children 1–3 years: 6 mg; *Children 4–8 years:* 7 mg; *Children 9–13 years:* 11 mg; *Adolescents ≥ 14 years and adults:* 15 mg.
   Vitamin E deficiency: Neonates: 25–50 units/day; *Children:* 1 units/kg/day water-miscible vitamin E; *Adults:* 60–75 units/day.

S/Sx of Deficiency: Deficiency more likely on low-fat diet (may need to supplement); erythrocyte hemolysis.

S/Sx of Toxicity: > 1000 units/day: Can result in bleeding (inhibits platelet aggregation); this effect may occur at lower doses on warfarin. Also fatigue, headache, nausea, diarrhea, flatulence, blurred vision, dermatitis.

Notes: Discontinue use before surgery due to effects on platelet aggregation and tendon healing; 1 unit vitamin E = 1 mg d-alpha tocopherol.

VITAMIN K (PHYTONADIONE)

Indications/Effects: Enhances production of clotting factors and healthy bone formation.

RDA/Dosage: Infants: 1–5 mcg/kg/day; *Adults:* 0.03 mcg/kg/day.

S/Sx of Deficiency: Rare, but more likely to occur in hospitalized patients, newborn infants, patients receiving tube feedings, and those taking antibiotics, especially sulfas; bruising; bleeding.

S/Sx of Toxicity: Usually not toxic in older children and adults.

Notes: Blocks pharmacologic effects of warfarin (as a supplement and in dietary intake).

5. TABLES

TABLE VIII–1. INSULINS

Type of Insulin	Onset (h)	Peak (h)	Duration (h)	Compatible to Mix With
Rapid-Acting				
Aspart (Novolog)	0.25	0.5–1.5	3–5	All
Lispro (Humalog)	0.25	0.5–1.5	3–4	All
Regular Iletin II	0.5–1	5–10	6–8	All
Humulin R	0.5–1	5–10	6–8	All
Novolin R	0.5–1	5–10	6–8	All
Intermediate-Acting				
NPH Iletin II	1–1.5	4–6	24	Regular
Humulin N	1–1.5	4–6	24	Regular
Novolin N	1–1.5	4–6	24	Regular
Lente Iletin II	1–2.5	7.5	24	Regular, Semilente
Long-Acting				
Humulin U	4–8	10–30	36	Regular
Ultralente	4–8	10–30	36	Regular
Insulin Glargine (Lantus)	1–1.5	Peakless	24	*Do not* mix with other insulins
Combinations				
Humulin 70/30	0.5	4–8	24	—
Novolin 70/30	0.5	4–8	24	—

From Haist SA, Robbins JB, eds. Internal Medicine On Call, 3rd ed. McGraw-Hill. Copyright © 2002.

TABLE VIII–2. COMPARISON OF GLUCOCORTICOIDS

Drug (Trade)	Equivalent Dose (mg)	Anti-inflammatory Potency	Mineralocorticoid Potency
Short-Acting			
Cortisone (Cortone)	25	0.8	2
Hydrocortisone (Cortef)	20	1	2
Intermediate-Acting			
Methylprednisolone (Medrol)	4	5	0
Prednisone (Deltasone)	5	4	1
Prednisolone (Delta-Cortef)	5	4	1
Triamcinolone	4	5	0
Long-Acting			
Betamethasone (Celestone)	0.6–0.75	20–30	0
Dexamethasone (Decadron)	0.75	20–30	0

From Haist SA, Robbins JB, eds. Internal Medicine On Call, 3rd ed. McGraw-Hill. Copyright © 2002.

TABLE VIII–3. FIRST-GENERATION CEPHALOSPORINS[a–c]

Drug (Trade)	Dose	Dosing Interval	Supplied	Notes
Cefadroxil (Duricef, Ultracef)	*Ped:* 30 mg/kg/day	2 times/day	Caps, tabs, suspension	
	Adult: 500 mg–1 g	12–24 h	Caps, tabs	
Cefazolin (Ancef, Kefzol)	*Ped:* 50–100 mg/kg/day	8 h	Injection	For surgical prophylaxis most widely used antibiotic
	Adult: 1–2 g	8 h	Injection	
Cephalexin (Keflex, Keftab)	*Ped:* 25–100 mg/kg/day	6–8 h	Caps, tabs, suspension	
	Adult: 250–500 mg	4 times/day	Caps, tabs	

cap = capsule; ped = pediatric; tab = tablet.

[a] ***Indications:*** Treatment of infections caused by susceptible strains of *Streptococcus*, *Staphylococcus*, *E coli*, *Proteus*, and *Klebsiella* involving the skin, bone and joints, upper and lower respiratory tract, and urinary tract.

[b] ***Actions:*** Bactericidal: inhibits cell wall synthesis.

[c] ***Dosage adjustments:*** Necessary in patients with renal impairment.

Modified from Haist SA, Robbins JB, eds. Internal Medicine On Call, 3rd ed. McGraw-Hill. Copyright © 2002.

TABLE VIII–4. SECOND-GENERATION CEPHALOSPORINS[a–d]

Drug (Trade)	Dose	Dosing Interval	Supplied	Notes
Cefaclor (Ceclor)	*Ped:* 20–40 mg/kg/day	8–12 h	Caps, tabs, suspension	
	Adult: 250–500 mg	8 h	Caps, tabs	
Cefoxitin (Mefoxin)	*Ped:* 80–160 mg/kg/day	6–8 h	Injection	Best activity against anaerobes
	Adult: 1–2 g	6 h	Injection	
Cefprozil (Cefzil)	*Ped:* 15–30 mg/kg/day	12–24 h	Tabs, suspension	Use higher doses for otitis media and pneumonia
	Adult: 250–500 mg	1–2 times/day	Tabs	
Cefuroxime[e] (Ceftin)	*Ped:* 20–30 mg/kg/day	12 h	Tabs, suspension	Ceftin should be taken with food
	Adult: 250–500 mg	2 times/day	Tabs	
Cefuroxime axetil[f] (Zinacef)	*Ped:* 75–200 mg/kg/day	8 h	Injection	
	Adult: 750 mg–1.5 g	8 h	Injection	

cap = capsule; ped = pediatric; tab = tablet.

[a] ***Indications:*** Treatment of infections caused by susceptible bacteria involving the upper and lower respiratory tract, skin, bone, urinary tract, abdomen, and female reproductive system.

[b] ***Actions:*** Bactericidal: inhibits cell wall synthesis.

[c] ***Notes:*** More active than first-generation agents against *H influenzae, E coli, Klebsiella spp,* and *Proteus mirabilis.* Risk of hypoprothrombinemia or bleeding has been associated with cephalosporins containing an N-methylthiotetrazole (NMTT) side chain. These agents include cefotetan, cefmetazole, and cefoperazone (third-generation). Administration of vitamin K will prevent clinical bleeding associated with these drugs for patients with vitamin K deficiency.

[d] ***Dosage adjustment:*** Necessary in renal impairment.

[e] PO formulation.

[f] IM or IV formulation.

Modified from Haist SA, Robbins JB, eds. Internal Medicine On Call, 3rd ed. McGraw-Hill. Copyright © 2002.

TABLE VIII-5. THIRD- AND FOURTH-GENERATION CEPHALOSPORINS[a–d]

Drug (Trade)	Dose	Dosing Interval	Supplied	Notes
Cefdinir (Omnicef)	*Ped:* 14 mg/kg/day *Adult:* 300–600 mg	12–24 h 12–24 h	Caps, suspension Caps	
Cefepime[e] (Maxipime)	*Ped:* 100–150 mg/kg per dose *Adult:* 1–2 g	8–12 h 12 h	Injection Injection	
Cefixime (Suprax)	*Ped:* 8 mg/kg/day *Adult:* 200–400 mg	12–24 h 12–24 h	Tabs, suspension Tabs, suspension	Use suspension for otitis media
Cefotaxime (Claforan)	*Ped:* 100–300 mg/kg/day *Adult:* 1–2 g	6–8 h 4–8 h	Injection Injection	Crosses the blood-brain barrier
Cefpodoxime (Vantin)	*Ped:* 10 mg/kg/day *Adult:* 200–400 mg	12 h 12 h	Tabs, suspension Tabs	Has drug interactions with agents that increase gastric pH
Ceftazidime (Fortaz, Ceptaz, Tazidime, Tazicef)	*Ped:* 100–150 mg/kd/day *Adult:* 1–2 g	8 h 8 h	Injection Injection	Best activity against *Pseudomonas;* crosses the blood-brain barrier
Ceftriaxone (Rocephin)	*Ped:* 50–100 mg/kg/day *Adult:* 1–2 g	12–24 h 12–24 h	Injection Injection	Treatment of choice for gonorrhea; crosses the blood-brain barrier

cap = capsule; ped = pediatric; tab = tablet.

[a] **Indications:** Treatment of infections caused by susceptible bacteria involving the respiratory tract, skin, bone and joints, and urinary tract; treatment of meningitis, febrile neutropenia, and septicemia.

[b] **Actions:** Bactericidal; inhibits cell wall synthesis.

[c] **Notes:** Less active against gram-positive cocci than first- and second-generation agents. Increased activity against gram-negative aerobes (*Enterobacteriaceae* including *Enterobacter and Serratia*) due to increased stability to beta-lactamases. May be used in combination with an aminoglycoside.

[d] **Dosage adjustment:** Necessary in renal impairment.

[e] Fourth-generation cephalosporin.

Modified from Haist SA, Robbins JB, eds. Internal Medicine On Call. 3rd ed. McGraw-Hill. Copyright © 2002.

TABLE VIII–6. OPHTHALMIC AGENTS

Drug (Trade)	Strength (%)	Dosing Schedule
Agents for Glaucoma		
α₂-Adrenergic Agonists		
Apraclonidine (Iopidine)	0.5, 1.0	1–2 drops 3 times/day (0.5%), 1 drop 1 h prior to surgery (1.0%)
Brimonidine (Alphagan)	0.2	1 drop 3 times/day
Dipivefrin (Propine)	0.1	1 drop q12h
β-Blockers		
Betaxolol (Betoptic-S, Betoptic)	0.25, 0.5	1 drop 2 times/day
Carteolol (Ocupress)	1.0	1 drop 2 times/day
Levobetaxolol (Betaxon)	0.5	1 drop 2 times/day
Levobunolol (Betagan Liquifilm)	0.25, 0.5	1 drop 1–2 times/day
Metipranolol (OptiPranolol)	0.3	1 drop 2 times/day
Timolol[a] (Timoptic)	0.25, 0.5	1 drop 1–2 times/day
Carbonic Anhydrase Inhibitors		
Brinzolamide (Azopt)	1.0	1 drop 3 times/day
Dorzolamide (Trusopt)	2.0	1 drop 3 times/day
Miotics, Cholinesterase Inhibitors		
Carbachol (Isopto Carbachol)	0.75–3	1–2 drops 3 times/day
Demecarium (Humorsol)	0.125, 0.25	1–2 drops twice weekly, up to 1–2 drops 2 times/day
Echothiophate iodine (Phospholine iodide)	0.03, 0.06, 0.125	1 drop 2 times/day
Physostigmine (Isopto Eserine)	0.25, 0.5	2 drops up to 4 times/day
Pilocarpine (Isopto Carpine, Pilocar)	0.25–10	1–2 drops up to 6 times/day
(Pilopine HS gel)	4.0	0.5 inch at bedtime
Prostaglandin Agonists		
Latanoprost[b] (Xalatan)	0.005	1 drop at bedtime
Combination Agents		
Dorzolamide and timolol (Cosopt)	2/0.5	1 drop 2 times/day
Antibiotics		
Bacitracin (see p. 610)		
Chloramphenicol (AK-Chlor)	Oint/sol	1–2 drops or 0.5 inch q3–4h
Ciprofloxacin (Ciloxan)	Solution	1–2 drops 4–6 times/day
Erythromycin (AK-Mycin, Ilotycin)	Ointment	0.5 inch 2–8 times/day
Gentamicin (Garamycin)	Oint/sol	1–2 drops or 0.5 inch 2–3 times/day, up to q3–4h
Neomycin, polymyxin B, hydrocortisone 1% (Cortisporin)	Suspension	1–2 drops q3–4h
Sulfacetamide sodium (Sodium Sulamyd, Bleph-10)	10–30% oint/sol	1–2 drops q1–3h or 0.5 inch 1–4 times/day
Tobramycin (Tobrex)	Oint/sol	1–2 drops or 0.5 inch 2–3 times/day, up to q3–4h
Anti-Inflammatory		
NSAIDs		
Flurbiprofen (Ocufen)	0.03	1 drop 4 times/day (post-op inflammation following cataract surgery)

TABLE VIII–6. OPHTHALMIC AGENTS (*Continued*)

Drug (Trade)	Strength (%)	Dosing Schedule
Ketoralac (Acular)	0.5	1 drop q4h for 3 days (ocular inflammation) 1 drop 4 times/day (relieves itching due to seasonal allergic conjunctivitis)
Corticosteroids		
Dexamethasone (AK-Dex, others)	0.05 (oint), 0.1 (sol)	1–2 drops or 0.5 inch 3–4 times/day
Fluorometholone[c] (FML, Flarex)	0.1, 0.25	1–2 drops 2–4 times/day
Prednisolone (AK-Pred, Pred Forte)	0.12, 0.125, 1.0	1–2 drops q1h (day), q2h (night) until response, then 1 drop q4h
Rimexolone (Vexol)	1	1–2 drops q1h to 4 times/day
Decongestant/Anti-allergy		
Ketotifen[d] (Zaditor)	0.025	1 drop 2–3 times/day
Levocabastine (Livostin)	0.05	1 drop 4 times/day
Lodoxamide (Alomide)	0.1	1–2 drops 4 times/day
Naphazoline and antazoline (Albalon-A)	0.05/0.5	1–2 drops 3–4 times/day
Naphazoline and pheniramine acetate (Naphcon A)	0.025/0.3	1–2 drops 3–4 times/day
Mast Cell Stabilizers		
Nedocromil sodium (Alocril)	2%	1–2 drops 2 times/day
Pemirolast potassium (Alamast)	0.1%	1–2 drops 4 times/day
Combination Agents (see also Glaucoma)		
Gentamicin and prednisolone (Pred-G)	Oint/sol	0.5 inch 2–3 times/day (oint), 1–2 drops q2–4h up to q2h (sol)
Neomycin and dexamethasone (Dex-Neo-Dex)	Oint/sol	0.5 inch 3–4 times/day (oint), 1–2 drops q3–4h (sol)
Neomycin, polymyxin, hydrocortisone (Cortisporin)	Oint/sol	0.5 inch 1–4 times/day (oint), 1–2 drops 2–4 times/day (sol)
Neomycin, polymyxin, and dexamethasone (Maxitrol)	Oint/sol	0.5 inch 3–4 times/day (oint), 1–2 drops q4–6h (sol)
Neomycin, polymyxin, and prednisolone (Poly-Pred)	Oint/sol	0.5 inch 3–4 times/day (oint), 1–2 drops q4–6h (sol)
Sulfacetamide and prednisolone (Blephamide)	Oint/sol	0.5 inch 1–4 times/day (oint), 1–3 drops q2–3h (sol)
Tobramycin and dexamethasone (TobraDex)	Solution	1–2 drops q4–6h

oint = ointment; sol = solution.
[a] Systemic absorption may cause bradycardia.
[b] May darken light irides.
[c] Not recommended in children younger than 2 years of age.
[d] Wait at least 10 minutes before putting in contact lens.
Modified from Haist SA, Robbins JB, eds. Internal Medicine On Call, 3rd ed. McGraw-Hill. Copyright © 2002.

Appendices

APPENDIX A. BLOOD CELL INDICES: AGE-SPECIFIC

TABLE A–1. AGE-SPECIFIC BLOOD CELL INDICES

Age	Hb (g%)[a]	HCT (%)[a]	MCV (fL)[a]	MCHC (g/% RBC)[a]	Reticulocytes	WBCs (× 10³/mm³)[b]	Platelets (10³/mm³)[b]
26–30 wk gestation[c]	13.4 (11)	41.5 (34.9)	118.2 (106.7)	37.9 (30.6)	—	4.4 (2.7)	254 (180–327)
28 wk	14.5	45	120	31.0	(5–10)	—	275
32 wk	15.0	47	118	32.0	(3–10)	—	290
Term[d] (cord)	16.5 (13.5)	51 (42)	108 (98)	33.0 (30.0)	(3–7)	18.1 (9–30)[e]	290
1–3 day	18.5 (14.5)	56 (45)	108 (95)	33.0 (29.0)	(1.8–4.6)	18.9 (9.4–34)	192
2 wk	16.6 (13.4)	53 (41)	105 (88)	31.4 (28.1)		11.4 (5–20)	252
1 mo	13.9 (10.7)	44 (33)	101 (91)	31.8 (28.1)	(0.1–1.7)	10.8 (4–19.5)	
2 mo	11.2 (9.4)	35 (28)	95 (84)	31.8 (28.3)			
6 mo	12.6 (11.1)	36 (31)	76 (68)	35.0 (32.7)	(0.7–2.3)	11.9 (6–17.5)	
6 mo–2 y	12.0 (10.5)	36 (33)	78 (70)	33.0 (30.0)	(0.5–1.0)	10.6 (6–17)	(150–350)
2–6 y	12.5 (11.5)	37 (34)	81 (75)	34.0 (31.0)	(0.5–1.0)	8.5 (5–15.5)	(150–350)
6–12 y	13.5 (11.5)	40 (35)	86 (77)	34.0 (31.0)	(0.5–1.0)	8.1 (4.5–13.5)	(150–350)
12–18 y							
Male	14.5 (13)	43 (36)	88 (78)	34.0 (31.0)	(0.5–1.0)	7.8 (4.5–13.5)	(150–350)
Female	14.0 (12)	41 (37)	90 (78)	34.0 (31.0)	(0.5–1.0)	7.8 (4.5–13.5)	(150–350)
Adult							
Male	15.5 (13.5)	47 (41)	90 (80)	34.0 (31.0)	(0.8–2.5)	7.4 (4.5–11)	(150–350)
Female	14.0 (12)	41 (36)	90 (80)	34.0 (31.0)	(0.8–4.1)	7.4 (4.5–11)	(150–350)

Hb = hemoglobin; HCT = hematocrit; MCHC = mean cell hemoglobin concentration; MCV = mean cell volume.
[a] Data are mean (−2 SD).
[b] Data are mean (±2 SD).
[c] Values are from fetal samplings.
[d] < 1 mo, capillary hemoglobin exceeds venous: 1 h: 3.6 g difference; 5 days: 2.2 g difference; 3 wk: 1.1 g difference.
[e] Mean (95% confidence limits).

From Gunn VL, Nechyba C. The Harriet Lane Handbook, 16th ed. Mosby, 2002:284–285. Data from Forestier F, et al. Pediatr Res 1986;20:342; Oski FA, Naiman JL. Hematological Problems in the Newborn Infant. Saunders, 1982; Nathan D, Oski FA. Hematology of Infancy and Childhood. Saunders, 1998; Matoth Y, Zaizov R, Varsano I. Acta Paediatr Scand 1971;60:317; and Wintrobe MM. Clinical Hematology. Williams and Wilkins, 1999.

APPENDIX B. BLOOD PRESSURE MEASUREMENT PERCENTILES (GIRLS AND BOYS): AGE SPECIFIC

TABLE B-1. MINIMUM SYSTOLIC BLOOD PRESSURE BASED ON AGE

Age	Heart Rate (beats/min)
0–1 mo	60 mm Hg
>1 mo–1 y	70 mm Hg
1–10 y	70 mm Hg + (2 × age in years)
>10 y	90 mm Hg

(*Source: American Heart Association.*)

APPENDIX C. BODY SURFACE AREA

Pediatric doses of medications are generally based on body surface area (BSA) or weight. To calculate a child's BSA using the West nomogram (Figure C–1), draw a straight line from the height (in the left-hand column) to the weight (in the right-hand column). The point at which the line intersects the surface area (SA) column is the BSA (measured in meters squared [m^2]). If the child is of roughly normal proportion, BSA can be calculated from the weight alone (in the enclosed are). The following formula can then be used to estimate the pediatric drug dose:

$$\frac{\text{BSA of child}}{\text{Mean BSA of adult}} \times \text{Adult dose} = \text{Estimated pediatric dose}$$

REFERENCE

Ball J, Bindler R, eds. *Pediatric Nursing: Caring for Children,* 2nd ed. Appleton & Lange, 1999.

APPENDIX D. CHILDHOOD IMMUNIZATION SCHEDULE

The Advisory Committee on Immunization Practices (ACIP) periodically reviews the recommended childhood and adolescent immunization schedule to ensure that it is current with changes in vaccine formulations and reflects revised recommendations for the use of licensed vaccines, including those newly licensed. The childhood and adolescent immunization schedule for 2005 is shown in Figure D–1. The current schedule can be viewed, downloaded, and printed from the Centers for Disease Control and Prevention website at http://www.cdc.gov/nip/acip.

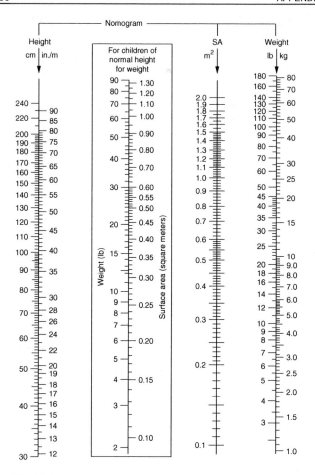

Figure C–1. West nomogram for calculation of body surface area. (*Modified from data of E Boyd by CD West; from Behrman RE, Kliegman RM, Jenson HB, eds. Nelson Textbook of Pediatrics, 17th ed. Saunders, 2004.*)

REFERENCE

Centers for Disease Control and Prevention. Recommended childhood and adolescent immunization schedule—United States, 2005. *MMWR Morb Mortal Wkly Rep* 2005;53(51–52):Q1–Q3.

Vaccine ▼ / Age ▶	Birth	1 month	2 months	4 months	6 months	12 months	15 months	18 months	24 months	4–6 years	11–12 years	13–18 years
Hepatitis B[1]	HepB #1		HepB #2			HepB #3					HepB series	
Diphtheria, tetanus, pertussis[2]			DTaP	DTaP	DTaP		DTaP			DTaP	Td	Td
Haemophilus influenzae type b[3]			Hib	Hib	Hib	Hib						
Inactivated poliovirus			IPV	IPV		IPV				IPV		
Measles, mumps, rubella[4]						MMR #1				MMR #2	MMR #2	
Varicella[5]							Varicella				Varicella	
Pneumococcal conjugate[6]			PCV	PCV	PCV	PCV			PCV	PPV		
Influenza[7]							Influenza (Yearly)			Influenza (Yearly)		
Vaccines below this line are for selected populations												
Hepatitis A[8]											Hepatitis a series	

This schedule indicates the recommended ages for routine administration of currently licensed childhood vaccines, as of December 1, 2004, for children through age 18 years. Any dose not administered at the recommended age should be administered at any subsequent visit when indicated and feasible.

■ Indicates age groups that warrant special effort to administer those vaccines not previously administered. Additional vaccines may be licensed and recommended during the year. Licensed combination vaccines may be used whenever any components of the combination are indicated and other components of the vaccine are not contraindicated. Providers should consult the manufacturers' package inserts for detailed recommendations. Clinically significant adverse events that follow immunization should be reported to the Vaccine Adverse Event Reporting System (VAERS). Guidance about how to obtain and complete a VAERS form is available at **www.vaers.org** or by telephone, **800-822-7967.**

Range of recommended ages | **Only if mother HBsAg(–)** | **Preadolescent assessment** | **Catch-up immunization**

Figure D–1. Recommended childhood and adolescent immunization schedule, by vaccine and age—United States, 2005. *(From Centers for Disease Control and Prevention. Recommended childhood and adolescent immunization schedule—United States, 2005. MMWR Morb Mortal Wkly Rep 2005;53(51–52):Q1–Q3.)*

APPENDIX E. DENVER DEVELOPMENTAL ASSESSMENT

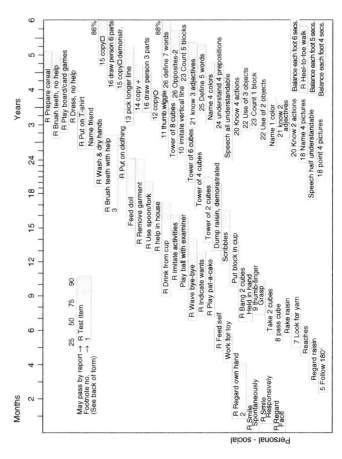

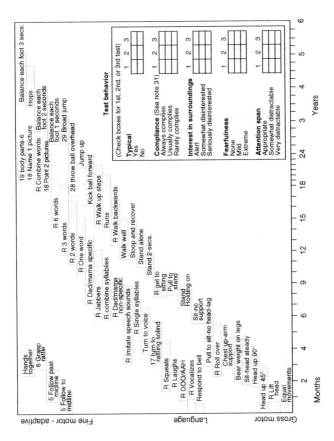

Figure E-1. Denver Developmental Assessment (Denver II). *(From WK Frankenburg, Denver, Colorado.)*

Directions for administration

1. Try to get child to smile by smiling, talking or waving. Do not touch him/her.
2. Child must stare at hand several seconds.
3. Parent may help guide toothbrush and put toothpaste on brush.
4. Child does not have to be able to tie shoes or button/zip in the back.
5. Move yarn slowly in an arc from one side to the other, about 8" above child's face.
6. Pass if child grasps rattle when it is touched to the backs or tips of fingers.
7. Pass if child tries to see where yarn went. Yarn should be dropped quickly from sight from tester's hand without arm movement.
8. Child must transfer cube from hand to hand without help of body, mouth, or table.
9. Pass if child picks up raisin with any part of thumb and finger.
10. Line can vary only 30 degrees or less from tester's line.
11. Make a fist with thumb pointing upward and wiggle only the thumb. Pass if child imitates and does not move any fingers other than the thumb.

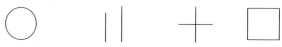

12. Pass any enclosed form. Fail continuous round motions.
13. Which line is longer? (Not bigger.) Turn paper upside down and repeat. (pass 3 of 3 or 5 of 6)
14. Pass any lines crossing near midpoint.
15. Have child copy first. If failed, demonstrate.

When giving items 12, 14, and 15, do not name the forms. Do not demonstrate 12 and 14.

16. When scoring, each pair (2 arms, 2 legs, etc.) counts as one part.
17. Place one cube in cup and shake gently near child's ear, but out of sight. Repeat for other ear.
18. Point to picture and have child name it. (No credit is given for sounds only.)
    If less than 4 pictures are named correctly, have child point to picture as each is named by tester.

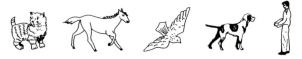

19. Using doll, tell child: Show me the nose, eyes, ears, mouth, hands, feet, tummy, hair. Pass 6 of 8.
20. Using pictures, ask child: Which one flies?... says meow?... talks?... barks?... gallops? Pass 2 of 5, 4 of 5.
21. Ask child: What do you do when you are cold?... tired?... hungry? Pass 2 of 3, 3 of 3.
22. Ask child: What do you do with a cup? What is a chair used for? What is a pencil used for?
    Action words must be included in answers.
23. Pass if child correctly places *and* says how many blocks are on paper. (1, 5).
24. Tell child: Put block **on** table; **under** table; **in front of** me, **behind** me. Pass 4 of 4.
    (Do not help child by pointing, moving head or eyes.)
25. Ask child: What is a ball?... lake?... desk?... house?... banana?... curtain?... fence?... ceiling? Pass if defined in terms of use, shape, what it is made of, or general category (such as banana is fruit, not just yellow). Pass 5 of 8, 7 of 8.
26. Ask child: If a horse is big, a mouse is_ ? If fire is hot, ice is_ ? If the sun shines during the day, the moon shines during the_ ? Pass 2 of 3.
27. Child may use wall or rail only, not person. May not crawl.
28. Child must throw ball overhand 3 feet to within arm's reach of tester.
29. Child must perform standing broad jump over width of test sheet (8 1/2 inches).
30. Tell child to walk forward, ⟋⟍⟋⟍⟋⟍→ heel within 1 inch of toe. Tester may demonstrate.
    Child must walk 4 consecutive steps.
31. In the second year, half of normal children are non-compliant.

Observations:

Figure E-1. (*Continued*)

APPENDIX F. GLASGOW COMA SCALE

TABLE F–1. GLASGOW COMA SCALE (GCS)

Score	Eye Opening	Best Verbal Response	Best Motor Response
6			Obeys verbal command
5		Oriented, converses	Localizes painful stimulus
4	Spontaneous	Disoriented, converses	Flexion withdrawal
3	To speech	Inappropriate words	Flexion abnormal (decorticate)
2	To pain	Incomprehensible sounds	Extension (decerebrate)
1	None	No response	No response

TABLE F–2. MODIFIED PEDIATRIC GLASGOW COMA SCALE: CHILDREN 4 YEARS OF AGE OR YOUNGER

Score	Eye Opening	Best Verbal Response	Best Motor Response
6			Obeys verbal command
5		Appropriate words or social smile, fixes and follows	Localizes painful stimulus
4	Spontaneous	Cries, but consolable	Flexion withdrawal
3	To speech	Persistently irritable	Flexion abnormal (decorticate)
2	To pain	Restless, agitated	Extension (decerebrate)
1	None	No response	No response

REFERENCES

American College of Surgeons Committee on Trauma. In: Krantz BE. *Advanced Trauma Life Support Student Course Manual*. ACS, 2002.

Nelson DS. Coma and altered level of consciousness. In: Fleisher GR, ed. *Textbook of Pediatric Emergency Medicine*. Lippincott Williams & Wilkins, 2000.

APPENDIX G. GROWTH CHARTS (GIRLS AND BOYS)

Growth charts for boys and girls are available from the Centers for Disease Control and Prevention (CDC). The charts have grids aligned to English units (lb, in), with metric units (kg, cm) on the secondary scale. A sample chart is shown in Figure G–1. The CDC provides the following individual charts:

A. Infants, Birth to 36 Months
1. Weight-for-age
2. Length-for-age
3. Weight-for-length
4. Head circumference-for-age

B. Children and Adolescents, 2 to 20 Years
5. Weight-for-age
6. Stature-for-age
7. Body mass index (BMI)-for-age

C. Preschoolers, 2 to 5 Years
8. Weight-for-stature

These charts are available in three sets:

- **Set 1:** 16 charts (8 each for boys and girls), with the 3rd, 5th, 10th, 25th, 50th, 75th, 90th, 95th, and 97th smoothed percentile lines for all charts, and the 85th percentile for BMI-for-age and weight-for-stature.
- **Set 2:** 16 charts (8 each for boys and girls), with the 5th, 10th, 25th, 50th, 75th, 90th, and 95th smoothed percentile lines for all charts, and the 85th percentile for BMI-for-age and weight-for-stature.
- **Set 3:** 16 charts (8 each for boys and girls), with the 3rd, 10th, 25th, 50th, 75th, 90th, and 97th smoothed percentile lines for all charts, and the 85th percentile for BMI-for-age and weight-for-statute.

Set 1 shows all of major percentile curves but may have limitations where curves are close together, especially at the youngest ages. Most users in the United States may wish to use the format shown in set 2 for the majority of routine applications. Pediatric endocrinologists and others dealing with special populations may wish to use the format in set 3 for selected applications.

All individual charts may be viewed, downloaded, and printed from the CDC website at http://www.cdc.gov/growthcharts.

REFERENCE

Centers for Disease Control and Prevention, National Center for Health Statistics. CDC Growth charts: United States.

CDC Growth Charts: United States

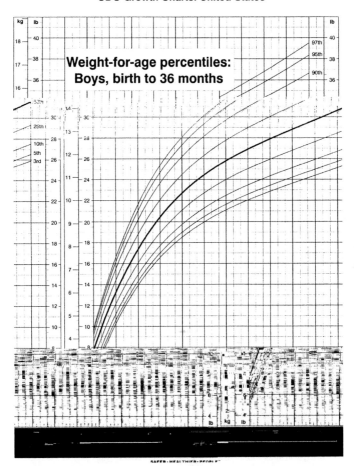

Figure G–1. Sample CDC growth chart. Weight-for-age percentiles: Boys, birth to 36 months. *(Developed by the National Center for Health Statistics in collaboration with the National Center for Chronic Disease Prevention and Health Promotion, 2000. Published May 30, 2000.)*

APPENDIX H. HEART RATES: AGE SPECIFIC

**TABLE H–1. NORMAL HEART RATE RANGES
FOR INFANTS AND CHILDREN**

Age	Heart Rate (beats/min)
Newborn	80–180
1 wk–3 mo	80–180
3 mo–2 y	80–160
2–10 y	65–130
10 y–adult	55–90

(*Source: American Heart Association.*)

APPENDIX I. SBE PROPHYLAXIS

TABLE I–1. GUIDELINES FOR PREVENTION OF SUBACUTE BACTERIAL ENDOCARDITIS

Dental procedures for which endocarditis prophylaxis is recommended[a]
  Dental extractions
  Periodontal procedures including surgery, scaling, and root planing, probing, and recall
    maintenance
  Endodontic (root canal) instrumentation or surgery only beyond the apex
  Subgingival placement of antibiotic fibers or strips
  Initial placement of orthodontic bands but not brackets
  Intraligamentary local anesthetic injections
  Prophylactic cleaning of teeth or implants where bleeding is anticipated

Other procedures for which endocarditis prophylaxis is recommended
  Respiratory tract
    Tonsillectomy and/or adenoidectomy
    Surgical operations that involve respiratory mucosa
    Bronchoscopy with a rigid bronchoscope
  Gastrointestinal tract[b]
    Sclerotherapy for esophageal varices
    Esophageal stricture dilation
    Endoscopic retrograde cholangiography with billiary obstruction
    Billiary tract surgery
    Surgical operations that involve intestinal mucosa
  Genitourinary tract
    Prostatic surgery
    Cystoscopy
    Urethral dilation

TABLE I–1. GUIDELINES FOR PREVENTION OF SUBACUTE BACTERIAL ENDOCARDITIS (*CONTINUED.*)

Prophylactic regimens for dental, oral, respiratory tract, or esophageal procedures. (Follow-up dose no longer recommended.) Total children's dose should not exceed adult dose.

I. Standard general prophylaxis for patients at risk:
Amoxicillin: Adults, 2.0 g (children, 50 mg/kg) given orally 1 h before procedure

II. Unable to take oral medications:
Ampicillin: Adults, 2.0 g (children 50 mg/kg) given IM or IV within 30 min before procedure

III. Amoxicillin/ampicillin/penicillin-allergic patients:
Clindamycin: Adults, 600 mg (children 20 mg/kg) given orally 1 h before procedure; or
Cephalexin or cefadroxil[c]: Adults, 2.0 g (children 50 mg/kg) orally 1 h before procedure; or Azithromycin or clarithromycin: Adults, 500 mg (children 15 mg/kg) orally 1 h before procedure

IV. Amoxicillin/ampicillin/penicillin-allergic patients unable to take oral medications:
Clindamycin: Adults, 600 mg (children 20 mg/kg) IV within 30 min before procedure; or
Cefazolin[c]: Adults, 1.0 g (children 25 mg/kg) IM or IV within 30 min before procedure

Cardiac conditions associated with endocarditis:

High-risk category:
Prosthetic cardiac valves, including bioprosthetic and homograft valves
Previous bacterial endocarditis
Complex cyanotic congenital heart disease (eg, single ventricle states, transposition of the great arteries, tetralogy of Fallot)
Surgically constructed systemic pulmonary shunts or conduits

Moderate-risk category
Most other congenital cardiac malformations (other than above)
Acquired valvar dysfunction (eg, rheumatic heart disease)
Hypertrophic cardiomyopathy
Mitral valve prolapse with valvar regurgitation and/or thickened leaflets

Prophylactic regimens for genitourinary/gastrointestinal procedures:

I. High-risk patients:
Ampicillin plus gentamicin: Ampicillin (adults, 2.0 g; children 50 mg/kg) plus gentamicin 1.5 mg/kg (for both adults and children, not to exceed 120 mg) IM or IV within 30 min before starting procedure; 6 h later, ampicillin (adults, 1.0 g; children, 25 mg/kg) IM or IV, or amoxicillin (adults, 1.0 g; children, 25 mg/kg) orally

II. High-risk patients allergic to ampicillin/amoxicillin:
Vancomycin plus gentamicin: Vancomycin (adults, 1.0 g; children, 20 mg/kg) IV over 1–2 h plus gentamicin 1.5 mg/kg (for both adults and children, not to exceed 120 mg) IM or IV; complete injection/infusion within 30 min before starting procedure

III. Moderate-risk patients:
Amoxicillin: Adults, 2.0 g (children 50 mg/kg) orally 1 h before procedure; or
Ampicillin: Adults, 2.0 g (children 50 mg/kg) IM or IV within 30 min before starting procedure

IV. Moderate-risk patients allergic to ampicillin/amoxicillin:
Vancomycin: Adults, 1.0 g (children 20 mg/kg) IV over 1–2 h; complete infusion within 30 min of starting procedure.

Note: For patients already taking an antibiotic, or for other special situations, please refer to the full statement referenced below.
[a]*Prophylaxis is recommended for patients with high- and moderate-risk cardiac conditions.*
[b]*Prophylaxis is recommended for high-risk patients; it is optional for medium-risk patients.*
[c]*Cephalosporins should not be used in patients with immediate-type hypersensitivity reaction to penicillins.*
Adapted from the Committee on Rheumatic Fever, Endocarditis, and Kawasaki Disease. Prevention of bacterial endocarditis: Recommendations by the American Heart Association. JAMA 1997, 277:1794–1801, Circulation 1997, 96:358–366, and JADA 1997;128:1142–1150.

APPENDIX J. SPECIMEN TUBES FOR PHLEBOTOMY

TABLE J–1. SPECIMEN TUBE IDENTIFICATION AND USES[a]

Tube Color	Additives	General Uses
Red	None	Clot tube to collect serum for chemistry, cross-matching, serology
Red and black (hot pink)	Silicone gel for rapid clot	As above, but not for osmolality or blood bank work
Blue	Sodium citrate (binds calcium)	Coagulation studies (best kept on ice, not for fibrin split products)
Blue/yellow label		Fibrin split products
Royal blue		Heavy metals, arsenic
Purple	Disodium EDTA (binds calcium)	Hematology, not for lipid profiles
Green	Sodium heparin	Ammonia, cortisol, ionized calcium (best kept on ice)
Green/glass beads		LE prep
Gray	Sodium fluoride	Lactic acid
Yellow	Transport medium	Blood cultures

EDTA = ethylenediamine tetra-acetic acid; LE = lupus erythematosus.
[a]Individual laboratories may vary slightly from these listings.
Reproduced with permission from Gomella LG, Lefor AT, eds. Surgery On Call, 3rd ed. McGraw-Hill, © 2001.

APPENDIX K. TEMPERATURE CONVERSION

TABLE K–1. FAHRENHEIT-TO-CENTIGRADE CONVERSION

°F	°C	°C	°F
95.0	35.0	35.0	95.0
96.0	35.5	35.5	95.9
97.0	36.1	36.0	95.8
98.0	36.6	36.5	97.7
98.6	37.0	37.0	98.6
99.0	37.2	37.5	99.5
100.0	37.7	38.0	100.4
101.0	38.3	38.5	101.3
102.0	38.8	39.0	102.2
103.0	39.4	39.5	103.1
104.0	40.0	40.0	104.0
105.0	40.5	40.5	104.9
106.0	41.1	41.0	105.8

$$°C = (°F - 32) \times 5/9 \qquad °F = (°C \times 9/5) + 32$$

Modified and reproduced with permission from Gomella LG, ed. Clinician's Pocket Reference, 10th ed. McGraw-Hill, © 2002.

APPENDIX L. TETANUS PROPHYLAXIS

I. **Clinical Manifestations.** Also known as *lockjaw,* tetanus is a neuro-logic disease that produces muscular spasms, including trismus. It is caused by a toxin produced by the anaerobic bacterium *Clostridium tetani.* Onset occurs over 1–7 days after an incubation period from 2 days to months (usually 14 days) and results in spasms that last for weeks if the patient recovers. Some localized manifestations exist.

II. **Etiology.** The spore-forming bacteria are present in contaminated wounds and produce an endotoxin. Exposure is more likely in wounds contaminated with dirt, feces, or saliva. Occurs worldwide but is more common in warmer climates and months, which is also when wounds are more likely. Wounds with devitalized tissue or deep punctures are more at risk. Also results from nonsterile umbilical cord care in new-borns from developing countries where women are not immunized. Approximately 90 cases occur annually in the United States, mostly in unimmunized individuals and two thirds in adults.

III. **Control Measures**
   A. **Care of Exposed People**
   1. Clean and debride all wounds, especially those contaminated with dirt, feces, and saliva and those resulting from frostbite, crush injury, and burns.
   2. If tetanus immunization is incomplete, administer vaccine at the time of wound treatment and complete the immunization series according to the accepted schedule. Patients with wounds at risk for tetanus and those infected with human immunodeficiency virus should be treated with human tetanus immune globulin (TIG). The dose of TIG is 250 units IM. Equine antitoxin is *not* advisable because of the risk of reactions, such as serum sick-ness, but may be used if human TIG is not available. If toxoid and TIG are both indicated (see Table L–1), different syringes and injection sites should be used.
   3. When vaccination with toxoid is required in a child 7 years of age or older, the adult type of toxoid vaccine (Td) should be used. This decreases the amount of diphtheria toxoid to avoid reac-tions, but maintains some immunity. For children 7 years of age or younger, DTaP (diphtheria and tetanus toxoids and acellular pertussis) should be given unless pertussis vaccination is con-traindicated, in which case DT should be used.
   4. See Tables L–1 and L–2 for details on wound prophylaxis.
   B. **Immunization**
   1. **Primary series.** Four shots are given at 2, 4, 5, and 15–18 months of age with a booster at 4–6 years of age, 11–12 years of age, and every 10 years thereafter. If series is not completed in childhood, 3 doses are required, 1–2 months between the first 2 doses and 6–12 months until the third.

TABLE L–1. GUIDE TO TETANUS PROPHYLAXIS IN WOUND MANAGEMENT

History of Toxoid Doses	Clean Wounds		Contaminated Wounds[a]	
	Toxoid	TIG	Toxoid	TIG
< 3 or unknown	Yes	No	Yes	Yes
≥ 3, last less than 10 y	No	No	Yes	No
≥ 3, last more than 10 y	Yes	No	Yes	No
≥ 3, last less than 5 y	No	No	No	No
≥ 3, last more than 5 y	No	No	Yes	No

[a]Contaminated with soil, feces, saliva, or from puncture, avulsion, crush, frostbite, or burn mechanism.
Modified from The Red Book: 2003 Report of the Committee on Infectious Disease, *26th ed. Committee on Infectious Diseases, American Academy of Pediatrics, 2003:611–616.*

2. **Booster.** If last tetanus immunization was given more than 5 years ago and patient has a wound at risk for contamination with tetanus, a booster dose should be given.
3. **Immunization status**
   a. **Fully immunized:** ≥ 3 vaccinations within 10 years.
   b. **Partially immunized:** ≥ 3 vaccinations more than 10 years prior.
   c. **Not adequately immunized:** < 3 vaccinations or unknown.

REFERENCES

Committee on Trauma, American College of Surgeons. *Advanced Trauma Life Support Program for Doctors Student Manual,* 6th ed. ACS, 1997:383–389.
The Red Book: 2003 Report of the Committee on Infectious Disease, 26th ed. Committee on Infectious Diseases, American Academy of Pediatrics, 2003:611–616.

TABLE L–2. WOUND CLASSIFICATION

Clinical Features	Clean Wounds, No Tetanus Risk	Wounds With Tetanus Risk
Age of wound	≤ 6 h	>6 h
Shape	Linear, abrasion	Stellate, avulsion
Depth	≤ 1 cm	>1 cm
Mechanism	Sharp surface	Missile, crush, burn, frostbite
Signs of infection	Absent	Present
Devitalized tissue	Absent	Present
Contaminants (soil, feces, saliva)	Absent	Present
Denervated or ischemic tissue	Absent	Present

Modified from Committee on Trauma, American College of Surgeons. Advanced Trauma Life Support Program for Doctors Student Manual, 6th ed. ACS, 1997:383–389.

US Dept of Health and Human Services, Centers for Disease Control and Prevention. Recommendation of the immunization practices advisory committee (ACIP): Diphtheria, tetanus, and pertussis—guidelines for vaccine prophylaxis and other preventive measures. *MMWR Morb Mortal Wkly Rep* 2001;34(27): 406–414, 419–426.

APPENDIX M. WEIGHT CONVERSION

TABLE M–1. POUNDS-TO-KILOGRAMS CONVERSION

lb	kg	kg	lb
1	0.5	1	2.2
2	0.9	2	4.4
4	1.8	3	6.6
6	2.7	4	8.8
8	3.6	5	11.0
10	4.5	6	13.2
20	9.1	8	17.6
30	13.6	10	22.0
40	18.2	20	44.0
50	22.7	30	66.0
60	27.3	40	88.0
70	31.8	50	110.0
80	36.4	60	132.0
90	40.9	70	154.0
100	45.4	80	176.0
150	68.2	90	198.0
200	90.8	100	220.0
kg = lb × 0.454		lb = kg × 2.2	

Modified and reproduced with permission from Gomella LG, ed. Clinician's Pocket Reference, 10th ed. McGraw-Hill, © 2002.

Index

Note: Page numbers followed by italic *f* or *t* denote figures or tables, respectively.